Step-by-Step
Medical Coding

Technical Collaborators

Karla R. Lovaasen, RHIA, CCS
Director of Patient Information Services
St. Francis Medical Center/Home
Breckenridge, Minnesota

Deborah L. Neville, RHIA, CCS-P, CPC
Coding Analyst
Revenue Recognition and Billing Compliance
Mayo Clinic
Rochester, Minnesota

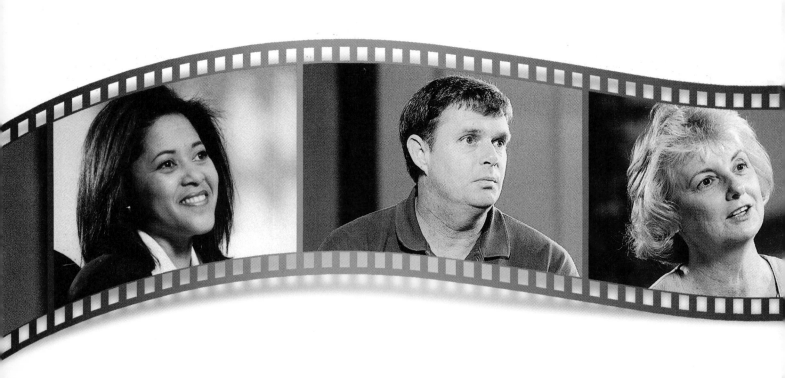

Step-by-Step Medical Coding

FOURTH EDITION

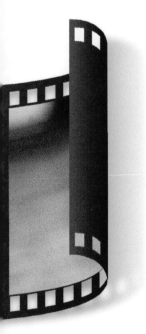

Carol J. Buck, BS, MS, CPC
Program Director
Medical Secretary Programs
Northwest Technical College
East Grand Forks, Minnesota

W.B. SAUNDERS COMPANY
An Imprint of Elsevier Science
Philadelphia   London   New York   St. Louis   Sydney   Toronto

W.B. SAUNDERS COMPANY
An Imprint of Elsevier Science

The Curtis Center
Independence Square West
Philadelphia, Pennsylvania 19106

Library of Congress Cataloging-in-Publication Data

Buck, Carol J.
    Step-by-step medical coding/Carol J. Buck; technical collaborators, Karla R. Lovaasen, Deborah L.
Neville.—4th ed.

p.   ; cm

Includes bibliographical references and index.

ISBN 0–7216–9333–4

1. Nosology—Code numbers.   I. Lovaasen, Karla R.   II. Neville, Deborah L.   III. Title.   [DNLM:
    1. Classification.   2. Terminology.   WB 15 B922s 2002]

RB115.B83 2002

616′.001′48—dc21   2001057594

Publishing Director: Andrew Allen
Senior Acquisitions Editor: Adrianne C. Williams
Developmental Editor: Elizabeth LoGiudice
Manuscript Editor: Amy Norwitz
Production Manager: Norman Stellander
Illustration Specialist: John Needles

Printed in the United States of America.

Last digit is the print number: 9 8 7 6 5 4 3 2

To the students, whose drive and determination to learn serve as my endless source of inspiration and enrichment.

To teachers, whose contributions are immense and workloads daunting. May this work make your preparation for class a little easier.

To DJ, for sharing the vision and the journey.

This book is dedicated in loving memory to my mother, Gladys E. Swen.

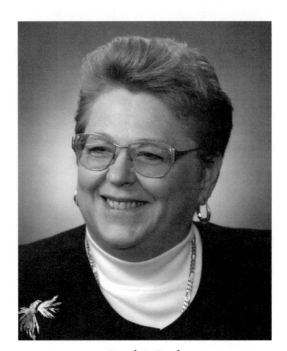

Carol J. Buck

Acknowledgments

This book developed from collaboration by educators and employers in their attempt to meet the needs of students preparing for a career in the medical coding allied health profession. Obtaining employers' input about the knowledge, skills, and abilities desired of entry-level coding employees benefits educators tremendously. This text is an endeavor to use this information to better prepare our students.

There are several other people who deserve special thanks for their efforts in making this text possible.

Karla R. Lovaasen and Deborah L. Neville, Technical Collaborators, for their immense technical knowledge and constant willingness to share that knowledge in the education of others.

Michelle A. Green, previous Technical Collaborator, for her continued support of this work. Her dedication to students and education is highly regarded.

Adrianne C. Williams, Senior Acquisitions Editor, Health Related Professions, W.B. Saunders Company, for her enthusiasm and encouragement. Elizabeth LoGiudice, Developmental Editor, W.B. Saunders Company, for her efficiency and patience.

Linda Krecklau, Provider Education and Communications Specialist, BCBS, Eagan, Minnesota, for translating the *Federal Register* into "ordinary words."

Senior Reviewers

Introduction

The number of people seeking health care services has increased as a result of an aging population, technologic advances, and better access to health care. At the same time, there is an increase in the use of outpatient facilities. This increase is due, in part, to the government's introduction of tighter controls over inpatient services. The government continues to increase its involvement in, and control over, health care through reimbursement of services for Medicare patients. Other insurance companies are following the government's lead and adopting reimbursement systems that have proven effective in reducing third-party payer costs.

Health care in America has undergone tremendous change in the recent past, and more changes are promised for the future. The outcome of these changes has resulted in an ever-increasing demand for qualified medical coders. The government predicts a growth in demand for medical coders of 32% during the 1996–2006 time period, with the average annual job openings due to growth and replacement at 11,730 nationally.[1] The national shortage has increased the salary for the coding occupation, and salaries in general show a solid upward trend.

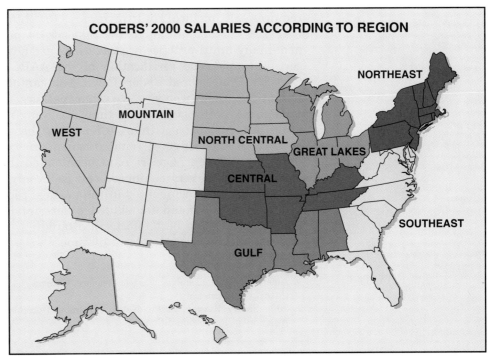

CODERS' 2000 SALARIES ACCORDING TO REGION

The regional averages for certified procedural coders from the 2000 Salary Survey[2] by the American Academy of Professional Coders (AAPC) are as follows*:

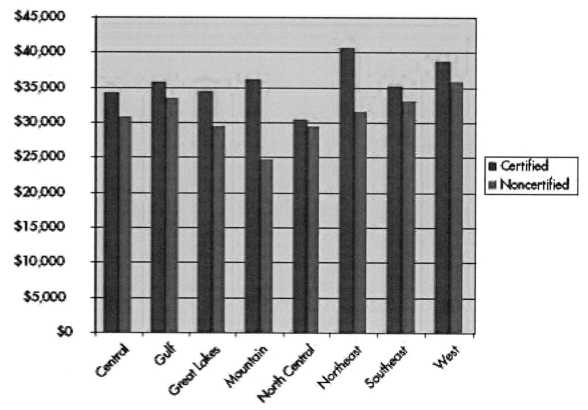

According to the AAPC, "Although tenure and geographical location have a rather large bearing on wages, one of the biggest factors is education . . . It is worth the effort to crack open those books and get an education."[2]

Certification for coders will continue to expand and will become the industry standard. According to the AAPC, "Hawaii has passed a bill that requires all medical bill reviewers to obtain certification through the AAPC."[2] Further, although the majority of practicing coders are not certified, many multi-practice organizations are now requiring their staff to have certification."[2] The certification of the AAPC for outpatient coders is the Certified Professional Coder (CPC). You can obtain information on certification at the AAPC web site, www.aapcnatl.org.

Medical coding is far more than assigning numbers to services and diagnoses. Coders abstract information from the patient record and combine it with their knowledge of reimbursement and coding guidelines to optimize physician payment. Coders have been called the "fraud squad" because they optimize, but never maximize, and code only for services provided to the patient that are documented in the medical record.

There is a demand for skilled coders, and you can be one of those in demand. Put your best efforts into building the foundation of your career and you will be rewarded for a lifetime.

REFERENCES

1. America's Career InfoNet: Fastest Growing Careers, U.S. Bureau of Labor Statistics, 2000. (http://www.acinet.org)
2. 2000 Salary Survey. AAPC News, November/December, 2000, Salt Lake City, American Academy of Professional Coders.

---

* American Academy of Professional Coders, published by permission.

Contents

unit I

Current Procedural Terminology (CPT)

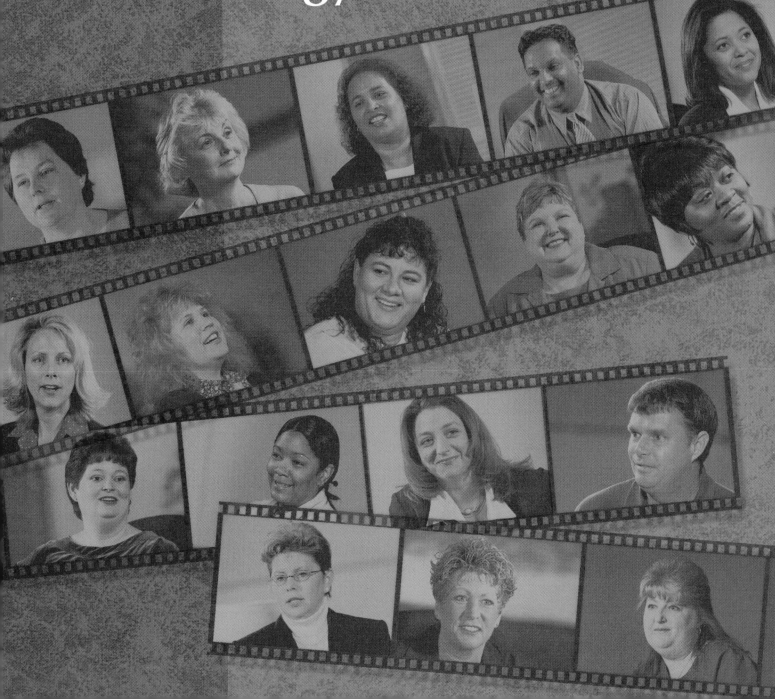

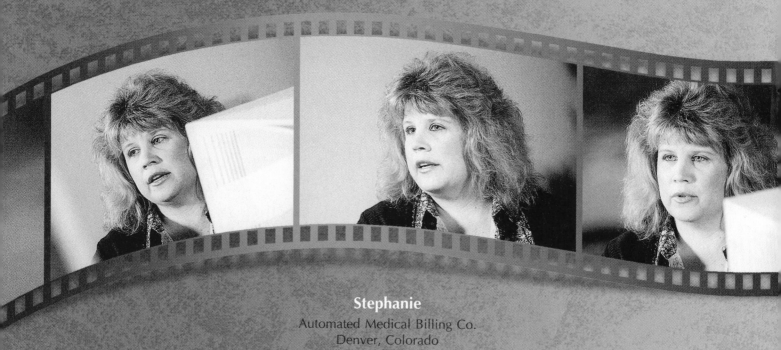

Stephanie
Automated Medical Billing Co.
Denver, Colorado

chapter 1

Introduction to the CPT

LEARNING OBJECTIVES

After completing this chapter you should be able to

1 Identify the purpose of the CPT manual.

2 State the importance of using the current-year CPT manual.

3 Recognize the symbols used in the CPT manual.

4 List the major sections found in the CPT manual.

5 Identify information in appendices of the CPT manual.

6 Interpret the information contained in section Guidelines.

7 Identify elements of the CPT manual format.

8 Understand modifiers.

9 Determine what is meant by unlisted procedures/services.

10 State the purposes of a special report.

11 Locate terms in the CPT manual index.

12 Define chapter terminology.

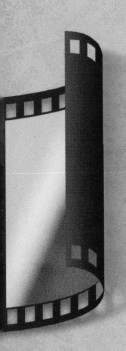

PURPOSE OF THE CPT MANUAL

Current Procedural Terminology (CPT), also known as CPT-4, is a coding system developed by the American Medical Association (AMA) to convert widely accepted, uniform descriptions of medical, surgical, and diagnostic services rendered by health care providers into five-digit numeric codes. The use of the CPT codes enables health care providers to communicate both effectively and efficiently with third-party payers (i.e., commercial insurance companies, Medicare, Medicaid) about the procedures and services provided to the patient. For example, on an insurance form you can report a service by typing 21182 rather than reconstruction of orbital walls, rims, forehead, nasoethmoid complex following intra- and extracranial excision of benign tumor of the cranial bone, with multiple autografts; with a total area of bone grafting less than 40 cm². By using 21182, you are able to communicate not only quickly but also exactly about a very detailed service.

A new section of codes appeared in the 2002 CPT—Category III codes. These are temporary codes that are used to help identify emerging technology, services, and procedures. The regular CPT codes are referred to as Category I codes. Category I codes have been approved by the Editorial Panel of the AMA, and they conform to standards established by the AMA. Let's begin the study of the CPT with the Category I codes.

Health care providers are reimbursed based on the codes submitted on a claim form for the procedures and services rendered. For an example of placement of the CPT codes on a claim form, refer to Figure 1–1. Reporting the correct code is essential because incorrect coding can result in a provider's being reimbursed incorrectly or in some cases being penalized by the government for submitting inappropriate claims. The CPT coding system is used by clinics, outpatient hospital departments, ambulatory surgery centers, and third-party payers to describe health care services. Although there are differences in the rules governing coding in various health care settings, CPT codes offer increased compatibility and comparability of data among users and providers, allowing for comparative analysis, research, and reimbursement.

The CPT coding system was first developed and published by the AMA in 1966 as a method of billing for medical and surgical procedures and services using standard terminology. Three editions of *Current Procedural Terminology* were published in the 1970s, and updates and revisions reflected changes in the technology and practices of health care. Use of the CPT manual was increased in 1983 when the Centers for Medicare and Medicaid Services (CMS), formerly the Health Care Financing Administration (HCFA), incorporated the CPT codes into HCFA's Common Procedure Coding System (HCPCS). CPT codes are Level I codes. Level II national codes (HCPCS) are alphanumeric codes that are used by providers to code for services, supplies, and equipment provided to Medicare and Medicaid patients for which no CPT codes exist.

Updating the CPT Manual

Because the practice of medicine is ever changing, the CPT manual is ever changing. It is updated annually to reflect technologic advances and editorial revisions. It is very important to use the most current CPT manual available to provide quality data and ensure appropriate reimbursement. In 2003, the AMA is anticipating the publication of the next generation of the CPT, CPT-5. The major changes in the CPT-5 will be the use of terminology that more clearly describes services and procedures. CPT-4 definitions include many vague terms such as "with or without," "and/or," and "by use of any method." This unclear terminology will be replaced with more precise definitions, making code selection a much easier process. The clarification of

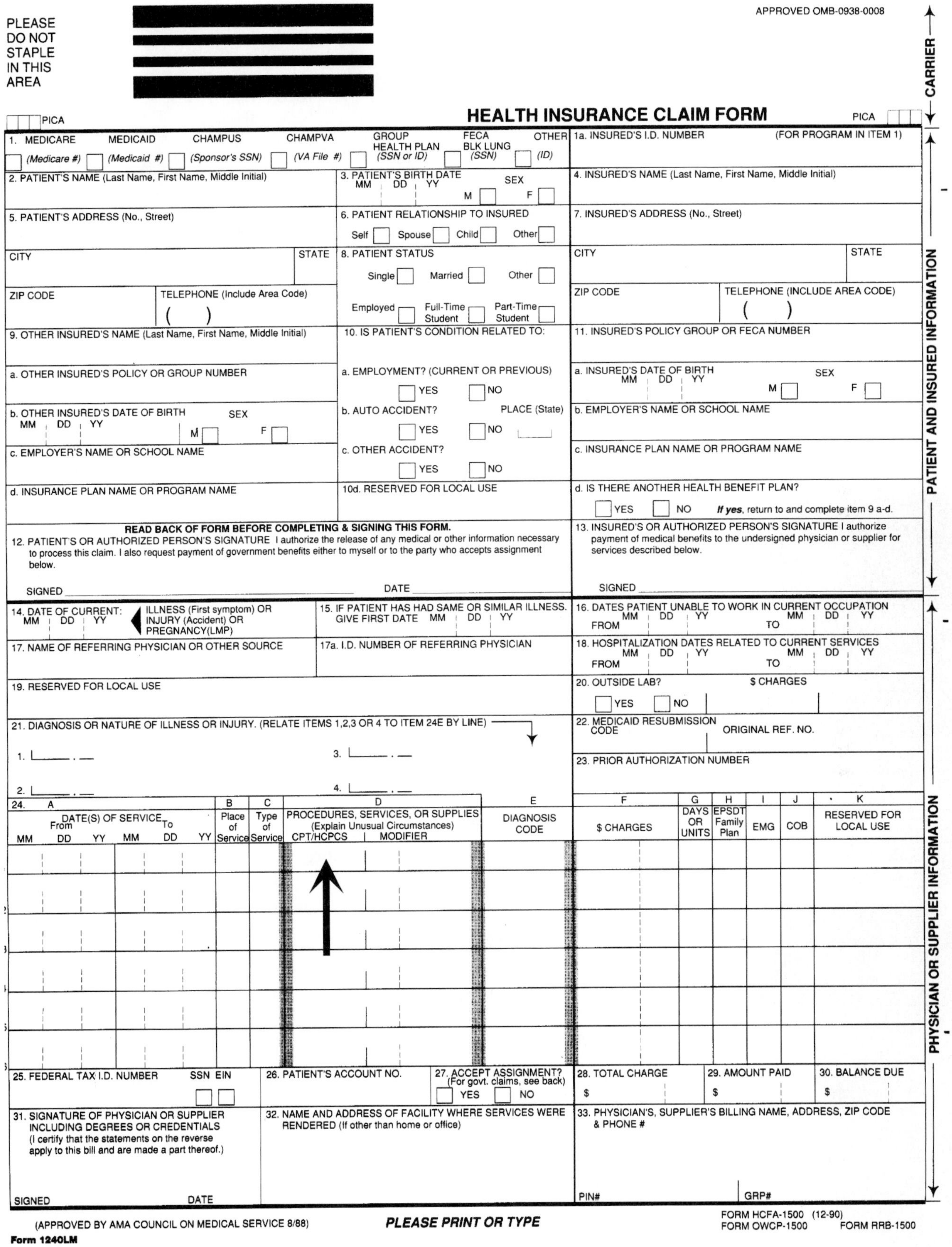

APPROVED OMB-0938-0008

PLEASE DO NOT STAPLE IN THIS AREA

PICA

HEALTH INSURANCE CLAIM FORM

PICA

CARRIER

1. MEDICARE (Medicare #) MEDICAID (Medicaid #) CHAMPUS (Sponsor's SSN) CHAMPVA (VA File #) GROUP HEALTH PLAN (SSN or ID) FECA BLK LUNG (SSN) OTHER (ID)

1a. INSURED'S I.D. NUMBER (FOR PROGRAM IN ITEM 1)

2. PATIENT'S NAME (Last Name, First Name, Middle Initial)

3. PATIENT'S BIRTH DATE MM DD YY SEX M F

4. INSURED'S NAME (Last Name, First Name, Middle Initial)

5. PATIENT'S ADDRESS (No., Street)

6. PATIENT RELATIONSHIP TO INSURED Self Spouse Child Other

7. INSURED'S ADDRESS (No., Street)

CITY STATE

8. PATIENT STATUS Single Married Other

CITY STATE

ZIP CODE TELEPHONE (Include Area Code) ( )

Employed Full-Time Student Part-Time Student

ZIP CODE TELEPHONE (INCLUDE AREA CODE) ( )

9. OTHER INSURED'S NAME (Last Name, First Name, Middle Initial)

10. IS PATIENT'S CONDITION RELATED TO:

11. INSURED'S POLICY GROUP OR FECA NUMBER

a. OTHER INSURED'S POLICY OR GROUP NUMBER

a. EMPLOYMENT? (CURRENT OR PREVIOUS) YES NO

a. INSURED'S DATE OF BIRTH MM DD YY SEX M F

b. OTHER INSURED'S DATE OF BIRTH MM DD YY SEX M F

b. AUTO ACCIDENT? PLACE (State) YES NO

b. EMPLOYER'S NAME OR SCHOOL NAME

c. EMPLOYER'S NAME OR SCHOOL NAME

c. OTHER ACCIDENT? YES NO

c. INSURANCE PLAN NAME OR PROGRAM NAME

d. INSURANCE PLAN NAME OR PROGRAM NAME

10d. RESERVED FOR LOCAL USE

d. IS THERE ANOTHER HEALTH BENEFIT PLAN? YES NO *If yes*, return to and complete item 9 a-d.

PATIENT AND INSURED INFORMATION

READ BACK OF FORM BEFORE COMPLETING & SIGNING THIS FORM.

12. PATIENT'S OR AUTHORIZED PERSON'S SIGNATURE I authorize the release of any medical or other information necessary to process this claim. I also request payment of government benefits either to myself or to the party who accepts assignment below.

SIGNED ____ DATE ____

13. INSURED'S OR AUTHORIZED PERSON'S SIGNATURE I authorize payment of medical benefits to the undersigned physician or supplier for services described below.

SIGNED ____

14. DATE OF CURRENT: MM DD YY ILLNESS (First symptom) OR INJURY (Accident) OR PREGNANCY(LMP)

15. IF PATIENT HAS HAD SAME OR SIMILAR ILLNESS. GIVE FIRST DATE MM DD YY

16. DATES PATIENT UNABLE TO WORK IN CURRENT OCCUPATION FROM MM DD YY TO MM DD YY

17. NAME OF REFERRING PHYSICIAN OR OTHER SOURCE

17a. I.D. NUMBER OF REFERRING PHYSICIAN

18. HOSPITALIZATION DATES RELATED TO CURRENT SERVICES FROM MM DD YY TO MM DD YY

19. RESERVED FOR LOCAL USE

20. OUTSIDE LAB? YES NO $ CHARGES

21. DIAGNOSIS OR NATURE OF ILLNESS OR INJURY. (RELATE ITEMS 1,2,3 OR 4 TO ITEM 24E BY LINE)

1. ___ . ___ 3. ___ . ___

2. ___ . ___ 4. ___ . ___

22. MEDICAID RESUBMISSION CODE ORIGINAL REF. NO.

23. PRIOR AUTHORIZATION NUMBER

24. A DATE(S) OF SERVICE From MM DD YY	To MM DD YY	B Place of Service	C Type of Service	D PROCEDURES, SERVICES, OR SUPPLIES (Explain Unusual Circumstances) CPT/HCPCS MODIFIER	E DIAGNOSIS CODE	F $ CHARGES	G DAYS OR UNITS	H EPSDT Family Plan	I EMG	J COB	K RESERVED FOR LOCAL USE

PHYSICIAN OR SUPPLIER INFORMATION

25. FEDERAL TAX I.D. NUMBER SSN EIN

26. PATIENT'S ACCOUNT NO.

27. ACCEPT ASSIGNMENT? (For govt. claims, see back) YES NO

28. TOTAL CHARGE $

29. AMOUNT PAID $

30. BALANCE DUE $

31. SIGNATURE OF PHYSICIAN OR SUPPLIER INCLUDING DEGREES OR CREDENTIALS (I certify that the statements on the reverse apply to this bill and are made a part thereof.)

SIGNED DATE

32. NAME AND ADDRESS OF FACILITY WHERE SERVICES WERE RENDERED (If other than home or office)

33. PHYSICIAN'S, SUPPLIER'S BILLING NAME, ADDRESS, ZIP CODE & PHONE #

PIN# GRP#

(APPROVED BY AMA COUNCIL ON MEDICAL SERVICE 8/88) ***PLEASE PRINT OR TYPE*** FORM HCFA-1500 (12-90) FORM OWCP-1500 FORM RRB-1500

Form 1240LM

Figure 1–1 HCFA-1500 Health Insurance Claim Form, also known as the "universal claim form," used by outpatient facilities for claims submission. (Courtesy of U.S. Department of Health and Human Services, Centers for Medicare and Medicaid Services.)

from the trenches

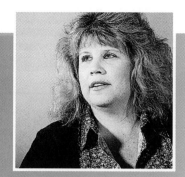

"*Medical coding is no longer a clerical field . . . other health professionals may not realize this. Just remember it's your responsibility if something is coded incorrectly as a result of following someone else's directive.*"

STEPHANIE

terminology is not the only change in the CPT-5. The revisions in the CPT-5 were necessary to address requirements of the Health Insurance Portability and Accountability Act of 1996 (HIPAA). HIPAA requires the Secretary of Health and Human Services to adopt national uniform standards for the electronic transmission of financial and administrative health information. These standards include a wide variety of health care information. One item that HIPAA requires is a common, concise coding system with clear, expandable definitions. If the AMA does not meet the challenge to make the code definitions precise, CPT may not continue to be the designated common code set for outpatient procedures. Most health care organizations in the United States use CPT to report services and procedures, and if these organizations stopped using the CPT, the AMA would lose an enormous revenue generator. So, enter the CPT-5 with clearer and more precise code descriptions.

Check This Out! ☞ HIPAA legislation at www.hcfa.gov/regs/hippaa-cer.htm.

Updated editions of the CPT manual are available for purchase in November for use beginning the following January 1.

Check This Out! ☞ The American Medical Association (AMA) has a Website located at http://www.ama-assn.org.

EXERCISE 1-1

PURPOSE OF THE CPT MANUAL

Complete the following:

1 The CPT manual was developed by the _____ .

2 CPT stands for _____ _____ _____ .

3 Providers of health care are paid based on the codes submitted for

   _____ and procedures provided to the patient.

4 The first CPT was published in this year: _____ .

5 In this year, HCFA incorporated CPT codes into HCPCS:

   _____ .

After completing Exercise 1–1, check your answers in Appendix B of this text.

THE CPT MANUAL FORMAT

Six Important Symbols

In the CPT manual, **new** codes for procedures and services are identified by the bullet (●) symbol that is placed in front of the code number. Note the location of this symbol in Figure 1–2.

A triangle (▲) placed in front of a code indicates that the description for the code has been **changed** or modified since the previous edition. Changes may be additions, deletions, or revisions in code descriptions (Fig. 1–3). When the text has changed, a right and a left triangle (▶ ◀) indicate the beginning and end of the text changes, as illustrated in Figure 1–4.

The plus symbol (+) placed in front of a code indicates an **add-on code** (Fig. 1–5). Add-on codes are never used alone; rather, they are used with another primary procedure or service code. For example, code 11000 describes a debridement (removal of contaminated tissue) of up to 10% of the body surface. Add-on code 11001 is used for each additional 10% of the body surface debrided. Code 11001 cannot be used unless code 11000 is used first. Also notice in Figure 1–5 that there is a note in parentheses that indicates that code 11001 can be used only in conjunction with code 11000. **Appendix E** in the CPT manual lists all add-on codes.

The circle with a line through it (⊘) identifies a **modifier -51 exempt code** (Fig. 1–6). Modifier -51 indicates multiple procedures. The symbol warns you to check the primary procedure code to see what is included in the primary procedure code before you use the modifier -51 exempt code. For example, when coding procedures in which a graft or implant is used, you will usually find that the primary procedure code includes the graft or implant performed during the procedure, making a separate graft or implant code unnecessary. Also note in Figure 1–6 that the category notes for

New code for service/procedure symbol

●3XXXX Exchange of a previously placed arterial catheter during thrombolytic therapy

Figure 1–2 New code symbol.

Changed code description

▲3XXXX Arteriovenous anastomosis, direct, any site (e.g., Cimino type)

Figure 1–3 Changed code symbol.

Pacemaker or ▶Pacing Cardioverter-◀ Defibrillator

A pacemaker system includes a pulse generator containing electronics and a battery, and one or more electrodes (leads). Pulse generators ▶are◀ placed in a subcutaneous "pocket" created in either a subclavicular site ▶or underneath the abdominal muscles just below the ribcage.◀ Electrodes may be inserted through a vein (transvenous) or ▶they may be placed◀ on the surface of the heart (epicardial).▶ The epicardial . . .

Figure 1–4 Changed text symbols.

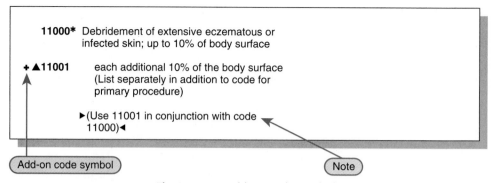

Figure 1–5   Add-on code symbol.

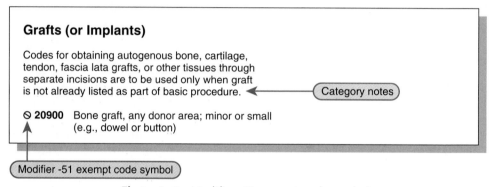

Figure 1–6   Modifier -51 exempt code symbol.

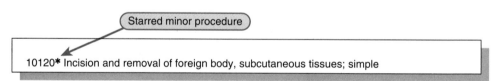

Figure 1–7   Minor procedure symbol.

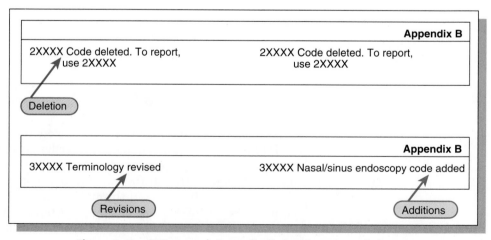

Figure 1–8   CPT manual Appendix B showing types of changes.

"Grafts (or Implants)" indicate that the codes in the category are used only when the graft is not a part of the basic procedure. **Appendix F** in the CPT manual contains the complete list of modifier -51 exempt codes.

A star (*) placed after a code number indicates that the service includes the **surgical procedure only** (Fig. 1–7). The starred minor procedure is discussed later in more detail along with the modifier -51 exempt code and the add-on code.

Appendix B of the CPT manual contains a complete list of the additions to, deletions from, and revisions of the previous edition of the CPT manual. When a code is listed in Appendix B, the type of change is listed beside the code number (Fig. 1–8). For example, if the procedure or service is still available but is to be reported with a different code, the deleted code is listed, followed by the new code to be used.

EXERCISE 1-2

SYMBOLS

Match the following code symbols with the correct definition:

1 ▲ _____   a. surgical procedure only

2 ✱ _____   b. modifier -51 exempt

3 ● _____   c. revised

4 ⊘ _____   d. add-on

5 + _____   e. new

6 Where is a complete list of additions, deletions, and revisions located in the CPT manual?

_____

7 Which CPT manual appendix contains a complete list of all modifier -51 exempt codes?

_____

8 Which CPT manual appendix contains a complete list of add-on codes?

_____

The Seven Sections

The CPT manual is composed of seven chapters into which all codes and descriptions are categorized. These chapters are called **sections.**

THE SECTIONS OF THE CPT MANUAL

- Evaluation and Management   99201–99499
- Anesthesia   00100–01999
- Surgery   10040–69990
- Radiology   70010–79999
- Pathology and Laboratory   80048–89399
- Medicine   90281–99199
- Category III Codes

The sections are further divided into subsections, subheadings, categories, and subcategories. A section is a chapter that covers one of the seven topics included in the CPT manual: Evaluation/Management (E/M), Anesthesia, Surgery, Radiology, Pathology/Laboratory, Medicine, and Category III codes. The CPT codes are arranged in numerical order in each section. For now, let's review the first six sections.

Sections are divided into subsections. For example, the Surgery section includes subsections of Integumentary, Musculoskeletal, Respiratory, Cardiovascular, and so forth.

Subsections, subheadings, categories, and subcategories are divisions of sections that are based on anatomy, procedure, condition, description, or approach.

E X A M P L E

Section:	Surgery
Subsection:	Cardiovascular System
Subheading:	Arteries and Veins
Category:	Embolectomy/Thrombectomy
Subcategory:	Arterial, With or Without Catheter
Section:	Surgery
Subsection:	Nervous System
Subheading:	Skull, Meninges, and Brain
Category:	Approach Procedures
Subcategory:	Anterior Cranial Fossa

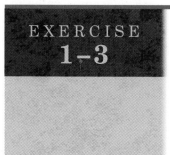

EXERCISE
1-3

SECTION, SUBSECTION, SUBHEADING, AND CATEGORY

To see an example of section, subsection, subheading, and category, locate the code 19000 Puncture aspiration of cyst of breast in the CPT manual in the Surgery section.

With a CPT manual beside you and open to the page on which CPT code 19000 is located, or referring to Figure 1–9, find the information on the top of page 11 on the CPT manual page:

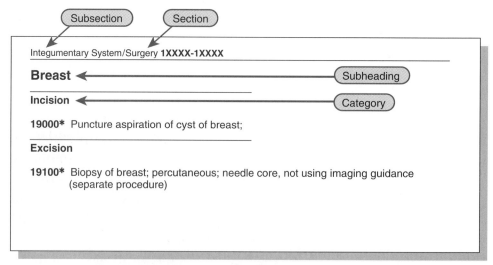

Figure 1–9 Section, subsection, subheading, and category.

Section. At the top of the page, the word "Surgery" indicates the section. Note that this word is followed by a range of numbers, which is a list of all the code numbers located on that page.

Subsection. Also at the top of the page, the phrase "Integumentary System" indicates the subsection.

Subheading. The word "Breast" indicates the subheading.

Category. The word "Incision" indicates the category.

In summary, the divisions for the previous example are

Section:	Surgery
Subsection:	Integumentary System
Subheading:	Breast
Category:	Incision

Now you try one.

With a CPT manual open to the page that contains code 30100, locate the following information for the 30100 code:

1 Section: _____

2 Subsection: _____

3 Subheading: _____

4 Category: _____

STOP *Using the section, subsection, subheading, and category information makes it much faster and easier to get around in the CPT manual.*

The Guidelines

Each section in the CPT manual includes Guidelines. The guidelines provide specific information about coding in that section and contain valuable information for the coder. Guidelines that are applicable to all codes in the section are found at the beginning of each section (Fig. 1–10). Notes pertaining to specific codes or groups of codes are listed before or after the codes (Fig. 1–11). The Guidelines and notes may contain definitions of terms, applicable modifiers, subsection information, unlisted services, special reports information, or clinical examples. Always read the Guidelines and notes before coding to help ensure accurate assignment of the CPT codes.

(Section Guidelines applicable to all Surgery codes)

Surgery Guidelines

Items used by all physicians in reporting their services are presented in the **Introduction**. Some of the commonalities are repeated here for the convenience of those physicians referring to this section on **Surgery**. Other definitions and items unique to Surgery are also listed.

Figure 1–10 Section guidelines.

Specific notes applicable to a group of codes

SURGERY OF SKULL BASE

The surgical management of lesions involving the skull base (base of anterior, middle, and posterior cranial fossae) often requires the skills of several surgeons of different surgical specialties working together or in tandem during the operative session. These operations are usually...

Figure 1–11 Specific notes.

EXERCISE 1-4

GUIDELINES

Using the Guidelines for each of the sections, answer the following questions:

1 Write the definition of a chief complaint using the E/M Guidelines._____

_____

_____

_____

2 According to the Surgery Guidelines, is surgical destruction usually considered part of a surgical procedure? _____

3 According to the Radiology Guidelines, who must sign a written report to have the report considered part of the radiologic procedure? _____

4 Under whose supervision are Pathology and Laboratory services provided? _____

5 What is the code listed in the Medicine Guidelines that is to be used to identify materials supplied by the physician that are beyond those ordinarily included in the service provided? _____

Code Format

Procedure and service descriptions are located after the code number (Fig. 1–12). They are commonly accepted descriptions of procedures or services that are provided to patients.

There are two types of codes: **stand-alone codes** and **indented codes** (Fig. 1–13). Only the stand-alone codes have the full description; indented codes are listed under associated stand-alone codes. It is understood that descriptions for indented codes include the portion of the stand-alone code

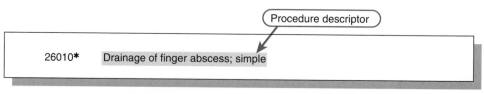

Procedure descriptor

26010*   Drainage of finger abscess; simple

Figure 1–12 Code and description format.

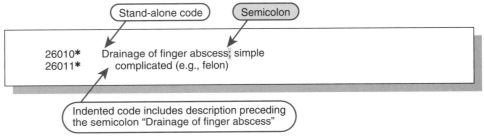

Figure 1–13 Stand-alone codes and indented codes.

description that precedes the semicolon. The purpose of the semicolon is to save space.

STOP *You may not have realized it, but you've just been given a critical clue to coding—the semicolon. The following information will help you understand why the semicolon is so important.*

In Figure 1–13, the code 26011 is an indented code—the indentation serves to represent the words "Drainage of finger abscess," which appear before the semicolon in CPT code 26010. The semicolon is a powerful tool in the CPT manual; when you see it, be sure to read the words before it carefully.

The words following the semicolon can indicate alternative anatomic sites, alternative procedures, or a description of the extent of the service.

E X A M P L E

Alternative Anatomic Site:

27705   Osteotomy; tibia

27707   fibula

27709   tibia and fibula

Alternative Procedure:

31505   Laryngoscopy, indirect; diagnostic (separate procedure)

31510   with biopsy

31511   with removal of foreign body

31512   with removal of lesion

Description of Extent of the Service:

20520*   Removal of foreign body in muscle or tendon sheath; simple

20525   deep or complicated

STOP *Before assigning an indented code, make sure you refer to the preceding stand-alone code and read the words that precede the semicolon. That is the only way to ensure a full description and select a correct code.*

EXERCISE
1-5

CODE FORMAT

Complete the following:

1 Describe a stand-alone code. _____

_____

2 Describe an indented code. _____

_____

_____

3 Words following the semicolon in stand-alone codes can indicate the following three things:

a. _____

b. _____

c. _____

Modifiers

Modifiers provide additional information to the third-party payer about services provided to a patient. At times, the five-digit CPT code may not reflect completely the service or procedure provided. Because numeric codes, not written procedure descriptions, are required by third-party payers, additional numbers or letters may be added to the basic five-digit code to modify the CPT code and thereby provide further specificity. These additional modifiers may be two numbers, two letters, or a letter and a number and are appended, or "tacked on," to the basic five-digit CPT code, or they may be five-digit numbers that are listed together with the basic code. In the HCPCS, two-place modifiers such as -RC and -F1 are used.

In the CPT system, a modifier can be either an appended two-digit number or an additional five-digit number.

EXAMPLE

> -62
> *or*
> 09962

The two-digit modifier is added to the five-digit CPT code.

EXAMPLE

> Code 43820 is the CPT procedure code for a gastrojejunostomy, without vagotomy. If two surgeons with different surgical skills participated as primary surgeons, each performing a specific part of the procedure, the procedure code 43820 could be altered by the addition of the modifier -62 to indicate co-surgeons (Fig. 1–14). The code would be 43820-62 for a gastrojejunostomy, without vagotomy, in which two surgeons participated as primary surgeons. Each physician would submit his or her own bill indicating code 43820-62.

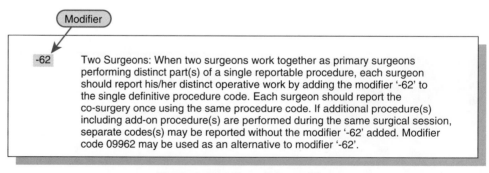

Figure 1–14 Two-digit modifier.

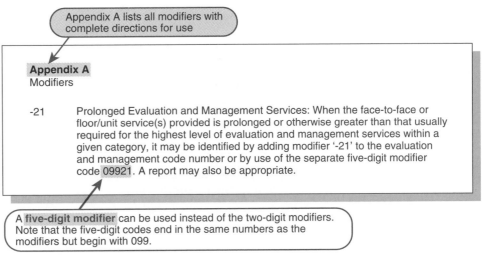

Figure 1–15 Modifiers in Appendix A.

The five-digit modifiers are used for some electronic billing. As illustrated in Figure 1–14, the five-digit modifier is composed of the prefix 099 plus the two-digit modifier.

EXAMPLE

The two-digit modifier -22 is used to indicate a more extensive or unusual procedure. The five-digit modifier is 09922. The code 27332 for an arthrotomy of the knee with complex excision of cartilage can be stated in two ways:

27332-22   Arthrotomy, with excision of semilunar cartilage (meniscectomy) knee; medial OR lateral

or

27332 and 09922   Arthrotomy, with excision of semilunar cartilage (meniscectomy) knee; medial OR lateral

For a complete listing of all modifiers, see Appendix A in the CPT manual. Refer to Figure 1–15 for an example of the information found in Appendix A. Further information regarding modifiers is presented throughout the following chapters of this text.

EXERCISE
1-6

MODIFIERS

Using Appendix A of the CPT manual and the information you just learned, fill in the blank with the correct number:

1 What is the five-digit modifier to indicate two primary surgeons?

Code(s): _____

2 If the CPT code is 43820 (gastrojejunostomy without vagotomy) and two primary surgeons performed the service, the service could be stated two ways:

_____ or _____

and _____

Use Appendix A of the CPT manual to list the correct two- and five-digit modifiers in the following examples. You do not have to supply the five-digit CPT procedure code, only the two- and five-digit modifiers.

3 Bilateral inguinal herniorrhaphy: _____ and _____ .

4 A postoperative ureterotomy patient needs to be returned to the operating room for a related procedure during the postoperative period:

_____ and _____

5 A decision to perform surgery was made during an evaluation, and management service is _____ and _____ .

6 There is a need for multiple procedures during the same surgical session:

_____ and _____ .

7 A surgical team is required: _____ and _____ .

8 Physician A assists physician B: _____ and _____ .

Unlisted Procedures

When developing the CPT manual, the AMA realized that not every surgical and diagnostic procedure could be listed. There may not be a code for many procedures that are considered experimental, newly approved, or seldom used. In addition, medical advancements often create a variation of procedures currently performed. A procedure or service not found in the CPT manual can be coded as an unlisted procedure. For example, when the first heart transplant was performed, there was no code to use to report the new surgical procedure. Until a code was available, the unlisted code for cardiac surgery was used to report this procedure (Fig. 1–16). The Surgery Guidelines have unlisted procedure codes listed by body site or type of procedure. Individually unlisted procedure codes are also at the end of the subsection or subheading to which they refer. For example, at the end of the Cardiovascular System subsection is the unlisted cardiac procedure code 33999, and at the end of the Respiratory System is the unlisted lungs/pleura code 32999.

Category III was a new addition to the 2002 CPT. Category III contains codes for emerging technology; they are temporary codes. If there is a Category III code for the service or procedure you are reporting, you must use the Category III code, not the Category I unlisted code.

Category I codes are those that are widely used to describe services and

from the trenches

What lets you take the most pride in your career?
"Knowing that I can assist in helping a practice to succeed in its business."

STEPHANIE

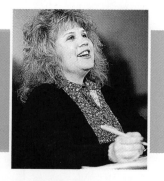

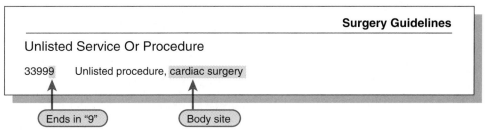

Figure 1-16 Unlisted service or procedure.

procedures that have been approved by the Food and Drug Administration (FDA), if appropriate. Category I codes also relate to services and procedures that been proven to have clinical effectiveness. Category III codes describe services and procedures that have not been approved by the FDA, if appropriate, may not be widely offered, and have not been proven to be clinically effective. The use of the Category III codes allows physicians, other health care professionals, third-party payers, researchers, and health policy experts to identify emerging trends in health care.

Format of Category III Codes

The codes have five digits—four numbers and a letter: for example, 0012T (Arthroscopy, knee, surgical, implantation of osteochondral graft(s) for treatment of articular surface defect, autografts) and the indented code that follows, 0013T (allografts). These two codes represent new procedures that are being performed to repair knee joints. Prior to the existence of Category III codes, you would have reported one of these procedures using an unlisted code, because there was no specific code that described the procedure. But because there now is a Category III code available that describes the procedure, you must report the procedure using the Category III code, not the unlisted code from Category I.

Category III codes may or may not eventually receive Category I code status and be placed in the main part of the CPT.

Publication of Category III Codes

New Category III codes are released twice a year (January and July) via the AMA Website. The full set of temporary codes is then published in the next edition of the CPT in a section following the Medicine section.

EXERCISE 1-7

UNLISTED PROCEDURES

Assuming there is no Category III code available for the procedure you are reporting, using the Guidelines in the front of the sections indicated below, locate the five-digit unlisted procedure code for each of the following:

1 Surgery

Unlisted procedure; middle ear: Code(s): _____

    arthroscopy: Code(s): _____

    esophagus: Code(s): _____

2 Pathology and Laboratory

Unlisted procedure; cytogenetic
study: Code(s): _____

    urinalysis procedure: Code(s): _____

    chemistry procedure: Code(s): _____

3 Medicine

Unlisted procedure; special ser-
vice, procedure, or report: Code(s): _____

4 Radiology

Unlisted procedure; clinical
brachytherapy: Code(s): _____

Unlisted miscellaneous procedures;
diagnostic nuclear medicine: Code(s): _____

Special Reports

Special reports must accompany claims when an unusual, new, seldom used, unlisted, or Category III procedure is performed. The special report should include an adequate definition or description of the **nature, extent,** and **need** for the procedure and the **time, effort,** and **equipment** necessary to provide the service. The special report helps the third-party payer determine the appropriateness of the care and the medical necessity of the service provided.

STARTING WITH THE INDEX

Locating the Terms

The CPT index is located at the back of the CPT manual and is arranged alphabetically. Index headings located at the top right and left corners of the index pages direct the coder to the entries that are included on that page, much like a dictionary. Use of index headings speeds location of the term (Fig. 1–17).

Code numbers are displayed in the CPT index in one of the ways shown in the example on page 19.

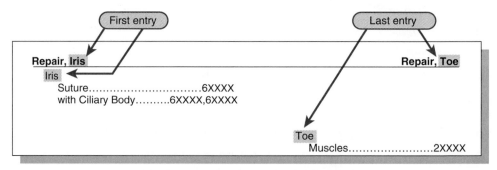

Figure 1–17   CPT manual index headings.

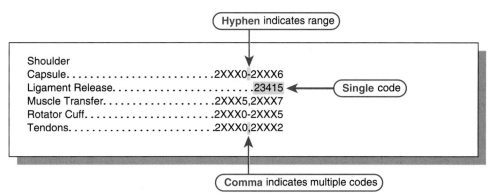

Figure 1–18   Code display.

EXAMPLE

single code:	38115
multiple codes:	26645, 26650
range:	22305–22325

See Figure 1–18 for an example of the display in the index using the single, multiple, and range formats.

Single Code

When only one code number is stated, you should verify the code in the main portion of the CPT manual to ensure its accuracy.

Multiple Codes

The use of a **comma** between code numbers indicates the presence of only those numbers displayed. If more than one code number is listed, then all codes must be referenced to make an accurate choice.

Range of Codes

A range is indicated by a **hyphen.** When a range is given in the index, you must look up each code within the range in the main portion of the CPT manual to select the appropriate code from the range.

CAUTION *Never code directly from the index. You can't be sure you have the right code until you have located the code in the main portion of the CPT manual and read the information presented there regarding the specifics of the code.*

The index is in alphabetic order by main terms and further divided by subterms. Figure 1–19 illustrates the main term and subterm as used in the index. Having identified the main term of the service or procedure, you can locate the term in the index. When you are just beginning to use the

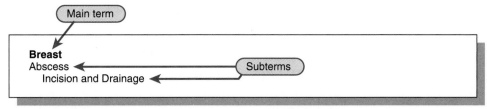

Figure 1–19   CPT manual index indicating main terms and subterms.

CPT manual, it may be difficult to locate the main term. Not being able to locate a term in the index can be very frustrating, but don't be discouraged if you don't identify the main term on the first try. This is a skill that is learned by practice, and part of the practice is making mistakes. Soon you'll be locating those main terms quickly. Just keep thinking about the service or procedure and looking up the words in the index.

Some basic location methods will help you to locate these main terms.

LOCATION METHODS
- Service or Procedure
- Anatomic Site
- Condition or Disease
- Synonym
- Eponym
- Abbreviation

Let's take these location methods and apply each one to locating "repair of a fracture of a femur."

EXERCISE 1-8

TERM PRACTICE

Service or Procedure

1   When using the service or procedure location method, "repair" would be the main term in "*repair* of a fracture of a femur."

   a. Locate "Repair" in the index of the CPT manual. Using this location method, "Repair" is the main term and the subterms are "Fracture" and "Femur."

   b. Under the main term "Repair," locate the subterm "Femur." If you were to look under "Repair" and then look for the term "Fracture," you wouldn't find "Fracture," because listed under "Repair" are the anatomic divisions that can be repaired. "Fracture" isn't an anatomic division, so it isn't located under "Repair." It can be just as difficult to locate the correct subterm as it is to find the main term.

   Right now, don't be concerned with looking up the codes in the main part of the CPT manual; we will come to that in Chapter 2. For now, concentrate on learning how to locate the main term and subterms in the index of the CPT manual.

Anatomic Site

2   The second method of locating an anatomic site uses the word "femur" as the main term, and the subterms are "fracture" and "repair."

   a. Locate "Femur" in the index of the CPT manual.

   b. Under the main term "Femur," locate the subterm "Fracture."

   c. Notice that the entry "Fracture" is further divided based on repair type or anatomic location.

Condition or Disease

3   The third location method focuses on the condition or disease. In this instance you would use the main term "fracture" as a condition.

a. Locate the main term "Fracture" in the index.

b. Locate the subterm "Femur."

The use of the first three location methods will usually get you to the applicable codes in the index. If you try each of the first three methods and still can't locate the codes in the index, don't despair; try one of the other location methods: synonym, eponym, and abbreviation.

Synonym

4 The fourth location method involves synonyms. Synonyms are words with similar meanings.

a. Toe joint is a synonym for interphalangeal joint or metatarsophalangeal joint. Suppose, then, you couldn't think of the correct medical term, but you could think of the word "toe." In that case, you could look up "Toe" in the CPT manual index, and that entry would direct you to:

See Interphalangeal Joint, Toe; Metatarsophalangeal Joint, Phalanx

Eponym

5 The fifth location method uses eponyms. Eponyms are things that are named after people. For example, the Barr Procedure—a tendon-transfer procedure—was named after the person who developed it.

a. Locate "Barr Procedure" in the CPT manual index. You are directed to:

See Tendon Transfer, Leg, Lower.

Abbreviation

6 The sixth location method uses abbreviations. Abbreviations are common in medicine for names of drugs, diseases, and procedures.

a. Locate the abbreviation "INH" in the index of the CPT manual. You are directed to:

See Drug Assay.

Medicine uses many synonyms, eponyms, and abbreviations. A good medical dictionary that contains the most common synonyms, eponyms, and abbreviations will be a necessity for you.

Locate each of the following main terms in the CPT manual index, and then locate the subterms and secondary subterms:

Main Term	Subterm	Secondary Subterm
Repair	Abdomen	Suture
Femur	Abscess	Incision
Fracture	Ankle	Lateral

CAUTION *Never code directly from the index. The index does not include the information necessary for appropriate code selection.*
Locate the code in the index and then verify the code in the main part of the CPT manual to ensure that the code is the correct one to apply to the given procedure.
Don't rely on memory.
Always follow the steps outlined for coding.

You are now ready to put your term location skills to work by doing the next exercise.

MAIN TERM LOCATION

Identify the main terms in the following examples and write the main term on the line provided. Then, locate the main terms and any subterms in the CPT manual index. Write the code listed in the index for that service or procedure on the line provided.

1   Description: Emergency Department Services, Physician Direction of Advanced Life Support

   a. Main term: _____

   b. Locate the code available in the index of the CPT manual for Emergency Department Services, Physician Direction of Advanced Life Support.

      Code(s): _____

2   Condition/Disease: intertrochanteric femoral fracture (closed treatment)

   a. Main term: _____

   b. Locate the code available in the index of the CPT manual for intertrochanteric femoral fracture (closed treatment).

      Code(s): _____

3   Procedure: removal of gallbladder calculi

   a. Main term: _____

   b. Locate the code available in the index of the CPT manual for removal of gallbladder calculi.

      Code(s): _____

4   Anatomic site: lung, bullae excision

   a. Main term: _____

   b. Locate the code available in the index of the CPT manual for excision of bullae of lung.

      Code(s): _____

STOP *As you can probably see from this exercise, there are often many ways to locate an item in the index. The same word can serve as a main term or a subterm, depending on the location method you are using. In addition, the annual updating of the CPT results in numerous changes within the index.*

You will be locating terms in the CPT manual index throughout your study of this text. For your ready reference, there is a guideline at the beginning of the index in the CPT manual that contains directions for the use of the CPT manual index. Beginning with Chapter 2 of this text, Appendix B will list not only the correct code answer, but also one index location for that code. For example, if the correct answer is 99203, the following appears in after the code: (Office and/or Other Outpatient Services, New Patient). It is difficult to locate items in the CPT index when you begin coding, so if you get stuck and just cannot locate the index entry, you will be able to find one location in Appendix B.

See

"*See*" is a cross-reference term found in the index of the CPT manual. The term directs you to another term or other terms.

"*See*" indicates that the correct code will be found elsewhere.

EXAMPLE

Anticoagulant   *See* Clotting Inhibitors

STOP *The coder must follow the instructions given in the index.*

EXERCISE 1–10

SEE

Complete the following:

1 Locate the term "Renal Disease Services" in the CPT index. You are directed to _____
_____ .

2 Locate the abbreviation "ANA" in the CPT index. The entry you find is
_____ .

3 Locate the term "Arm" in the CPT index. You are directed to _____
_____ .

CAUTION *Never code directly from the index. To ensure correct coding, the code number must be located in the main portion of the CPT manual.*

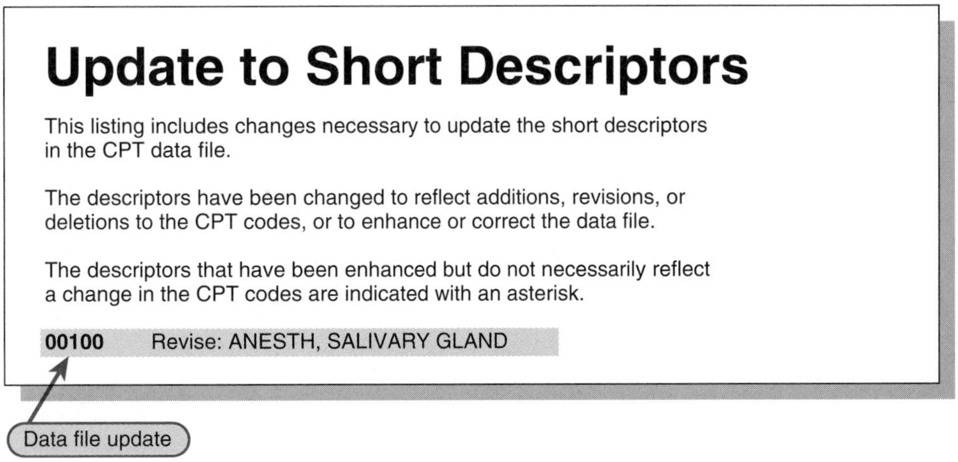

Update to Short Descriptors

This listing includes changes necessary to update the short descriptors in the CPT data file.

The descriptors have been changed to reflect additions, revisions, or deletions to the CPT codes, or to enhance or correct the data file.

The descriptors that have been enhanced but do not necessarily reflect a change in the CPT codes are indicated with an asterisk.

| 00100 | Revise: ANESTH, SALIVARY GLAND |

(Data file update)

Figure 1–20 Appendix C of the CPT manual contains electronic updating information.

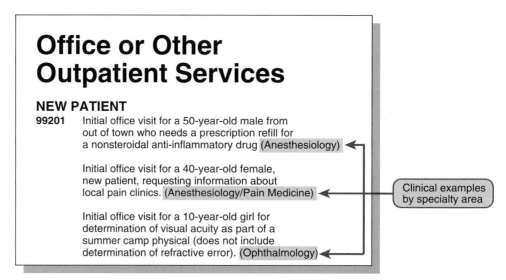

Figure 1–21 Appendix D of the CPT manual contains clinical examples of the use of E/M codes.

Two More CPT Appendices

The CPT is available on computer diskettes. **Appendix C** of the CPT manual contains a listing of the updates of the electronic data file to reflect all the additions, revisions, and deletions that have been made in the manual since the last edition (Fig. 1–20). With these updates, the data files can remain current without your having to purchase a new set of diskettes. Although the electronic version saves the coder time, it is not a replacement for the skill and knowledge of the coder—it is only a tool to be used by a skillful and knowledgeable coder.

Appendix D of the CPT manual contains clinical examples of many of the Evaluation and Management (E/M) service codes (Fig. 1–21). The examples are meant to offer a broad idea of the type of presenting problem that each code could represent. But a word of caution: only the patient's record and the particular services rendered by the physician to a particular patient can determine the level of service provided. Appendix D is not meant to be an exhaustive list of E/M services.

CHAPTER GLOSSARY

Appendix A: located near the back of the CPT manual; lists all modifiers with complete explanations for use

Appendix B: located near the back of the CPT manual; contains a complete list of additions to, deletions from, and revisions of the previous edition

Appendix C: located near the back of the CPT manual; contains the list of updates to the electronic version of the CPT

Appendix D: located near the back of the CPT manual; presents clinical examples of Evaluation and Management (E/M) Procedures

Appendix E: located near the back of the CPT manual; contains a listing of the CPT add-on codes

Appendix F: located near the back of the CPT manual; contains a list of modifier -51 exempt codes

CPT (Current Procedural Terminology): a coding system developed by the American Medical Association (AMA) to convert widely accepted, uniform descriptions of medical, surgical, and diagnostic services rendered by health care providers into five-digit numeric codes

Guidelines: provide specific instructions about coding for each section; the Guidelines contain definitions of terms, applicable modifiers, explanation of notes, subsection information, unlisted services, special reports information, and clinical examples

modifiers: two- or five-digit numbers added to CPT codes to supply more specific information about the services provided to the patient

sections: the seven major areas into which all CPT codes and descriptions are categorized

See: a cross-reference system within the index of the CPT manual used to direct the coder to another term or other terms. The *See* indicates that the correct code will be found elsewhere

special reports: detailed reports that include adequate definitions or descriptions of the nature, extent, and need for the procedure and the time, effort, and equipment necessary to provide the services

subsections: the further division of sections into smaller units, usually by body systems

symbols: special guides that help the coder compare codes and descriptors with the previous edition. A bullet (●) is used to indicate a new procedure or service code added since the previous edition of the CPT manual. A solid triangle (▲) placed in front of a code number indicates that the code has been changed or modified since the last edition. A star (*) placed after a code number indicates a minor procedure. A plus (+) is used to indicate an add-on code. A circle with a line through it (⊘) is used to identify a modifier -51 exempt code. A right and left triangle (► ◄) indicate the beginning and end of the text changes.

term location methods: service/procedure, anatomic site/body organ, condition/disease, synonym, eponym, and abbreviation

unlisted procedures: procedures that are considered unusual, experimental, or new and do not have a specific code number assigned; unlisted procedure codes are located at the end of the subsections or subheadings and may be used to identify any procedure that lacks a specific code

CHAPTER REVIEW

CHAPTER 1, PART I, THEORY

Do not use your CPT manual for this part of the review.

1 CPT stands for _____ .

2 The CPT manual often reflects the technologic advances made in medicine with _____ .

3 The CPT manual is divided into how many sections? _____

4 What type of five-digit code begins with 099?

_____

5 Coding information that pertains to an entire section is located in the _____ .

6 Procedures that include variable preoperative or postoperative services are noted in the CPT manual with what symbol?

_____

7 What is the name of the two-digit code number that is located after the CPT code number and provides more detail about the code?

_____

8 Where is a list of all the modifiers located?

_____

9 When using an unlisted or Category III code, third-party payers usually require the submission of what?

_____

10 Additions, deletions, and revisions are listed in which Appendix?

_____

11 A listing of all add-on codes is located in which Appendix?

_____

12 The symbol used between two code numbers to indicate that a range is available is a

_____ .

Using Figure 1–22, identify the category, section, subheading, and subsection.

13 _____

14 _____

15 _____

16 _____

CHAPTER 1, PART II, PRACTICAL

Use your CPT manual for this part of the review. Using Appendix A of the CPT manual, list the correct two- and five-digit modifiers for the following services:

17 Repeat procedure by the same physician:

_____ or _____

18 Surgical care only: _____ or _____

19 Anesthesia by the surgeon: _____ or _____

20 Bilateral procedure: _____ or _____

Assuming there is no Category III code for the unlisted procedure you are reporting, locate the following unlisted procedure codes using the Surgery Guidelines:

21 Orbit: Code(s): _____

22 Rectum: Code(s): _____

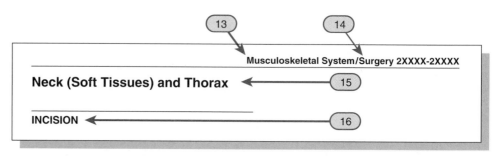

Figure 1–22 Identify the section, subsection, subheading, and category.

23 Lips: Code(s): _____

24 General musculoskeletal: Code(s): _____

Using the index of the CPT manual, locate an example of each of the following types of code display:

25 Single code _____

26 Multiple code _____

27 Range _____

Using the index of the CPT manual, locate the following terms and write what the index note directs you to do:

28 Td Shots _____

29 SHBG _____

30 Radius _____

31 Physical Therapy _____

Using the index of the CPT manual, locate the code(s) for the following:

32 Repair, abdomen _____

33 Bypass graft, excision, abdomen _____

34 Catheterization, arteriovenous shunt _____

35 Cystotomy, with drainage _____

36 Fracture, femur, intertrochanteric, closed treatment _____

37 Alveoloplasty _____

38 Duodenotomy _____

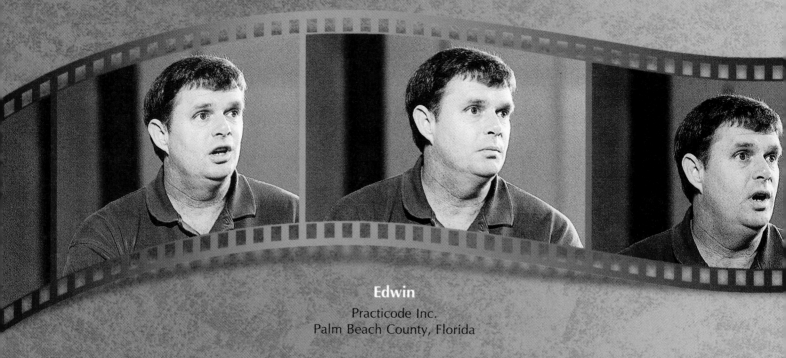

Edwin
Practicode Inc.
Palm Beach County, Florida

chapter 2

The Evaluation and Management (E/M) Section

LEARNING OBJECTIVES

After completing this chapter you should be able to

1 Identify and explain the three factors of E/M code assignment.

2 Analyze the key components.

3 Explain the levels of E/M service.

4 List contributing factors.

5 Analyze code information.

6 Assign E/M codes.

7 Identify Documentation Guidelines.

8 Define chapter terminology.

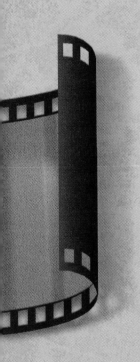

CONTENTS OF THE E/M SECTION

The information in Chapter 1 described the basic format of the CPT manual. The information and exercises in this chapter will familiarize you with the first section of the CPT manual, Evaluation and Management (E/M). The E/M section has 18 subsections.

1. Office or Other Outpatient Services   99201–99215
2. Hospital Observation Services   99217–99220
3. Hospital Inpatient Services   99221–99239
4. Consultations   99241–99275
5. Emergency Department Services   99281–99288
6. Patient Transport   99289–99290
7. Critical Care Services   99291–99292
8. Neonatal Intensive Care   99295–99298
9. Nursing Facility Services   99301–99316
10. Domiciliary, Rest Home, or Custodial Care Services   99321–99333
11. Home Services   99341–99350
12. Prolonged Services   99354–99360
13. Case Management Services   99361–99373
14. Care Plan Oversight Services   99374–99380
15. Preventive Medicine Services   99381–99429
16. Newborn Care   99431–99440
17. Special Evaluation and Management Services   99450–99456
18. Other Evaluation and Management Services

THREE FACTORS OF E/M CODES

Code assignment in the E/M section varies according to three factors.

1. Place of service
2. Type of service
3. Patient status

Place of Service

The first factor you must consider in code assignment is the place of service (Fig. 2–1). Place of service explains the setting in which the services were provided to the patient. Codes vary depending on the place of the service. Places of service can be a physician's office, hospital, emergency department, nursing home, and so on.

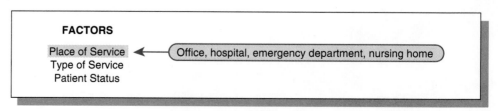

FACTORS

Place of Service ◄—— Office, hospital, emergency department, nursing home
Type of Service
Patient Status

Figure 2–1   Place of service.

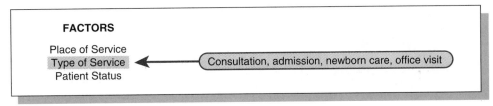

Figure 2-2 Type of service.

Type of Service

The second factor in code assignment is the type of service (Fig. 2-2). Type of service is the reason the service is requested or performed. Examples of types of service are consultation, admission, newborn care, and office visit.

- *Consultation* is requested to obtain an opinion or advice about a diagnosis or management option from another physician.

- *Admission* is attention to an acute illness or injury that results in admission to a hospital.

- *Newborn care* is the evaluation and determination of care management of a newly born infant.

- *Office visit* is a face-to-face encounter between a physician and a patient to allow for primary management of the patient's health care status.

Patient Status

The third factor in code assignment is patient status (Fig. 2-3). The four types of patient status are new patient, established patient, outpatient, and inpatient. Codes are often grouped in the CPT manual according to the type of patient involved.

- *New patient* is one who has not received professional services from the physician or another physician of the same specialty in the same group within the past 3 years.

- *Established patient* is one who has received professional services from the physician or another physician of the same specialty in the same group within the past 3 years.

- *Outpatient* is one who has not been formally admitted to a health care facility.

- *Inpatient* is one who has been formally admitted to a health care facility.

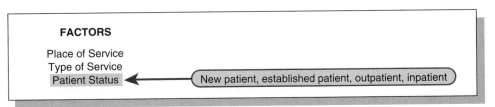

Figure 2-3 Patient status.

EXERCISE 2-1

THREE FACTORS OF E/M CODES

Using a CPT manual, locate the subsection Office and Other Outpatient Services and then the category New Patient in the E/M section to answer the following questions:

1 Where is the place of service? _____

2 What is the type of service? _____

3 What is the patient status? _____

4 What is the first code number listed under the subheading New Patient?

   Code: _____

5 Each code represents a different level of service. How many codes are

   listed under Office or Other Outpatient Services for a new patient? _____

6 How many codes are listed for the established patient in the Office or

   Other Outpatient Services category? _____

VARIOUS LEVELS OF E/M SERVICE

The levels of E/M service are based on documentation located in the patient's medical record supporting various amounts of skill, effort, time, responsibility, and medical knowledge used by the physician to provide the service to the patient. The levels of service are based on **key components** (history, examination, and medical decision-making complexity) and **contributing factors** (counseling, coordination of care, nature of presenting problem, and time). The components contain a great deal of information that you need to know before you learn about factors. Let's look at each of these components and factors individually.

Key Components

- History
- Examination
- Medical decision-making

The key components of history, examination, and medical decision-making reflect the clinical information that is recorded by the physician in the patient's medical record. Key components are present in every patient case except counseling encounters, which are discussed later in the chapter. Key components enable you to choose the appropriate level of service. New patient encounters, consultations, emergency department visits, and admissions require documentation of all three of the key components. Subsequent visits such as daily hospital visits or outpatient visits for an established patient require that only two of the three key components be present for assignment to a given code. For example, to assign code 99214—established patient, office visit—at least two of the three key components must be documented in the patient's medical record.

EXAMPLE

99214	Office or other outpatient visit for the evaluation and management of an established patient, which requires **at least two of these three key components:**

  • **a detailed history**

  • **a detailed examination**

  • **medical decision-making of moderate complexity**

History

The history is the *subjective* information the patient tells the physician based on the four elements of a history—chief complaint (CC); history of present illness (HPI); review of systems (ROS); and past, family, and/or social history (PFSH). The history contains the information the physician needs to appropriately assess the patient's condition. Not all histories have all elements. The inclusion of each of the elements and the extent to which each of the elements is contained in a history are determined by the physician based on the need for more or less subjective information and will determine the history level. The documentation of the history is found in the patient's medical record and is recorded by the physician.

Ancillary staff (nurses, physician assistants, and so forth) are allowed to document some of the history, such as chief complaint and past, family, and social histories. Also, a physician can have the patient complete a form composed of questions concerning the review of systems; however, the physician must evaluate the form and indicate in the medical record that the form has been reviewed.

THE FOUR ELEMENTS OF A HISTORY

■ Chief Complaint (CC)

■ History of Present Illness (HPI)

■ Review of Systems (ROS)

■ Past, Family, and/or Social History (PFSH)

History Elements

You need to be able to identify the various elements and levels of a history by reading the notes entered into the medical record by the physician.

1. **Chief Complaint (CC)** is a concise statement describing the symptom, problem, condition, diagnosis, physician-recommended return, or other factor that is the reason for the encounter, usually stated in the patient's words.

2. **History of Present Illness (HPI)** is a chronological description of the development of the patient's present illness from the first sign and/or symptom or from the previous encounter to the present. The HPI may include the following elements:

  • Location   • Timing

  • Quality   • Context

  • Severity   • Modifying factors

  • Duration   • Associated signs and symptoms

   The HPI must be documented in the medical record by the physician.

3. **Review of Systems (ROS)** is an inventory of body systems obtained through a series of questions seeking to identify signs and/or symptoms that the patient may be experiencing or has experienced. According to Huffman's *Health Information Management,** the "ROS is an inventory of systems to reveal subjective symptoms that the patient either forgot to describe or which at the time seemed relatively unimportant. In general, an analysis of the subjective findings will indicate the nature and extent of the examination required." The inventory of systems may be asked by means of a questionnaire filled out by the patient or ancillary staff; but the physician *must* evaluate the questionnaire and document in the medical record that the questionnaire has been reviewed in order for it to qualify as an ROS. For purposes of ROS, the following systems are recognized*:

- Constitutional symptoms

    Usual weight, recent weight changes, fever, weakness, fatigue

- Eyes (Ophthalmologic)

    Glasses or contact lenses, last eye examination, visual glaucoma, cataracts, eyestrain, pain, diplopia, redness, lacrimation, inflammation, blurring

- Ears, Nose, Mouth, Throat (Otolaryngologic)

    Ears: hearing, discharge, tinnitus, dizziness, pain

    Nose: head colds, epistaxis, discharges, obstruction, postnasal drip, sinus pain

    Mouth and Throat: condition of teeth and gums, last dental examination, soreness, redness, hoarseness, difficulty in swallowing

- Cardiovascular

    Chest pain, rheumatic fever, tachycardia, palpitation, high blood pressure, edema, vertigo, faintness, varicose veins, thrombophlebitis

- Respiratory

    Chest pain, wheezing, cough, dyspnea, sputum (color and quantity), hemoptysis, asthma, bronchitis, emphysema, pneumonia, tuberculosis, pleurisy, last chest radiograph

- Gastrointestinal

    Appetite, thirst, nausea, vomiting, hematemesis, rectal bleeding, change in bowel habits, diarrhea, constipation, indigestion, food intolerance, flatus, hemorrhoids, jaundice

- Genitourinary

    Urinary: frequent or painful urination, nocturia, pyuria, hematuria, incontinence, urinary infection

    Genito-reproductive: male—venereal disease, sores, discharge from penis, hernias, testicular pain or masses; female—age at menarche and menstruation (frequency, type, duration, dysmenorrhea, menorrhagia; symptoms of menopause), contraception, pregnancies, deliveries, abortions, last Papanicolaou smear

- Musculoskeletal

    Joint pain or stiffness, arthritis, gout, backache, muscle pain, cramps, swelling redness, limitation in motor activity

---

* Definitions from Huffman E: Health Information Management, 10th ed. Revised by the American Medical Record Association. Berwyn, IL, Physician's Record Company, 1994, pp. 57–62.

- Integumentary (skin and/or breast)

    Rashes, eruptions, dryness, cyanosis, jaundice, changes in skin, hair, or nails

- Neurologic

    Faintness, blackouts, seizures, paralysis, tingling, tremors, memory loss

- Psychiatric

    Personality type, nervousness, mood, insomnia, headache, nightmares, depression

- Endocrine

    Thyroid trouble, heat or cold intolerance, excessive sweating, thirst, hunger, or urination

- Hematologic/Lymphatic

    Anemia, easy bruising or bleeding, past transfusions

- Allergic/Immunologic

    Sneezing, itching eyes, rhinorrhea, nasal obstruction, or recurrent infections

4. **Past, Family, and/or Social History (PFSH)***

- *Past history* is the patient's past experience with illnesses, operations, injuries, and treatments; specifically

    Prior major illnesses and injuries

    Prior operations

    Prior hospitalizations

    Current medications

    Allergies (e.g., drug, food)

    Age appropriate immunization status

    Age appropriate feeding/dietary status

- *Social history* is an age appropriate review of past and current activities that includes significant information about

    Marital status and/or living arrangements

    Current employment

    Occupational history

    Use of drugs, alcohol, and tobacco

    Level of education

    Sexual history

    Other relevant social factors

    Exercise habits or other activities

- *Family history* is a review of medical events in the patient's family that includes significant information about

    The health status or cause of death of parents, siblings, and children

    Specific diseases related to problems identified in the Chief Complaint or History of the Present Illness, and/or System Review

    Diseases of family members which may be hereditary or place the patient at risk

---

* Definitions from 2001 CPT, Evaluation and Management Guidelines, pp. 3–4. CPT codes, descriptions, and materials only are © 2001 American Medical Association.

Three of the elements of a history (HPI, ROS, and PFSH) are included to varying degrees in all patient encounters. The degree or level of HPI, ROS, and PFSH is determined by the chief complaint or presenting problem of the patient.

History Levels

Now that you have reviewed the elements of a history you are prepared to choose a history level. There are four history levels; the level is based on the extent of the history during the history-taking portion of the physician-patient encounter.

HISTORY LEVELS

- Problem focused
- Expanded problem focused
- Detailed
- Comprehensive

1. **Problem focused:** The physician focuses on the chief complaint and a brief history of the present problem of a patient.

   A *brief* history would include a review of the history regarding pertinent information about the present problem or chief complaint. Brief history information would center around the severity, duration, and symptoms of the problem or complaint. The brief history does not have to include the past, family, or social history or a review of systems.

2. **Expanded problem focused:** The physician focuses on a chief complaint, obtains a *brief* history of the present problem, and also performs a *problem pertinent* review of systems. The expanded problem focused history does not have to include the past, family, or social history.

   This history would center around specific questions regarding the system involved in the presenting problem or chief complaint. The review of systems for this history would cover the organ system most closely related to the chief complaint or presenting problem and any related or associated organ system. For example, if the presenting problem or chief complaint is a red, swollen knee, the system reviewed would be the musculoskeletal system.

3. **Detailed:** The physician focuses on a chief complaint, obtains an *extended* history of the present problem, an *extended* review of systems, and a *pertinent* PFSH.

   The system review in this history is "extended," which means that positive responses and pertinent negative responses relating to multiple organ systems should be documented.

4. **Comprehensive:** This is the most complex of the history types: the physician documents the chief complaint, obtains an *extended* history of the present problem, does a *complete* review of systems, and obtains a *complete* PFSH.

For a summary of the elements required for each level of history, see Figure 2–4.

Some third-party payers have established standards for the number of elements that must be documented in the medical record to qualify for a given level of service. For example, a third-party payer may state that to qualify as a comprehensive history the medical record must document that an extended HPI was conducted and that it included four of the eight elements (e.g., location, quality, severity, duration), a complete ROS, including a review of at least 10 of the 14 organ systems, and a complete review of all three areas of the PFSH.

History Elements

Chief Complaint (CC)
Reason for the encounter in the patient's words

History of Present Illness (HPI)
Location
Quality
Severity
Duration
Timing
Context
Modifying factors
Associated signs and symptoms

Review of Systems (ROS)
Constitutional symptoms
Ophthalmologic (eyes)
Otolaryngologic (ears, nose, mouth, throat)
Cardiovascular
Respiratory
Endocrine
Gastrointestinal
Genitourinary
Musculoskeletal
Integumentary
Neurologic
Psychiatric
Hematologic/Lymphatic
Allergic/Immunologic

Past, Family, and/or Social History (PFSH)
Past illnesses, operations, injuries, and treatments
Family medical history for heredity and risk
Social activities, both past and current

Elements Required for Each Level of History

	Problem Focused	Expanded Problem Focused	Detailed	Comprehensive
History	CC	CC	CC	CC
	Brief HPI	Brief HPI	Extended HPI	Extended HPI
		Problem-pertinent ROS	Extended ROS	Complete ROS
			Pertinent PFSH	Complete PFSH

Figure 2–4   History elements and elements required for each level of history.

EXERCISE
2-2

HISTORY LEVELS

Using the CPT manual, locate the Office or Other Outpatient Services subsection, New Patient category, to identify the history level on each of the following codes:

	Code	History Level
1	99201	_____
2	99202	_____
3	99203	_____
4	99204	_____
5	99205	_____

Examination

The patient has presented the physician with the **subjective** information regarding the complaint or problem in the history portion of the encounter; now the physician will do an examination of the patient to provide **objective** information (those findings observed by the physician) about the complaint or problem. The physician then documents the objective findings in the patient record.

Examination Levels

The examination levels have the same titles as the history levels—problem focused, expanded problem focused, detailed, and comprehensive. The four levels are used to indicate the extent and complexity of the patient examination.

EXAMINATION LEVELS

- Problem focused
- Expanded problem focused
- Detailed
- Comprehensive

Examination Elements

General
    Constitutional

Body Areas (BA)
    Head (including the face)
    Neck
    Chest (including breasts and axillae)
    Abdomen
    Genitalia, groin, buttocks
    Back
    Each extremity

Organ System (OS)
    Ophthalmologic (eyes)
    Otolaryngologic (ears, nose, mouth, throat)
    Cardiovascular
    Respiratory
    Endocrine
    Gastrointestinal
    Genitourinary
    Musculoskeletal
    Integumentary
    Neurologic
    Psychiatric
    Hematologic/Lymphatic
    Allergic/Immunologic

Elements Required for Each Level of Examination

	Problem Focused	Expanded Problem Focused	Detailed	Comprehensive
Examination	Limited to affected BA or OS	Limited to affected BA or OS and other related OS(s)	Extended of affected BA(s) and other related OS(s)	General multi-system or complete single OS

Figure 2–5   Examination elements and elements required for each level of examination.

1. **Problem focused:** Examination is limited to the affected body area or organ system identified by the chief complaint.

2. **Expanded problem focused:** A limited examination is made of the affected body area or organ system and other related body area(s)/organ system(s).

3. **Detailed:** An extended examination is made of the affected body area(s) or related organ system(s).

4. **Comprehensive:** This is the most extensive examination; it encompasses a complete single-specialty examination or a complete multisystem examination.

Figure 2–5 summarizes the elements required for each level of examination. These elements include various body areas (BAs) and organ systems (OSs). The elements also include an assessment of a patient's general condition, which is indicated by the patient's general appearance, vital signs, and the like. The three elements—general, BAs, and OSs—are as follows:

General
- Constitutional (vital signs, general appearance)

Body Areas
- Head (including the face)
- Neck
- Chest (including breasts and axillae)
- Abdomen
- Genitalia, groin, buttocks
- Back
- Each extremity

Organ Systems
- Ophthalmologic (eyes)
- Otolaryngologic (ears, nose, mouth, throat)
- Cardiovascular
- Respiratory
- Endocrine (In the CPT Guidelines, the endocrine system is not listed as an organ system.)
- Gastrointestinal
- Genitourinary
- Musculoskeletal
- Integumentary (skin)
- Neurologic
- Psychiatric
- Hematologic/Lymphatic
- Allergic/Immunologic (In the CPT Guidelines, the term "Allergic" is not listed as an organ system, and the term "Immunologic" is listed as a part of the Hematologic/Lymphatic system.)

EXERCISE 2-3

EXAMINATION LEVELS

Using the CPT manual, locate the Office or Other Outpatient Services subsection, New Patient category, to identify the examination levels for each of the following codes:

	Code	Examination Levels
1	99201	_____
2	99202	_____
3	99203	_____
4	99204	_____
5	99205	_____

The patient's medical record will reflect the number of systems examined in a brief statement of the findings. The examination would include the examination elements in the number and extent of elements required for the physician to arrive at the diagnosis. For example, if a patient came to a physician with the complaint of a small foreign object lodged in the eye, the physician would not need to do a cardiologic examination. The extent of the examination is based on what needs to be done to treat the patient.

Now you need to pull all the information on history and examination together so that it is usable information. What better way to do that than to use the information in the practical application of an exercise?

EXERCISE 2-4

EXAMINATION ELEMENTS

Label each of the following as body area (BA) or organ system (OS):

1 Skin _____
2 Head _____
3 Eyes _____
4 Ears _____
5 Nose _____
6 Mouth _____
7 Throat _____
8 Neck _____
9 Thorax, anterior and posterior _____
10 Breasts _____
11 Lungs _____
12 Heart _____
13 Abdomen _____
14 Genitourinary _____

15 Vaginal _____

16 Arm _____

17 Musculoskeletal _____

18 Lymphatics _____

19 Blood vessels _____

20 Neurologic _____

Read the following patient record:

21 A new patient, an 8-year-old female, is brought into the office by her mother, who states that the child has an earache in the right ear. Mother reports that the child has been complaining of aching and ringing in right ear of increasing severity for the past 2 days. Child appears to be in only minor distress. Temperature, 101°F. Examination: ears, eyes, and nose. Tympanic membrane red, fluid noted in right ear. Health history reviewed. Diagnosis: Otitis media.

From the patient record, we can identify the history elements—chief complaint (CC), history of present illness (HPI), past, family, and/or social history (PFSH), and review of symptoms (ROS)—as in the following:

History Elements	Patient Record
CC:	*Earache in the right ear*
HPI:	*Aching and ringing in right ear of increasing severity for the past 2 days* (Note: This HPI indicates location, severity, and duration.)
PFSH:	*Review of child's health history* (The patient information form completed by the mother contains the information that the physician reviewed, along with questions to the patient.)
ROS:	*Ears, eyes, and nose* (two organ systems)
	Head (The complaint involves only one body area.)

In this case, the physician focused on the chief complaint and did a brief history centered on gathering information about the present illness. Referring to the description of history levels summarized in Figure 2–4 or discussed in the E/M Guidelines, answer the following question:

a. What is the history level for this case? _____

Now let's establish the level of the examination:

Examination	Patient Record
General Survey:	*Child appears to be in only minor distress*
Vital Signs:	*Temperature, 101°F*
Body Areas/ Organ Systems:	*Head* (one body area)/*ears, eyes, and nose* (two organ systems)

In this case, the physician focused on one affected body area and two organ systems. Referring to the description of examination levels summarized in Figure 2–5 or discussed in the E/M Guidelines, answer the following question:

b. What is the examination level for this case? _____

That wasn't so difficult, was it? Okay, now you do one.

Read the following patient record:

22 A 68-year-old female established patient presents to the office today with a "cold" of 9 days' duration. Patient reports that she has had a dry, hacking cough and nasal congestion for the past 6 days and a fever for the past 3 days. She states that she is unable to sleep due to the cough, fever, and aching. She appears to be in minor distress. Personal and family history are negative for respiratory problems. Temperature is 100°F; blood pressure 150/90; pulse 93 and regular. Lungs clear to percussion and auscultation. Examination of head and ears, normal; nose, mucous membranes inflamed with postnasal phlegm. Diagnosis: Sinusitis. Plan: Patient was advised to drink fluids, take aspirin as needed for pain, obtain bed rest, and to return if symptoms have not improved in 5 days.

Locate the information in the patient record that matches the history element and place the information on the lines provided:

History Elements	Patient Record
CC:	_____
	_____
	_____
HPI:	_____
	_____
	_____
PFSH:	_____
	_____
	_____
ROS:	_____
	_____
	_____

With the information you placed on the preceding lines, choose the correct history level:

a. What is the history level for this case? _____

Locate the information in the patient record that matches the examination and place the information on the lines provided:

Examination	Patient Record
General Survey:	_____
Vital Signs:	_____
	_____
	_____
	_____
Body Areas/ Organ Systems:	_____

With the information you placed on the preceding lines, choose the correct examination level:

b. What is the examination level for this case? _____

Medical Decision-Making

The key component of medical decision-making (MDM) is based on the complexity of the decision the physician must make about the patient's diagnosis and care. Complexity of decision-making is based on three elements:

1. Number of diagnoses or management options. The options can be minimal, limited, multiple, or extensive.

2. Amount or complexity of data to review. The data can be minimal or none, limited, moderate, or extensive.

3. Risk of complication or death if the condition goes untreated. Risk can be minimal, low, moderate, or high.

Levels

The extent to which each of these elements is considered determines the levels of MDM complexity.

MEDICAL DECISION-MAKING COMPLEXITY LEVELS

- Straightforward
- Low
- Moderate
- High

1. **Straightforward decision-making:** *minimal* diagnosis and management options, *minimal or none* for the amount and complexity of data to be reviewed, and *minimal* risk to the patient of complications or death if untreated.

2. **Low-complexity decision-making:** *limited* number of diagnoses and management options, *limited* data to be reviewed, and *low* risk to the patient of complications or death if untreated.

3. **Moderate-complexity decision-making:** *multiple* diagnoses and management options, *moderate* amount and complexity of data to be reviewed, and *moderate* risk to the patient of complications or death if untreated.

4. **High-complexity decision-making:** *extensive* diagnoses and management options, *extensive* amount and complexity of data to be reviewed, and *high* risk to the patient for complications or death if the problem is untreated.

Management Options. Some basic guidelines for documentation of management options in the medical record are as follows:

1. For each encounter, an assessment, clinical impression, or diagnosis should be documented. It may be explicitly stated or implied in documented decisions regarding management plans or further evaluation.

   - For a presenting problem with an established diagnosis the record should reflect whether the problem is (a) improved, well controlled, resolving, or resolved; or (b) inadequately controlled, worsening, or failing to change as expected.

- For a presenting problem without an established diagnosis, the assessment or clinical impression may be stated in the form of differential diagnoses or as a "possible," "probable," or "rule out" (R/O) diagnosis.

2. The initiation of, or changes in, treatment should be documented. Treatment includes a wide range of management options, including patient instructions, nursing instructions, therapies, and medications.

3. If referrals are made, consultations requested, or advice sought, the record should indicate to whom or where the referral or consultation is made or from whom the advice is requested.

Data to Be Reviewed. The following are some basic documentation guidelines for the amount and complexity of data to be reviewed:

1. If a diagnostic service (test or procedure) is ordered, planned, scheduled, or performed at the time of the E/M encounter, the type of service (e.g., laboratory or radiology) should be documented.

2. The review of laboratory, radiology, or other diagnostic tests should be documented. An entry in a progress note such as "WBC elevated" or "chest x-ray unremarkable" is acceptable. Alternatively, the review may be documented by initializing and dating the report containing the test results.

3. A decision to obtain old records or to obtain additional history from the family, caregiver, or other source to supplement that obtained from the patient should be documented.

4. Relevant findings from the review of old records or the receipt of additional history from the family, caregiver, or other source should be documented. If there is no relevant information beyond that already obtained, that fact should be documented. A notation of "old records reviewed" or "additional history obtained from family" without elaboration is insufficient.

5. The results of discussion of laboratory, radiology, or other diagnostic tests with the physician who performed or interpreted the study should be documented.

TABLE 2–1   Levels of Risk

Level of Risk	Presenting Problem or Problems
Minimal	One self-limited or minor problem (e.g., insect bite, tinea corporis)
Low	Two or more self-limited or minor problems
	One stable chronic illness (e.g., well-controlled hypertension or non–insulin dependent diabetes, cataract, benign prostatic hypertrophy)
	Acute, uncomplicated illness or injury (e.g., cystitis, allergic rhinitis, simple sprain)
Moderate	One or more chronic illnesses with mild exacerbation, progression, or side effects of treatment
	Two or more stable chronic illnesses
	Undiagnosed new problem with uncertain prognosis (e.g., lump in breast)
	Acute illness with systemic symptoms (e.g., pyelonephritis, pneumonitis, colitis)
High	One or more chronic illnesses with severe exacerbation, progression, or side effects of treatment
	Acute or chronic illnesses or injuries that pose a threat to life or body function (e.g., multiple trauma, acute myocardial infarction, pulmonary embolus, severe respiratory distress, progressive severe rheumatoid arthritis, psychiatric illness with potential threat to self or others, peritonitis, acute renal failure)
	An abrupt change in neurologic status (e.g., seizure, transient ischemic attack, weakness, or sensory loss)

Medical Decision-Making Elements

Number of Diagnoses or Management Options
Minimal
Limited
Multiple
Extensive

Amount or Complexity of Data to Review
Minimal/None
Limited
Moderate
Extensive

Risk of Complications or Death if Condition Goes Untreated
Minimal
Low
Moderate
High

Elements Required for Each Level of Medical Decision-Making

	Straightforward	**Low**	**Moderate**	**High**
Number of diagnoses or management options	Minimal	Limited	Multiple	Extensive
Amount or complexity of data to review	Minimal/None	Limited	Moderate	Extensive
Risk	Minimal	Low	Moderate	High

Figure 2–6 Medical decision-making elements and elements required for each level of medical decision-making.

6. The direct visualization and independent interpretation of an image, tracing, or specimen previously interpreted by another physician should be documented.

Risk. Some basic documentation guidelines for risk of significant complications, morbidity, or mortality include the following:

1. Comorbidities, underlying diseases, or other factors that increase the complexity of medical decision-making by increasing the risk of complications, morbidity, or mortality should be documented.

2. If a surgical or invasive diagnostic procedure is *ordered*, *planned*, or *scheduled* at the time of the E/M encounter, the type of procedure (e.g., laparoscopy) should be documented.

3. If a surgical or invasive diagnostic procedure is *performed* at the time of the E/M encounter, the specific procedure should be documented.

4. The referral for or decision to perform a surgical or invasive diagnostic procedure on an urgent basis should be documented or implied.

Examples of the levels of risk may be found in Table 2-1.

When you select one of the four types of complexity of medical decision-making—straightforward, low, moderate, or high—the documentation in the medical record must support the selection in terms of the number of diagnoses or management options, amount and/or complexity of data to be reviewed, and risks.

Refer to Figure 2–6 for an overview of medical decision-making. Given the information in the medical record, you would consider the information in the context of the complexity of the diagnosis and management options, data to be reviewed, and risks to the patient in order to choose the complexity of MDM. Let's look at an example of choosing the MDM level.

EXAMPLE 1

An established patient's office medical record states the following: Female patient fell and scraped arm; problem focused history and examination were done. The patient states that she slipped on the ice on the walk outside her home approximately 3 hours earlier. The area of abrasion appears to be relatively clean, with no noted foreign materials imbedded. There appears to be only minimal cutaneous damage. The area was washed and a dressing applied.

1. **Diagnosis and management options** for an abrasion (clean and dress). (Options can be minimal, limited, multiple, or extensive.)

    How many various options are open to the physician to diagnose the problem and decide how to manage this patient's care—minimal, limited, multiple, extensive? The management of an abrasion is fairly clear—clean and dress the wound; therefore, the diagnosis and management options are minimal.

2. **Data to review** to provide service. (Data can be minimal/none, limited, moderate, or extensive.)

    How much and how complex would the information (data) be that the physician must obtain, review, and analyze to care for this patient—minimal/none, limited, moderate, or extensive? The amount of data to review would be minimal/none for the abrasion.

3. **Risk** of infection if not treated. (Risk can be minimal, low, moderate, or high.)

    How great a risk is there that the patient would die or encounter severe complications if the abrasion were not treated—minimal, low, moderate, or high? The risk of death or of complications is minimal.

The diagnosis and management options are minimal, data are minimal/none, and risk is minimal. Consideration of these three elements has placed this patient's care into a straightforward MDM complexity level.

The history level is stated to be problem focused and the examination level is problem focused. The patient was an established patient seen as an outpatient. Carefully look at each of the items set in boldface type in code 99212 below for an established patient. The place of service, type of service, type of history, type of examination, and complexity level of the MDM are identified in the description of the code.

99212   **Office or other outpatient** visit for the evaluation and management of an **established patient,** which requires at least two of these three key components:

- **a problem focused history**
- **a problem focused examination**
- **straightforward medical decision-making**

CPT code 99212 is where this service to the patient fits.

Now let's establish the MDM level for a more complex case.

EXAMPLE 2

The patient's record states the following: Unknown (new) patient presenting in the office with chest pain. A comprehensive history was taken and an examination immediately performed.

Again, the MDM complexity level must be chosen:

1. **Diagnosis and management options** for cardiac origin of possible myocardial infarction, angina, or heart block. Gastrointestinal origin could be reflux or an ulcer. Respiratory origin could be a pulmonary embolism or pleuritis. (Diagnosis and management options can be minimal, limited, multiple, or extensive.)

What do you think it would take for the physician to decide on the diagnosis or management options of this patient? There are many possibilities of origin for the chest pain; therefore, the diagnosis and management options are extensive.

2. **Data to review** in order to provide service. (Data can be minimal/none, limited, moderate, or extensive.) How much data would the physician have to obtain through current tests on the patient and how much review and analysis of previous records would be necessary to provide services to the patient—minimal/none, limited, moderate, extensive? In this case, the patient's care requires moderate data review, including laboratory, radiology reports, and ECG. You very well may have chosen the data review level of extensive rather than moderate. But this is a new patient and there is no time to request medical records from the patient's previous physician. The physician will be able to analyze only the current medical tests, so the review of data is less extensive than it would be if the patient's previous records had been available.

3. **Risk** if left untreated. (Risk can be minimal, low, moderate, or high.) If the patient's condition were untreated, what do you think the risk of death or serious complication would be—minimal, low, moderate, or high? This patient would have a high risk of death or of severe complications if untreated.

The extensive diagnosis and management options and high risk to the patient if this condition is not treated mean that the necessary standard of two of the three elements' being present has been met. So this patient's care is considered to have a high level of MDM complexity. A new patient with a comprehensive history and examination together with a high MDM complexity places this case in the category of 99205.

EXERCISE 2-5

MEDICAL DECISION-MAKING COMPLEXITY

A patient's record states that an initial office visit was made for the evaluation and management of a 48-year-old male with recurrent low back pain from a herniated disk, with pain radiating to the leg. A detailed history was obtained from this new patient and a physical examination was performed.

Using the information given for this patient, identify the following factors in the case:

1 Diagnosis and management options for recurrent low back pain radiating to the leg. (Options can be minimal, limited, multiple, or extensive.)

_____

2 Data to review in order to provide service. (Data can be minimal/none, limited, moderate, or extensive.) Current record available.

_____

3 Risk if left untreated. (Risk can be minimal, low, moderate, or high.)

_____

4 Two of the three elements have been met to qualify this patient for what level of MDM complexity? (Complexity can be straightforward, low, moderate, or high)

_____

5 The patient record indicates that a detailed history was taken and a detailed examination was performed. When this is combined with the level of MDM complexity you arrived at for this patient, what is the correct CPT code for the case?

Code: _____

Now, let's look again at two cases for which you previously established the history and examination levels:

6 A new patient, an 8-year-old female, is brought into the office by her mother, who states that the child has an earache in the right ear. Mother reports that the child has been complaining of aching and ringing in right ear of increasing severity for the past 2 days. Child appears to be in only minor distress. Temperature, 101°F. Examination: ears, eyes, and nose. Tympanic membranes red, fluid noted in right ear. Health history reviewed. Diagnosis: Otitis media.

What is the MDM level for this patient? _____

7 A 68-year-old female established patient presents to the office today with a "cold" of 9 days' duration. Patient reports that she has had a dry, hacking cough and nasal congestion for the past 6 days and a fever for the past 3 days. She states that she is unable to sleep due to the cough, fever, and aching. She appears to be in minor distress. Personal and family history are negative for respiratory problems. Temperature is 100°F; blood pressure 150/90; pulse 93 and regular. Lungs clear to percussion and auscultation. Examination of head and ears, normal; nose, mucous membranes inflamed with postnasal phlegm. Diagnosis: Sinusitis. Plan: Patient was advised to drink fluids, take aspirin as needed for pain, obtain bed rest, and return if symptoms have not improved in 5 days.

What is the MDM level for this patient? _____

TABLE 2-2 Elements of the Key Components

History Elements

Chief Complaint (CC)
Reason for the encounter in the patient's words

History of Present Illness (HPI)
Location
Quality
Severity
Duration
Timing
Context
Modifying factors
Associated signs and symptoms

Review of Systems (ROS)
Constitutional symptoms
Ophthalmologic (eyes)
Otolaryngologic (ears, nose, mouth, throat)
Cardiovascular
Respiratory
Endocrine
Gastrointestinal
Genitourinary
Musculoskeletal
Integumentary
Neurologic
Psychiatric
Hematologic/Lymphatic
Allergic/Immunologic

Past, Family, and/or Social History (PFSH)
Past illnesses, operations, injuries, and treatments
Family medical history for heredity and risk
Social activities, both past and current

Elements Required for Each Level of History

	Problem Focused	Expanded Problem Focused	Detailed	Comprehensive
History	CC	CC	CC	CC
	Brief HPI	Brief HPI	Extended HPI	Extended HPI
		Problem-pertinent ROS	Extended ROS	Complete ROS
			Pertinent PFSH	Complete PFSH

TABLE 2–2   Elements of the Key Components *Continued*

Examination Elements

General
  Constitutional

Body Areas (BA)
  Head (including the face)
  Neck
  Chest (including breasts and axillae)
  Abdomen
  Genitalia, groin, buttocks
  Back
  Each extremity

Organ System (OS)
  Ophthalmologic (eyes)
  Otolaryngologic (ears, nose, mouth, throat)
  Cardiovascular
  Respiratory
  Endocrine
  Gastrointestinal
  Genitourinary
  Musculoskeletal
  Integumentary
  Neurologic
  Psychiatric
  Hematologic/Lymphatic
  Allergic/Immunologic

Elements Required for Each Level of Examination

	Problem Focused	Expanded Problem Focused	Detailed	Comprehensive
Examination	Limited to affected BA or OS	Limited to affected BA or OS and other related OS(s)	Extended of affected BA(s) and other related OS(s)	General multi-system or complete single OS

Medical Decision-Making Elements

Number of Diagnoses or Management Options
  Minimal
  Limited
  Multiple
  Extensive

Amount or Complexity of Data to Review
  Minimal/None
  Limited
  Moderate
  Extensive

Risk of Complications or Death if Condition Goes Untreated
  Minimal
  Low
  Moderate
  High

Elements Required for Each Level of Medical Decision-Making

	Straightforward	Low	Moderate	High
Number of diagnoses or management options	Minimal	Limited	Multiple	Extensive
Amount or complexity of data to review	Minimal/None	Limited	Moderate	Extensive
Risk	Minimal	Low	Moderate	High

There is certainly a great amount of information that must be considered in order to choose the correct E/M code! Only with practice can you expect to remember all of the various elements and levels within each component. Each medical facility has its own procedure for identifying the level of E/M service; some facilities require the physician to identify all the components of service, whereas other facilities require the component information to be abstracted from the medical record by support personnel. Either way, you need to be knowledgeable about all components of E/M codes (Table 2–2).

from the trenches

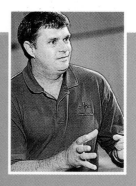

"*Don't compromise. Ever. When it feels wrong, it is wrong. I can be 98% sure about a coding call, but that 2% will keep me up all night. Ideally, you want to be 100% sure on every call.*"

EDWIN

STOP *You have examined each of the three key components and seen how they apply to the assignment of a code. You will be referring to the information as you are presented with additional cases. Make note of the important points and remember that the information about the key components is in the E/M Guidelines at the beginning of the E/M section in the CPT manual.*

Now that you are familiar with the key components of history, examination, and medical decision-making, let's review the contributing factors.

Contributing Factors

There are four contributing factors: counseling, coordination of care, the nature of the presenting problem, and time. Contributing factors are those conditions that help the physician to determine the extent of history, examination, and decision-making (key components) necessary to treat the patient. Contributing factors may or may not be considered in every patient case.

CONTRIBUTING FACTORS

- Counseling
- Coordination of care
- Nature of presenting problem
- Time

Counseling

Counseling is a service that physicians provide to patients and their families. It involves discussion of diagnostic results, impressions, and recommended diagnostic studies; prognosis; risks and benefits of treatment; instructions for treatment; importance of compliance with treatment; risk factor reduction; and patient and family education. Some form of counseling usually takes place in all physician and patient encounters, and this was factored into the codes when they were developed by the AMA. Only when counseling is the reason for the encounter or consumes most of the visit time (more than 50% of the total time) is counseling considered a component of code assignment. The following statement is made often within the codes in the E/M section:

Counseling and/or coordination of care with other providers or agencies are provided consistent with the nature of the problem(s) and the patient's and/or family's needs.

Coordination of Care

Coordination of care with other health care providers or agencies may be necessary for the care of a patient. In coordination of care, a physician might arrange for other services to be provided to the patient, such as arrangements for admittance to a long-term nursing facility.

Nature of the Presenting Problem

The presenting problem is the patient's chief complaint or the situation that leads the physician into determining the level of care necessary to diagnose and treat the patient. The CPT describes the **presenting problem** as a disease, condition, illness, injury, symptom, sign, finding, complaint, or other reason for the encounter, with or without a diagnosis being established at the time of the encounter. There are five types of presenting problems.

- Minimal

- Self-limited

- Low severity

- Moderate severity

- High severity

1. **Minimal:** A problem may not require the presence of the physician, but service is provided under the physician's supervision. A minimal problem is a blood pressure reading, a dressing change, or another service that can be performed without the physician's being immediately present.

2. **Self-limited:** Also called a minor presenting problem, a self-limited problem runs a definite and prescribed course, is transient (it comes and goes), and is not likely to permanently alter health status, or the presenting problem has a good prognosis with management and compliance.

3. **Low severity:** The risk of complete sickness (morbidity) without treatment is low, there is little or no risk of death without treatment, and full recovery without impairment is expected.

4. **Moderate severity:** The risk of complete sickness (morbidity) without treatment is moderate, there is moderate risk of death without treatment, and an uncertain prognosis or increased probability of impairment exists.

5. **High severity:** The risk of complete sickness (morbidity) without treatment is high to extreme, there is a moderate to high risk of death without treatment, or there is a strong probability of severe, prolonged functional impairment.

The patient's medical record should contain the physician's observation of the complexity of the presenting problem(s). Your responsibility is to identify the words that correctly indicate the type of presenting problem.

EXERCISE
2-6

PRESENTING PROBLEM

Match the presenting problem to the severity level in the patient:

1   Four-year-old female established patient presents with persistent pain in right ear, of 2 days' duration.

   Physician prescribes medication. _____

2   Eighty-six-year-old woman who has a history of chronic obstructive pulmonary disease (COPD) and is oxygen-dependent comes in today because of dizziness and weakness. _____

3   Established patient, 71 years old, with shortness of breath on exertion and a history of left ventricular dysfunction with cardiomyopathy. _____

4   Fourteen-year-old presents with moderate pain in left thumb after a fall from his skateboard. _____

5   Established patient, 34 years old, presents for a blood pressure check. _____

a. minimal

b. self-limited

c. low

d. moderate

e. high

Time

Time was not included in the CPT manual before 1992 but was incorporated to assist with the selection of the most appropriate level of E/M services. The times indicated with the codes are only averages and represent a simple estimate of the possible duration of a service.

Direct face-to-face and **unit/floor time** are two measures of time. Outpatient visits are measured as direct face-to-face time. Direct face-to-face time is the time a physician spends directly with a patient during an office visit obtaining the history, performing an examination, and discussing the results. Inpatient time is measured as unit/floor time and is used to describe the time a physician spends in the hospital setting dealing with the patient's care. Unit/floor time includes care given to the patient at the bedside as well as at other settings on the unit or floor (e.g., the nursing station). It is an often-heard comment that physicians get paid a great deal of money just for stopping in to see a hospitalized patient. However, what is not realized is that the physician spends additional time reviewing the patient's records and writing orders for the patient's care.

Time in the E/M section is referred to in statements such as this one that is located with code 99203:

> Usually, the presenting problem(s) is (are) of moderate severity. Physicians typically spend 30 minutes face to face with the patient and/or family.

These statements concerning time are used when counseling or coordination of care represent more than 50% of the time spent with a patient. The times referred to in these statements are the basis of the selection of the correct E/M code. For example: An established patient returns for an office visit to get results of previous tests. The physician spends 25 minutes going over the unfavorable results of the tests. The physician discusses various treatment options, the prognosis, and the risks of treatment and of treatment refusal. The correct code would be 99214, in which the time statement is, "Physician typically spends 25 minutes face to face with the patient and/or family."

AN E/M CODE EXAMPLE

With the CPT manual open to the first page of the E/M section, locate the notes above the 99201 code. These notes highlight the incidents in which codes in that particular category are appropriate for assignment. The notes above 99201 indicate that the codes that follow the notes are appropriate for use in coding services provided in a "physician's office or in an outpatient or other ambulatory facility."

The information also directs you to other code subsections if the patient classification is not correct. As an example of this directional feature, the notes above 99201 state, "For services provided by physicians in the Emergency Department, *see* 99281–99285."

Figure 2–7 shows the first code for a new patient under the category New Patient under subsection Office or Other Outpatient Services. Review Figure 2–7 carefully before continuing. Note the location of each important piece of information.

Locate the following items in Figure 2–7:

1. Three contributing factors

2. Three key components

3. Number of key components required

4. Place of service

5. Category of the code

USING THE E/M CODES

Now you are going to use the information you have learned about codes in the E/M services section as you continue to identify the differences among the code numbers.

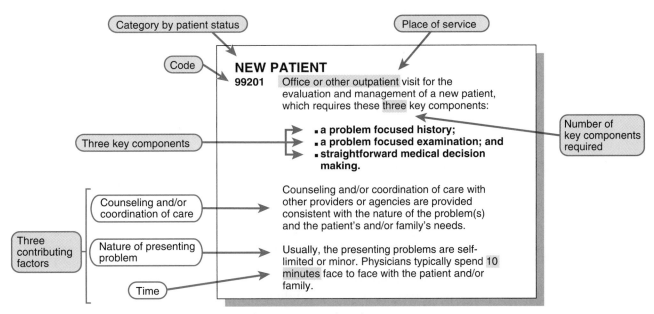

Figure 2–7   Code information.

Office and Other Outpatient Services

New Patient

The first subsection in the E/M section is Office and Other Outpatient Services, New Patient Category.

You will recall from information presented earlier that a new patient is defined as one that has not seen the physician or another physician with the same specialty in the same group within the past 3 years. A physician must spend more time with a new patient—obtaining the history, conducting the examination, and considering the data—than with an established patient. Consider that the established patient is probably known to the physician and the person's medical records are available. For these reasons, the cost of a new patient office visit is higher, so third-party payers reimburse the physician at a higher rate for new patient services than for the same type of service when it is provided to an established patient.

EXERCISE 2-7

NEW PATIENT SERVICES

Using the CPT manual, fill in the blanks with the correct words:

1 For code 99203, the history level is _____ , the examination is _____ , and the MDM is of _____ complexity.

2 For code 99204, the history level is _____ , the examination is _____ , and the MDM complexity is

_____ .

3 For code 99205, the history level is _____ , the examination is _____ , and the MDM complexity is

_____ .

Code the following cases:

4 A 53-year-old new patient presents for an initial office visit to discuss a surgical vasectomy for sterilization. The history and examination was detailed and the MDM was of low complexity.

Code(s): _____

5 A 4-year-old new patient presents for the removal of sutures made for an appendectomy 10 days earlier in another city. The physician conducts a brief history and examination prior to removing the stitches.

Code(s): _____

6 A 23-year-old man who is a new patient has an initial office visit for severe depression that has led to frequent thoughts of suicide in the past several weeks and is acute today. More than an hour is spent discussing the patient's problems and options. Past medical history is negative. The social history reveals that the patient suffers from sleeplessness; smokes between two and two and a half packs of unfiltered cigarettes a day; drinks 10 to 12 cups of coffee; and denies current use of drugs. (The actual patient record continues and indicates that a comprehensive examination was conducted; high MDM complexity.)

Code(s): _____

7 A new patient, a 10-year-old boy, is brought in by his father for a knee injury sustained in a hockey game. The knee is swollen and the patient is in apparent pain. A detailed history and examination are obtained. A diagnosis of probable meniscus tear is made. Low MDM complexity.

Code(s): _____

8 A 41-year-old woman, who is a new patient, complains of headache and rhinitis of 4 days' duration. The patient states that she has had a problem with her allergies during this season for years. An expanded problem focused history and examination are done. Straightforward MDM complexity.

Code(s): _____

Established Patient

The second category of codes in subsection Office and Other Outpatient Services is for the established patient in an outpatient setting. You will recall that the definition of an established patient is one who has received professional services from the physician or another physician of the same specialty in the same group within the past 3 years.

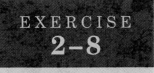

EXERCISE
2-8

ESTABLISHED PATIENT SERVICES

Fill in the blanks with information from codes in the Established Patient category:

1 99211: This minimal service level does not exist in the New Patient category because a new patient is usually seen by the physician. The established patient may or may not be seen by the physician. Read the description and information for code 99211 in the CPT manual. Would an established patient returning for a simple blood pressure check be appropriately reported as 99211?

_____

2 A 42-year-old established patient presents for an office visit with complaints of severe vaginal itching and moderate pain. During the problem focused history, the patient states that several weeks ago she had noted a slight itching, which has increased in severity. Yesterday, she noted a lesion on her genitalia. Burning and painful urination have increased over the past 5 days accompanied by rectal itching. She has tried a variety of over-the-counter ointments and creams, which induced no improvement. The patient states that she has had several yeast infections in the past that had been successfully treated by her previous physician. Personal history indicates several prior urinary infections. No discharge noted. A problem focused examination of the external genitalia revealed a lesion, which had previously ruptured, located on the vulva. Bacterial and viral smears were done. The MDM complexity was straightforward. The patient was advised that the smears would be back in 24 hours and that a treatment plan would be developed based on the reports. (The smear was positive for a bacterial infection, for which antibiotics were prescribed.)

Code(s): _____

3   A 17-year-old football player comes to the clinic for a gold injection by the nurse. Only the nurse saw this established patient. (Code only the E/M service.)

Code(s): _____

4   A 53-year-old established patient complains of frequent fainting. The history and examination were comprehensive, and the MDM was of high complexity.

Code(s): _____

5   A 61-year-old established patient is seen for medication management of fatigue produced by hypertensive medication. An expanded problem focused history and examination were done, and the MDM was of moderate complexity.

Code(s): _____

6   An established 31-year-old patient presents with an irritated skin tag. A problem focused history and examination were done. MDM complexity was low.

Code(s): _____

7   A 48-year-old woman has had diarrhea for the past 5 days. Her temperature is 101°F. An expanded problem focused history and examination were done. MDM complexity was low.

Code(s): _____

STOP *Remember, it takes a lot of practice to learn to code. It is not a skill that is quickly acquired. You need to have patience and know that practice, practice, practice is the only thing that will make this skill yours.*

Hospital Observation Services

The codes in the Hospital Observation subsection are used to identify initial observation care or observation discharge services. The services in the observation subsection are for patients who are in a hospital on observation status.

Observation is a status used for the classification of a patient who does not have an illness severe enough to meet acute inpatient criteria and does not require resources as intensive as an inpatient but does require hospitalization for a short period of time. Patients are also admitted to observation so further information can be obtained about the severity of the condition and so it can be determined whether the patient can be treated on an outpatient basis. In some parts of the country, observation status is conducted in the temporary care unit (TCU).

The observation codes are for new or established patients. There are no time components with observation codes, as codes are based on the level of service.

If a patient is admitted to the hospital as an inpatient after having been admitted earlier the same day as an observation patient, you do not report the observation status separately. The services provided during observation become part of (are bundled into) the initial inpatient hospital admission code.

Observation Care Discharge Services

The Observation Care Discharge Services code includes the final examination of the patient upon discharge from observation status. Discussion of the hospital stay, instructions for continued care, and preparation of discharge records are also bundled into the Observation Care Discharge Services code. The code is used only with patients who are discharged on a day that follows the first day of observation.

Initial Observation Care

Initial Observation Care codes (99218–99220) are used to designate the beginning of observation status in a hospital. Again, the hospital does not need to have a formal observation area, since the designation of observation status is dependent on the severity of illness of the patient. These codes also include development of a care plan for the patient and periodic reassessment while on observation status. Observation admission can be reported only for the first day of the service. If the patient is admitted and discharged on the same day, a code from the range 99234–99236, Observation or Inpatient Care Services, is used to report the service. If the patient is in the hospital overnight but remains there for a period that is **less than 48 hours,** the first day's service is coded with a code from the range 99218–99220, Initial Observation Care, and the second day's service is coded 99217, Observation Care Discharge Services. If the patient is on observation status for *longer than 48 hours,* the first day is coded with a code from the range 99218–99220, Initial Observation Care; the second day is coded with a code from the range 99211–99215, Established Office or Other Outpatient Services; and the third day is coded 99217, Observation Care Discharge Services.

Services performed in sites other than the observation area (e.g., clinic, nursing home, emergency department) and that precede admission to observation status are included in (bundled into) the Initial Observation Care codes and are not to be coded separately.

For example, an established patient was seen in the physician's office for frequent fainting of unknown origin. The history and examination were comprehensive and the MDM complexity was moderate. The code for the office visit would be 99215. But the physician decided to admit the patient immediately on observation status until a further determination could be made as to the origin of the fainting. You would chose a code from the Hospital Inpatient Services subsection, Initial Observation Care subheading, in order to report the physician's service of admission on observation status (99219) and would not separately report the office visit.

If a patient is admitted to observation status and then becomes ill enough to be admitted to the hospital, an initial hospital care code (99221–99223), not an observation code, is used to report services.

CAUTION *Observation or Inpatient Care Services, codes 99234–99236, have a very specific purpose: they code for services to a patient who is admitted to and discharged from observation or inpatient status on the same day. All the services provided to the patient—same-day office services, observation care, and discharge—are covered by the use of one code from the 99234–99236 range.*

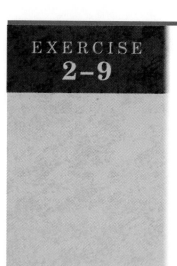

HOSPITAL OBSERVATION SERVICES

Using the CPT manual, locate the correct information about the Hospital Observation codes:

1 A patient was in an automobile accident and is complaining of a minor headache and no other apparent injuries. History gathered from bystanders states that patient was not wearing a seat belt and hit his head on the windshield. A 15-minute loss of consciousness was noted. The patient was then admitted for 24-hour observation to rule out head injury. A comprehensive history and examination were done. The MDM was of moderate complexity.

Code(s): _____

EXERCISE 2-9

Hospital Inpatient Services

Hospital Inpatient Services codes (99221–99239) are used to indicate a patient's status as an inpatient in a hospital or partial hospital setting and, therefore, to identify the hospital setting as the place where the physician renders service to the patient. An **inpatient** is one who has been formally admitted to an acute health care facility.

Note that within the subsection Hospital Inpatient Services, all the subheadings except Hospital Discharge Services are divided primarily on the basis of the three key components of history, examination, and MDM complexity. Further, within this subsection only Subsequent Hospital Care codes do not require all three key components to be at the level described in the code. For example, the key components for code 99222 are a comprehensive history, a comprehensive examination, and a moderate level of MDM complexity. If the case you are coding has a comprehensive history and a comprehensive examination but a low complexity of MDM, you cannot assign code 99222 to the case; instead, you would have to assign the lower level code of 99221.

The subsection of Hospital Inpatient Services is divided into three subheadings.

1. Initial Hospital Care
2. Subsequent Hospital Care
3. Hospital Discharge Services

Initial Hospital Care

Initial Hospital Care codes are used to code for the initial service of admission to the hospital by the admitting physician. Only the admitting physician can use the Initial Hospital Care codes. These codes reflect services in any setting (office, emergency department, nursing home) that are provided in conjunction with the admission to the hospital. For example, if the patient is seen in the office and subsequently is admitted to the hospital, the office visit is considered bundled into the initial hospital care service. All services provided in the office may be taken into account when selecting the appropriate level of hospital admission.

EXERCISE 2-10

INITIAL HOSPITAL CARE

Fill in the missing words or codes for the following:

1   Which Initial Hospital Care code has a comprehensive history with a straightforward or low complexity of MDM?

Code: _____

2   Which code has a time component of 70 minutes?

Code: _____

3   Code 99222 has a _____ history and examination level

and a _____ MDM complexity.

4   An 80-year-old woman has inflammation of the kidneys and renal pelvic area. She is complaining of hematuria, dysuria, and pyuria. She is in good general health other than this condition. She has had some previous workup for this condition as an outpatient but is now being admitted for a cystoscopy. In the patient's history, the physician noted the patient's chief complaints and described the bright red nature of the hematuria, the severe discomfort associated with the dysuria, including burning and itching, and her other symptoms of frequency and urgency. The patient had stated that her symptoms had begun gradually over the past 2 weeks but had become more intense in the past 48 hours. The physician documented the patient's positive responses and pertinent negative responses in his review of her cardiovascular, respiratory, genitourinary, musculoskeletal, neurologic, and endocrine systems. Her past history relating to urinary and renal problems was reviewed. The physical examination noted the complete findings relative to her reproductive system as well as to her urinary system. An examination of her back and related musculoskeletal structures was included because she complained of mild back pain as well. After completing the detailed history and examination, the physician concluded with a provisional diagnosis of cystitis and pyelitis, possibly associated with endometritis. The MDM complexity was low. The patient was reassured and told to expect a short stay once the exact problem was pinpointed.

Code(s): _____

Subsequent Hospital Care

Subsequent Hospital Care codes (99231–99233) are the second subheading of codes in the Hospital Inpatient Services subsection. The Subsequent Hospital Care codes are used by physicians to report daily hospital visits while the patient is hospitalized.

The first Subsequent Hospital Care code is 99231. Typically, the 99231 level implies that the patient is in stable condition and is responding well to treatment. Subsequent codes in the subsection indicate (in the "Usually, the patient . . ." area) the status of the patient, such as stable/unstable or recovering/unresponding. Be certain to read the contributing factors area for each code in this subheading.

More than one physician can use the subsequent care codes on the same day. This is called concurrent care. **Concurrent care** is being provided when more than one physician provides service to a patient on the same day for different conditions. An example of concurrent care is a circumstance in which physician A, a cardiologist, treats the patient for a heart condition and at the same time physician B, an oncologist, treats the patient for a cancer condition. The patient's attending physician maintains the primary responsibility for the overall care of the patient, no matter how many other physicians are providing services to the patient, unless a formal transfer of care has occurred.

An **attending physician** is a doctor who, on the basis of education, training, and experience, is granted medical staff membership and clinical privileges by a health care organization to perform diagnostic or therapeutic procedures. An attending physician is legally responsible for the care and treatment provided to a patient. The attending physician may be a patient's personal physician or may be a physician assigned to a patient who has been admitted to a hospital through the emergency department. The attending physician is usually a provider of primary care, such as a family practitioner, internist, or pediatrician, but the attending physician may also be a surgeon or another type of specialist. In an academic medical center, the attending physician is a member of the academic or medical school staff who is responsible for the supervision of medical residents, interns, and medical school students and oversees the care the residents, interns, or students provide to the patients.

STOP *Note that there is no comprehensive history or comprehensive examination level in the codes in the Subsequent Hospital Care subheading because the comprehensive level of service would have been provided at the time of admission.*

Hospital Discharge Services

Inpatient Hospital Discharge Services are reported on the final day of services for a multiple-day stay in a hospital setting. The service reflects the final examination of the patient as appropriate, follow-up instructions to the patient, and arrangements for discharge, including completion of discharge records. The codes are based on the time spent by the physician in handling the final discharge of the patient.

The Hospital Discharge Services codes are not used if the physician is a consultant. If a consulting physician is following the patient for a separate condition, those services would require a subsequent hospital care code. Only the attending physician, not the consultant, is responsible for completion of the final examination, follow-up instructions, and arrangements for discharge and discharge records. Because these additional services are included in the Hospital Discharge codes, only the attending physician's services can be reported using the codes.

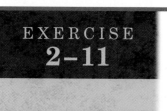

EXERCISE 2-11

HOSPITAL DISCHARGE SERVICES

Fill in the blanks:

1   What are the times indicated for each of the Hospital Discharge Services codes? _____

2   According to the category notes in Hospital Discharge Services, does the time spent by the physician arranging for the final hospital discharge of the patient have to be continuous? _____

Consultation Services

We all need advice once in a while—maybe for a problem or situation that we cannot find a solution to. Perhaps we think we are doing the right thing but want another person's advice or view to make certain we are following the best course of action. Physicians need opinions and advice, too, and when they do, they ask another physician for an opinion or advice on the treatment, diagnosis, or management of a patient. The physician asking for the advice or opinion is making a **request for consultation** and is the **requesting** physician. The physician giving the advice is providing a consultation and is the **consultant.** Consultations can be done for both outpatients and inpatients. The CPT manual has different codes for each of the three types of patient consultation—outpatient, inpatient, and confirmatory.

"Request for consultation" used to be termed "referral"; making a referral meant that the referring physician was asking for the advice or opinion of another physician (a consultation). However, some third-party payers have chosen to define "referral" to mean a total transfer of the care of a patient. In other words, if a patient is referred by physician A to physician B, physician A is expecting physician B to evaluate and treat the patient for the condition for which the patient is being referred. The services of physician B would **not** be reported using consultation codes. On the other hand, if physician A makes a **request for a consultation** to physician B, it is expected that physician B will provide physician A with his or her advice or opinion and that the patient will return to physician A for any necessary treatment. Physician B would then report his or her services using consultation codes. Although these semantics (uses of words) may seem unimportant, they make a difference in the codes you use to report the services.

In the Consultation subsection, there are four subheadings of consultations.

1. Office or Other Outpatient Consultations

2. Initial Inpatient Consultations

3. Follow-up Inpatient Consultations

4. Confirmatory Consultations

The first three subheadings—Office or Other Outpatient Consultations, Initial Inpatient Consultations, and Follow-up Inpatient Consultations—define the location in which the service is rendered; the patient is either an outpatient or an inpatient. The fourth subheading—Confirmatory Consultations—can be provided on either an outpatient or an inpatient basis. All the subheadings are for new or established patients, except the Follow-up Inpatient Consultations subheading.

Only one initial consultation is reported by a consultant for the patient on each admission, and any subsequent service is reported using codes from the Follow-up Inpatient subheading or subsequent hospital codes (99231–99233), depending on the circumstances.

A **consultation** is a service provided by a physician whose opinion or advice regarding the management or diagnosis of a specific problem has been requested. The consultant provides a written report of the opinion or advice to the attending physician and documents the opinion and services provided in the medical record; the care of the patient is thus complete. Sometimes the attending physician will request the consultant to assume responsibility for a specific area of the patient's care. For example, a consultant may be asked by the attending physician to see an inpatient regarding the care of the patient's diabetes while the patient is hospitalized for gallbladder surgery. After the initial consultation, the attending physician may ask the consultant to continue to monitor the patient's diabetic condition. The consultant assumes responsibility for management of the patient in the specific area of diabetes. Subsequent visits made by the consultant would then be coded using the codes from the subheading Subsequent Hospital Care.

Documentation in the medical record for a consultation must show a request from the attending physician for an opinion or the advice of a consultant on a specific condition. Findings and treatments rendered during the consultation must be documented in the medical record by the consultant and communicated to the attending physician. A consultant can order tests and services for an inpatient, but the medical necessity of all tests and services must be indicated in the medical record.

Office or Other Outpatient Consultations

The Office or Other Outpatient Consultations codes (99241–99245) are used to code consultative services provided a patient in an office or other ambulatory patient setting, including hospital observation services, home services, custodial care, and services that are provided in a domiciliary, rest home, or emergency department. Outpatient consultations include consultations provided in the emergency department because the patient is considered an outpatient in the emergency department setting. The codes are for both new and established patients. The codes in this subsection are of increasing complexity, based on the three key components and any contributing factors.

Initial Inpatient Consultations

The codes in the Initial Inpatient Consultations subheading (99251–99255) are used to report services by physicians in inpatient settings. This subheading is used for both new and established patients and can be reported only one time per patient admission per consulting physician.

After the initial consultation report, the subsequent hospital visit codes would be used to report services, unless documentation meets the criteria for a follow-up consultation (discussed in the next paragraph).

Follow-up Inpatient Consultations

The follow-up inpatient consultation (99261–99263) is used only for inpatients. These codes are used only when the consultant must see the patient again so as to complete the initial consultation or if the attending physician requests another evaluation and the consultant has not already assumed responsibility for part of the patient's care.

from the trenches

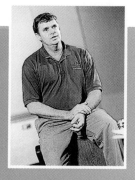

"*While most payers have customer service lines, most patients don't know what questions to ask. A lot of people are out there who don't know anything about insurance or coding . . . they just pay the bill without checking into it.*"

EDWIN

Confirmatory Consultations

Various persons request consultations. Patients may request a confirmation of a diagnosis or recommended treatment such as surgery. Insurance companies and other third-party payers may request a consultation for confirmation of a diagnosis, prognosis, or treatment plan for a patient. These consultations are **confirmatory consultations** (99271–99275). Patients and third-party payers often seek more than one confirmatory consultation. The consultant should document that he or she is providing a second or third opinion. The Confirmatory Consultations codes for New or Established Patient are used to report services provided when the consulting physician is aware of the confirmatory nature of the opinion sought. Confirmatory consultations can be for inpatients or outpatients. Services after the initial confirmatory consultation are coded using the appropriate level of office visit, established patient, or subsequent hospital care. If the confirmatory consultation is required, the Mandated Service modifier (-32) is used with the correct five-digit code.

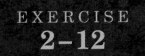

EXERCISE
2-12

CONSULTATION SERVICES

Using the CPT manual, code the following scenarios:

1 A 56-year-old female was sent by her primary care physician (PCP) to the oncologist for his opinion regarding the treatment options. The patient had had a right breast carcinoma 6 years earlier but over the past 4 months had developed progressively more painful back pain. In the physician's HPI it was noted that the pain was in the mid-back, with the patient rating it an 8 on a scale of 1 to 10 in intensity. However, when the pain started, she thought it was about a 4 on the same scale. The pain has caused her to have neck and leg pains as well, as she has adjusted her walking stance in order to alleviate the pain. She responded to the physician's questions in the review of seven of her organ systems. Her past medical and surgical history was noted, including the fact that her mother and one sister had also had breast cancer. A comprehensive history was taken. She had worked as a legal secretary up until 2 weeks ago but was on sick leave now. The comprehensive physical examination performed by the physician was a complete multisystem review of 12 organ systems. The physician ordered a series of radiographic and laboratory tests and reviewed her recent spine x-ray series, which revealed multiple vertebral compression fractures. The MDM complexity was moderate.

   Code(s): _____

2 A 45-year-old man was sent by his PCP to an orthopedic surgeon's office for acute pain and stiffness in his right elbow. In his problem focused history, the physician noted that the man was a farmer and used his right hand and arm repeatedly, lifting heavy objects. The patient had no other complaints and reported to be in otherwise excellent health. The farmer described the pain as severe and unrelenting, and it prevented him from using the arm. The problem focused physical examination noted the man's slightly swollen right elbow, with marked pain on movement. No other problems were noted with his right upper extremity. The physician diagnosed the problem as elbow tendinitis and bursitis, recommended warm compresses, and gave the patient a pre-

scription for an anti-inflammatory medication. The MDM complexity was straightforward.

Code(s): _____

3   A 72-year-old man was seen in the internal medicine clinic as an outpatient for medical clearance prior to the replacement of his right knee. The patient had a history of essential hypertension and mild coronary artery disease. The internist noted, during the expanded problem focused history, that the patient had no complaints relative to his hypertension or heart disease. His blood pressure appeared to be controlled by his medication and low-salt diet. The patient denied any chest pain or discomfort either while working or at rest. The physician's review of his cardiovascular and respiratory systems appeared to be unremarkable. The physician performed an expanded problem focused physical examination of his head, neck, chest, and abdomen but found no major problems related to his cardiovascular or respiratory system. The internist confirmed the diagnoses previously established and made no changes in the management of either condition. The MDM complexity was straightforward.

Code(s): _____

4   A 52-year-old patient was sent to a surgeon for an office consultation concerning hemorrhoids. A problem focused history and examination were performed. The consultant recommended treating with medication after a straightforward MDM.

Code(s): _____

5   A 60-year-old man was seen in consultation by a cardiologist for complaints of dyspnea, fatigue, and lightheadedness. His history included the insertion of a pacemaker 6 years earlier. He also had a history of mitral regurgitation. The cardiologist performed a comprehensive cardiology physical examination, including cardiac monitoring, pacemaker evaluation, and review of his associated respiratory status. Noted in the comprehensive history were a variety of complaints the patient had in addition to the past pacemaker insertion and mitral valve regurgitation diagnosed by cardiac catheterization. The physician reviewed the patient's medical history, from the first signs of problems 6 years earlier until the present. His review of systems elicited positive findings in the cardiovascular, respiratory, gastrointestinal, genitourinary, musculoskeletal, and neurologic systems. The other systems had negative responses. The physician had multiple management options concerning the pacemaker function but also had to consider new valvular problems that might have been present as well as related gastrointestinal symptoms. Extensive tests that had been performed recently were reviewed, and additional testing was ordered. The MDM complexity was moderate.

Code(s): _____

6   A 65-year-old man had recently undergone a prostatectomy for prostate cancer. Since the surgery, his previously controlled atrial fibrillation had become a problem again. A cardiologist was called in for an inpatient consultation; he reviewed the patient's present status, including the duration and severity of his symptoms. The cardiologist's review of systems related strictly to the cardiovascular system during an expanded problem focused history. The expanded problem focused physi-

cal examination concentrated on the man's neck, chest, and abdomen and attempted to elicit all cardiovascular pathology. The consultant suggested that the atrial fibrillation could be controlled better with a newer medication. The MDM complexity was straightforward.

Code(s): _____

7 An internist requested an inpatient consultation from an orthopedic surgeon to evaluate and manage a 35-year-old female who had been in a motor vehicle accident. After reviewing the multiple x-ray reports and the documentation generated by the emergency department physicians, the paramedics' progress notes from the scene of the accident, and the history and physical examination produced by the internist, the orthopedist performed a complete review of systems; complete past, family, and social history; and extended details of the history of the present illness in a comprehensive history review. The comprehensive physical examination was a complete musculoskeletal and neurologic examination with a review of all other organ systems. Based on the patient's multiple fractures and internal injuries, the orthopedist concluded that the patient needed immediate surgery to repair and control the life-threatening conditions that existed. The MDM complexity was high. A neurosurgeon and a general surgeon were also asked to see the patient immediately and possibly to assist in surgery. (Code only the orthopedic consultation.)

Code(s): _____

8 A 55-year-old patient was injured at work when he fell from a house roof and struck his head. He was admitted for a right frontal parietal craniotomy with removal of a subdural hematoma. After 5 days of rapid recovery from this surgery, a consultation was requested regarding a drug reaction that produced a rash on the upper torso. The physician conducted a brief HPI during the expanded problem focused history, in addition to an ROS focused on the patient's condition. The expanded problem focused examination included three body areas and one organ system. The MDM complexity was straightforward.

Code(s): _____

9 A 10-year-old was admitted 4 days ago for tympanotomy. Postsurgically the child developed fever and seizures of unknown origin. A pediatric consultation was requested. The HPI was extended with a complete ROS. A complete PFSH was elicited from the mother as part of a comprehensive history. A comprehensive examination was conducted on all body areas and organ systems. The MDM complexity was high.

Code(s): _____

10 A cardiologist was asked by a family practitioner to see an 80-year-old male patient a second time. One week prior, the patient, who has multiple other medical problems, suffered an anterior wall myocardial infarction. Despite following the medical management suggested by the cardiologist, the patient continued to have angina and ventricular arrhythmias. The cardiologist closely examined all of the documentation and test results that had been generated in the past week and performed a complete ROS and an extended HPI during the detailed interval history. The detailed physical examination performed was a complete cardiovascular system examination. Based on the subjective and objective findings, the cardiologist concluded that more aggressive med-

ical management was in order. Given the patient's multiple problems coupled with the new threat of cardiorespiratory failure, the patient was immediately transferred to the intensive care unit. The MDM was of high complexity.

Code(s): _____

11 The attending physician had requested an inpatient consultation on a 10-year-old admitted 7 days earlier for tympanotomy. Postsurgically, the patient developed fever and seizures. An initial consultation diagnosis was febrile seizure. Now, on day 7, the child's temperature had returned to normal but the child had had a recurrence of seizures of increased severity. A follow-up consultation was requested. The consultant performed a detailed history and physical examination. The MDM was of high complexity.

Code(s): _____

12 Dr. Jones asked Dr. Williams to confirm the diagnosis of tetralogy of Fallot in a 6-day-old male infant prior to cardiovascular surgery. Dr. Williams performed a comprehensive history and physical examination on the infant and reviewed the results of the extensive tests already performed. The consultant concluded that the child's problem was of moderate to high severity and recommended immediate surgery. The MDM complexity was moderate.

Code(s): _____

13 The 45-year-old female's insurance company required a second opinion regarding the degenerative disk disease of her lumbar spine. One orthopedic surgeon had recommended a laminectomy. A second orthopedic surgeon was consulted and performed an expanded problem focused history and physical examination, particularly of her musculoskeletal and neurologic systems. Based on his findings and the conclusive findings of a recent myelogram, the second orthopedic surgeon was quick to conclude that the laminectomy was a reasonable course to follow. The MDM complexity was straightforward.

Code(s): _____

14 A third-party payer sought confirmatory consultation for an opinion about a patient's ability to return to work after the removal of a subdural hematoma 2 months previously. The patient's primary physician had stated that the patient was not yet able to return to his employment, and the third-party payer wanted a second opinion. The patient stated that he continued to have severe and incapacitating headaches and was unable to return to work. A comprehensive history and physical examination were performed. The MDM was of moderate complexity, based on physician findings.

Code(s): _____

Emergency Department Services

Emergency Department Services codes (99281–99285) are used for new or established patients when services are provided in an emergency department that is a part of a hospital and available 24 hours a day. These patients are presenting for immediate attention. The codes are used for patients without appointments. Emergency Department Services codes are not used for patients at the hospital on observation status even if the observation unit is located at or near the emergency department.

The codes in the Emergency Department Services subsection are based on the type of service the physician performs in terms of the history, the examination, and the complexity of the MDM. In addition to this information within each code, note that the paragraph at the end of each code that begins with "Usually, the presenting problem(s) are of . . ." identifies the immediacy of the care. For example, 99283 indicates that the presenting problem is of "moderate severity," whereas 99285 indicates that the presenting problem is of "high severity and poses an immediate significant threat to life. . . ." Sometimes the patient's clinical condition poses an immediate threat to life, making it possible for the physician to use the higher level code even if it may not be possible to perform the required history and physical examination.

Critical care provided to the patient in the emergency department is reported using additional codes from the Critical Care Service code section.

Other Emergency Department Services

The Other Emergency Department Services subheading is at the end of the Emergency Department Services subsection, and the code located there is used to report the services of a physician based at the hospital who provides two-way communication with the ambulance or rescue team. This physician provides direction and advice to the team as they attend the patient en route to the emergency department.

The subheading notes contain examples of the types of medical services the physician might direct. Be certain to read these notes so you understand the types of services the code refers to.

EXERCISE 2-13

EMERGENCY DEPARTMENT SERVICES

Use the information contained in the code descriptions from the Emergency Department Services subsection to answer the questions in this exercise.

1 Key components: problem focused history, problem focused examination, straightforward MDM complexity. The severity of the presenting problem would usually be _____ .

2 Key components: detailed history, detailed examination, and moderate MDM complexity. The severity of the presenting problem would usually be _____ .

3 Key components: expanded problem focused history, expanded problem focused examination, low MDM complexity. The severity of the presenting problem would usually be _____ .

4 Key components: expanded problem focused history, expanded problem focused examination, moderate MDM complexity. The severity of the presenting problem would usually be _____ .

Code the following:

5 A patient in the emergency department has extreme acute chest pains and goes into cardiac arrest. The emergency department physician is

unable to obtain a history or perform a physical examination because the patient's condition is critical. The MDM is of high complexity.

Code(s): _____

6 A patient in the emergency department has a temperature of 105°F and is in acute respiratory distress. Symptoms include shortness of breath, chest pain, cyanosis, and gasping. The physician is unable to obtain a history or perform a comprehensive physical examination because the patient's condition is critical. The MDM complexity is high.

Code(s): _____

7 A child presents to the emergency department with his parents after being bitten by a dog. The child is in extreme pain and bleeding from a wound on the forearm. The animal has not been located to quarantine for rabies. An expanded problem focused history is obtained and an expanded problem focused physical examination is performed. The MDM complexity is moderate because of the possibility of rabies.

Code(s): _____

8 The physician directs the emergency medical technicians via two-way communications with an ambulance en route to the emergency department with a patient in apparent cardiac arrest.

Code(s): _____

Patient Transport

Patient Transport codes are time-based codes used to report physician services provided to critically ill patients being transported from one medical facility to another. If the physician is in physical attendance for less than 30 minutes, the service is not reported. The codes are divided based on the first 30 to 74 minutes and each additional block of 30 minutes beyond 74. Bundled into the Patient Transport codes are routine monitoring and evaluation, such as of heart rate and blood pressure. Other services provided by the physician before transport or nonroutine services provided during the transport can be reported separately.

Critical Care Services

Critical Care Services codes are used to identify services that are provided during medical emergencies to patients who are either critically ill or injured. These service codes require the physician to be constantly available to the patient and providing services exclusively to that patient. For example, a patient who is in shock or cardiac arrest would require the physician to provide bedside critical care services. Critical care is often, but not required to be, provided in an acute care setting of a hospital. Acute care settings are intensive care units, coronary care units, emergency departments, pediatric intensive care units, and similar critical care units of a hospital. Codes in this subsection are listed according to the time the physician spends providing critical care to the patient.

The total critical care time, per day, the physician spends in care of the patient is stated in one amount of time, even if the time was not concurrent. Code 99291 is used only once a day. As an example, if a physician sees a critical care patient for 74 minutes and then leaves and returns for 30 minutes of critical care at a later time in the same day, the coding would be for 104 minutes of care. The coding for 104 minutes would be

99291 for the 74 minutes
99292 for the additional 30 minutes

Code 99291 is reported for the first 30 to 74 minutes of critical care and code 99292 is used for the time beyond 74 minutes. If the critical care is less than 30 minutes, an E/M code would be used to report the service.

There are service codes that are bundled into the Critical Care Services codes. These services are normally provided to stabilize the patient. An example of this bundling is as follows: A physician starts ventilation management (94656) while providing critical care services to a patient in the intensive care unit of a hospital. The ventilator management is not reported separately but, instead, is considered to be bundled into the Critical Care Services code. The notes preceding the critical care codes in the CPT manual list the services and procedures bundled into the codes. If the physician provided a service at the same time as critical care and that service is not bundled into the code, the service could be reported separately. You will know what is bundled into the codes because this information is listed either in the extensive description of the code or in the notes preceding the code. Be certain to read these notes, as they contain many exclusions and inclusions for these codes.

If the patient is in a critical care unit but is stable, you report the services using codes from the Hospital Inpatient Services subsection, Subsequent Hospital Care subheading or from the Consultations subsection, Initial Inpatient or Follow-up Inpatient subheadings.

EXERCISE 2-14

CRITICAL CARE SERVICES

Fill in the information for the following:

1 Critical care is provided to the patient for 70 minutes.

   Code(s): _____

2 Can code 99292 be reported without code 99291? _____

3 A physician is called to the intensive care unit to provide care for a patient who has received second-degree burns over 50% of his body. The physician provides support for 2 hours. After leaving the unit, the physician returns later that day to provide an additional hour of critical care support to the patient.

   Code(s): _____

Neonatal Intensive Care Services

Neonatal Intensive Care Services (99295–99298) are provided by the physician in a neonatal intensive care unit. The newborns being cared for are of very low birth weight (VLBW), below 1500 grams. Once the neonate has reached 1500 grams, use codes from Subsequent Hospital Care, 99231–99233.

The codes from the Neonatal Intensive Care subsection are reported only once in every 24-hour period (same day). There are no hourly service codes as there are in other critical care codes. If an infant older than 30 days is admitted to an intensive care unit and is critically ill, the services would be coded using the Critical Care Service codes 99291 and 99292, which are based on hourly service.

The name of the intensive care unit does not matter in the application of the Neonatal Intensive Care codes. The services can be provided in a pediatric intensive care unit, neonatal critical care unit, or any of the many other names that these types of intensive care units have. What is important in the use of Neonatal Intensive Care codes is that the neonate is less than 30 days old and has a weight of less than 1500 grams, or is critically ill.

Bundled into the Neonatal Intensive Care codes are many services you would anticipate would be used in the support of a critically ill neonate. For example, umbilical arterial catheters, nasogastric tube placement, endotracheal intubation, and invasive electronic monitoring of vital signs. The notes preceding the codes list bundled services, descriptions, and codes for services, for example, blood transfusion, 36440. As you are coding Neonate Intensive Care services, you will need to refer back to the list of services and codes that are bundled into the codes in this subsection. If the physician performed a service not listed in the notes, you would code for the service separately. Other notes indicating bundled services appear in the code descriptions. Refer to code 99295 and see that the description indicates that cardiac and/or respiratory support as well as many other services are bundled into the code. So extensive reading is mandatory in this complicated subsection. The codes here are based on whether the infant is critically ill or critically ill *and* unstable.

EXERCISE 2-15

NEONATAL INTENSIVE CARE SERVICES

Answer the following:

1 What does the abbreviation VLBW mean? _____

2 Once a neonate is no longer considered to be critically ill and has attained a birth weight of 1500 grams, the codes from what subheading

   would be used to report services? _____

3 Which code is the only code in the Neonatal Intensive Care subsection

   for reporting services on the admission date? _____

4 According to the Neonatal Intensive Care notes, may you report a code from the subheading Physician Standby Services with a Neonatal Intensive Care code? _____

5 A neonate is admitted to neonatal intensive care in critical condition and requires respiratory support, which includes ventilation. The physician directs the health care team in an attempt to stabilize the infant.

   Code(s): _____

Nursing Facility Services

A **nursing facility** is not a hospital but does have inpatient beds and a professional health care staff that provides health care to persons who do not require the level of service provided in an acute care facility.

A **skilled nursing facility** (SNF) is one that has a professional staff that often includes physicians and nurses. The patients of a skilled nursing facility require less care than that given in an acute care hospital, but more care than that provided in a nursing home. Skilled nursing facilities are also called skilled nursing units, skilled nursing care, or extended care facilities. Professional and practical nursing services are available 24 hours a day. Rehabilitation services, such as occupational therapy, physical therapy, and speech therapy, are available on a daily basis. A skilled nursing facility may previously have been called an extended care facility. Patients may stay for several weeks in a skilled nursing facility before returning home or being transferred to an intermediate care facility for long-term care. Skilled nursing facilities provide care for individuals of all ages, even though the majority of services are provided to geriatric patients.

An **intermediate care facility** provides regular, basic health services to individuals who do not need the degree of care or treatment provided in a hospital or a skilled nursing facility. Residents, because of their mental or physical conditions, require assistance with their activities of daily living, such as bathing, dressing, eating, and ambulating. Intermediate care facilities generally provide long-term care, usually over several years. Professional and practical nursing services are available on a 24-hour basis. Activities, social services, and dietary and other therapies are available on a daily basis. The majority of residents of intermediate care facilities are geriatric individuals or individuals of any age with mental retardation or developmental disabilities.

The phrase **long-term care facility** describes health and personal services provided to ill, aged, disabled, or retarded individuals for an extended period of time. Other types of facilities are better described as skilled or intermediate care facilities.

Three subheadings of nursing facility services are available as codes: Comprehensive Nursing Facility Assessment, Subsequent Nursing Facility Care, and Nursing Facility Discharge Services.

Comprehensive Nursing Facility Assessment

Comprehensive Nursing Facility Assessment codes do not distinguish between new and established patients. These codes are used to report services provided by the physician at the time of admission or at a time during the resident's stay when his or her condition substantially changes and a reassessment is warranted. These assessments by physicians play a central role in the development of the resident's individualized care plan. The care plan is developed by an interdisciplinary care team using the Resident Assessment Instrument (RAI) and the Minimum Data Set (MDS).

Subsequent Nursing Facility Care

Subsequent Nursing Facility Care codes do not distinguish between a new and an established patient. These codes reflect services provided by a physician on a periodic basis when a resident does not need a comprehensive assessment. Typically, such a resident has not had a major change in his or her condition since the previous physician visit but requires ongoing management of a chronic condition or treatment of an acute short-term problem.

Nursing Facility Discharge Services

The Nursing Facility Discharge Services codes are used to report the services the physician renders to the patient on the day of discharge. The time spent is counted in increments of 30 minutes and need not be continuous or spent entirely with the patient. The physician may conduct a final physical examination, give instructions to the patient's caregivers, and prepare all necessary discharge documentation, referral forms, and prescriptions.

Additional Nursing Facility Circumstances

As with many subheadings throughout the E/M section, if a patient is admitted to a nursing facility but the service was started elsewhere, such as a physician's office or emergency department, all the evaluation and management services provided to the patient are considered part of the nursing facility code. For example, a patient was seen in the hospital emergency department, where a comprehensive history and examination were performed for a condition that required high MDM complexity, coded 99285, Emergency Department Services. The physician made the decision to admit the patient to a nursing facility on the same day. Rather than coding the 99285, you would code the same level service from the subheading Comprehensive Nursing Facility Assessment, code 99303.

Nursing Facility Services codes are also used for coding services in a type of place you would not think would apply—psychiatric residential treatment centers. The center must be a stand-alone facility or a separate part of a facility that provides group living facilities and it must have 24-hour staffing. Nursing Facility Services codes are used to identify evaluation and management services. If a physician also provides medical psychotherapy, you would code those services separately.

When a patient has been in the hospital and is discharged from the hospital to a nursing facility all on the same day, you can code the hospital discharge (99238–99239) and nursing facility admission (99301–99303) separately. This is also true for same-day services for patients who are discharged from observation status (99234–99236) and admitted to a nursing facility (99301–99303).

EXERCISE 2-16

NURSING FACILITY SERVICES

Answer the following:

1   What is the time indicated in code 99303 as a typical time spent with a patient? _____

2   A 72-year-old male patient is transferred to a nursing facility from a hospital after suffering a cerebrovascular accident. The patient needs a comprehensive assessment before his active rehabilitation plan can be started. A comprehensive history is gathered by the internist, including the patient's chief complaint of paralysis and weakness, an extended HPI, and a complete ROS. Details of the patient's past, family, and social history add information to the care-planning process. The internist performs a comprehensive multisystem physical examination. After much deliberation with the multidisciplinary rehabilitation team, the physician determines that the patient is ready for active rehabilitation. The physician also writes orders to continue treatment of the patient's other medical conditions, including hypertension and diabetes. The MDM complexity is high.

Code(s): _____

Using the following information within the code descriptions in the Subsequent Nursing Facility Care subheading, match the time in the description of the code with the stated current status of the patient:

3 Responding inadequately to therapy _____   a. 35

4 Stable, recovering, improving _____   b. 25

5 Significant new problem _____   c. 15

Code the following:

6 Subsequent follow-up care is provided for a comatose patient transferred to a long-term care center from the hospital. The resident shows no signs of consciousness on examination but appears to have developed a minor upper respiratory tract infection with a fever and cough. The physician performs an expanded problem focused interval history and physical examination, including neurologic status, respiratory status, and status of related organ systems. Because the physician is concerned that the respiratory infection could progress to pneumonia, appropriate treatment is ordered. The MDM complexity is moderate.

Code(s): _____

Domiciliary, Rest Home (e.g., Boarding Home), or Custodial Care Services

These codes are divided into subheadings based on the patients' status as new or established. The codes are arranged in levels based on the documentation in the patients' medical records. No time estimates are established for codes in this category.

These codes are used for the evaluation and management of residents who reside in a domiciliary, rest home, or custodial care center. Generally, health services are not available on site, nor are any medical services included in the codes. These facilities provide residential care, including lodging, meals, supervision, personal care, and leisure activities, to persons who, because of their physical, mental, or emotional condition, are not able to live independently. Such facilities might include alternative living residences, retirement centers, community-based living units, group homes, or residential treatment centers. These facilities provide custodial care for residents of all ages.

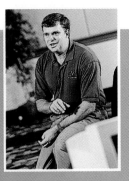

from the trenches

What has been your most embarrassing moment as a professional coder?
"Going into a radiology practice and surviving the initial barrage of questions. . . . I was certified but not experienced in radiology. I excused myself to the restroom and called a fellow coder for guidance."

EDWIN

Home Services

Health care services can also be provided to patients in their homes. Times have been established for this category of services. Note that there is a statement about typical time located under the code description in the paragraph that begins, "Usually, the patient is . . . ." The codes for these services are also divided into categories for new and for established patients.

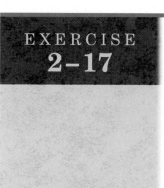

**EXERCISE
2-17**

HOME SERVICES

Code the following scenario:

1 A 64-year-old established female patient has diabetes mellitus and has been having problems adjusting her insulin doses. She has had an onset of dizziness and sensitivity to light. The physician makes a home visit during which he gathers a brief HPI and a problem-pertinent ROS during the problem focused history. The problem focused physical examination focuses on the body systems currently affected by the diabetes. The physician finds the patient's condition to be moderately severe and the MDM complexity is straightforward.

Code(s): _____

Prolonged Services

In the Prolonged Services subsection there are three subheadings:
- Prolonged Physician Services *With* Direct (Face-to-Face) Patient Contact
- Prolonged Physician Services *Without* Direct (Face-to-Face) Patient Contact
- Physician Standby Services

Prolonged Physician Services With or Without Direct Patient Contact

Prolonged Physician Services codes are all add-on codes, except for the codes in the Physician Standby Services subheading. Note the plus symbol (+) beside all codes in the range 99354 to 99359. Because add-on codes can be used only with another code, all Prolonged Physician Services codes are intended to be used only in addition to other codes to show an extension of some other service. The following example illustrates the use of these codes.

EXAMPLE

An established patient with a history of asthma presents, in an office visit, with acute bronchospasm and moderate respiratory distress. The physician conducts a problem focused history followed by a problem focused examination, which shows a respiratory rate of 30, and labored breathing and wheezing are heard in all lung fields. Office treatment is initiated; it includes intermittent bronchial dilation and subcutaneous epinephrine. The service requires the physician to have intermittent face-to-face contact with the patient over a 2-hour period. The MDM complexity is low.

The office visit service would be reported using the office visit code 99212; but the additional time the physician spent providing service to the patient over and above that which is indicated in code 99212 would have to be coded using a prolonged service code.

CAUTION *If you hadn't carefully read the notes preceding the Prolonged Services codes, you would not know that there are many rules that govern the calculation of time when determining the codes.*

As the notes indicate, the first 30 minutes of prolonged services are not even counted but are considered part of the initial service. So you cannot use a prolonged services code until after the first 30 minutes of the prolonged services have been provided. The physician, therefore, has to spend 60 minutes with the patient in prolonged services before it is possible to code for 30 minutes using code 99354. That takes care of 1 hour of our physician's time for the case above. Now, what about the next hour?

Read the description for the indented code 99355. The description states that 99355 is to be used for each additional 30 minutes; but this is where the second time rule comes in. You can use 99355 only if the physician has spent at least 15 minutes providing service over and above the first 60 minutes. The physician in this example spent 1 hour beyond the first 60 minutes providing service, so we can claim 99355 twice. The coding for the case is 99212 for the office visit; 99354 for the first hour of prolonged services; and 99355 × 2 for the next hour.

The time the physician spends providing the prolonged services does not have to be continuous, as is the situation in this example; the physician monitored the patient on an intermittent basis, coming into the room to check on the patient and then leaving the room.

But, let's change this case a bit and see how the coding changes. If the physician spent 70 minutes with the patient, you could code only the first hour at 99354. The additional 10 minutes beyond the first 60 are not coded separately. Remember that you would need at least 15 minutes beyond the first hour to code for the time beyond the first hour. For help in applying these codes, note the table preceding the codes; there you can locate the total time your physician spent with the patient and see an example of the correct coding.

The face-to-face Prolonged Physician Services codes describe services that require the physician to have direct contact with the patient; but the Prolonged Physician Services Without Direct (Face-to-Face) Patient Contact codes describe services during which the physician is not in direct contact with the patient. For example, a physician evaluates an established patient, a 70-year-old female with dementia, in an office visit. The physician then spends an extensive amount of time discussing the patient's condition, her treatment plan, and other recommendations with the daughter of the patient. The services would be reported by using an office visit code for the patient evaluation and the appropriate prolonged service without face-to-face contact code for the time spent with the daughter.

Prolonged Physician Services codes are most often used with the higher level E/M codes, which themselves carry longer time frames.

Prolonged Physician Services With Direct Patient Contact codes are divided on the basis of whether the services were provided to an outpatient or an inpatient.

Physician Standby Services

The codes for Physician Standby Services are used when a physician, at the request of the attending physician, is standing by in case his or her services are needed. The standby physician cannot be rendering services to another patient during this time. The standby codes are reported in increments of 30 minutes. The 30-minute increments referred to here really mean from the 1st minute to the 30th minute and do not have any of the complicated rules for reporting time that exist for reporting prolonged or critical services.

An important note concerning the standby codes is that these codes are used only when no service is performed and there is no face-to-face contact with the patient. These codes are not used when a standby status ends in the physician's providing a service to a patient. The service the physician provides is reported as any other service would be, even though it began as a physician standby service.

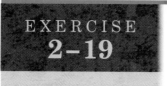

PROLONGED AND PHYSICIAN STANDBY SERVICES

Using the notes in the subsections, answer the following:

1 Does the time the physician spends with the patient in prolonged, direct contact have to be continuous? _____

2 Can a code from the Prolonged Services subsection be reported alone?

   _____

3 If the prolonged contact with the patient lasts less than 30 minutes, is the time reported separately? _____

4 The codes in the Prolonged Physician Services With Direct Patient Contact subheading are based not only on the time the physician spends with the patient, but also on another factor. What is that other factor?

   _____

5 Are the codes in the subheading Prolonged Physician Services Without Direct Patient Contact categorized according to the place of service?

   _____

6 According to the notes in the Physician Standby Services subsection, can a physician report the time spent in proctoring (monitoring) another physician? _____

Case Management Services

The Case Management Services subsection consists of codes used by physicians to report coordination of care services with other health care professionals. These services may include team conferences and telephone calls for the purpose of coordinating the medical care of a patient. Telephone calls are based on complexity of service but are not usually paid by most third-party payers.

CASE MANAGEMENT SERVICES

Complete the following:

1 What are the two time components specified in the Team Conference codes from the Case Management Services subsection? _____

   _____

2 Telephone call codes are based on the complexity of service. What are the three measurements? _____

_____

Care Plan Oversight Services

At times, a physician is asked to manage a complex case that involves an individual such as a hospice patient or a patient who is homebound and receives the majority of his or her health care from visiting nurses. When regular communication is necessary between the nurses and the physician to discuss revising the care plan, coordinating the treatment plan with other professionals, or adjusting the therapies, codes from the Care Plan Oversight Services subsection may be used to report these additional services. The codes are divided according to whether the physician is supervising a patient being cared for by home health workers or a patient in a hospice or nursing facility. The codes are also divided based on the length of time of the service—either 15 to 29 minutes or 30 minutes or more. Reporting is by time over a month-long period.

Preventive Medicine Services

Use Preventive Medicine Services codes to report the routine evaluation and management of a patient who is healthy and has no complaint or when the patient has a chronic condition or disease that is controlled but involves yearly routine physicals. The codes in this subsection would be used to report a routine physical examination done at the patient's request, such as a well-baby check-up. Preventive Medicine codes are intended to be used to identify comprehensive services, not a single-system examination, such as an annual gynecologic examination. The codes are used for infants, children, adolescents, and adults; they differ according to the age of the patient and whether the patient is a new or an established patient.

coding shot

If the physician should encounter a problem or abnormality during the course of a preventive service, and the problem or abnormality requires significant additional service, you can also code an office visit code with a modifier -25 added. The modifier -25 is used to indicate that a significant, separately identifiable E/M service was performed by the physician on the same day as the preventive medicine service. If you did not add the modifier -25, the third-party payer would think that you had made an error and were reporting both a preventive medicine service code and an office visit code for the same service. Only with the use of the modifier -25 can you convey that the services were indeed separate.

Note that in the code descriptions for both the New Patient and the Established Patient categories, the terms "comprehensive history" and "comprehensive examination" are used. These terms are not the same as the ones used with other E/M codes (99201–99350). Here, "comprehensive" means a complete history and a complete examination, as is conducted during an annual physical. The comprehensive examination performed as part of the preventive medicine E/M service is a multisystem examination, but the extent of the examination is determined by the age of the patient and the risk factors identified for that individual.

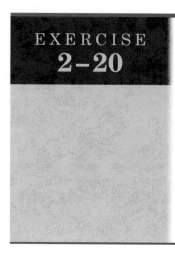

PREVENTIVE MEDICINE SERVICES

EXERCISE 2-20

Complete the following:

1   According to the notes in the Preventive Medicine Services subsection, the extent and focus of the services provided, whether to a new or to an established patient, will depend largely upon what factor?

_____

2   If, during the preventive medicine evaluation, a problem is encountered that requires the physician to perform a problem focused E/M service,

what modifier would be appended to the code? _____

Counseling and/or Risk Factor Reduction Intervention

Counseling and/or Risk Factor Reduction Intervention codes are for both new and established healthy patients. The services are based on whether individual or group counseling is provided to the patient and on the amount of time the service requires. These codes can be used in conjunction with preventive medicine services. Codes in this category would be used to report a physician's services to a patient for risk factor interventional counseling, such as a diet and exercise program, smoking cessation, or contraceptive management.

Besides preventive counseling for individuals or groups, there are also two additional codes under the category for Other Preventive Medicine Services that include unlisted preventive procedures and administration and interpretation of a health risk assessment. A special report would accompany the unlisted code.

Newborn Care Services

The Newborn Care Services subsection has codes used to identify services provided to normal or high-risk newborns. The codes are for services provided to a newborn in several settings. Note that there are two history and examination codes; one is specifically for a newborn assessment and **discharge** from a hospital or birthing room on the same date, and one is for birthing room **deliveries.**

If the physician provides a discharge service to a newborn who is discharged subsequent to the admission date, you would choose a code from the Hospital Inpatient Services subsection, Hospital Discharge Services subheading.

Special Evaluation and Management Services

The codes in this subsection are used to report evaluations for life or disability insurance baseline information. The services can be performed in any setting for either a new or an established patient. The codes vary, based on whether the service is for an examination for life or disability insurance and whether the examination is done by the physician treating the patient's disability or by someone other than the treating physician.

EXERCISE 2-21

SPECIAL EVALUATION AND MANAGEMENT SERVICES

Answer the following:

1 An insurance examination was conducted by the physician for a new patient for a term life insurance policy. From what subheading would you select a code to report this service?

_____

2 A 50-year-old man was referred for a disability examination. The patient had been injured when he slipped off a ladder and fell from a height of 10 feet, landing on his back. He had not returned to work since that time 6 months ago. The patient had been under the care of a physician from another state and was referred by the insurance company for the assessment of the patient's ability to return to work. His primary physician had stated that this patient will be unable to return to his previous work as a bricklayer. From what subheading would you select a code to report this service?

_____

3 What is the difference between the two codes in the Work Related or

Medical Disability Evaluation Services codes? _____

_____

_____

4 A 58-year-old man was seen by his private physician for an examination as part of his claim for long-term medical disability. The patient has chronic obstructive lung disease with severe emphysema and has been unable to work during the past year. The physician completed all the necessary documentation required by the insurance company, including his opinion that the patient would be unable to work in the future, as his pulmonary function is markedly impaired, in spite of continual respiratory and pharmacologic therapy.

Code(s): _____

Other Evaluation and Management Services

Other Evaluation and Management Services is the last subsection in the E/M section. It is used to report unlisted services. Use of this code indicates that there is no code in the E/M section that accurately represents the services provided to the patient. A special report would accompany the unlisted E/M service code.

Coding Practice

Good job! You have been through all of the E/M codes and are now familiar with the basics of CPT code arrangement. Can you imagine how well you would know your favorite novel if you read it several times a month? Well, coders use their CPT manuals every day and become very familiar with the information in the guidelines, notes, and descriptions of the codes. Please be sure to locate the code in the CPT manual and read all notes, guidelines, and descriptions about each code you work with. In this way, you will build a solid knowledge foundation.

Now let's begin to do some coding that will require you to combine all the information you have learned in Chapters 1 and 2 as you begin to code patient cases.

EXERCISE 2-22

CODING PRACTICE

Code the following:

1   A new patient is seen in the office for an earache (otalgia). The history and examination are problem focused and the MDM complexity is straightforward.

Code(s): _____

2   An established patient is seen in the office of an ENT (ear-nose-throat) specialist with the chief complaint of otalgia. The physician completes a problem focused history and physical examination of the head, eyes, ears, nose, and throat. To the physician, this is a straightforward case of acute otitis media, and prescription medications are ordered. The MDM complexity is straightforward.

Code(s): _____

3   An established patient is seen in the office for suture removal, which is done by the physician's nurse.

Code(s): _____

4   Lilly Wilson, a new patient, is seen by the physician in the skilled nursing facility for an initial nursing facility assessment. Mrs. Wilson recently suffered a cerebral thrombosis with residual dysphagia and paresis of the left extremities. She was transferred from the acute care hospital to the skilled nursing facility for concentrated rehabilitation. Mrs. Wilson also has arteriosclerotic heart disease with a permanent pacemaker in place, rheumatoid arthritis, urinary incontinence, and macular degeneration in her right eye. The physician, who did not know Mrs. Wilson prior to her transfer, performs a comprehensive history and physical examination. Given the patient's multiple diagnoses and the moderate amount of data the physician has to review, the MDM is of a high level of complexity.

Code(s): _____

5   John Taylor is a 16-year-old outpatient who is a new patient to the office. John complains of severe facial acne. The history and physical examination are expanded problem focused. The physician must consider related organ systems in addition to the integumentary system in order to treat the condition properly. With the minimal number of

diagnoses to consider and the minimal amount of data to review, the physician's decision-making is straightforward with regard to the plan of care.

Code(s): _____

6 Jan Sharp, an established patient, has an office appointment because she needs a new dressing on the laceration on her arm. The physician's nurse changes the dressing.

Code(s): _____

7 Anna Rall is seen in the emergency department, complaining of pressure in her chest and the feeling that her heart is racing. After her vital signs are taken, an immediate electrocardiogram is performed, and her heart rate is found to be in excess of 160 beats per minute, with increased activity at the atrioventricular junction. After performing a comprehensive history and physical examination, the physician continues to evaluate the patient, who has been placed on continuous electrocardiographic monitoring. The emergency department physician considers the diagnosis of paroxysmal nodal tachycardia and calls a cardiologist for a consultation and possible admission of the patient to the hospital. Given the uncertainty of the diagnosis and the various other possible options, the physician's decision-making is at a highly complex level. (Code only the emergency department physician's services.)

Code(s): _____

8 A physician is called to the intensive care unit at the local hospital to care for Joe West, a patient in coronary crisis. The physician spends an hour at the patient's bedside, stabilizing him.

Code(s): _____

9 The physician is preparing to leave the hospital after seeing Joe West but is called back to the intensive care unit to see and stabilize another patient, Ted Keel. The service to the patient takes 1½ hours.

Code(s): _____

10 An established patient, Harriet Turner, comes into the office for a follow-up visit. She had been prescribed medication for her recent onset of depression, but since her last visit, when the dosage was increased, she has felt that the medication is making her sleepy and lethargic. Considering the other factors such as other medical problems and drug interactions, the physician spends 25 minutes with the patient performing a detailed history and physical examination. After reviewing the details as well as recent laboratory work, the physician concludes that a different medication should be prescribed. The physician's decision-making is moderately complex, given the possible medical complications that could arise.

Code(s): _____

11 Dr. Welton calls Dr. Stouffer to perform a consultation on Carol Jones for advice on the management of her diabetes. Mrs. Jones is hospitalized for a hysterectomy, which had been an uncomplicated procedure, but is experiencing a slow recovery four days post op. Her abdominal wound does not appear to be healing well and her blood sugar has been fluctuating each day. Dr. Stouffer, who has never met Mrs. Jones be-

fore, performs a comprehensive, multisystem physical examination as well as completing a comprehensive history with a complete review of systems and extensive past medical history review. Dr. Stouffer recommends a new insulin regimen in addition to other medications to manage what might be a postoperative wound infection. Dr. Stouffer's medical decision-making is of high complexity because he has to consider multiple diagnoses, a moderate amount of data, and the moderate risk of complications that Mrs. Jones could develop.

Code(s): _____

Congratulations   Now you're coding! Be sure to check your answers as you complete each activity. If you identify a code incorrectly, go back and read the CPT manual information again.

DOCUMENTATION GUIDELINES

Medicare recipients account for the majority of patients receiving services in the American health care system. Thus, any change by the third-party payer, Medicare, has dramatic effects on the health care system. One such change that currently is in development is the documentation necessary when submitting a claim for Evaluation and Management services provided to a Medicare patient. The Medicare program is the responsibility of the Centers for Medicare and Medicaid Services (CMS), formerly the Health Care Financing Administration (HCFA). Several years ago, CMS determined that there should be a nationally uniform requirement for documentation contained in the patient record when submitting charges for E/M services. The CMS developed a set of standards for documentation of E/M services. The standards are informational items that must be in the patient record to

---

GENERAL MULTISYSTEM EXAMINATION

To qualify for a given level of multisystem examination, the following content and documentation requirements should be met:

- **Problem Focused Examination**—should include performance and documentation of one to five elements identified by a bullet (•) in one or more organ system(s) or body area(s).

- **Expanded Problem Focused Examination**—should include performance and documentation of at least six elements identified by a bullet (•) in one or more organ system(s) or body area(s).

- **Detailed Examination**—should include at least six organ systems or body areas. For each system/area selected, performance and documentation of at least two elements identified by a bullet (•) is expected. Alternatively, a detailed examination may include performance and documentation of at least twelve elements identified by a bullet (•) in two or more organ systems or body areas.

- **Comprehensive Examination**—should include at least nine organ systems or body areas. For each system/area selected, all elements of the examination identified by a bullet (•) should be performed, unless specific directions limit the content of the examination. For each area/system, documentation of at least two elements identified by a bullet is expected.

Figure 2–8 Documentation guidelines for a general multisystem examination. (Courtesy of U.S. Department of Health and Human Services, Centers for Medicare and Medicaid Services.)

General Multisystem Examination

System/Body Area	Elements of Examination
Constitutional	• Measurement of **any three of the following seven** vital signs: (1) sitting or standing blood pressure, (2) supine blood pressure, (3) pulse rate and regularity, (4) respiration, (5) temperature, (6) height, (7) weight (may be measured and recorded by ancillary staff) • General appearance of the patient (e.g., development, nutrition, body habitus, deformities, attention to grooming)
Eyes	• Inspection of conjunctivae and lids • Examination of pupils and irises (e.g., reaction to light and accommodation, size and symmetry) • Ophthalmoscopic examination of optic disks (e.g., size, C/D ratio, appearance) and posterior segments (e.g., vessel changes, exudates, hemorrhages)
Ears, Nose, Mouth, and Throat	• External inspection of ears and nose (e.g., overall appearance, scars, lesions, masses) • Otoscopic examination of external auditory canals and tympanic membranes • Assessment of hearing (e.g., whispered voice, finger rub, tuning fork) • Inspection of nasal mucosa, septum, and turbinates • Inspection of lips, teeth, and gums • Examination of oropharynx: oral mucosa, salivary glands, hard and soft palates, tongue, tonsils, and posterior pharynx
Neck	• Examination of neck (e.g., masses, overall appearance, symmetry, tracheal position, crepitus) • Examination of thyroid (e.g., enlargement, tenderness, mass)

Figure 2–9 Documentation guidelines for the elements of a general multisystem examination. (Courtesy of U.S. Department of Health and Human Services, Centers for Medicare and Medicaid Services.)

substantiate a given level of service. The standards are called the **Documentation Guidelines.** These guidelines apply only to E/M services and only to patients covered by Medicare and Medicaid. E/M services represent 40% of all services provided to these patients. The importance of the guidelines cannot be underestimated. Whatever guidelines the CMS institutes for patients, they have a dramatic effect on the systems in health care and will soon spread to other third-party payers, who will then begin to require the same or similar documentation.

The CMS published the first set of documentation guidelines in 1995, but did not require compliance for payment of claims. A new set of guidelines was published in July 1997 for implementation January 1, 1998. The 1998 set of guidelines were intended to be the standard used when reviewing claims for payment. If the physician did not have the documentation required in the guidelines, payment would be adjusted based on what was actually in the medical record. The guidelines were so complex and required such extensive revision of medical record-keeping practices that the AMA (American Medical Association), on behalf of its physician members, requested an extension of the implementation date to allow time for education about the guidelines and for the CMS to meet with representatives of the AMA to reconsider the guidelines. Although the CMS rescinded the requirement for strict compliance with the guidelines, they continue random review of claims, based on whichever set of guidelines (1995 or 1997) the provider has elected to use.

The Documentation Guidelines specify the information that must be documented in the medical record for an E/M service to qualify for a given level of service. Figure 2–8 illustrates the examination requirements for a general multisystem examination under the 1997 Documentation Guidelines. Note that for an examination to qualify as an expanded problem focused examination, the medical record must document that the physician performed at least six of the elements identified by a bullet (•) in Figure 2–9. If the medical record documents that only five of the elements identified by a bullet were performed, the examination would have to be reported at the lower problem focused examination level.

A revised set of guidelines, published in 2000, took into consideration some of the suggestions put forth by the AMA. At the time of the publication of this text, the CMS and the AMA were still in discussions regarding which set of documentation guidelines would become the standard for documenting E/M services.

Check This Out! ☞ The CMS has its own Website: http://www.hcfa.gov
You'll find the Documentation Guidelines under the Medicare information, Professional/Technical option.

Although the guidelines will change before implementation and will continue to be revised, guidelines will be a part of the standard for the medical record now and in the future for Medicare and Medicaid patients. You can anticipate that, as a coder, you will be required to learn about these Documentation Guidelines.

CHAPTER GLOSSARY

admission: attention to an acute illness or injury resulting in admission to a hospital

attending physician: the physician with the primary responsibility for care of the patient

concurrent care: the provision of similar services (e.g., hospital visits) to the same patient by more than one physician on the same day. Each physician provides services for a separate condition, not reasonably expected to be managed by the attending physician. When concurrent care is provided, the diagnosis must reflect the medical necessity of different specialties

consultation: includes those services rendered by a physician whose opinion or advice is requested by another physician or agency concerning the evaluation and/or treatment of a patient; a consultant is not an attending physician

contributing factors: counseling, coordination of care, nature of the presenting problem, and time of an E/M service

counseling: a discussion with a patient and/or family concerning one or more of the following areas: diagnostic results, impressions, and/or recommended diagnostic studies; prognosis; risks and benefits of treatment; instructions for treatment; importance of compliance with treatment; risk factor reduction; and patient and family education

critical care: the care of critically ill patients in medical emergencies that requires the constant attendance of the physician (e.g., cardiac arrest, shock, bleeding, respiratory failure); critical care is usually, but not always, given in a critical care area, such as the coronary care unit (CCU) or the intensive care unit (ICU)

emergency care services: services that are provided by the physician in the emergency department for unplanned patient encounters; no distinction is made between new and established patients who are seen in the emergency department

established patient: a patient who has received professional services from the physician or another physician of the same specialty in the same group within the past 3 years

inpatient: one who has been formally admitted to a health care facility

key components: the history, examination, and medical decision-making complexity of an E/M service

new patient: a patient who has not received any professional services from the physician or another physician of the same specialty in the same group within the past 3 years

newborn care: the evaluation and determination of care management of a newly born infant

office visit: a face-to-face encounter between a physician and a patient to allow for primary management of a patient's health care status

outpatient: a patient who receives services in an ambulatory health care facility and is currently not an inpatient

referral: the transfer of the total or a specific portion of care of a patient from one physician to another that does not constitute a consultation

systemic: affecting the entire body

CHAPTER REVIEW

CHAPTER 2, PART I, THEORY

Without using the CPT manual, complete the following:

1 How many subsections are there in the E/M section? _____

2 The four types of patient status are

_____ , _____ ,

_____ , and _____ .

3 The first visit is called the _____ visit, and the second visit is called the

_____ visit.

4 The first three factors a coder must consider when coding are patient

_____ , _____ ,

and _____ .

5 How many types of histories are there?

_____

6 Which history is more complex: the problem focused history or the expanded problem focused history?

_____

7 The four types of examinations, in order of difficulty (from least difficult to most difficult), are as follows:

a. _____

b. _____

c. _____

d. _____

8 The examination that is limited to the affected body area is the

_____ .

9 What does VLBW stand for? _____

_____

10 What medical decision-making involves a situation in which the diagnosis and management options are minimal, data amount and complexity that must be reviewed are minimal/none, and there is a minimal risk to the patient of complications or death?

_____

11 What term is used to describe a patient who has been formally admitted to a hospital?

_____

CHAPTER 2, PART II, PRACTICAL

Using the CPT manual, identify the codes for the following cases:

12 The physician provides initial intensive care service for the evaluation and management of a critically ill newborn for one day.

Code(s): _____

13 A 55-year-old man is seen by the dermatologist for the first time and complains of two cystic lesions on his back. Considering that the patient is otherwise healthy and has a primary care physician caring for him, the dermatologist focuses the history of the present illness on the skin lesions (problem focused history) and focuses the problem focused physical examination on the patient's trunk. The physician concludes with straight-forward decision-making that the lesions are sebaceous cysts. The physician advises the patient that the lesions should be monitored for any changes but that no surgical intervention is warranted at this time.

Code(s): _____

14 A 68-year-old woman visits her internist again complaining of angina that seems to have worsened over the past 3 days. The patient had had an acute anterior wall myocardial infarction (MI) 2 months earlier. One month after the acute MI, she began to have angina pectoris. The patient also states that she thinks the medications are causing her to have gastrointestinal problems while not relieving her symptoms. She had refused a cardiac catheterization after her MI to evaluate the extent of her coronary artery disease. The physician performs a detailed history and a detailed physical examination of her cardiovascular, respiratory, and gastrointestinal systems. The physician indicates that the decision-making process is moderately complex, given the number of conditions it is necessary to consider.

Code(s): _____

15 A 22-year-old woman visits the gynecologist for the first time since relocating from another state last year. The patient wants a gynecologic examination and wants to discuss contraceptive options with the physician (Think Preventive Medicine Services!). The physician collects pertinent past and social history related to the patient's reproductive system and performs a pertinent systems review extended to a limited number of additional systems. The physician completes the history with an extended history of her present physical state. A physical examination includes her cardiovascular and respiratory systems with an extended review of her genitourinary system. Given the patient's history of not tolerating certain types of oral contraceptives in the past, the physician's decision-

making involves a limited number of management options, all with low risk of morbidity to the patient.

Code(s): _____

16 An established patient is admitted on observation status for influenza symptoms and extreme nausea and vomiting. The patient is severely dehydrated and has been experiencing dizziness and mental confusion for the past 2 days. Prior to this episode the patient was well but became acutely ill overnight with these symptoms. Given the abrupt onset of these symptoms, the physician has to consider multiple possible causes and orders a variety of laboratory tests to be performed. The patient is at risk for a moderate number of complications. The MDM complexity is moderate. A comprehensive history is collected, and a comprehensive head-to-toe physical examination is performed.

Code(s): _____

17 A physician visits a patient on observation status who has severe influenza. The decision is made to admit the patient, whose condition has worsened and who is not responding to the therapy initiated on the observation unit. The physician performs a detailed history and a detailed physical examination to reflect the patient's current status. The patient's problem is of low severity but requires ongoing active management, with possible surgical consultation. The MDM complexity is low.

Code(s): _____

18 An 8-month-old infant, who is a new patient, is brought in by her mother for diaper rash. The physician focuses on the problem of the diaper rash for the problem focused history and examination. The MDM complexity is straightforward.

Code(s): _____

19 A 33-year-old man is brought to his private physician's office by his wife. The man, who is an established patient, has been experiencing severe leg pain of 2 weeks' duration. In the past 2 days, the patient has experienced fainting spells, nausea, and vomiting. The patient has had multiple other vague complaints over the past month that he dismissed as unimportant, but his wife is not so sure, and she describes his general health as deteriorating. The physician performs a comprehensive multisystem physical examination after performing a complete review of systems and a complete past medical, family, and social history, with an extended history of the present illness (comprehensive history). The physician has to consider an extensive number of diagnoses, orders a variety of tests to be performed immediately, and indicates the MDM complexity to be high.

Code(s): _____

20 A 42-year-old woman, who is an established patient, visits her family practitioner with the chief complaint of a self-discovered breast lump. She describes a feeling of fullness and tenderness over the mass that has become more pronounced in the past 2 weeks. Because the patient is otherwise healthy and has had a physical within the past 6 months, the physician focuses his attention on the breast lump during the taking of a problem focused history and the performance of a problem focused physical examination. The physician orders an immediate mammography to be performed and a follow-up appointment in 5 days. The physician has given the patient no other options and indicates that the MDM complexity is straightforward.

Code(s): _____

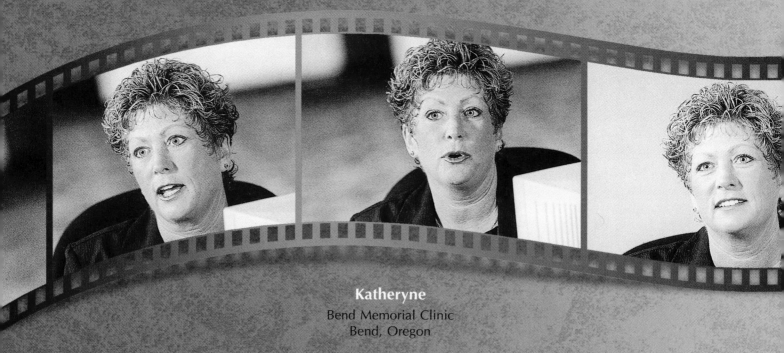

Katheryne
Bend Memorial Clinic
Bend, Oregon

chapter 3

The Anesthesia Section and Modifiers

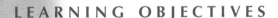

LEARNING OBJECTIVES

After completing this chapter you should be able to

1. Explain the Anesthesia section and subsection format.

2. Recognize the elements of the anesthesia formula.

3. Identify the modifiers used in the Anesthesia section.

4. Accurately report unlisted anesthesia procedures.

5. Calculate anesthesia service payment.

6. Analyze cases and apply the correct CPT codes.

7. Understand the use of modifiers.

8. Identify the modifiers used throughout the CPT manual.

9. Correctly apply modifiers.

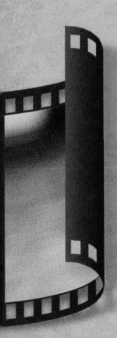

PART I: Learning About the Anesthesia Section

TYPES OF ANESTHESIA

The Anesthesia section is a specialized section that is used by an anesthesiologist, anesthetist, or other physician to report the provision of anesthesia services, usually during surgery. **Anesthesia** means induction or administration of a drug to obtain partial or complete loss of sensation. **Analgesia** (absence of pain) is achieved so that a patient may have surgery or a procedure performed without pain. Types of anesthesia may be general, regional, or local.

The practice of anesthesiology is not limited to administration of anesthesia for the surgical patient. The American Society of Anesthesiologists (ASA) defines the practice of anesthesiology as follows:

- The management of procedures for rendering a patient insensible to pain and emotional stress during surgical, obstetrical, and certain medical procedures.

- The evaluation and management of life functions under the stress of anesthetic and surgical manipulations.

- The clinical management of the patient unconscious from whatever cause.

- The evaluation and management of problems in pain relief.

- The management of problems in cardiac and respiratory resuscitation.

- The application of specific methods of respiratory therapy.

- The clinical management of various fluid, electrolyte, and metabolic disturbances.*

Conscious Sedation

Conscious sedation is a type of sedation that can be provided by a physician performing a procedure; it provides a decreased level of consciousness that does not put the patient completely to sleep. This level of consciousness allows the patient to breathe without assistance and to respond to stimulation and verbal commands. A trained observer is required to be present during the use of the conscious sedation to assist the physician in monitoring the patient. The codes used to report this type of conscious sedation are located in the Medicine section (99141–99142), not in the Anesthesia section. If the sedation is provided by a physician other than the physician performing the procedure, you would use the appropriate anesthesia code.

coding shot

The conscious sedation codes 99141 or 99142 from the Medicine section are used only when the physician performing the procedure administers the sedation.

---

* Definitions excerpted from the *2000 Relative Value Guide,* American Society of Anesthesiologists, p. iv. A copy of the full text can be obtained from ASA, 520 N. Northwest Hwy., Park Ridge, IL 60068-2573.

The conscious sedation codes in the Medicine section are divided based on the method by which sedation is achieved. Code 99141 is for intravenous, intramuscular, or inhalation sedation methods, whereas code 99142 is for oral, rectal, or intranasal sedation methods. These sedation methods are much less invasive than is the complete loss of consciousness. For example, for a colonoscopy, a physician could administer an intravenous sedation, such as meperidine (Demerol), morphine, or diazepam (Valium). The patient would be monitored closely as the medication is administered so that the appropriate level of sedation is reached. After the procedure, the physician may administer a drug such as naloxone (Narcan) intravenously to reverse the effects of the sedation. The patient would have this procedure in an outpatient setting and be able to go home after the procedure.

ANESTHESIA SECTION FORMAT

Anesthesia procedure codes are divided first by anatomic site and then by specific type of procedure, as shown in Figure 3–1.

The last three subsections in Anesthesia—Radiologic Procedures, Burn Excisions or Debridement, and Other Procedures—are *not* by anatomic division. The CPT codes in the Radiologic Procedures subsection of the Anesthesia section are used to report anesthesia service when radiologic services are provided to the patient for diagnostic or therapeutic reasons.

EXAMPLE

Therapeutic reason:	01921	Anesthesia for angioplasty
Diagnostic reason:	01922	Anesthesia for noninvasive imaging or radiation therapy

---

EXERCISE 3-1

ANESTHESIA FORMAT

Complete the following exercise:

1 Using the CPT manual, list each subsection in the Anesthesia section.

_____

_____

_____

_____

_____

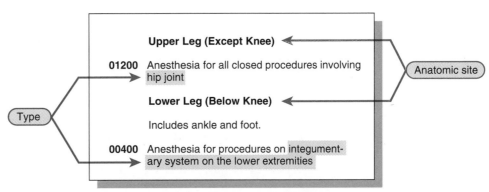

Figure 3–1   Anatomic divisions in Anesthesia section.

_____

_____

_____

_____

_____

_____

_____

_____

_____

_____

_____

_____

_____

_____

_____

2 Which subsections are *not* divided by anatomic site? _____

_____

3 What is analgesia? _____

4 What is anesthesia? _____

5 Name the three types of anesthesia: _____ , _____ , and

_____

6 What is the type of sedation that enables the patient to maintain

breathing for himself/herself? _____

7 In what section of the CPT are the sedation codes identified in Question 6 located? _____

FORMULA FOR ANESTHESIA PAYMENT

When an anesthesiologist provides an anesthesia service to a patient, the preoperative, intraoperative (care during surgery), and postoperative care are all included in the CPT code. If the anesthesiologist provides care that is unusual or beyond that which would usually be provided, you can report those services in addition to the basic anesthesia service. For example, if the patient requires intraoperative fluid management, the anesthesiologist might insert a Swan-Ganz catheter, as illustrated in Figure 3–2. Central venous catheter insertion such as the Swan-Ganz catheter is not a normal service provided during a surgery, so it could be reported using a code from the Surgery section for placement of a central venous catheter (36488–36491).

What makes anesthesia coding different from any other coding is the way in which anesthesia services are billed. There is a standard formula for payment of anesthesia services that is, for the most part, nationally accepted. The formula is basic units + time units + modifying units (B + T + M). Let's look at each of these elements in more detail.

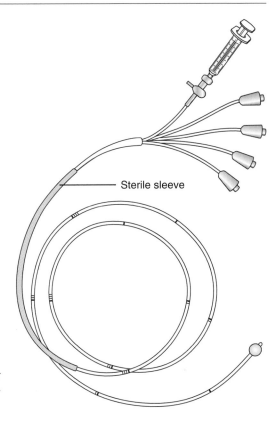

Figure 3–2 The Swan-Ganz catheter is the most commonly used central venous catheter.

B Is for Basic Unit

The ASA publishes a *Relative Value Guide* (RVG), which contains codes for anesthesia services. The CPT manual contains most of these anesthesia service codes in the Anesthesia section. The RVG includes about 23 anesthesia service codes that are not included in the CPT manual (Fig. 3–3) and several codes that have components of the service that vary from the CPT description for the code (Fig. 3–4).

The ASA's RVG is not a fee schedule (a list of the charges for services) but instead compares anesthesia services with each other. For example, anesthesia services provided for a biopsy of a sinus are less complicated than services provided for a radical sinus surgery. A team of physicians with expertise in anesthesiology developed the comparisons and assigned numerical values to each service, termed the **basic unit value** (Fig. 3–5). The ASA's basic unit is accepted as the standard in the United States.

One coding circumstance unique to anesthesia coding occurs when multi-

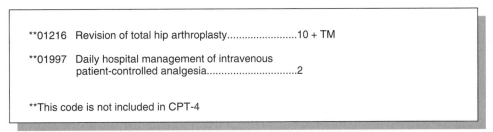

**01216   Revision of total hip arthroplasty........................10 + TM

**01997   Daily hospital management of intravenous
         patient-controlled analgesia...............................2

**This code is not included in CPT-4

Figure 3–3 *Relative Value Guide* codes not included in the CPT manual. (Based on the *2000 Relative Value Guide* of the American Society of Anesthesiologists, pp. viii and xiv. A copy of the full text can be obtained from ASA, 520 N. Northwest Hwy., Park Ridge, IL 60068-2573.)

*00918   Anesthesia for transurethral procedures (including urethrocystoscopy); with fragmentation, manipulation and/or removal of ureteral calculus...5 + TM

*In CPT, "manipulation" was not included in this code until the 2000 CPT.

Figure 3–4 *Relative Value Guide* code whose description differs from that in the CPT manual. (Based on the *2000 Relative Value Guide* of the American Society of Anesthesiologists, p. vii. A copy of the full text can be obtained from ASA, 520 N. Northwest Hwy., Park Ridge, IL 60068-2573.)

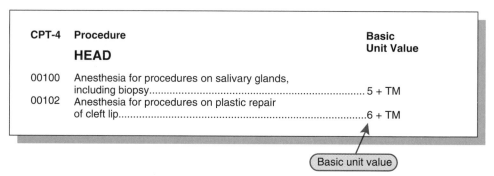

CPT-4	Procedure	Basic Unit Value
	HEAD	
00100	Anesthesia for procedures on salivary glands, including biopsy...........................	5 + TM
00102	Anesthesia for procedures on plastic repair of cleft lip.................................	6 + TM

Basic unit value

Figure 3–5 Base unit value. (Based on the *2000 Relative Value Guide* of the American Society of Anesthesiologists, p. i. A copy of the full text can be obtained from ASA, 520 N. Northwest Hwy., Park Ridge, IL 60068-2573.)

ple surgical procedures are performed during the same session. In this case the procedure with the highest unit value is the basic unit value. For example, if during the same surgical procedure session a clavicle biopsy (basic unit value of 3) and a radical mastectomy (basic unit value of 5) are done, the basic unit value for both procedures becomes 5.

Another coding circumstance unique to anesthesia coding applies when there is a second attending anesthesiologist (one who performs the same types of services as the first attending physician). In this case a basic value of 5 units is added to report the additional physician's service. A special report must accompany the submission to the third-party payer explaining why the procedure required the services of two anesthesiologists. The time for both anesthesiologists is also reported.

T Is for Time

Anesthesia services are provided based on the time during which the anesthesia was administered, in hours and minutes. The timing is started when the anesthesiologist begins preparing the patient to receive anesthesia, continues through the procedure, and ends when the patient is no longer under the personal care of the anesthesiologist. The hours and minutes during which anesthesia was administered are recorded in the patient record. Carriers independently determine the amount of time in a unit. Usually, 15 minutes equals a unit.

M Is for Modifying Unit

As the name implies, modifying units reflect circumstances or conditions that change or modify the environment in which the anesthesia service is provided. There are two basic modifying characteristics: qualifying circumstances and physical status modifiers.

from   the   trenches

"*Don't set your goals too high at first. Coding is a learned science, and experience grows with time. Be patient with yourself.*"

KATHERYNE

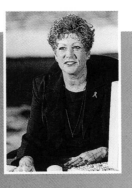

Qualifying Circumstances

At times, anesthesia is provided in situations that make the administration of the anesthesia more difficult. These types of cases include those that are performed in emergency situations and those dealing with patients of extreme age; they also include services performed during the use of controlled hypotension or the use of hypothermia. The Qualifying Circumstances codes begin with the number 99 and are considered **adjunct codes,** which means that the codes cannot be used alone but must be used in addition to another code and are used to provide additional information only. The Qualifying Circumstances code is used in addition to the anesthesia procedure code. The Qualifying Circumstances codes are located in two places in the CPT manual: the Medicine section and the Anesthesia section guidelines. In both locations the plus symbol is located next to the codes (99100–99140), indicating their status as add-on codes only.

STOP *You were just presented with some very important information about the use of certain codes in the CPT manual. The plus (+) symbol next to any CPT code—not just next to Qualifying Circumstances codes—indicates that that code cannot be used alone. Throughout the remaining sections of the CPT manual, the plus symbol will appear to caution you to use the code only as an adjunct code (with other codes).*

When used, the Qualifying Circumstances code is listed separately in addition to the primary anesthesia procedure code. For example, if anesthesia was provided for an 80-year-old patient during a corrective lens procedure, the coding would be

> 00142   Anesthesia for procedure on eye; lens surgery
>
> 99100   Anesthesia for 80-year-old patient

The RVG lists the qualifying circumstances along with the relative value for each code (Fig. 3–6). The CPT index lists the qualifying circumstances coded under Anesthesia, Special Circumstances.

Physical Status Modifiers

The second type of modifying unit used in the Anesthesia section is the physical status modifier. These modifiers are used to indicate the patient's condition at the time anesthesia was administered. The physical status modifier not only indicates the patient's condition at the time of anesthesia but also serves to identify the level of complexity of services provided to the patient. For instance, anesthesia service to a gravely ill patient is much more complex than the same type of service to a normal, healthy patient. The physical status modifier is not assigned by the coder but is determined

Qualifying Circumstances

Code	Description	Relative Value
+99100	Anesthesia for patient of extreme age, under one year and over seventy	1
+99116	Anesthesia complicated by utilization of total hypothermia	5
+99135	Anesthesia complicated by utilization of controlled hypotension	5
+99140	Anesthesia complicated by emergency conditions (specify)	2

Figure 3–6 Qualifying circumstances with relative value. (Based on the *2000 Relative Value Guide* of the American Society of Anesthesiologists, p. xii. A copy of the full text can be obtained from ASA, 520 N. Northwest Hwy., Park Ridge, IL 60068-2573.)

by the anesthesiologist and documented in the anesthesia record. The physical status modifier begins with the letter "P" and contains a number from 1 to 6 (Fig. 3–7). Note that the relative value for P1, P2, and P6 is zero because these conditions are considered not to affect the service provided. A physical status modifier is used after the five-digit CPT code and is illustrated in Figure 3–8.

Summing It Up!

Let's put the elements of the equation to practical use by applying the equation (B + T + M) to a specific case.

An 84-year-old female (qualifying circumstance for extreme age, value 1) with severe hypertension has a 4-cm malignant lesion removed from her right knee (basic value of 3). The total time of anesthesia service was 60 minutes (4 units). The anesthesiologist indicates in the medical record that

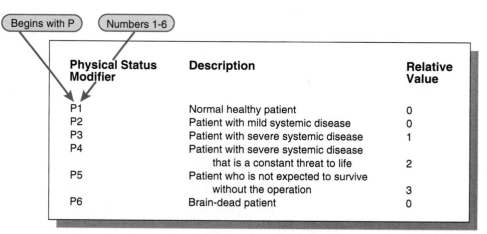

Physical Status Modifier	Description	Relative Value
P1	Normal healthy patient	0
P2	Patient with mild systemic disease	0
P3	Patient with severe systemic disease	1
P4	Patient with severe systemic disease that is a constant threat to life	2
P5	Patient who is not expected to survive without the operation	3
P6	Brain-dead patient	0

Figure 3–7 Physical status modifiers. (Based on the *2000 Relative Value Guide* of the American Society of Anesthesiologists, p. x. A copy of the full text can be obtained from ASA, 520 N. Northwest Hwy., Park Ridge, IL 60068-2573.)

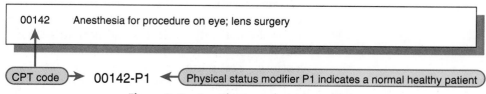

00142	Anesthesia for procedure on eye; lens surgery

CPT code ► 00142-P1 ◄ Physical status modifier P1 indicates a normal healthy patient

Figure 3–8 Anesthesia code and modifier.

Locality Name	Anesthesia Conversion Factor
Manhattan, NY	20.48
NYC suburbs/Long I., NY	20.01
Queens, NY	19.79
Rest of state	16.84
North Carolina	16.01
North Dakota	15.77

Figure 3–9 1999 HCFA anesthesia conversion factors.

the patient's physical status at the time of the procedure was P3 for a severe systemic disease (relative value of 1).

3	basic value
4	time units
2	modifiers: physical status = 1; extreme age = 1
9	total units

The coding that identifies all elements of this case would be

00400-P3	Anesthesia for procedure of integumentary system of knee
99100	Anesthesia for an 84-year-old patient
9	Units at the third-party payer established rate per unit

Conversion Factors

A conversion factor is the dollar value of each unit. Each third-party payer issues a list of conversion factors. The lists vary with geographic location because the cost of practicing medicine varies from one region to another. Figure 3–9 shows an example of a third-party payer's anesthesia conversion factors. Note that North Dakota is $15.77 per unit and Manhattan, NY, is $20.48 per unit, as it is much less expensive to provide anesthesia services in Grand Forks, ND, than it is to provide the same services in Manhattan, NY.

The conversion factor for your locale is multiplied by the number of units in the procedure. For example, the case above has 9 units. If the anesthesiologist were located in Manhattan, NY, which has a conversion factor of $20.48, the total for the procedure would be $184.32 (9 × $20.48). If the same services were provided in North Dakota, with the conversion factor of $15.77, the total for the procedure would be $141.93 (9 × $15.77).

Modifiers in the Anesthesia Section

The CPT two-digit modifiers are used with anesthesia service codes. Modifier -51, multiple procedures, is not usually used with anesthesia codes because when multiple services are provided during the same anesthesia session, the value assigned to the highest valued service is used to report all services. If services for a value of 10 and 5 were done during the same session, the value of 10 would report all services for that session. In coding within other sections of the CPT, the modifier -51 is added to the second procedure, and usually the third-party payer pays that second service at a reduced rate, but this is not the case in anesthesia.

EXERCISE 3-2

MODIFIERS

Using Appendix A of the CPT manual, identify the following CPT modifiers:

1 Unusual Procedural Services _____

2 Unusual Anesthesia _____

Using the descriptions for the preceding modifiers, answer the following questions. Which modifier would be used to identify

3 A service greater than that usually provided? _____

4 A service that required general anesthesia when usually a local anesthesia would be used? _____

The preceding modifiers you identified are the most commonly used modifiers in the Anesthesia section.

5 In addition to modifier -51, Appendix A of the CPT manual identifies one modifier that is not to be used with anesthesia procedures. Identify this "not-to-be-used" modifier.

_____

Concurrent Care Modifiers

Some third-party payers require additional modifiers to indicate how many cases an anesthesiologist is performing or supervising at one time. Certified registered nurse anesthetists (CRNAs) may administer anesthesia to patients under the direction of a licensed physician, or they may work independently. When an anesthesiologist is directing the provision of anesthesia in more than one case at a time, modifiers are used to indicate the context and number of cases that are being reported concurrently. The following modifiers are among the most commonly used:

AA   Anesthesia services performed personally by anesthesiologist

AD   Medical supervision by a physician: more than four concurrent anesthesia procedures

QX   Certified registered nurse anesthetist (CRNA) service, with medical direction by a physician

QY   Anesthesiologist medically directs one CRNA

QZ   CRNA service, without medical direction by a physician

These modifiers are not CPT modifiers but HCPCS modifiers. These modifiers further define the services provided. As a coder, you will need to become familiar with numerous coding systems that are used in addition to the CPT codes.

EXERCISE 3-3

MODIFIERS IN ANESTHESIA

Complete the following:

1 If the anesthesia service was provided to a patient who had mild systemic disease, what would the physical status modifier be likely to be?

_____

2 If the same service was provided to a patient who had severe systemic disease, what would the physical status modifier be likely to be?

_____

3 Anesthesia complicated by utilization of total body hypothermia

Code(s): _____

UNLISTED ANESTHESIA CODE

In the Anesthesia section, an unlisted procedure code number is available. The unlisted procedure code is located under the Other Procedures subsection in the Anesthesia section.

When a new surgical procedure is used, there is no CPT code to indicate the surgical procedure or the anesthesia services provided during the procedure. The anesthesia services are reported using the lone unlisted anesthesia code—01999.

EXERCISE 3-4

ANESTHESIA CODES

Complete the following:

1 What is the unlisted anesthesia procedure code number?

Code: _____

Locate anesthesia procedures in the CPT manual index under the entry "Anesthesia" and then subtermed by the anatomic site. Write the CPT index location on the line provided (e.g., Anesthesia, Thyroid). Then locate the code(s) identified in the Anesthesia section of the CPT manual. Choose the correct code(s) and write the code(s) on the line provided.

2 Needle biopsy of the thyroid (neck)

Index location: _____

Code(s): _____

3 Cesarean section

Index location: _____

Code(s): _____

4 Transurethral resection of the prostate

Index location: _____

Code(s): _____

5 Repair of cleft palate

Index location: _____

Code(s): _____

6 Repair of ruptured Achilles tendon without graft

Index location: _____

Code(s): _____

Using the following information and the B + T + M formula, calculate the payment for the anesthesia services.

For the following questions a time unit will be 15 minutes. Basic unit value for each case is provided within the questions. Refer to Figure 3–9 for the conversion factors used in these questions; to Figure 3–6 for the value of the Qualifying Circumstances; and to Figure 3–7 for value of the Physical Status Modifiers.

7 A needle biopsy lasting 15 minutes was conducted in North Dakota on a normal healthy 75-year-old patient. The basic unit value for the service is 3.*

Anesthesia payment: _____

8 A patient with diabetes mellitus, controlled by diet and exercise, undergoes a 60-minute anesthesia period for a transurethral resection of the prostate (basic unit value of 5).* Calculate the anesthesia rate if the procedure were performed in the following locales:

a. Manhattan _____

b. North Carolina _____

9 A cesarean section was conducted in Alfred, NY, on a patient with preeclampsia. The basic unit value for the service is 7.* Calculate the anesthesia rates for procedures lasting two different lengths of time:

a. 30-minute procedure _____

b. 45-minute procedure _____

The Anesthesia section is a very specialized section used to code services provided to patients.

PART II: Modifiers Used with CPT Codes

THE CPT MODIFIERS

Modifiers are used to tell the third-party payer of circumstances that may affect the way payment is made. Remember that a modifier may be a two-digit code added to the five-digit code or may be listed as its own five-digit modifier. Five-digit modifiers are used when the computer system will not accept a five-digit CPT code with a two-digit modifier added. Each third-party payer has a preference for the modifier—two or five digit—it wants providers to use, so always check with the payer for the preferred method. The CPT manual's Appendix A lists all modifiers and the circumstances for their use.

Modifiers are used to indicate the following types of information:

- altered service

    prolonged service

    service greater than usually required

    unusual circumstances

    part of a service

---

* Excerpted from *2000 Relative Value Guide,* American Society of Anesthesiologists, 520 N. Northwest Hwy., Park Ridge, IL 60068-2753.

Usually Affects Reimbursement	May Affect Reimbursement	Added Information Only
-21	-23	-24
-22	-47	-25
-26	-78	-32
-50		-57
-51		-58
-52		-59
-53		-76
-54		-77
-55		-79
-56		-90
-62		-99
-66		
-80		
-81		
-82		
-91		

Figure 3–10 The effect of modifiers on reimbursement.

- bilateral procedure
- multiple procedures
- professional part of the service/procedure, only
- more than one physician/surgeon

Some modifiers add information and have no effect on reimbursement; others may or may not have an effect; and still others do have an effect on reimbursement. All modifiers are displayed in Figure 3–10, along with their usual effects on reimbursement.

Because the use of modifiers can have a dramatic effect on the amount of the reimbursement received for services, each modifier and its use must be reviewed.

MODIFIERS THAT USUALLY AFFECT REIMBURSEMENT

-21 Prolonged Evaluation and Management Services

As is indicated by the title of modifier -21, the purpose of this modifier is to indicate an extended E/M service, and it is not used with codes other than E/M codes. The full description of the modifier is as follows:

> When the face-to-face or floor/unit service(s) provided is prolonged or otherwise greater than that usually required for the highest level of E/M service within a given category, it may be identified by adding modifiers -21 to the E/M code or by the use of the separate five digit modifier code 09921. A report may be appropriate.

CAUTION *Modifier -21 should be used only with the highest level E/M code. For example, 99205 is the highest level for a new patient office visit. If an extended service above that described in 99204 were provided you would move up to code 99205 to report the service. Therefore, it is never correct to report modifier -21 with anything but the highest level code. This rule applies to both outpatient and inpatient services.*

The use of modifier -21 in the E/M section is limited to the codes in the range 99205–99397. Codes in the ranges 99291–99292 (critical care) and

99295–99298 (neonatal intensive care) are based on time units, so additional time would be reported by using additional codes or units rather than by adding the prolonged service modifier -21.

For an example of the use of modifier -21, review the following case:

A 34-year-old male patient is admitted to the hospital with acute chest pains. The physician conducts a comprehensive history and examination. The decision-making complexity is high. The physician spends 90 minutes at the bedside of the patient, on the unit with the patient's family, and in the development of a plan for the patient's care.

You would code this case as a 99233, initial hospital care, the highest level code available. But the code description indicates the typical time for a 99233 is 70 minutes. To fully describe the service provided to this patient you would have to add modifier -21. The code for the service would be 99233-21.

The use of the modifier -21 does not always have an effect on third-party reimbursement. For example, Medicare does not pay additionally for the use of modifier -21. But you still want to be as specific as possible when coding all services, and this includes the use of modifiers to fully explain a service.

-22 Unusual Procedural Service

Modifier -22 indicates that a service was provided that was greater than usual, and a special report would accompany the use of the code to explain exactly in which ways the service was greater. A description of modifier -22 is as follows:

> When the service(s) provided is greater than that usually required for the listed procedure, it may be identified by adding modifier -22 to the usual procedure number or by using the separate five digit modifier 09922. A report may also be appropriate.

The use of modifier -22 indicates that the service provided was significantly more than the service described in the CPT code. A few additional minutes spent on a procedure do not warrant the use of this modifier. The medical record must contain documentation that substantiates the claim that the service was unusual in some way. The medical record would contain statements about the increased risk to the patient, the difficulty of the procedure, excessive blood loss, or other statements to indicate the occurrence of an unusually difficult situation. Modifier -22 is overused, so it comes under particularly close scrutiny by third-party payers, especially as there is a payment increase of 20% to 30% for services that qualify for the use of modifier -22. So when using it, you have to be sure that you have the documentation to support your claim. When the third-party payer receives a claim that includes a service to which modifier -22 has been added, the claim is sent to an individual who reviews the claim. Appropriate documentation must, therefore, accompany the claim—an operative report, a pathology report, office notes, hospital chart notes, and so forth.

-26 Professional Component

Modifier -26 is used to designate a physician and a technical part of a service. The description of modifier -26 is as follows:

> Certain procedures are a combination of a physician component and a technical component. When the physician component is reported separately, the service

> may be identified by adding the modifier -26 to the usual procedure number or the service may be reported by using the five digit modifier code 09926.

Modifier -26 is usually used with radiology service. An example of the technical component is an independent radiology facility that takes the x-rays (the technical component) and sends them to a private radiologist who reads the x-rays and writes a report of the findings (the professional component). The physician's services would be reported with the modifier -26 added to the code for the x-ray, indicating that only the professional component of the x-ray service was provided.

-50 Bilateral Procedures

If the same procedure is performed on a mirror-image part of the body, modifier -50, indicating a bilateral procedure, would be submitted. The description of the modifier is as follows:

> Unless otherwise identified in the listings, bilateral procedures that are performed at the same operative session should be identified by adding the modifier -50 to the appropriate five digit code or by use of the separate five digit modifier code 09952.

For example, an arthroplasty (total knee replacement, 27447 and 27447-50) for both left and right knees at the same operative session would be coded using the -50 modifier.

Another example in which the same services may be performed on two sides would be a bilateral breast procedure (i.e., bilateral, simple complete mastectomy, 19180 and 19180-50).

Be sure to find out whether your third-party payer wants the surgical code used once with the modifier (code plus modifier -50) or used twice (code alone and code plus modifier -50), or whether the procedure should be listed twice. For hospital outpatient coding, the code is usually listed twice. As of 1999, some modifiers were allowed for hospital outpatient coding. Appendix A of the CPT manual contains a section that lists all modifiers approved for hospital outpatient coding.

CAUTION *Some CPT codes are for bilateral procedures and do not require a bilateral modifier. For example, 27395 is for a bilateral lengthening of the hamstring tendon, and it would be incorrect to place a bilateral modifier on the code.*

-51 Multiple Procedures

During any given operative session, more than one procedure may be performed. This is referred to as "multiple procedures" and is indicated by modifier -51. The description of the modifier is as follows:

> When multiple procedures, other than E/M services, are performed at the same session by the same provider, the primary procedure or service may be reported as listed. The additional procedure(s) or service(s) may be identified by appending the modifier -51 to the additional procedure or service code(s) or by the use of the separate five digit modifier 09951. Note: This modifier should not be appended to designated "add-on" codes.

CAUTION *You have to be careful when coding multiple procedures because CPT codes include many different procedures bundled together in one code. For example, code 58200 is a total abdominal hysterectomy, but it also includes a partial vaginectomy (removal of the vagina) with para-aortic and pelvic lymph node sampling, with or without removal of tube(s), and with or without removal of ovary(ies). It would be incorrect to code separately for each service because they are included (bundled) in the description for code 58200. Listing the subsequent procedures separately (unbundling) may be considered fraud by a third-party payer. **Unbundling** is assigning multiple codes when one code would fully describe the service or procedure. The assigning of multiple codes results in increased reimbursement.*

However, if one code does not describe all of the procedures performed, and the secondary procedure is not considered a minor procedure that is incidental to the major procedure, each procedure may be billed by using the multiple-procedure modifier (-51). For example, if a patient has a laminectomy with lumbar disk removal (for a herniated disk)—code 63030—and also has an arthrodesis (stabilization of the area where the disk was removed)—code 22612—they are multiple procedures. Both services would be coded, and modifier -51 would be used after the lesser of the two codes (services).

Multiple Procedures

Now that you know the basics about modifier -51, let's look more closely at the use of this important modifier. There are three significant times when multiple procedures are coded:

1. Same Operation, Different Site
2. Multiple Operation(s), Same Operative Session
3. Procedure Performed Multiple Times

Same Operation, Different Site

Multiple procedures are coded using modifier -51 when the same procedure is performed on different sites. For example, a patient has an excision of a 1.5-cm benign lesion from the forearm and at the same time has an excision of a 3-cm benign lesion from the neck. In this case the coding would be 11423 for the 3-cm lesion and 11402-51 for the 1.5-cm lesion. The third-party payer usually pays for the second procedure at 50% of the usual full cost of the procedure. Therefore, the code after which you place the -51 modifier is very important. Always list the most costly procedure first, without a modifier.

Multiple Operation(s), Same Operative Session

Multiple procedures (-51) are also coded when more than one procedure is performed during the same operative session.

The primary procedure during the surgical session would be paid at the full fee, the second procedure during the same session would usually be paid at 50% of the fee, and the third procedure would usually be paid at 25% of the fee. Therefore, when you are coding procedures for payment, it is important that you put the most costly procedure first, without a modifier, and then list the subsequent procedures in order of complexity, remembering to use the -51 modifier on all subsequent procedures. This process of assigning the -51 modifier helps to ensure that optimal reimbursement occurs. For example, an abdominal hysterectomy (58150) may be performed along with a posterior (rectocele) repair (57250-51). The hysterectomy is the most costly procedure, so it is listed first, without the modifier, to be paid at the full fee. The posterior repair is less costly so it is listed second, with the modifier, to be paid at 50% of the fee.

Procedure Performed Multiple Times

Multiple procedures are also coded when the same procedure code is used to identify a service performed more than once during a single operative session. There are two ways to report procedures performed multiple times, depending on the requirements of the third-party payer. One way is to use the code number only once but to list the number of times it is performed (number of units). For example, if a patient needs a repair of two flexor tendons of the leg, you would use 27658 × 2 units. Units are identified because the code description states "each" tendon, and two tendons were repaired. The other way to code this would be to list 27658 once without a modifier and again with modifier -51 (i.e., 27658-51). Remember, check with the payer to determine the preferred method of billing.

EXERCISE 3-5

MULTIPLE PROCEDURES

Using the CPT manual, code the following:

1 Destruction of malignant lesion of neck (most resource intensive), 4 cm in diameter, with destruction of malignant lesion of arm, 4 cm in diameter

   Code(s): _____

2 Abdominal hysterectomy with posterior (rectocele) repair

   Code(s): _____

3 Treatment of two tarsal bone fractures, without manipulation

   Code(s): _____

4 What would the code and/or modifier(s) be for an established patient who received the highest level outpatient service available for an office visit, and the time that was required for the service, as indicated in the medical record, exceeded the time indicated in the code by 25 minutes?

   Code(s) and/or modifier(s): _____

5 What would the code and/or modifier(s) be if an established patient received the next to the highest level outpatient service available for an office visit (99214), and the time that was required for the service, as indicated in the medical record, exceeded the time indicated in the code by 25 minutes?

   Code and/or modifier(s): _____

6 A 60-year-old female patient is referred to a radiology laboratory by her general physician. The laboratory takes the x-rays requested and sends them on to a radiologist to interpret and to develop the written report that is sent to the general physician. If you were coding for the radiologist, what modifier would you use to indicate the service provided by the radiologist?

   Modifier: _____

7 A patient has bilateral carpal tunnel surgery. When you code the case, what modifier would you be certain to use?

Modifier: _____

8 What is the code for a single arthroplasty, knee (total knee replacement)?

Code(s): _____

9 What are the codes for bilateral arthroplasties of the knees?

Codes: _____ and _____

10 The code for a radical mastectomy is 19200. List two ways the bilateral modifier could be used to indicate that a bilateral procedure was performed, depending on the third-party payer's preferences.

Codes _____ and _____

CAUTION *Modifier -51 is not used with add-on codes that specify "each additional. . . ." For example, 19290 is for placement of one wire into a breast lesion. If two wires were placed, the first wire would be coded 19290 from the subheading Breast and the category Introduction, and the second wire would be coded 19291 for an additional wire.*

-52 Reduced Services

Modifier -52 is used to indicate a service that was provided but was reduced in comparison to the full description of the service.

The description of the modifier is as follows:

> Under certain circumstances a service or procedure is partially reduced or eliminated at the physician's discretion. Under these circumstances the service provided can be identified by its usual procedure number and the addition of the modifier -52, signifying that the service is reduced. This provides a means of reporting reduced services without disturbing the identification of the basic service. Modifier code 09952 may be used as an alternative for modifier -52. Note: For hospital outpatient reporting of a previously scheduled procedure/service that is partially reduced or canceled as a result of extenuating circumstances or those that threatened the well-being of the patient prior to or after administration of anesthesia, see modifiers -73 and -74

An example of a circumstance in which modifier -52 would be used is a surgical procedure for the removal of an abdominal carcinoma in which the patient was anesthetized and the procedure begun but then terminated by the physician because the metastasis was too far advanced. When modifier -52 is used, additional documentation, such as operative reports and/or physician explanation of the reason for the reduced service, will facilitate the reimbursement process, as the third-party payer usually wants to know the reason for the reduction before making payment.

-53 Discontinued Procedure

Modifier -52 is used to describe circumstances in which services were reduced at the direction of the physician, whereas modifier -53 describes circumstances in which a procedure is stopped because of the patient's condition.

The description of the modifier is as follows:

> Under certain circumstances, the physician may elect to terminate a surgical or diagnostic procedure. Due to extenuating circumstances or those that threaten the well-being of the patient, it may be necessary to indicate that a surgical or diagnostic procedure was started but discontinued. This circumstance may be reported by adding the modifier -53 to the code reported by the physician for the discontinued procedure or by use of a separate five digit modifier code 09953. Note: This modifier is not used to report the elective cancellation of a procedure prior to the patient's anesthesia induction and/or surgical preparation in the operating suite. For outpatient hospital/ambulatory surgery centers (ASC) reporting of a previously scheduled procedure/service that is partially reduced or canceled as a result of extenuating circumstances or those that threaten the well-being of the patient prior to or after administration of anesthesia, see modifiers -73 and -74.

An example of the correct use of modifier -53 is a situation in which a patient was undergoing a surgical procedure and during the procedure developed arrhythmia that could not be controlled. The physician discontinued the procedure due to the risk that continuation presented to the patient and then stabilized the patient. The code for the surgical procedure would be reported along with modifier -53 to indicate that although the procedure was begun, it was discontinued. The key to proper use of modifier -53 is that the patient had been prepared for surgery and anesthetized.

Modifier -53 is **not** used to report services

- when the patient cancels the procedure

- with E/M codes

- with any code that is based on time (i.e., critical care codes)

Modifiers -54, -55, and -56

There may be times when a surgeon performs the surgery only (modifier -54) and asks another physician to perform the preoperative evaluation (modifier -56) and/or the postoperative care (modifier -55). When billing for his or her own individual services, each physician would use the same procedure code for the surgery, letting the modifier indicate to the third-party payer the part of the surgical package that each personally performed.

EXAMPLE

19180	Mastectomy, simple, complete
19180-54	Mastectomy, simple, complete, surgery only
19180-56	Mastectomy, simple, complete, preoperative evaluation only
19180-55	Mastectomy, simple, complete, postoperative care only

Let's take a closer look at each of these important modifiers.

-54 Surgical Care Only

Modifier -54 is used to indicate the surgical care portion of a surgical procedure (intraoperative). Use modifier -54 only with codes from the Surgery section (10040–69990). The description of the modifier is as follows:

> When one physician performs a surgical procedure and another provides preoperative and/or postoperative management, surgical services may be identified by adding the modifier -54 to the usual procedure number or by use of the separate five digit modifier code 09954.

Modifier -54 is used correctly only when there has been transfer of responsibility for care from one physician to another. This transfer takes place by means of a transfer order that is signed by both physicians and kept in the patient's medical record. Modifier -54 is not used for minor surgical procedures but for major procedures that involve follow-up care as a part of the service of the surgery (a surgery package). Although third-party payers vary, the payment for only the surgical procedure is usually about 70% of the total payment for the procedure, with 10% going to the physician who provided the preoperative service, and 20% to the physician who provided the postoperative care.

-55 Postoperative Management Only

Another part of a surgical procedure is the postoperative care. The amount of postoperative care that is considered part of a surgery varies according to the complexity of the surgery, with zero, 10, or 90 days being the most commonly used number of postoperative days. The description of the modifier -55 is as follows:

> When one physician performs the postoperative management and another physician has performed the surgical procedure, the postoperative component may be identified by adding the modifier -55 to the usual procedure number or by use of the separate five digit modifier code 09955.

Modifier -55 is used only for services provided to the patient after discharge from the hospital. To report services provided while the patient is still in the hospital, you would use E/M codes because the payment to the operating physician (70%) assumes that the operating physician provides the care until the patient is discharged from the hospital.

You report the postoperative services by adding modifier -55 to the surgical code. For example, a patient had a nephrolithotomy (calculus removed from kidney), coded 50060, and the operating physician transferred to a second physician the postoperative care after the patient's discharge from the hospital. The operating physician would report services using 50060-54, and the physician providing the postoperative care would report 50060-55. The physicians use the same surgery code (50060) and also report the date of service as the date of the surgical procedure. In this way, the third-party payer knows that the two physicians are splitting the care of the patient into surgical care and postoperative care after discharge.

CAUTION *For Medicare patients, care must be officially transferred from the physician providing the surgical care to the physician providing the postoperative care by way of a transfer order that is kept in the medical record.*

-56 Preoperative Management Only

The third part of a surgical service is the preoperative care. If a physician provides only the preoperative management to a patient in preparation for surgery, the service is reported with modifier -56 added to the surgical code. The description of the modifier is as follows:

> When one physician performs the preoperative care and evaluation and another physician performs the surgical procedure, the preoperative component may be identified by adding the modifier -56 to the usual procedure number or by use of the separate five digit modifier code 09956.

Before patients undergo surgery, a physical examination is performed to determine whether they are physically able to withstand the surgery. This examination is the *preoperative workup*. When one physician performs the preoperative workup and another physician performs the surgery, both physicians report the services using the surgical procedure code and adding the correct modifier. For example, in preparation for a nephrolithotomy, the patient's general medicine physician provides the preoperative workup (50060-56) at the surgeon's request, and the surgeon provides the surgery (50060-54).

STOP *Modifier -56 is never used for services reported to Medicare, as Medicare considers the preoperative service to be part of the surgery.*

At the present time, not all modifiers are recognized by all third-party payers. Some third-party payers have agreed to pay a physician separately from the surgical package for the initial evaluation of a condition during which the decision to perform surgery was made. Under the conditions of a global package, this visit would have become part of the preoperative care if performed the day of or the day before major surgery. When this initial visit occurs within the time requirements of the preoperative portion of the global surgical package, modifier -57 is used to let the payer know that payment for this initial evaluation should be made in addition to payment for surgery. E/M services provided the day before or on the day of a major surgery, or on the day of a minor procedure, are included in the global package unless it is the patient's initial visit to the physician. To receive payment for these initial visits, modifier -57 is added to the E/M services with major procedures and -25 to the E/M services with minor procedures.

EXAMPLE

99215-57   Office visit for established patient at which a decision for surgery was made.

EXERCISE 3-6

ADDITIONAL MODIFIERS THAT AFFECT REIMBURSEMENT

Code the following:

1 The surgical care only for a total esophagectomy without reconstruction

Code(s): _____

2 The postoperative care only for a radical mastectomy including pectoral muscles, axillary, and internal mammary lymph nodes

Code(s): _____

3 The procedure in Question 2 when the preoperative service only is provided

Code(s): _____

4 Which modifier describes a procedure that was reduced at the direction of the physician?

_____

-62 Two Surgeons

Modifier -62 is used to indicate that two surgeons acted as co-surgeons. The description of the modifier is as follows:

> When two surgeons work together as primary surgeons performing distinct part(s) of a single reportable procedure, each surgeon should report his/her distinct operative work by adding the modifier -62 to the single definitive procedure code. Each surgeon should report the co-surgery once using the same procedure code. If additional procedure(s) including add-on procedure(s) are performed during the same surgical session, separate code(s) may be reported without the modifier -62 added. Modifier code 09962 may be used as an alternative to modifier -62. Note: if a co-surgeon acts as an assistant in the performance of additional procedure(s) during the same surgical session, those services may be reported using separate procedure code(s) with the modifier -80 or modifier -81 added, as appropriate.

from the trenches

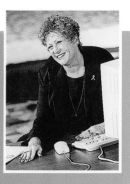

"The most difficult part of the job is organizing the workload and setting priorities."

KATHERYNE

To use modifier -62 correctly, two physicians of different specialties must work together as co-surgeons. If one physician assists another physician, the service **cannot** be reported using modifier -62. The co-surgeons use different skills during the surgery. Many third-party payers require documentation showing the medical necessity of co-surgeons. The operative report should clearly show the distinct services each surgeon provided. Modifier -62 is correctly used when two physicians are necessary to complete one surgical procedure, each completing a distinct portion of the procedure. For example, a cardiologist and a general surgeon may install a pacemaker, with the general surgeon preparing the implantation site, the cardiologist inserting and activating the pacemaker, and the general surgeon closing the site. Each physician would report his/her service using pacemaker insertion code with the modifier -62 added.

-66 Surgical Team

Modifier -66 is used with very complex surgical procedures that require several physicians, each with a different specialty, to complete the procedure. The description of the modifier is as follows:

> Under some circumstances, highly complex procedures (requiring the concomitant services of several physicians often of different specialties, plus other highly skilled, specially trained personnel, various types of complex equipment) are carried out under the "surgical team" concept. Such circumstances may be identified by each participating physician with the addition of the modifier -66 to the basic procedure number used for reporting services. Modifier code 09966 may be used as an alternative to modifier -66.

A surgical team consists of physicians, technicians, and other trained personnel that function together to complete a complex procedure. Teams are usually used in organ transplant surgeries, with each member of the team completing the same function at each surgery. Third-party payers will often increase the total reimbursement for a team to 50% higher than the usual reimbursement for the procedure. The reimbursement is then divided among the physicians on the basis of a prearranged agreement.

-80 Assistant Surgeon

A surgical assistant is one who provides service to the primary surgeon during a surgical procedure. The description of the modifier is as follows:

> Surgical assistant services may be identified by adding the modifier -80 to the usual procedure number(s) or by use of the separate five digit modifier code 09980.

The assistant surgeon's services are reported using the same code as the primary surgeon's, but modifier -80 is added to alert the third-party payer to the assistant surgeon status. Usually, the assistant receives only 15% to 30% of the usual charge for a surgery when acting in the assistant capacity. Some third-party payers do not reimburse for the presence of a surgical assistant during procedures. You will need to work closely with your third-party payer to know what assistant charges the payer will reimburse. For example, Medicare has a list of surgeries for which it will pay for an assistant surgeon.

-81 Minimum Assistant Surgeon

Modifier -81 is used to indicate an assistant surgeon who provides services that are less extensive than those described by modifier -80. The description of the modifier is as follows:

> Minimum surgical assistant services are identified by adding the modifier -81 to the usual procedure number or by use of the separate five digit modifier code 09981.

Some procedures require **more than one assistant;** those additional assistant services are reported by using the surgical procedure code with modifier -81 added. In other instances, the first assistant is required to be in attendance for only a portion of the procedure, and this lesser service would be reported by using modifier -81. Many third-party payers do not pay for a minimum assistant surgeon. For example, Medicare will pay for a minimum assistant only on rare occasions in which medical necessity can be proven. Usually, the minimum assistant surgeon receives 10% of the usual charge for a surgery.

CAUTION *Do not use modifier -81 to report nonphysician service assistance during a surgical procedure. Modifier -81 is limited to a physician serving in the capacity of an assistant.*

-82 Assistant Surgeon (When Qualified Resident Surgeon Not Available)

Modifier -82 is used when the hospital in which the procedure was performed has an affiliation with a medical school and has a residency program, but no resident was available to serve as an assistant surgeon. Residents are medical students who are completing a required surgical training period in the hospital. The description of the modifier is as follows:

> The unavailability of a qualified resident surgeon is a prerequisite for use of modifier -82 appended to the usual procedure code number(s) or by the use of the separate five digit modifier code 09982.

Do not confuse modifier -80 with -82 when reporting services. Medicare does not pay for an assistant surgeon if the hospital has a residency program because the residents serve as employees of the hospital who are there to receive training and provide assistance to physicians as part of the hospital's agreement with the medical school. Hospitals that have affiliations with medical schools are considered teaching facilities. Modifier -82 has very limited use and requires supporting documentation that the patient's condition was so severe that it required an assistant and that a qualified resident was not available.

-91 Repeat Clinical Diagnostic Laboratory Test

Modifier -91 is used to report a laboratory test that was performed on the same day as the original laboratory test. The description of the modifier is as follows:

> In the course of treatment of a patient, it may be necessary to repeat the same laboratory test on the same day to obtain subsequent (multiple) test results. Under these circumstances, the laboratory test performed can be identified by its usual procedure number and the addition of the modifier -91. Note: This modifier may not be used when tests are rerun to confirm initial results; due to testing problems with specimens or equipment; or for any other reason when a normal, one-time, reportable result is all that is required. This modifier may not be used when other code(s) describe a series of test results (e.g., glucose tolerance tests, evocative/suppression testing). This modifier may only be used for laboratory test(s) performed more than once on the same day on the same patient.

This modifier is correctly used when a laboratory test has been repeated so as to produce multiple test results. It cannot be used if the equipment malfunctioned or there was a problem with the specimen, which would result in third-party payers' paying for laboratory errors. Nor can you use the modifier to report services performed because a subsequent test was done to confirm the results of the initial test. The modifier cannot be used when there is a series of test results, such as those found in allergy testing.

EXERCISE 3-7

MORE MODIFIERS THAT AFFECT REIMBURSEMENT

Using your knowledge about modifiers, complete the following:

1 The medical record indicated that the physician had an established patient go to the lab for a blood panel in the morning, and in the afternoon had the patient return to the lab for another blood panel so as to produce multiple test results. What modifier would you add to the code for the panel?

_____

2 Dr. Edwards, a cardiologist, and Dr. Mathews, a general surgeon, worked together as primary surgeons on a complex surgical case. What modifier would be added to the CPT surgery codes for the services of both Dr. Edwards and Dr. Mathews?

_____

3 A team of physicians with different specialties, along with a highly skilled team of technical personnel, performed a liver transplant. The surgical team concept would be indicated by using which modifier?

_____

4 Dr. Stenopolis served as an assistant to Dr. Edwards in a quadruple bypass procedure. Dr. Stenopolis' services were reported by using this modifier:

_____

5 In the middle of the bypass procedure in Question 4, the patient experienced severe complications. Dr. Edwards asked Dr. Loren to come into the operating room to temporarily assist in stabilizing the patient. What modifier would be used when reporting the service Dr. Loren provided?

_____

MODIFIERS THAT MAY AFFECT REIMBURSEMENT

-23 Unusual Anesthesia

Modifier -23 is used by an anesthesiologist to indicate a service for which general anesthesia was used when normally the anesthesia would have been local or regional. The description of the modifier is as follows:

> Occasionally, a procedure, which usually requires either no anesthesia or local anesthesia, because of unusual circumstances must be done under general anesthesia. This circumstance may be reported by adding the modifier -23 to the procedure code of the basic service or by use of the separate five digit modifier code 09923.

This modifier can be used only with codes in the Anesthesia section (00100–01999) and only by the physician providing the general anesthesia, usually an anesthesiologist. When the modifier is used, the claim must be accompanied by a written report explaining the unusual circumstance that required general anesthesia instead of the normally used local or regional anesthesia.

-47 Anesthesia by Surgeon

Modifier -47 is used to report a surgical procedure in which the surgeon administered regional or general anesthesia to the patient. The description of the modifier is as follows:

> Regional or general anesthesia provided by the surgeon may be reported by adding the modifier -47 to the basic service or by use of the separate five digit modifier code 09947. (This does not include local anesthesia.) Note: Modifier -47 or 09947 would not be used as a modifier for the anesthesia procedures 00100–01999.

There are times, although they occur infrequently, when a physician acts as both the anesthesiologist and the surgeon. This usually occurs during procedures that require a regional anesthetic. For example, a surgeon places a tourniquet on an arm, administers a regional anesthetic, and performs a surgical procedure. The physician is acting as the anesthesiologist and would report the time spent administering the block (regional anesthetic). If the third-party payer allowed payment for modifier -47, payment would be made based on the time spent administering the regional anesthetic. Modifier -47 is added only to surgery codes and is never added to anesthesia codes. The surgeon acting as anesthesiologist would therefore report modifier -47 added to a surgery code.

-78 Return to the Operating Room for a Related Procedure During the Postoperative Period

Modifier -78 is used to explain a circumstance in which a patient is taken back to the operating room for surgical treatment of a complication resulting from the first procedure. The description of the modifier is as follows:

> The physician may need to indicate that another procedure was performed during the postoperative period of the initial procedure. When this subsequent procedure is related to the first, and requires the use of the operating room, it may be reported by adding the modifier -78 to the related procedure, or by using the separate five digit modifier 09978. (For repeat procedures on the same day, see -76.)

Modifier -78 is placed after the subsequent procedure code to indicate to the third-party payer that the second surgery was necessary because of complications resulting from the first operation. For many third-party payers, only the surgery portion (intraoperative) of the surgical package is paid when the -78 modifier is used. The patient remains within the postoperative period of the first operation for any further preoperative or postoperative care. For example, if the patient were to develop a second set of complications stemming from the original surgery, you would again report the procedure performed to treat the second complication and add modifier -78 to the code. In this way, the third-party payer continues to know that the complication requiring surgery originated from the original surgery.

CAUTION *Do not use modifier -78 to report the same physician repeating the same procedure on the same patient. If a repeat procedure was done by the same physician, you would report those services using modifier -76, Repeat Procedure by Same Physician.*

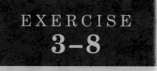

EXERCISE
3-8

MODIFIERS THAT MAY AFFECT REIMBURSEMENT

Using your knowledge of modifiers, complete the following:

1 A patient has a hernia repair and two days later must be returned to the operating room for a related repair. When coding the hernia repair, which modifier would you add onto the surgical code?

_____

2 Dr. Ramus administers regional anesthesia by intravenous injection (a.k.a. Bier's local anesthesia) for a surgical procedure on the patient's arm below the elbow. Dr. Ramus then performs the surgical procedure. What modifier would be added to the surgical code?

_____

3 A extremely anxious elderly man is admitted to the hospital for a gastroscopy for which he will receive general anesthesia. The patient is unable to cooperate in the outpatient same-day surgery unit. The physician determines that, because of the patient's advanced dementia, general anesthesia during this procedure, which usually does not require anesthesia, is the best approach to use with the patient. What modifier would you use when coding this case?

_____

4 Mr. Williams has an appendectomy on March 4 and is taken back to surgery on March 6 for evacuation of a hematoma of the wound site (a complication of the original procedure). What modifier would be used?

_____

MODIFIERS THAT PROVIDE ADDED INFORMATION ONLY

-24 Unrelated Evaluation and Management Service by the Same Physician During a Postoperative Period

Modifier -24 is also used only with E/M codes. The full description of the modifier is as follows:

> The physician may need to indicate that an evaluation and management service was performed during a postoperative period for a reason(s) unrelated to the original procedure. This circumstance may be reported by the addition of the modifier -24 to the appropriate level of E/M service, or the separate five digit modifier 09924 may be used.

The most common use for modifier -24 is to report services that were preformed during a postoperative period. As you will learn in Chapter 4, surgical procedures come with a package of services, such as preoperative, the procedure, and normal follow-up care. If an E/M service unrelated to the surgical procedure is provided to a patient during the postoperative period, the third-party payer would think that the service was part of the surgical care. Modifier -24 is added to indicate that the E/M service was not a part of the surgical care but was an unrelated service. The postoperative period of a major surgical procedure is usually 90 days, of minor surgery, 10 days. Payment for the surgical procedure includes postoperative care of the patient during these periods.

You can also use modifier -24 with the General Ophthalmological Services codes 92002–92014 even though these codes are located in the Medicine section. Ophthalmologists report their new and established patient services for medical examination using these services codes.

-25 Significant, Separately Identifiable E/M Service by the Same Physician on the Same Day of the Procedure or Other Service

Modifier -25 is used to report an E/M service on a day when another service was provided to the patient by the same physician. The description of the modifier is as follows:

> The physician may need to indicate that on the day a procedure or service identified by a CPT code was performed, the patient's condition required a significant, separately identifiable E/M service above and beyond the other service provided or beyond the usual preoperative and postoperative care associated with the procedure that was performed. The E/M service may be prompted by the symptom or condition for which the procedure and/or service was provided. As such, different diagnoses are not required for reporting of the E/M services on the same date. This circumstance may be reported by adding the modifier -25 to the appropriate level of E/M service, or the separate five digit modifier 09925 may be used. Note: This modifier is not used to report an E/M service that resulted in a decision to perform surgery. See modifier -57.

For modifier -25 to be used correctly, there must be a medical necessity to provide a separate, additional E/M service on the same day a procedure was performed or another service was provided. The medical necessity for this additional E/M service must be documented in the patient's medical record. If you do not add the modifier -25 to the separate, additional E/M code for service on the day of a procedure, the third-party payer would disallow the charge because it would be thought to be the evaluation/management portion of the procedure. By adding modifier -25 you are stating that the service was separate from the procedure or original service and thereby increasing the potential of receiving payment for the service. For example, if a physician provided a dialysis service to a hospital inpatient and then, in addition, provided a separate E/M service for that patient, you would report the dialysis service (the procedure) and also report an inpatient service (E/M service), adding the modifier -25. The use of modifier -25 is not limited to procedures; it can also be used when other E/M services are provided on the same day to the same patient. For example, if a patient came into the office for a visit early in the day and then later in the day needed to return for a separate service, you would report both services using E/M codes and add modifier -25 to the second code.

-32 Mandated Services

Modifier -32 indicates a service that was required by some entity. The description of the modifier is as follows:

> Services related to *mandated* consultation and/or related services (e.g., PRO, third party payer, governmental, legislative or regulatory requirement) may be identified by adding the modifier -32 to the basic procedure or the service may be reported by the use of the five digit modifier 09932.

This modifier is not used to indicate a second opinion requested by a patient, a family member, or another physician. Modifier -32 is used only when a service is required. For example, the police require a suspected rape or abuse victim to have certain tests. Another common use of modifier -32 is to indicate that a third-party payer or workers' compensation requires a physical examination of a covered patient. The third-party payer usually waives the deductible and copayment for the patient and usually pays 100% of the service.

-57 Decision for Surgery

Modifier -57 is used with an E/M code to indicate the day the decision to perform a surgery was made. The description of the modifier is as follows:

> An E/M service that resulted in the initial decision to perform the surgery may be identified by adding the modifier -57 to the appropriate level of E/M service, or the separate five digit modifier 09957 may be used.

Modifier -57 can be used not only with E/M codes (99201–99499) to indicate the initial decision to perform a procedure or service but also with the ophthalmological codes (92002–92014) located in the Medicine section.

CAUTION *Don't make the all too common mistake of adding -57 to codes from the Surgery section. Modifier -57 is never added to surgical codes.*

coding shot

Note that the description of modifier -57 does not indicate whether the decided-upon procedure is diagnostic or therapeutic, minor or major. But Medicare guidelines direct that modifier -57 be used only with E/M or ophthalmologic codes to indicate when the decision to perform a **major** procedure was made.

-58 Staged or Related Procedure or Service by the Same Physician During the Postoperative Period

Modifier -57 explains that the subsequent surgery was planned or staged at the time of the first surgery. The description of the modifier is as follows:

> The physician may need to indicate that the performance of a procedure or service during the postoperative period was: a) planned prospectively at the time of the original procedure (staged); b) more extensive than the original procedure; or c) for therapy following a diagnostic surgical procedure. This circumstance may be reported by adding the modifier -58 to the staged or related procedure, or the separate five digit modifier 09958 may be used. Note: This modifier is not used to report the treatment of a problem that requires a return to the operating room. See modifier -78.

The procedure as a whole must have been intended to include the original procedure plus one or more subsequent procedures. For example, multiple skin grafts are often done in stages to allow adequate healing time between procedures. Modifier -58 can also be used if a therapeutic procedure is performed because of the findings of a diagnostic procedure. For example, a patient may have a surgical breast biopsy, and if the pathology report indicates that the specimen was malignant, the patient may elect to have an immediate radical mastectomy. The mastectomy may be performed during the postoperative period of the biopsy. Modifier -58 indicates to the third-party payer that the second surgery was therapeutic treatment that followed the original diagnostic procedure, and full payment would usually be made for the mastectomy. A new postoperative period would start after the mastectomy, and any postoperative care provided to the patient would be part of the surgical package for the mastectomy.

-59 Distinct Procedural Service

Modifier -59 is used to indicate that services that are usually bundled into one payment were provided as separate services. The description of the modifier is as follows:

> Under certain circumstances, the physician may need to indicate that a procedure or service was distinct or independent from other services performed on the same day. Modifier -59 is used to identify procedures/services that are not normally reported together, but are appropriate under the circumstances. This may represent a different session or patient encounter, different procedure or surgery, different site or organ system, separate incision/excision, separate

lesion, or separate injury (or area of injury in extensive injuries) not ordinarily encountered or performed on the same day by the same physician. However, when another already established modifier is appropriate it should be used rather than modifier -59. Only if no more descriptive modifier is available, and the use of modifier -59 best explains the circumstances, should modifier -59 be used. Modifier code 09959 may be used as an alternative to modifier -59.

As the code description notes, modifier -59 is used to identify the following:

- Different session or patient encounter
- Different procedure or surgery
- Different site or organ system
- Separate incision/excision
- Separate lesion
- Separate injury or area of injury in extensive injuries

Modifier -59 is used with codes from all sections of the CPT manual except E/M codes. Medicare has lists of codes that cannot be billed together; they are called edits. These edits have been established to ensure that providers do not bill for services that are included in the bundle for a given code. For example, you would not bill for a standard preoperative visit related to a major surgical procedure and bill separately for the surgery and follow-up care. All three services—preoperative, intraoperative, postoperative—are packaged together in one major surgical CPT code. The use of modifier -59 indicates that the service was not a part of another service but, indeed, was a distinct service.

-76 Repeat Procedure by Same Physician

Modifier -76 is used to report services or procedures that are repeated and are provided by the same physician. The description of the modifier is as follows:

The physician may need to indicate that a procedure or service was repeated subsequent to the original procedure or service. This circumstance may be reported by adding the modifier -76 to the repeated procedure/service, or the separate five digit modifier code 09976 may be used.

The modifier is used to indicate to third-party payers that the services are not duplicate services and, therefore, the bill is not a duplicate bill. Sometimes these repeat services are provided on the same day as the previous service, and without the use of modifier -76, the third-party payer would assume a duplicate bill had been submitted. If only a portion of the original service or procedure has been repeated, you would use modifier -52 to indicate a reduced service. When modifier -76 has been used, documentation must accompany the claim in order to establish medical necessity.

-77 Repeat Procedure by Another Physician

Modifier -77 is used to report services or procedures that are repeated and are provided by a physician other than the physician who originally provided the service or procedure. The description of the modifier is as follows:

The physician may need to indicate that a basic procedure or service performed by another physician had to be repeated. This situation may be reported by adding modifier -77 to the repeated procedure/service, or the separate five digit code 09977 may be used.

The modifier is used to indicate to third-party payers that the services are not duplicate services and, therefore, the bill is not a duplicate bill. Sometimes these repeat services are provided on the same day as the original service, and without the use of modifier -77, the third-party payer would assume a duplicate bill had been submitted. If only a portion of the original service or procedure is repeated, you would use modifier -52 to indicate a reduced service. When modifier -77 has been used, documentation must accompany the claim in order to establish medical necessity.

-79 Unrelated Procedure or Service by the Same Physician During the Postoperative Period

Modifier -79 is used to explain that a patient requires surgery for a condition totally unrelated to the condition for which the first operation was performed. The description of the modifier is as follows:

The physician may need to indicate that the performance of a procedure or service during the postoperative period was unrelated to the original procedure. This circumstance may be reported by using the modifier -79 or by using the separate five digit modifier 09979. (For repeat procedures on the same day, see -76.)

For example, the patient may have had an appendectomy and 2 weeks later has a gallbladder episode that necessitates removal of the gallbladder. The modifier -79 would be placed on the cholecystectomy code, indicating that the subsequent procedure was unrelated to the first procedure. The diagnosis codes for the two procedures would also be different, thus substantiating that the two procedures were unrelated.

CAUTION *Do not use modifier -79 with staged procedures (use modifier -58) or with procedures that are related to the original procedure. If the service is provided during the postoperative period of a major surgical procedure, billing separately for services included in the surgical package is fraudulent.*

-90 Reference (Outside) Laboratory

Modifier -90 is used to indicate that services of an outside laboratory were used. The description of the modifier is as follows:

When laboratory procedures are performed by a party other than the treating or reporting physician, the procedure may be identified by adding the modifier -90 to the usual procedure number or by use of the separate five digit modifier code 09990.

This modifier is used with codes in the Pathology and Laboratory section to report that the procedures were performed by someone other than the treating or reporting physician. Medicare does not allow physicians to bill for outside laboratory services and then reimburse the outside laboratory for those services. If the outside laboratory provides the services, the outside laboratory must report the services.

-99 Multiple Modifiers

Modifier -99 is needed only if the third-party payer does not accept the addition of multiple modifiers to a code. This is the case with some computerized insurance submissions. The description of the modifier is as follows:

> Under certain circumstances two or more modifiers may be necessary to completely delineate a service. In such situations modifier -99 should be added to the basic procedure, and other applicable modifiers may be listed as part of the description of the service. Modifier code 09999 may be used as an alternative to modifier -99.

Services that require that more than one modifier be added to the code can be displayed either by the use of the multiple modifiers (19220-22-23) or by the use of modifier -99 (19220-99) and the modifiers listed in item 19 of the HCFA-1500 insurance form. Figure 3–11 illustrates correct placement of the multiple modifiers. Third-party payers vary in terms of how they require multiple modifiers to be reported, so be certain to check with the payer before submitting multiple modifiers.

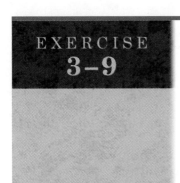

MODIFIERS THAT ADD INFORMATION

EXERCISE 3-9

Fill in the blanks:

1 If Mr. Smith undergoes an appendectomy on June 8, and then a cholecystectomy is performed on August 16, what modifier would be placed on the cholecystectomy code?

Code(s): _____

2 Mrs. Knight has a diagnostic surgical biopsy of deep cervical lymph nodes on May 8, and the pathology report comes back showing malig-

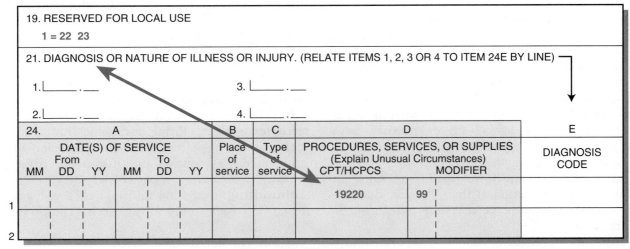

Figure 3–11   Using modifier -99.

nancy. Mrs. Knight elects to have a lymphadenectomy on May 11. What modifier would be used with the lymphadenectomy code?

Code(s): _____

3 What is the modifier that indicates that multiple modifiers apply?

_____

4 What modifier would be added to the laboratory procedure code to indicate testing by an outside laboratory?

_____

5 Dr. Foster admits a patient to a skilled nursing facility because of the patient's advanced dementia, shortly after a herniorrhaphy. What modifier would be added to the admission service?

_____

6 A patient came to the office twice in one day to see the same physician for unrelated problems. What modifier would be added to the second office visit code?

_____

7 What modifier would you add to a code to indicate that a basic procedure performed by another physician was repeated?

_____

8 Workers' compensation referred a patient to a physician for a mandatory examination to determine the legitimacy of a claim. What modifier would be added to the code for the examination service?

_____

CHAPTER GLOSSARY

conscious sedation: a decreased level of consciousness in which the patient is not completely asleep

CRNA: certified registered nurse anesthetist

Demerol: a narcotic analgesic

distinct procedure: one service or procedure that has no relationship to another service or procedure

hypotension: abnormally low blood pressure

hypothermia: low body temperature; sometimes induced during surgical procedures

intraoperative: period of time during which a surgical procedure is being performed

mandated service: a service required by an agency or organization to be performed for a patient; usually the agency or organization pays all or a portion of the patient's medical bills

morphine: a narcotic analgesic

physical status modifiers: modifying units in the Anesthesia section of the CPT that describe a patient's condition at the time anesthesia is administered

postoperative: period of time after a surgical procedure

preoperative: period of time prior to a surgical procedure

professional component: term used in describing radiology services provided by a radiologist

qualifying circumstances: five-digit CPT codes that describe situations or conditions that make the administration of anesthesia more difficult than is normal

Relative Value Guide: comparison of anesthesia services; published by the American Society of Anesthesiologists (ASA)

Swan-Ganz catheter: central venous catheter

technical component: term used in describing radiology services provided by a technician

transfer order: official document that transfers the care of a patient from one physician to another, often required by third-party payers to transfer the care of a patient legally

unbundling: assigning multiple CPT codes when one CPT code would fully describe the service or procedure

Valium: a sedative

CHAPTER REVIEW

CHAPTER 3, PART I, THEORY

Complete the following:

1 Anesthesia time is listed in _____

   and _____ . Units of time are
   determined by the third-party payer.

2 Anesthesia time begins when the anesthesiol-

   ogist _____ ,

   continues _____

   the procedure, and ends when _____

   _____ .

3 According to the Anesthesia Guidelines, what
   is the one modifier that is not used with anesthesia procedures?

   _____

4 "P1" is an example of what type of modifier?

   _____

5 What word means "in a dying state"?

   _____

6 What word means "affecting the body as a

   whole"? _____

7 The letter "P" in combination with what number indicates a brain-dead patient?

   _____

8 What type of circumstance identifies a component of anesthesia service that affects the
   character of the service?

   _____

9 Anesthesia procedures are divided by what
   type of site?

   _____

10 When several physicians, with technicians
   and specialized equipment, work together to
   complete a complicated procedure and each
   physician has a specific portion of the surgery
   to complete, they are termed what?

   _____

11 Is it true that a physician who personally administers the anesthesia to the patient upon
   whom he or she is operating cannot bill the
   third-party payer?

   _____

12 What is the name of the guide that is published by the American Society of Anesthesiologists and provides the weights of various anesthesia services?

   _____

CHAPTER 3, PART II, PRACTICAL

*Using your CPT manual, identify the modifier for
the following descriptions:*

13 Repeat procedure by same physician

   _____

14 Two surgeons _____

15 Professional component _____

16 Multiple modifiers _____

17 Distinct procedural service _____

18 Mandated service _____

19 Prolonged E/M service _____

20 Minimum assistant surgeon _____

21 Repeat procedure by another physician

   _____

22 Unrelated procedure or service by the same
   physician during the postoperative period

   _____

23 Unusual anesthesia _____

24 Return to the operating room for a related
   procedure during the postoperative period

   _____

25 Surgical care only _____

26 Reduced service _____

27 Surgical team _____

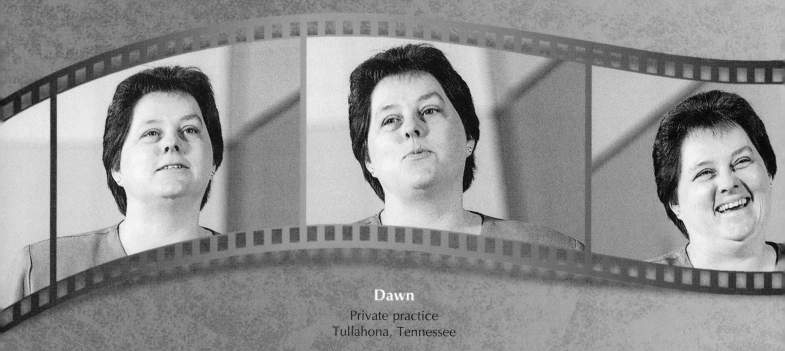

Dawn
Private practice
Tullahona, Tennessee

chapter 4

Introduction to the Surgery Section and Integumentary System

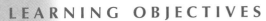

CHAPTER TOPICS

Part I: Introduction to the Surgery Section

Format

Separate Procedures

Starred Procedures

Surgical Package

Part II: General and Integumentary System

Format

Skin, Subcutaneous and Accessory Structures

Repair (Closure)

Burns

Destruction

Breast Procedures

Chapter Glossary

Chapter Review

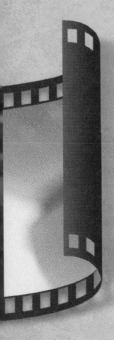

LEARNING OBJECTIVES

After completing this chapter you should be able to

1 Understand the Surgery section and subsection formats.

2 Define Surgery section and subsection terminology.

3 Analyze unique Surgery subsection characteristics.

4 Examine the Integumentary System subsection.

5 Review each Integumentary System subheading and category.

6 Understand the unique terminology in the subsection.

7 Apply coding knowledge to integumentary cases.

PART I: Introduction to the Surgery Section

FORMAT

The Surgery section is the largest in the CPT manual. The codes range from 10021 to 69990. Surgery is divided into 18 subsections. Most Surgery subsections are according to anatomic site (e.g., integumentary or respiratory).

EXERCISE 4-1

THE SECTION FORMAT

To help you become familiar with the format of the Surgery section, write the names of the Surgery subsections on the lines provided in the order in which they are found in the CPT manual.

List the Surgery subsections:

1 _____

2 _____

3 _____

4 _____

5 _____

6 _____

7 _____

8 _____

9 _____

10 _____

11 _____

12 _____

13 _____

14 _____

15 _____

16 _____

17 _____

18 _____

Within the Surgery section, some of the more complex subsections are the Integumentary, Musculoskeletal, Respiratory, Cardiovascular, Digestive, and Female Genital subsections. These subsections have extensive notes, and each is covered in this text. Before we get into the details of the subsections, let's look at the general information that is pertinent to the entire Surgery section.

Notes and Guidelines

Guidelines are found at the beginning of each of the CPT sections. The section Guidelines define terms that are necessary for appropriately interpreting and reporting the procedures and services contained in that section. For example, the Surgery Guidelines contain the following information:

- *Physicians' Services:* when to use an E/M code with surgery codes
- *Surgical Package Definitions:* what is included in a procedure
- *Follow-up Care for Diagnostic Procedures:* how to list services when procedures such as an endoscopy are performed
- *Follow-up Care for Therapeutic Surgical Procedures:* what is included in therapeutic services
- *Materials Supplied by Physician:* when code 99070 is used
- *Reporting More Than One Procedure/Service:* identifies situations in which it may be appropriate to use modifiers
- *Add-on Codes:* what an add-on code is and how it is used
- *Separate Procedure:* how to use codes with this designation
- *Subsection Information:* lists subsections that have instructional notes
- *Unlisted Service or Procedure:* all unlisted service codes from the Surgery section
- *Special Reports:* what to include in and when to submit a special report
- *Starred Procedures or Items:* what a star next to a code means and how to use starred codes
- *Surgical Destruction:* when destruction is part of a surgery

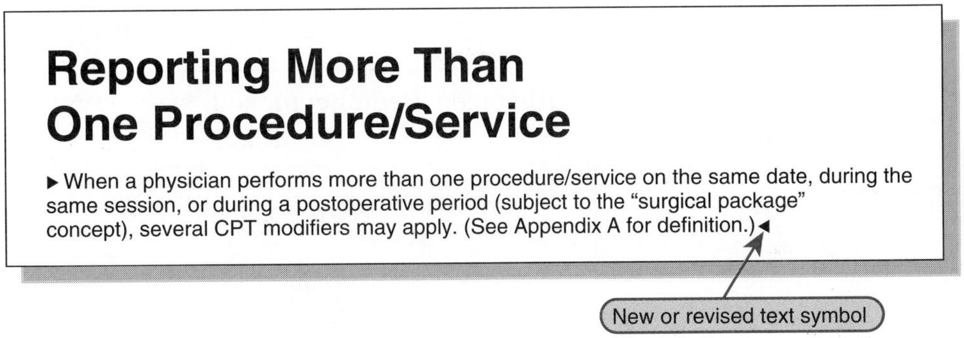

Reporting More Than One Procedure/Service

▶ When a physician performs more than one procedure/service on the same date, during the same session, or during a postoperative period (subject to the "surgical package" concept), several CPT modifiers may apply. (See Appendix A for definition.) ◀

New or revised text symbol

Figure 4–1   New or revised text symbol.

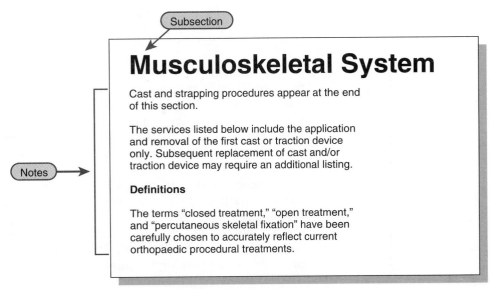

Subsection

Musculoskeletal System

Cast and strapping procedures appear at the end of this section.

The services listed below include the application and removal of the first cast or traction device only. Subsequent replacement of cast and/or traction device may require an additional listing.

Notes

Definitions

The terms "closed treatment," "open treatment," and "percutaneous skeletal fixation" have been carefully chosen to accurately reflect current orthopaedic procedural treatments.

Figure 4–2   Subsection notes.

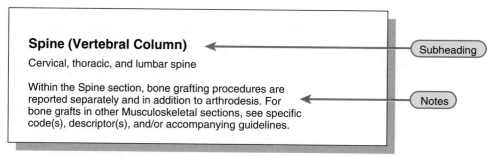

Figure 4–3   Subheading notes.

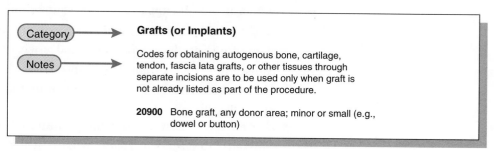

Figure 4–4   Category notes.

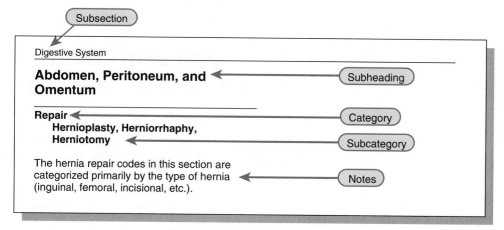

Figure 4–5   Subcategory notes.

The Guidelines contain information that you will need to know in order to correctly code in the section, and most of the information is not repeated elsewhere in the section. So always review the Guidelines before coding in the section. Remember that with each new edition of the CPT manual, you will need to review the Guidelines for any changes. The changes are indicated by the "New or Revised Text" symbols used throughout the CPT manual (Fig. 4–1).

Common throughout the CPT manual are notes. Notes may appear before subsections (Fig. 4–2), subheadings (Fig. 4–3), categories (Fig. 4–4), and subcategories (Fig. 4–5). The information in the notes indicates the special instructions unique to particular codes or unique to particular groups of codes. The notes are extremely important because the information contained in them is not usually available in the Guidelines of the CPT manual. Always make it a practice to read any notes available before coding. If notes are present, they must be followed if the coding is to be accurate.

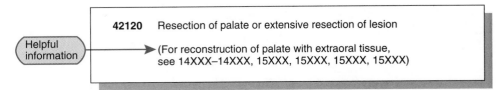

Figure 4–6 Additional helpful information.

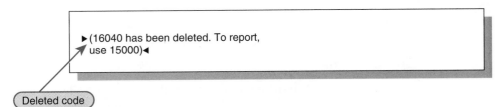

Figure 4–7 Deleted codes.

STOP *Additional information is enclosed in parentheses. Called parenthetical phrases, they sometimes follow the code or group of codes, and they provide further information about codes that may be applicable. For example, 42120, for the resection of the palate or extensive resection of a lesion, is followed by information about the codes you would use if reconstruction of the palate followed the resection (Fig. 4–6). Deleted codes are also indicated in the CPT manual, enclosed in parentheses. Often the code that is to be used in place of the deleted code will be listed (Fig. 4–7). Also note in Figure 4–7 that the arrows at the beginning and end of the information indicate that the information is new or has been revised for the current edition.*

Unlisted Procedures

The Surgery Guidelines contain many unlisted procedure codes, presented by anatomic site. These unlisted codes are presented in alphabetical order by their location in the Surgery section and in the subsections by body system. For example, the unlisted procedure code for procedures of the forearm or wrist, 25999, is located at the end of the subheading Forearm and Wrist. The unlisted codes are used to identify procedures or services throughout the Surgery section for which there is no CPT code. If a Category III code is available for the unlisted service you are reporting, you must use the Category III code, not the unlisted Category I code.

EXERCISE
4–2

UNLISTED PROCEDURES

Using the CPT manual, locate the unlisted procedure codes in the Surgical Guidelines, and identify the unlisted procedure codes for the following anatomic areas:

1 Musculoskeletal system

Code(s): _____

2 Inner ear

Code(s): _____

3 Skin, mucous membranes, and subcutaneous tissue

Code(s): _____

4 Leg or ankle

Code(s): _____

5 Nervous system

Code(s): _____

6 Eyelids

Code(s): _____

Special Reports

When using an unlisted procedure code for surgery, a special report describing the procedure must accompany the claim. According to the CPT manual, "Pertinent information [in the special report] should include an adequate definition or description of the nature, extent, and need for the procedure, and the time, effort, and equipment necessary to provide the service." Unlisted codes are used only after thorough research fails to reveal an existing code.

SEPARATE PROCEDURES

Some procedure codes will have the words "separate procedure" after the descriptor. This term, "separate procedure," does not mean that the procedure was the only procedure that was performed; rather, it is an indication of how the code can be used. Locate code 19100 in the CPT manual. The breast biopsy code 19100 has the words "separate procedure" after the description. Procedures followed by the words "separate procedure" (in parentheses) are minor procedures that are coded only when they are the only services performed or when a procedure is performed on a body area different from the area at which another procedure was performed during the same operative session. When the same minor procedure is performed in conjunction with a related major procedure, the minor procedure is considered incidental and is bundled into the code with the major procedure.

EXAMPLE

Separate procedure bundled into the major procedure: Breast biopsy (19100) has "separate procedure" after it. If a breast biopsy was performed in conjunction with a modified radical mastectomy (19240), only the mastectomy would be coded. Because the breast biopsy and the mastectomy were conducted on the same body area, the breast biopsy would be considered a minor procedure that was incidental and would be bundled into the major procedure of the mastectomy.

from the trenches

"The ultimate goal is to help the patients. They're getting treated because they are sick . . . they don't want to have to worry about the bill and whether it will get paid."

DAWN

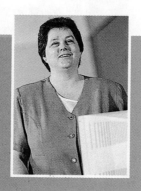

EXAMPLE

> *Two separate procedures:* If a breast biopsy (19100—separate procedure) was performed in conjunction with an esophagoscopy (43200), both the breast biopsy and esophagoscopy would be coded. Because the breast biopsy and the esophagoscopy were conducted on different body areas, the breast biopsy is considered a separate procedure, not a minor procedure incidental to a major procedure.

EXAMPLE

> *Separate procedure bundled into the major procedure.* Salpingo-oophorectomy (58720—removal of tubes and ovaries) has "separate procedure" after it. If a salpingo-oophorectomy was performed in conjunction with an abdominal hysterectomy (58150), only the hysterectomy would be coded. Because the salpingo-oophorectomy and the abdominal hysterectomy were conducted on the same body area, the salpingo-oophorectomy would be considered a minor procedure that was incidental and would be bundled into the major procedure of the hysterectomy.

EXAMPLE

> *Two separate procedures:* If a salpingo-oophorectomy (58720—separate procedure) was performed in conjunction with an esophagoscopy (43200), both the salpingo-oophorectomy and the esophagoscopy would be coded. Because the salpingo-oophorectomy and the esophagoscopy were conducted on different body areas, the salpingo-oophorectomy is considered a separate procedure, not a minor procedure incidental to a major procedure.

STARRED PROCEDURES

The CPT manual includes many procedures that are considered minor surgical procedures requiring varying amounts of preoperative or postoperative services or both.

Figure 4–8 illustrates a CPT code with a star after the code, which indicates the code is subject to the starred procedure guideline. If the 10080 procedure (incision and drainage of pilonidal cyst; simple) was done at the time of the initial visit of a new patient, the procedure would be coded 10080 along with code 99025 (initial new patient visit when a starred surgical procedure constitutes the major service). If the visit was for evaluation of a condition other than the pilonidal cyst, the appropriate visit code, 99201–99215, would be reported, with the addition of modifier -25 (significant, separate identifiable E/M service by the same physician on the same day as the procedure), to the procedure code.

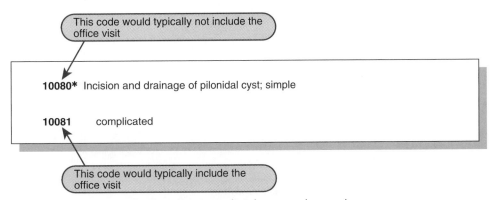

Figure 4–8   Starred and unstarred procedures.

SURGICAL PACKAGE

Often, the time, effort, and services rendered when accomplishing a procedure are bundled together to form a surgical package. Payment is made for a package of services and not for each individual service provided within the package. The CPT manual describes the surgical package as including the operation itself, local anesthesia, and "typical follow-up care, one related E/M encounter prior to the procedure, and written orders." Local anesthesia is defined as local infiltration, metacarpal/digital block, or topical anesthesia. The CPT manual further states that follow-up care for complications, exacerbations, recurrence, and the presence of other diseases that require additional services is not included in the surgical package. General anesthesia for surgical procedures is not part of the surgical package; general anesthesia services are billed separately by the anesthesiologist.

Third-party payers have varying definitions of what constitutes a surgical package and varying policies about what is to be included in the surgical package. Surgical packages also define the services for which you can or cannot submit additional charges because the rules of the surgical package define what is and is not included with the surgical procedure. Included in the definition of the surgical package are routine preoperative and postoperative care—including usual complications—up to a predefined number of days before and after the surgery. For example, in the case of a Medicare patient, the treatment of all complications is bundled into the package—with the exception of complications that require surgery. The period of time following each surgery that is included in the surgery package is established by the third-party payer and is referred to as the **global (postoperative) surgery** period. The global surgery period is usually 90 days for major surgery and 10 days for minor surgery.

Figure 4–9 shows CPT codes 10080 and 10081 for incision and drainage of a cyst. Code 10080 is starred and has no surgical package, so you would usually charge for any additional services that were provided after the initial incision and drainage. But CPT code 10081 would include routine follow-up care and services (such as removal of sutures) at no charge because these services are considered part of the surgical package.

One last item that you have to know about before you begin to code surgical procedures with and without surgical packages is the materials and supply codes.

When **materials or supplies** over and above those usually used in an office visit have been used, you code and charge for these materials and supplies in addition to charging for the office visit. For example, when a physician does a wound repair during an office visit and uses a surgical

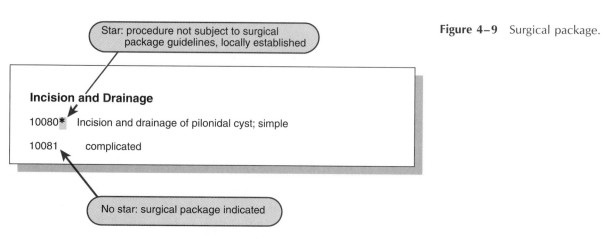

Star: procedure not subject to surgical package guidelines, locally established

Incision and Drainage

10080*   Incision and drainage of pilonidal cyst; simple

10081   complicated

No star: surgical package indicated

Figure 4–9   Surgical package.

tray, the surgical tray is identified by CPT code 99070. Code 99070 is listed in the Medicare section, Special Services, Procedures, and Reports subsection, Miscellaneous subheading.

coding shot

HCPCS code A4550 is also used to report the use of a surgical tray. Third-party payers who pay separately for a surgical tray usually want the HCPCS A code to be used to report the tray. Many third-party payers do not pay separately for a surgical tray. For example, Medicare does not pay separately for a surgical tray.

There are five major guidelines relating to the surgical package located in the Surgery section.

1. Unstarred surgical procedures usually include the preoperative service, the procedure, and the postoperative service.

EXAMPLE

An established patient, Mary Smith, is referred to a surgeon for excessive bleeding. The surgeon decides a hysterectomy is necessary and schedules the surgical procedure for 2 weeks later. The surgeon plans to recheck Mary in the office the day before surgery. The initial visit, at which the decision was made to perform surgery, is billable, but the follow-up visit on the day before surgery is bundled into the surgical package.

2. If the surgical procedure is starred, preoperative and postoperative services are variable and are usually billed separately.

EXAMPLE

Jane, an established patient with a history of breast cysts (fibrocystic breasts) comes into the office because of a breast lump found during self-examination. On the basis of her past history, Dr. Green performs a needle biopsy (19100*) in the office surgical suite, and the specimen is sent to the lab for analysis. The results are benign. The office visit for an established patient (99214) and the needle biopsy (19100*) are billed separately. The breast biopsy was the major service provided during the office visit and therefore would be billed. The office visit would be listed with modifier -25, Significant, Separately Identifiable E/M Service by the Same Physician on the Same Day of the Procedure or Other Service, to indicate that both the office visit and the procedure were provided on the same day. The billing for Jane would be

99214-25	Office visit, established patient	$xx.xx
19100	Needle biopsy, right breast	$xx.xx
99070	Surgical tray	$xx.xx

3. When a surgical procedure is starred, services for preoperative and postoperative care, in addition to complications, are added on a service-by-service basis. When the procedure is not starred, preoperative and postoperative care and care of the usual complications are often included in the surgical package. Have you noticed how the words "usual" and "usually" keep appearing in the sentences about surgical packages? That is because third-party payers vary greatly in terms of what is and is not included in each surgical package for each code.

When a procedure is starred, the preoperative services are considered to be one of the following:

a. The starred procedure is carried out at the time of the initial visit of a **new patient** and the starred procedure is the **major service** provided during the visit. Instead of the E/M code for an office visit for a new patient, the Medicine code 99025 is used in addition to the procedure code. The description for 99025 is "Initial (new patient) visit when starred (*) surgical procedure constitutes major service at that visit." Note that the phrase "new patient" is specified for use of code 99025; therefore, the code cannot be used with an established patient service.

EXAMPLE

Sally, a new patient, sees the physician during an office visit and undergoes a breast biopsy of the right breast. The coding would be

19100	Needle biopsy, right breast (starred procedure)	$xx.xx
99025	New patient, office visit	No Charge
99070	Surgical tray	$xx.xx

b. The starred procedure is carried out at the time of the visit for a **new or established patient,** and the starred procedure is a **significant service** for the office visit. The office visit, procedure, and any follow-up care are billed separately.

EXAMPLE

Deb, a 42-year-old established patient, sees her physician for a physical. During the examination, the physician notes a mass in the right breast and does a needle biopsy. Deb returns for a follow-up visit a week later. The billing would be

99396	Routine physical examination	$xx.xx
19100	Needle biopsy, right breast (starred procedure)	$xx.xx
99070	Surgical tray	$xx.xx
99213	Subsequent office visit, established	$xx.xx

c. The starred procedure is carried out at the time of the follow-up visit of an **established patient** and the starred procedure is the **major service.** Therefore, only the procedure is coded. No E/M code is assigned.

EXAMPLE

| 19100 | Needle biopsy, right breast (starred procedure) | $xx.xx |
| 99070 | Surgical tray | $xx.xx |

d. When the starred procedure requires hospitalization, the hospital visit(s), procedure, and follow-up are billed.

EXAMPLE

Adele (new patient) is admitted to the hospital for a biopsy of a breast lump in the left breast immediately after an office visit with Dr. Green. Dr. Green does a comprehensive history and examination, and the medical decision-making complexity is at a moderate level. Adele is taken into surgery, Dr. Green does a needle biopsy, and the pathology report is negative. No further procedure needs to be done. Adele remains overnight in the observation unit at the hospital because she is experiencing severe nausea and vomiting due to the administration of anesthesia. By morning, her condition has improved, and after Dr. Green talks with her, the decision is made that she is well enough to be released. She returns to Dr. Green's office a week later for a follow-up visit. The billing would be

99219	Initial observation care	$xx.xx
19100	Breast biopsy, left breast (starred procedure)	$xx.xx
99217	Discharge service	$xx.xx
99213	Office visit, established patient	$xx.xx

4. For starred procedures, preoperative services are added on a service-by-service basis.

5. Complications are added on a service-by-service basis.

Even though the routine follow-up care is not billed for, the service is still coded to indicate that the service was provided. The CPT code 99024 (Postoperative follow-up visit, included in global service) alerts the third-party payer that the services were rendered to the patient but were included in a surgical package and not charged.

EXAMPLE

A patient undergoes a wound repair that is coded 12014 (unstarred code) and shortly afterward sees the physician for routine follow-up care. The fee statement for the office visit at which the routine follow-up care is provided would be

| 99024 | Postoperative follow-up visit | No charge |

But if a patient undergoes the repair of a 7.9-cm wound that is coded 12004 (starred code) and sees the physician a few days later for routine follow-up care, the service is coded and charged for.

12004	Wound repair, 7.9 cm	$xx.xx
99070	Surgical tray	$xx.xx
99212	Office visit	$xx.xx

The code 99025 is used to identify a patient visit when a surgical procedure is the major service of the visit.

EXAMPLE

If a new patient visits the physician for the simple repair of a scalp wound (2.4 cm) coded 12001 (starred code), only the wound repair is charged for.

99025	Office visit, new patient	No charge
12001	Wound repair, 2.4 cm	$xx.xx
99070	Surgical tray	$xx.xx

Inclusion or exclusion of a procedure in the CPT manual does not imply any health insurance coverage or reimbursement policy. Although the CPT manual includes guidelines on usage, third-party payers may interpret and accept the use of CPT codes and the guidelines in any manner they choose.

EXERCISE 4-3

SURGICAL PACKAGE

Answer the following:

1 What are the three things bundled into a surgical package?

a. _____

b. _____

c. _____

2 Is general anesthesia included in the surgical package? _____

3 Do all third-party payers follow the same reimbursement guidelines for the global packages? _____

PART II: General and Integumentary System

The subsection General contains codes for fine needle aspirations, excluding bone marrow aspirations (see code 38220). The codes are divided based on whether imaging guidance was used during the aspiration.

The Integumentary System subsection of the Surgery section includes codes used by many different physician specialties. There is no restriction on who uses the codes from this or any other subsection. You may find a family practitioner using the incision and drainage, debridement, or repair codes; a dermatologist using excision and destruction codes; a plastic surgeon using skin graft codes; or a surgeon using breast procedure codes.

You will learn about the Integumentary System subsection by first reviewing the subsection format and then learning about coding the services and procedures in the subsection.

FORMAT

The subsection is formatted on the basis of anatomic site and category of procedure. For example, an anatomic site is "neck" and a category of procedure is "repair."

The subsection Integumentary contains the subheadings Skin, Subcutaneous and Accessory Structures; Nails; Repair; Destruction; and Breast. Each subheading is further divided by category. For example, the subheading Skin, Subcutaneous and Accessory Structures is divided into the following categories:

from the trenches

"It's important to educate the physicians . . . let them know they need to document everything."

DAWN

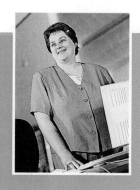

- Incision and Drainage
- Excision—Debridement
- Paring or Cutting
- Biopsy
- Removal of Skin Tags
- Shaving of Epidermal or Dermal Lesions
- Excision—Benign Lesions
- Excision—Malignant Lesions

SKIN, SUBCUTANEOUS AND ACCESSORY STRUCTURES

Incision and Drainage

Incision and Drainage (I&D) codes are divided according to the type of I&D being done. Acne surgery, abscess, carbuncle, boil, cyst, hematoma, and wound infection are just some of the conditions for which a physician uses I&D. The physician opens the lesion, cutting into it to allow drainage. Also included under this heading is a puncture aspiration code, which describes inserting a needle into a lesion and withdrawing the fluid (aspiration). Whichever method is used—incision or aspiration—the contents of the lesion are drained. Packing material may be inserted into the opening or the wound may be left to drain freely. A tube or strip of gauze, which acts as a wick, may be inserted into the wound to facilitate drainage.

The I&D codes are first divided according to the condition and then according to whether the procedure was simple or complicated/multiple. The medical record would indicate the number and complexity of the I&D.

Excision—Debridement

Codes in this category describe services of debridement based on depth, body surface, and condition. **Debridement** is the cleaning of an area or wound. The first debridement codes (11000 and 11001) are used for eczematous debridement. **Eczema** is a skin condition that blisters and weeps. The dead tissue may have to be cut away with a scalpel or scissors or, in less severe cases, washed with saline solution. Code 11000 is used to report debridement of 10% of the body surface or less, and add-on code 11001 is used to report each additional 10%.

Debridement cleans surface areas and removes necrotic tissue. Some codes in this category are based on the extent of the cleansing—skin, subcutaneous tissue, muscle fascia, muscle, or bone.

coding shot

You may report a debridement as a separate service when the medical record indicates that a greater than usual debridement was provided. For example, if an extensive debridement was done when usually a simple debridement would be done, you would report the additional service using a debridement code from the 11040–11044 range.

Introduction to Lesions

Before you learn about coding the various methods of lesion destruction and excision, you need to review a few rules that apply broadly to this commonly performed procedure. After you have learned the general lesion information, you will review each of the destruction and excision methods individually.

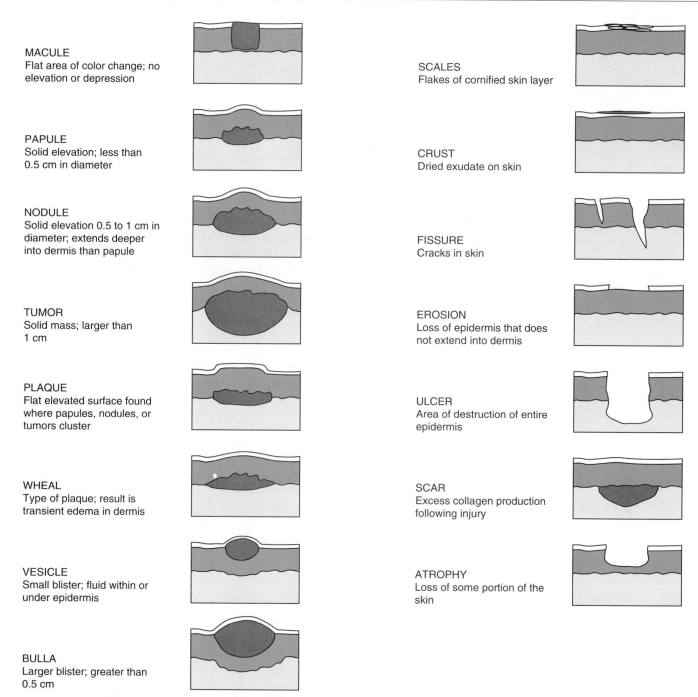

MACULE
Flat area of color change; no elevation or depression

PAPULE
Solid elevation; less than 0.5 cm in diameter

NODULE
Solid elevation 0.5 to 1 cm in diameter; extends deeper into dermis than papule

TUMOR
Solid mass; larger than 1 cm

PLAQUE
Flat elevated surface found where papules, nodules, or tumors cluster

WHEAL
Type of plaque; result is transient edema in dermis

VESICLE
Small blister; fluid within or under epidermis

BULLA
Larger blister; greater than 0.5 cm

SCALES
Flakes of cornified skin layer

CRUST
Dried exudate on skin

FISSURE
Cracks in skin

EROSION
Loss of epidermis that does not extend into dermis

ULCER
Area of destruction of entire epidermis

SCAR
Excess collagen production following injury

ATROPHY
Loss of some portion of the skin

Figure 4–10   Lesions of the skin.

Lesion Excision and Destruction

There are many types of lesions of the skin (Fig. 4–10) and many types of treatment for lesions. Types of treatment include paring, shaving, excision, and destruction. To code these procedures properly, you must know the **site, number,** and **size** of the lesion(s), as well as whether the lesion is malignant or benign.

A pathology report includes margins (extra skin) taken from around the lesion, so the stated size is inaccurate for the purpose of coding. Also, the preserving fluids in which the specimen is placed for processing may shrink the tissue sample. Thus, the pathology report is used to identify the size of the lesion only if no other record of the size can be documented.

coding shot

The size of the lesion should be taken from the physician's notes, not the pathology report.

The malignant lesion codes (11600–11646) are the same whether the lesion is malignant melanoma or basal cell carcinoma. The codes reflect only the size of the lesion. All lesions that are excised will have a pathology report for diagnosing the removed tissue as malignant or benign; and since the codes are divided based on whether the excised lesion is malignant or benign, the billing for the excision is not submitted to the third-party payer until the pathology report has been completed.

CAUTION *Destruction of lesions destroys all tissue, leaving none available for biopsy; therefore, there will be no pathology report for lesions that have been destroyed by laser, chemicals, electrocautery, or other methods. In these cases you will have to take the type and size of the destroyed lesion from the medical record.*

Codes in the Integumentary System subsection differ greatly in their descriptions. Some codes indicate only one lesion per code, others are for the second and third lesions only, and still others indicate a certain number of lesions (e.g., up to 15 lesions). When coding multiple lesions, you must read the description carefully to prevent incorrect coding.

If multiple lesions are treated, code the most complex lesion procedure first and the others using modifier -51 to indicate that multiple procedures were performed. Remember that the third-party payer will usually reduce the payment for the services identified with modifier -51; so you want to be certain that you place the service with the highest dollar cost first, without the modifier. If the code description includes multiple lesions (a stated number of lesions), the -51 is not necessary.

Closure of Excision Sites

Included in the codes for lesion excision is the direct, primary, or simple closure of the operative site. The notes following the category for the exci-

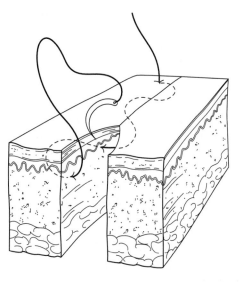

Figure 4–11   Simple subcuticular closure.

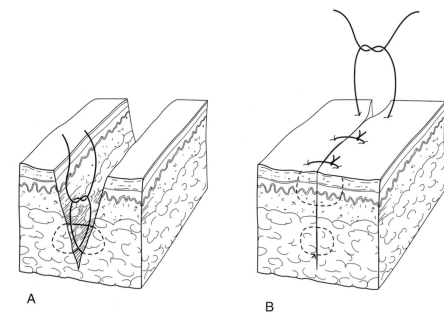

Figure 4–12 *A* and *B*, Intermediate two-layer closure.

sion of a benign lesion define a simple excision as being full thickness (through the dermis) and a simple closure as one that is nonlayered (Fig. 4–11). Closures can also be intermediate (layered; Fig. 4–12) or complex (greater than layered). The codes in the Excision—Benign Lesions category are based on the size and location of the lesion excised. The local anesthesia is also included in the excision codes. Any closure other than a simple closure can be billed separately.

There are several codes at the end of the category (11450–11471) for excision of the skin and subcutaneous tissue in cases of hidradenitis, which is the chronic abscessing and subsequent infection of a sweat gland. The abscess is excised and the wound left open to heal. The hidradenitis codes are based on the abscess location (axillary, inguinal, perianal, perineal, or umbilical) and the complexity of the repair (simple, intermediate, or complex).

Three final notes on treatment of lesions:

1. The shaving of lesions requires no closure because no incision has been made.

2. Excision includes simple closure but may require more complex closure. If more complex closure is required, follow the notes in the CPT manual to appropriately code for these services.

3. Destruction may be by any method, including freezing, burning, chemicals, and so on.

Paring

Paring codes are used to report the services provided when a physician removes a benign hyperkeratotic skin lesion such as a callus or corn. Paring codes include removal by peeling or scraping. A small ring-shaped instrument (curette), blade, or similar sharp instrument is used for paring. Bleeding is usually controlled by a chemical that is applied to the surface after removal of the lesion. The codes are divided based on the number of lesions removed.

STOP *The codes 11100–11646 that you will now review include the biopsy, removal, shaving, and excision of lesions and, with the exception of the*

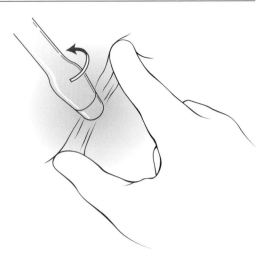

Figure 4–13   Punch biopsy.

removal codes (11200–11201), are intended to be used to report lesion removal by a sharp instrument, not by electrosurgical destruction of tissue. Lesion removal by electrosurgical destruction is coded by using codes from the 17000–17286 range, which you will soon learn about.

Biopsy

Biopsy of the skin includes subcutaneous tissue and mucous membranes. The tissue removed during the biopsy is being removed for microscopic study. Not all of the lesion is removed. If all of the lesion is removed, the service is an excision. In a biopsy, only a portion of the lesion and some of the surrounding tissue is removed. The section of surrounding tissue is included so the pathologist can compare the normal tissue to the lesion tissue and note differences.

> *coding shot*
>
> Included in the Biopsy codes are the codes that are to be used for biopsies of mucous membranes. A mucous membrane is the kind of tissue that covers a variety of body parts, such as the tongue and the nasal cavities.

Many methods are used to obtain biopsies; the method chosen is determined by the size and type of the lesion and the physician's preference. Common biopsy methods are scraping, cutting, and the punch. A punch biopsy is illustrated in Figure 4–13; it is used to excise a disk of tissue. A punch can also be used in the excision of the entire lesion, so just because the medical record refers to the use of a punch, it does not necessarily mean that only a biopsy was done.

Biopsy sites do not necessarily have to be closed; some are so small that they will close readily by themselves. Other sites are large enough that closure is required, and simple closure is included in the biopsy codes. If closure of the biopsy site was more than a simple closure, you would code separately for the more extensive closure. You will learn more about closure later in this chapter.

On the HCFA-1500 claim form, report the number of lesions treated in column 24G, Days or Units.

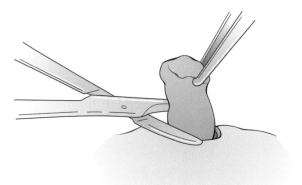

Figure 4–14   Scissors removal.

CAUTION *Do not use modifier -51 with these biopsy codes, as 11100 is used to report a single lesion, and 11101 is used to report two or more lesions. The correct coding for three lesions would be to use 11100 for lesion number one and 11101 × 2 for lesions two and three.*

Skin Tags

Skin tags are flaps of skin (benign lesions) that can appear anywhere, but most often appear on the neck or trunk, especially in older people. Skin tags are removed in a variety of ways—scissors, blades, ligatures, electrosurgery, or chemicals. **Scissors removal** is illustrated in Figure 4–14. Scissoring is often used for tissue column lesions. The forceps grasps the column, and the physician snips the lesion off at its base. Closure is achieved by using sutures. In **ligature strangulation,** a thread is tied at the base of the lesion and left there until the tissue dies. The lesion then drops off. Whatever method of removal is used, simple closure is included in the skin tag codes, as is any anesthesia that is used. Also, note that the codes are based on the first 15 lesions and then on each additional 10 lesions after the first 15.

On the HCFA-1500 claim form, report the number of lesions treated in 24G, Days or Units (Fig. 4–15).

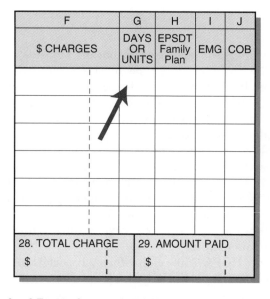

Figure 4–15   Units column (G) of the HCFA-1500. (Courtesy of U.S. Department of Health and Human Services, Centers for Medicare and Medicaid Services.)

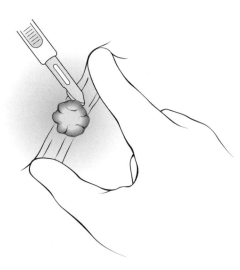

Figure 4–16 Shaving of a lesion.

CAUTION *Do not use modifier -51 (multiple procedure) with skin tag codes, as the codes are based on the number of lesions removed.*

Shaving of Lesions

The **shaving** of a lesion can be performed by using a scalpel blade or other sharp instrument. The shaving of a lesion is illustrated in Figure 4–16. The blade is held horizontal to the skin and an epidermal or dermal lesion is sliced off. Cauterization (electrocautery or chemical cautery) to control bleeding and anesthesia are included in the lesion-shaving codes.

Electrocautery is sometimes used to finish the edges of the shaving, but if electrocautery is the main method by which the lesion was removed, you would use codes from the Destruction, Benign or Premalignant Lesions category (17000–17250), not from the Shaving category.

The Shaving codes are further defined according to the location of the lesion—trunk, neck, nose—and the size of the lesion. If more than one lesion was removed, you would add modifier -51 (multiple procedures) to any codes after the first code. For example, if one 2.0-cm lesion was removed from the trunk, and a 1.0-cm lesion was removed from the hand, you list the 2.0-cm lesion first and the 1.0-cm lesion second, with modifier -51 added. Many third-party payers reimburse 100% for the first lesion and 50% for the second lesion, so by placing the more expensive procedure first, you optimize the amount of the reimbursement.

Excision of Benign Lesions

The CPT divides the category of excision of lesions on the basis of whether a lesion is benign or malignant. Although at the time of excision it is not known for certain whether the lesion is benign or malignant, the physician makes an assessment of the lesion's status and usually plans the extent of the excision based on that assessment. The codes in the Excision—Benign Lesions category are used for all benign lesions *except* skin tags, which you learned about earlier.

The codes include local anesthesia, so do not code for local anesthesia separately, as that would be unbundling. The excision codes also include simple closure (see Fig. 4–11) of the excision site. If the closure is noted in the medical record as being more than simple (intermediate or complex) you would code the more complicated closure using a separate code from Repair subheading (12001–13160).

In the material about the shaving category, you were instructed not to use the shaving codes if the shaving had penetrated through the dermis (full thickness). Full-thickness shavings are to be coded using the excision codes found in the Excision—Benign Lesions or Excision—Malignant Lesions categories.

> *coding shot*
>
> For unusual or complicated excisions, you will use a code from the Musculoskeletal section.

The codes in the Excision—Benign Lesions category are based on the location of the excision (e.g., trunk, scalp, ears, etc.) and the size of the lesion (e.g., 0.6–1.0 cm, 1.1–2.0 cm).

Excision of Malignant Lesions

Codes in the Excision— Malignant Lesions subheading are used for malignant lesions and include local anesthesia and simple closure. As with the benign lesion codes, these codes refer to *each* lesion removed and are divided according to the lesion's location and size. If you are coding a lesion removal that has been performed by a method other than excision (e.g., electrosurgery), the notes preceding the excision codes direct you to the Destruction codes (17000–17999). If the closure is more than simple you would also use a repair code.

> *coding shot*
>
> If the excision is of a malignant lesion on the eyelid, and the excision involves more than the skin of the eyelid (lid margin, tarsus, or conjunctiva), do *not* use malignant lesion excision codes. Instead, you would use a surgery code from the subsection Eye and Ocular Adnexa, Excision category (67800–67850).

NAILS

Within the category Nails are codes for the trimming of fingernails and toenails, debridement of nails, removal of nails, drainage of hematomas, biopsies of nails, repair of nails, reconstruction of nails, and excision of cysts of the nails. **Podiatrists** are physicians who specialize in the care of the foot; as such, these physicians use this category of codes extensively. However, all physicians can and do use these codes when providing nail care services to both the feet and the hands.

The first code in the Nails category is 11719, used for the trimming of nails that are not defective. This is a minimal service and the code covers trimming one fingernail/toenail or many fingernails/toenails. Debridement (11720) is a more complex service—the manual cleaning of up to five nails—and it includes the use of various tools, cleaning materials/solutions, and files. You would not charge separately for the supplies used for a nail debridement service, as these supplies are included in the codes. The two debridement codes are divided according to the number of nails attended to during the service.

Avulsion is the separation and removal of the nail plate, leaving the root so the nail will grow back. An anesthetic is administered, the nail lifted away from the nail bed, and a portion or all of the nail plate is removed.

Place the number of nails treated in the units column (G) of the HCFA-1500.

coding shot

Do not use modifier -51 (multiple procedures) with nail removal codes, as there are two codes available: one for a single nail and one for each additional nail. Often, third-party payers require the use of HCPCS modifiers (F1-FA to indicate the finger and T1-TA to indicate the toe [Fig. 4–17]; and the separate reporting of each digit treated.

A subungual hematoma (blood trapped under the nail) is evacuated by puncturing the nail with an electrocautery needle. The trapped blood and fluid are drained by applying pressure to the top of the nail.

Onychocryptosis (ingrown toenail) is the most common condition of the great toe. The nail grows down and into the soft tissue of the nail fold, causing extreme pain and often infection. Treatment for severe cases is a partial onychectomy (removal of the nail plate and root). The toe is anesthetized and a portion of the nail plate and root is removed. The nail will not grow back where the base has been removed.

coding shot

Code 11755 is used for any number of nail biopsies performed during one session, and no modifier is needed if several biopsies have been done. For example, if biopsies of three nails were performed in one session, you would report 11755 for the service and in 24G, Days or Units on the HCFA-1500, you enter the number of nails biopsied—three.

There is one group of codes in the Nails category that you would not expect—the codes for the excision of a pilonidal cyst or sinus (11770–11772). A pilonidal cyst is located in the sacral area and is most often caused by an ingrown hair. The codes are divided according to the complexity of the excision—simple, extensive, or complicated. For a simple cyst, the

Figure 4–17 HCPCS modifiers used to indicate digits of hands and feet.

F1	Left hand, second digit	T1	Left foot, second digit
F2	Left hand, third digit	T2	Left foot, third digit
F3	Left hand, fourth digit	T3	Left foot, fourth digit
F4	Left hand, fifth digit	T4	Left foot, fifth digit
F5	Right hand, thumb	T5	Right foot, great toe
F6	Right hand, second digit	T6	Right foot, second digit
F7	Right hand, third digit	T7	Right foot, third digit
F8	Right hand, fourth digit	T8	Right foot, fourth digit
F9	Right hand, fifth digit	T9	Right foot, fifth digit
FA	Left hand, thumb	TA	Left foot, great toe

physician would excise the cyst and suture the skin together. A cyst larger than 2 cm is considered complicated and requires more extensive excision and closure. A complicated excision is very extensive and requires reconstructive repair.

Introduction

Within the Introduction category of codes you will find lesion injection, tattooing, tissue expansion, contraceptive capsule insertion/removal, and hormone implantation services. Lesions are injected with medication to treat conditions such as acne, keloids (scar tissue), and psoriasis. Lesion injection codes are divided according to the number of lesions injected (1–7 or 8+).

STOP *Lesion injection code 11901 is not an add-on code! You use 11900 to report lesion injections numbering one through seven, and you use 11901 to report injections eight and above. For example, if seven lesions are injected in one patient, the service is reported using 11900. If eight lesions are injected in another patient, the service is reported using 11901. The number of lesions injected is reported in the units column (G) of the HCFA-1500.*

Tattooing codes are also located in the Introduction category. Tattooing is coded on the basis of square centimeters covered. Sometimes physicians use tattooing as a way to disguise birthmarks or scars.

Codes for subcutaneous injection of filling material are located in the Introduction category and are used for services such as collagen or silicone injections (injectable dermal implants), which are used as a wrinkle treatment. The codes are based on the amount of material injected. The procedure is usually repeated at 2- to 3-week intervals until the results are those desired.

Tissue-expander codes are also located in the Introduction category. A tissue expander is an elastic material formed into a sac that is then filled with fluid or air so it expands like a balloon. The expander is placed under the skin and then it is filled, stretching the skin. Expanders are most often used to prepare a site for a permanent implant. Expanders are also used to assist in the repair of scars and the removal of tattoos by stretching the skin, removing the expander, removing the scar or tattoo, and suturing the skin edges together. The codes are divided according to whether the service is an insertion, a removal, or an expander removal with replacement of a prosthesis.

CAUTION *Do not use an expander code from the Introduction category after a mastectomy in which a temporary expander has been inserted. Code 19357 from the reconstruction section of the Integumentary subsection is a combination of mastectomy and the insertion of an expander. If at a later date the expander was replaced with a permanent prosthesis, you would assign 11970, replacement of tissue expander with permanent prosthesis.*

You will also find insertion of implantable contraceptive capsules in the Introduction category. Implantable contraceptive capsules such as Norplant are inserted under the skin by means of a small incision on the upper arm. A capsule is effective for a number of years; at the end of that time, it must be removed. Read the descriptions in the implantable contraceptive capsule codes (11975–11977) carefully, as there are codes for insertion, removal, and removal with insertion.

coding shot

In addition to reporting the service of the introduction of the implantable contraceptive capsule, you report the supply of the contraceptive system using HCPCS code A4260.

Subcutaneous hormone pellet implantation is commonly used for the insertion of a hormone in a time-release capsule into the buttocks of women needing hormone replacement therapy after menopause, and the code for this implantation is in the Introduction category. The implantation area is anesthetized and the pellet is inserted through a tube. The pellet is completely absorbed into the system and so does not need to be removed, as does a contraceptive capsule. However, a new pellet must be inserted every 6 to 9 months, and each reinsertion is reported.

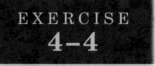

EXERCISE 4-4

SKIN, SUBCUTANEOUS AND ACCESSORY STRUCTURES

Apply the information about lesion procedures by coding the following:

1 Paring of three warts

   Code(s): _____

2 Removal of 15 skin tags

   Code(s): _____

3 Shaving of 1-cm lesion of face

   Code(s): _____

REPAIR (CLOSURE)

Repair Factors

When coding wound repair, the following three factors must be considered:
1. Length of the wound in centimeters
2. Complexity of the repair
3. Site of the wound repair

Remember **length, complexity,** and **site.** Figure 4–18 illustrates an example from the CPT manual of these three factors in the wound repair codes.

There are many different types of wounds (Fig. 4–19). Wound repair is classified by the type of repair necessary to repair the wound. There are three types of repair:

- Simple
- Intermediate
- Complex

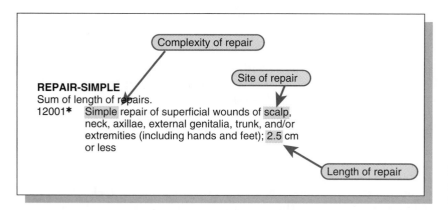

Figure 4–18 Wound repair. Note that metric measure is used throughout the CPT.

1. **Simple:** superficial wound repair that involves epidermis, dermis, and subcutaneous tissue and requiring only simple, one-layer suturing. If the simple wound repair is accomplished with tape or adhesive strips, the charge for the closure is included in the E/M service code and would not be coded separately with a Repair code. The repair codes are for suture closure.

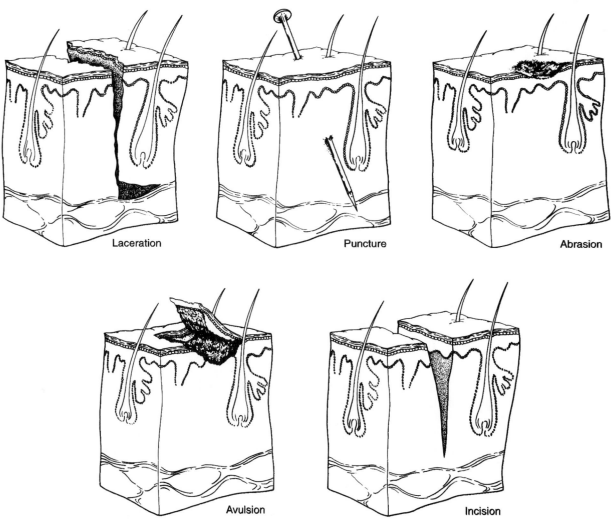

Figure 4–19 Types of wounds.

coding shot

Medicare has a HCPCS code to report skin closures using adhesives: G0168. All other third-party payers use the simple repair code to report these skin closures using adhesives.

2. **Intermediate:** requires closure of one or more layers of subcutaneous tissue and superficial fascia, in addition to the skin closure. You can use the codes for intermediate closure when the wound has to be extensively cleaned, even if the closure was a single-layer closure.

3. **Complex:** involves complicated wound closure including revision, debridement, extensive undermining, stents or retention sutures, and more than layered closure.

The lengths of wounds are totaled together by complexity (simple, intermediate, complex) and anatomic site (that is, all the simple wounds of the same site grouping are reported together; all the intermediate wounds of the same site grouping are reported together; and all the complex wounds of the same site grouping are reported together). The codes group together sites that require similar techniques to repair. For example, 12001 groups superficial scalp, neck, axillae, external genitalia, trunk, and extremities. When there is more than one repair type, the *most complex* type is listed as the first, or primary, procedure. The secondary procedure is then reported using modifier -51 (multiple procedure). Remember that the placement of the -51 indicates a discounted service to the payer.

STOP *Do not add together repairs*
- *from different groupings of anatomic sites such as face and hand.*
- *of different classifications such as simple and intermediate.*

The CPT manual notes that are found under the subheading Repair include extensive definitions of each of these levels of repair. These notes must be read carefully before you code repairs.

Repair Components

Three things are considered components (parts) of wound repair:
- Ligation
- Exploration
- Debridement

1. Simple **ligation** (tying) of vessels is considered part of the wound repair and is not listed separately.

2. Simple **exploration** of surrounding tissue, nerves, vessels, and tendons is considered part of the wound repair process and is not listed separately.

3. Normal **debridement** (cleaning and removing skin or tissue from the wound until normal, healthy tissue is exposed) is not listed separately.

If the wound is grossly contaminated and requires extensive debridement, a separate debridement procedure may be coded. (CPT codes 11000–11044 are used for extensive debridement.) Figure 4–20 illustrates a nonsurgical type of debridement.

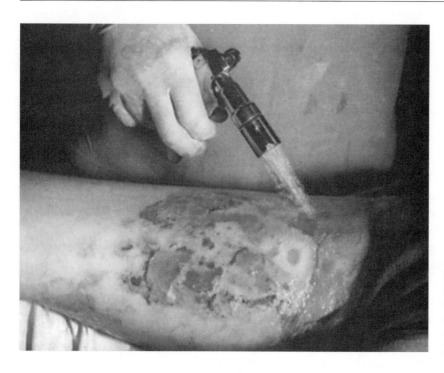

Figure 4–20 Burn debridement. (From Converse JM [ed]: Reconstructive Plastic Surgery: Principles and Procedures in Correction, Reconstruction and Transplantation, vol. 1. Philadelphia, WB Saunders, 1964, p 241.)

Tissue Transfers, Grafts, and Flaps

There are many types of grafting procedures that can be performed to correct a defect (e.g., adjacent tissue transfers or rearrangements, free skin grafts, flaps). To understand skin grafting, you must know that the **recipient site** is the area of defect that receives the graft, and the **donor site** is the area from which the healthy skin has been taken for grafting. (If a skin graft is required to close the donor site, the closure is coded as an additional procedure.) A brief description of some different types of skin grafting and coding guidelines specific to their use follows.

Adjacent Tissue Transfer or Rearrangement

There are many types of adjacent tissue transfers. Some of them are Z-plasty (Fig. 4–21), W-plasty, V-Y plasty, rotation flaps (Fig. 4–22), and advancement flaps. These procedures are various methods of moving a segment of skin from one area to an adjacent area, while leaving at least one side of the flap (moved skin) intact. At least one side of the flap is left

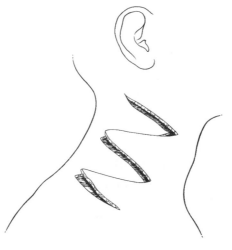

Figure 4–21 Z-plasty is named for the shape of the incision.

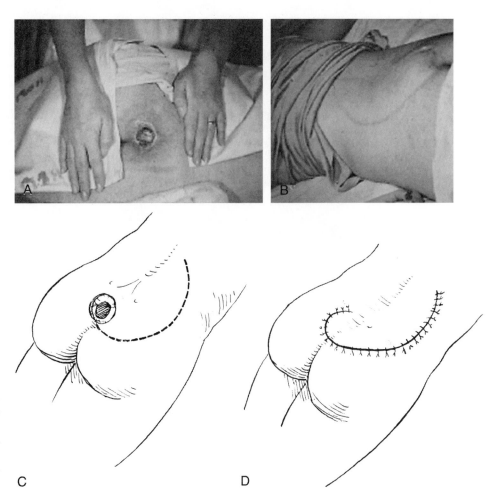

Figure 4–22 *A,* Sacral ulcer. *B,* Closure by a large rotation flap based superiorly. *C* and *D,* Outline of flap and rotation downward and medially. (From Converse JM [ed]: Reconstructive Plastic Surgery: Principles and Procedures in Correction, Reconstruction and Transplantation, vol. 5. Philadelphia, WB Saunders, 1964, p 1988.)

connected to retain some measure of blood supply to the graft. Incisions are made, and the skin is undermined and moved over to cover the defective area, leaving the base, or connected portion, intact. The flap is then sutured into place.

Adjacent tissue transfers are coded according to the size of the recipient site. The size is measured in square centimeters. Simple repair of the donor site is included in the tissue transfer code and is not coded separately. If there is a complex closure, or grafting of the donor site, this could be coded separately. Adjacent Tissue Transfer or Rearrangement in the CPT manual is divided based on the location of the defect (trunk or arm) and the size of the defect. In addition, there are codes at the end of the category for coding defects that are extremely complicated.

Any excision of a lesion that is repaired by adjacent tissue transfer is included in the tissue transfer code. If you bill for the excision in addition to the transfer, it would be considered unbundling.

Adjacent tissue transfer codes can be located in the CPT manual index under the term "Skin."

Free Skin Grafts

Free skin grafts are pieces of skin that are either split thickness, which consists of epidermis and part of the dermis, or full thickness, which consists of the epidermis and all of the dermis. The grafts are completely freed from the donor site and placed over the recipient site. There is no connection left between the graft and the donor site (Fig. 4–23).

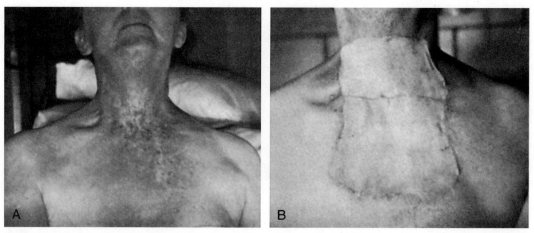

Figure 4–23   *A,* Chronic radiodermatitis of skin of the neck and sternal area following radiation treatment for hyperthyroidism 25 years previously. *B,* The irradiated skin was excised and covered with split-thickness skin grafts. (From Converse JM [ed]: Reconstructive Plastic Surgery: Principles and Procedures in Correction, Reconstruction and Transplantation, vol. 1. Philadelphia, WB Saunders, 1964, p 321.)

Free skin grafts are coded by recipient site, size of defect, and type of repair. The size is measured in square centimeters. Several codes (15000/15001, 15100/15101, and 15120/15121) have a special rule for determining the skin area involved in the repair. The measurement of 100 square centimeters (cm²) is applied to adults and to children 10 years and older, but the

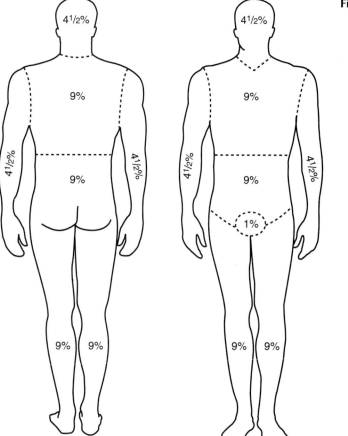

Figure 4–24   The Rule of Nines.

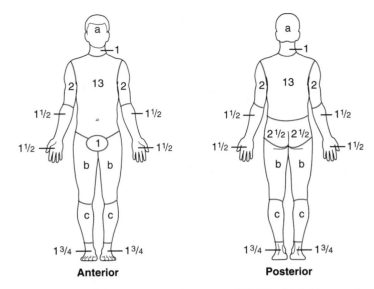

Anterior   **Posterior**

Relative percentage of body surface areas (% BSA) affected by growth

	0 yr	1 yr	5 yr	10 yr	15 yr
a − 1/2 of head	9 1/2	8 1/2	6 1/2	5 1/2	4 1/2
b − 1/2 of 1 thigh	2 3/4	3 1/4	4	4 1/4	4 1/2
c − 1/2 of lower leg	2 1/2	2 1/2	2 3/4	3	3 1/4

Figure 4–25 Lund-Browder chart for estimating the extent of burns in children.

measurement for children under age 10 years is by percentage of body area. For example, if in an adult a 100-cm² area on the trunk is prepared for a free skin graft, the preparation would be coded 15100. If in a child 1% of the trunk is prepared for a free skin graft, the preparation would be coded 15100. Figure 4–24 illustrates the Rule of Nines, which is used to calculate percentage of burns in adults. Figure 4–25 illustrates the Lund-Browder

Figure 4–26 Split-thickness and full-thickness skin grafts.

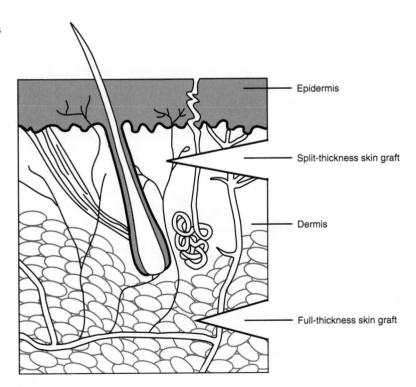

Epidermis

Split-thickness skin graft

Dermis

Full-thickness skin graft

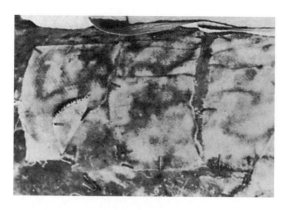

Figure 4–27 Three sheets of cultured epithelial autograft are in place on the left anterior thigh, which 3 weeks before was excised down to muscle fascia and covered with cadaver allograft. (From Gallico GG, O'Connor NE: Cultured epithelium as a skin substitute. Clin Plast Surg 12:155, 1985.)

classification of burns, which is often used to calculate percentage of burns in infants. Although the Lund-Browder approach is similar to the Rule of Nines, adjustments are made in the percentages because an infant's head is larger in proportion to the rest of his or her body. If the donor site for the graft requires repair by grafting, an additional graft code is used. Simple repair (closure) of the donor site is included in the graft code.

The category of Free Skin Grafts contains several different types of grafts: a **pinch graft** is a small, split-thickness repair; a **split graft** is a repair that involves the epidermis and some of the dermis; and a **full-thickness graft** is a repair that involves the epidermis and all of the dermis (Fig. 4–26). Often a split-thickness graft is referred to in the patient record as STSG and a full-thickness skin graft as FTSG.

Autografts are grafts taken from the patient's body. There are also several codes for grafts that include the application of grafts from other persons **(allografts)** or other species **(xenografts),** such as pigskin grafts in humans. These grafts are used as temporary grafts to help protect defect sites while healing is taking place (Figs. 4–27 and 4–28). A permanent graft may be placed over the site at a later date to complete the repair process.

CPT code 15000 is to be used to identify the additional procedure of preparing the recipient for grafting. Preparation of the site would also include removing or excising scar tissue or lesions. Codes in the range 15050–15261 are used to report the appropriate skin graft. The multiple procedure modifier -51 is not used with the preparation of site codes 15000–15001 or with the skin graft codes 15050–15621.

Free skin grafts can be located in the CPT manual index under Skin Grafts and Flaps or under Grafts.

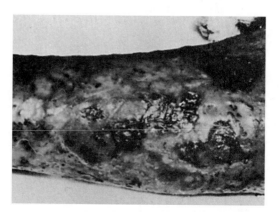

Figure 4–28 The same area of left anterior thigh as is seen in Figure 4–27, 1 month after grafting. (From Gallico GG, O'Connor NE: Cultured epithelium as a skin substitute. Clin Plast Surg 12:155, 1985.)

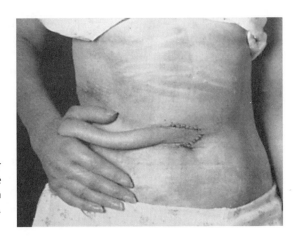

Figure 4–29 Transfer of an upper abdominal tube flap that was later used to reconstruct a nose. (From Converse JM [ed]: Reconstructive Plastic Surgery: Principles and Procedures in Correction, Reconstruction and Transplantation, vol. 5. Philadelphia, WB Saunders, 1964, p. 1956.)

Flaps

A physician may decide to develop a donor site at a location far away from the recipient site. The graft may have to be accomplished in stages. The graft code can be assigned more than once when the surgery is done in stages. Notes specific to this group of codes state that when coding transfer flaps (in stages), the donor site is used when a **tube graft** (Fig. 4–29) is formed for later use and when a **delayed flap** is formed before transfer (Fig. 4–30). The recipient site is used for coding when the graft is attached to its final site.

In a **delayed graft,** a portion of the skin is lifted and separated from the tissue below, but it stays connected to blood vessels at one end. This keeps the skin viable while it is being moved from one area to another, and at the same time, it lets the graft get used to living on a small supply of blood. It is hoped that living on a small blood supply will help to give the graft a better chance of survival when it is inset into the recipient site.

There are two categories of codes for flaps. The first category, Flaps (Skin and/or Deep Tissues), is subdivided based on the type of flap (i.e., pedicle, cross finger, delayed, or muscle flaps) and then by the location of the flap (scalp, trunk, or lips). The codes for procedures 15570–15738 do not include any extensive immobilization that may be necessary, such as a large plaster

Figure 4–30 *A,* Compound fracture of the elbow. A resection of the joint is necessary. Adequate soft tissue covering must be provided. *B,* A direct abdominal flap has been applied after complete excision of the scarred and infected tissues. Note the generous size of the flap and also the position of the upper extremity against the trunk. *C,* The flap after healing. The donor area on the abdomen has been partly closed by direct approximation. The remainder of the defect has been skin grafted. (From Converse JM [ed]: Reconstructive Plastic Surgery: Principles and Procedures in Correction, Reconstruction and Transplantation, vol. 1. Philadelphia, WB Saunders, 1964, p. 66.)

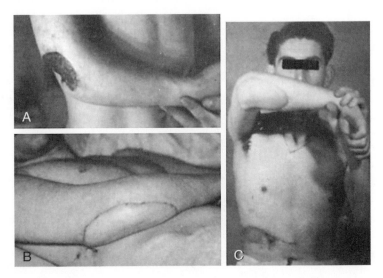

cast or other immobilizing device. Extensive immobilization would be coded in addition to the flap procedure. Also not included in the flap procedure codes is the closure of a donor site, which would be reported in addition to the flap procedure.

The second category, Other Flaps and Grafts, is subdivided based on the type of flap (free muscle, free skin, fascial, or hair transplant).

Other Procedures

The Other Procedures category contains codes for a wide variety of repair services, such as abrasion, chemical peel, and blepharoplasty. The codes are often divided based on the site or extent of repair.

Dermabrasion is used to treat acne, wrinkles, or general keratoses. The skin area is anesthetized by a chemical that freezes the area (a cryogen), and the area is sanded down using a motorized brush. The facial dermabrasion codes (15780–15787) are divided according to the surface area of the face treated (total, segment, region).

A tattoo can be removed by dermabrasion. The process involves the use of a high-speed mechanical wheel to remove the epidermis and part of the papillary dermis. The service is reported with code 15783.

The **abrasion** codes 15786–15787 are used to report the use of abrasion to remove a lesion, such as scar tissue, a wart, or a callus. This technique is often used to remove areas of sun-damaged skin. The first abraded lesion is reported with 15786, and each additional four or fewer lesions are reported with 15787.

Chemical peels, also known as chemexfoliation, are treatments in which a chemical is applied to the skin and then removed. The skin surface will then shed its outer layer, much as it does after a sunburn. The treatment is used for cosmetic purposes, such as smoothing the wrinkles around the mouth or removing liver spots (lentigines). The chemical peel codes (15788–15793) are divided according to whether the peel is on the face or not on the face, in addition to the depth of the peel (epidermal or dermal).

Salabrasion treatment codes are also located in the Other Procedures category. **Salabrasion** is the use of a saline (salt) solution to cause the skin to peel; it is not used often. Dermabrasion and laser treatments are more commonly used. Salabrasion used to be a popular method of removing tattoos.

Cervicoplasty, 15819, is the surgical procedure whereby the physician removes excess skin from the neck, usually for cosmetic reasons. **Blepharoplasty** (codes 15820–15823), also performed predominantly for cosmetic purposes, is the removal of excess skin and the support of the muscles of the upper eyelid. **Rhytidectomy** is the removal of wrinkles by pulling the skin tight and removing the excess. Rhytidectomy codes 15824–15829 are used to report these cosmetic services. Excision of excess skin elsewhere on the body—thigh, leg, hip, buttock, arm, and so forth—is reported by using codes in the range 15831–15839.

coding shot

If the excision of skin is done bilaterally, be certain to add modifier -50.

Grafts for facial nerve paralysis (15840–15845) are procedures in which the physician harvests a graft from some location on the body and grafts the area damaged by facial paralysis.

There are also codes in the Other Procedures category for the removal of sutures and for dressing changes performed under anesthesia. **Lipectomy** (commonly called liposuction) codes are divided according to the body area that is being treated—head, trunk, upper extremities, and so forth. Again, if the procedure is done bilaterally, add modifier -50.

Pressure Ulcers

Pressure ulcers are also known as decubitus ulcers or bedsores. Pressure ulcers are found on areas of the body that have bony projections, such as the hips and the area above the tailbone. Pressure on these areas causes decreased blood flow, and sores form. With continued pressure, the sores ulcerate, and deeper layers of tissue, such as fascia, muscle, and bone, may be affected. Pressure ulcers commonly occur in patients who are unable to change position or have devices that prevent mobility (splints, casts).

Although a pressure ulcer can be seen, the depth to which the ulceration has penetrated cannot be seen. The ulcer may involve only superficial skin or may affect deeper layers. The treatment for a pressure ulcer is excision of the ulcerated area to the depth of unaffected tissue, fascia, or muscle (see Fig. 4–22).

coding shot

Only an adjacent tissue transfer is included in the pressure ulcer codes. If the medical record indicates a myocutaneous flap closure or a muscle flap, use codes from both the Pressure Ulcer category and from the Flaps (Skin and/or Deep Tissue) category. Also, if a free skin graft is used to close the ulcer, that closure would be coded separately too, using a code from the Free Skin Grafts category.

You will note that many of the Pressure Ulcer codes have "with ostectomy" as the indented code. An ostectomy is the removal of the bone that underlies the ulcer area. The bony prominences are chiseled or filed down to alleviate future pressure.

Read the code descriptions carefully when coding from the ulcer repair category, as the codes are divided based on the location, type, and extent of closure needed.

Burns

Burn treatment is unique in that it is common for a patient to undergo multiple dressing changes or debridements (see Fig. 4–20) during the healing period. Dressing and debridement codes are either initial or subsequent treatments. Burn dressing and/or debridement codes are divided based on whether the dressing or debridement was accomplished with or without anesthesia and on the amount of body surface involved. The CPT codes are divided based on small, medium, and large body surface areas. Although not stated, an approximation is as follows: small is less than 4½%; medium, 4½% to 9%; large, more than 9%. The Rule of Nines is used to estimate the percentage of body surface (see Fig. 4–24). For example, a 4½% to 9% surface includes the whole face and one extremity.

Excision of burns using **alloplastic dressings** is listed by percentage of body surface area. These dressings are synthetic coverings used in the healing process and are not skin grafts.

The Burn category contains a code for **escharotomy,** a procedure in which the physician cuts through the dead skin that covers the surface when there is a full-thickness burn. The crust covers the surface and diminishes blood flow and healing.

**EXERCISE
4–5**

REPAIR (CLOSURE) AND BURNS

Pay special attention to the following descriptions of main terms. The main term, as introduced in Chapter 1, is the primary word or phrase that identifies the service or procedure, anatomic site, condition, or disease. In this example, the patient record states: **"simple wound repair 12-cm wound, left hand."**

To locate the code for the repair in the CPT manual index using the *condition method,* you first locate the main term, "Wound," and then the subterm, "Repair." Wound is the condition and Repair is the procedure. Finally, you identify the type (i.e., complex, simple).

To locate the code using the *service* or *procedure method,* you would first locate the main term, Repair. Repair is the service or procedure. The subterm, Wound, is located next, and finally the type (i.e., complex, simple). These are just two of the ways to locate this service in the index.

From the main term, Wound, subterm of Repair, simple, you are directed to a range of codes, 12001–12021. Locate this range in the CPT manual. The notes under the subheading Repair (Closure) are "must" reading. Also, read the description of the first code in the category (12001*). The description specifies that the code includes the term "hands," which is what you are looking for. Now locate the correct length (12 cm), and you will have the correct code—12004.

Now you do some:

The patient record states: "complex wound repair on leg, 3.1 cm."

1   What is the correct code?

Code(s): _____

2   After an assault with a knife, a patient requires simple repair of a 3-cm laceration of the neck, simple repair of a 4-cm laceration of the back, simple repair of a 5-cm laceration of the forearm, and complex repair of a 3-cm laceration of the abdomen.

Code(s): _____

3   Harry Torgerson, a 42-year-old construction worker, is injured at work when a box containing wood scraps and shingles falls from a second-story scaffolding and strikes him on the left forearm, causing multiple lacerations. Forearm repairs: 5.1-cm repair of the subcutaneous tissues and a 5.6-cm laceration, with particles of shingles and wood materials deeply embedded, both requiring intermediate closure. There is also a superficial wound of the scalp of 3.1 cm requiring simple closure.

Code(s): _____

4   A patient with multiple healed scars requests that they be removed and repaired for cosmetic reasons. The defects include a 100-cm² scar of the

right cheek and a 200-cm² defect of the left upper chest. Several split-thickness skin grafts totaling 300 cm² are harvested from the left and right thighs. The scar tissue is cut away, and the sites are prepared for grafting.

Code(s): _____

5 The patient had a 20-cm² defect of the right cheek that was repaired with a rotation flap.

Code(s): _____

6 The patient had a 10-cm² malignant neoplasm removed from the forehead. Z-plasty was used to repair this site. How would the excision and repair be coded?

Code(s): _____

7 A patient has had a portion of his mandible removed due to excision of a malignant tumor. Repair of the site is now performed by use of a myocutaneous flap graft.

Code(s): _____

8 A patient incurs second- and third-degree burns of the abdomen and thigh (10%) when she pulls a pan of boiling water off the stove. She requires daily debridements or dressing changes for the first week (Monday through Friday). She is in severe pain and requires anesthesia during these treatments. During the following 2 weeks she will be receiving dressing changes every other day (Monday, Wednesday, Friday), and it is expected that enough healing will have taken place that anesthesia will not be necessary. What codes would be reported for services during the 3-week treatment period?

Code(s): _____

coding shot

Some third-party payers allow you to submit charges for burn care using the first date of service to the last date of service. This allows you to indicate multiples of the same service (e.g., 16015, burn debridement, ×5). Other payers require you to list each date of service and to code each service separately. So if the patient received five burn debridements on five separate days, you would report 16015 five separate times, once for each day of service.

DESTRUCTION

The next subheading in the subsection of the Integumentary System is Destruction. The codes are for destruction of lesions by means **other than excision.** The codes in this subsection are for benign, premalignant, or malignant lesions destroyed by means of electrosurgery (use of various forms of electrical current to destroy the lesion), cryosurgery (use of extreme cold), laser (**l**ight **a**mplification by **s**timulated **e**mission of **r**adiation), or

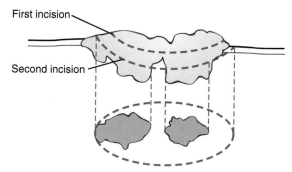

First incision

Second incision

Figure 4–31   Mohs' micrographic surgical technique.

chemicals (acids). Read the notes under the Destruction subsection heading; they contain a list of types of lesions. Destruction codes state "any method" and are divided according to type of lesion (benign or malignant). Further divisions are based on the number of lesions destroyed or the size of the area destroyed. The malignant lesions are divided based on location (nose, ear, and so forth) and size (0.6 cm to 1.0 cm, and so forth), regardless of the method used.

Mohs' Micrographic Surgery

One sophisticated destruction procedure is Mohs' micrographic surgery. The **Mohs microscope** is used by the surgeon during the surgical procedure to view the lesion and assess its pathology. If the lesion is malignant, it is immediately removed. Mohs' micrographic surgery is especially useful in cases of large tumors. The procedure involves mapping the exact contour of the tumor and removing tissue down to the level at which cancerous cells are no longer found. The process involves stages, whereby the surgeon removes a layer of skin and examines it under a microscope for cancerous cells, then returns to the lesion to remove another layer of skin, again examining it under a microscope (Fig. 4–31). This process is continued until cancerous cells are no longer identified in the layers being removed. The surgeon acts as both the pathologist and the surgeon.

The codes in the category include the removal of the lesion(s) and pathologic evaluation of the lesion(s). These codes are also divided based on the stage (first, second, third) of the surgery and the number of specimens the surgeon takes during the surgery for pathologic examination.

from the trenches

"You have to love the profession. I've been in the medical field since high school . . . it gets into your blood. Just have patience and don't give up."

DAWN

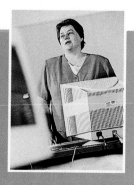

EXERCISE 4-6

DESTRUCTION

1 Electrosurgical destruction of a herpetic lesion.

Code(s): _____

2 Cryosurgical destruction of 14 actinic keratoses.

Code(s): _____

3 Mohs' micrographic surgery by a single physician removing and examining six specimens.

Code(s): _____

BREAST PROCEDURES

Breast procedures are divided according to category of procedure (e.g., incision, excision, introduction, repair). You must read the documentation to identify the procedure used, such as incisional versus excisional biopsies. In an **incisional biopsy,** an incision is made into the lesion and a small portion of the lesion is taken out. In an **excisional biopsy,** the entire lesion is removed for biopsy. In some cases it may be necessary to mark the lesion preoperatively by placing a thin wire (radiologic marker) down to the lesion to identify its exact location (Fig. 4–32). The placement of the wire is coded, and the excision of the lesion identified by the marker is coded.

Multiple codes are used to identify mastectomies. You should carefully review the operative report to confirm whether pectoral muscles, axillary

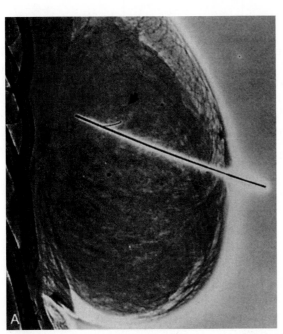
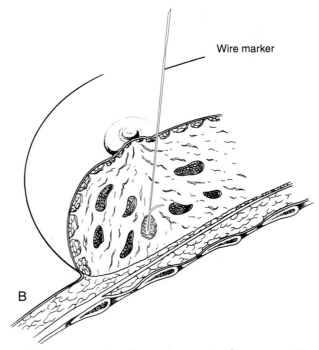

Figure 4–32 Wire marker used to mark breast lesion. *A,* Mammography allows placement of a preoperative needle that marks a lesion. (From Bland KI, Copeland EM [eds]: The Breast: Comprehensive Management of Benign and Malignant Diseases. Philadelphia, WB Saunders, 1991 p. 530; *B,* The wire marker serves as a guide for the surgeon when performing the biopsy. *B,* redrawn from Bland KI, Copeland EM [eds]: The Breast: Comprehensive Management of Benign and Malignant Diseases. Philadelphia, WB Saunders, 1991, p. 531.)

lymph nodes, or internal mammary lymph nodes were also removed. This information will be necessary to determine the correct mastectomy code.

CAUTION *Remember, any breast procedure done on* **both** *breasts must be coded as a bilateral procedure (modifier -50).*

EXERCISE 4-7

BREAST PROCEDURES

Locate the correct code for the following procedures. Be sure to read all notes in the CPT manual and the description of the code before applying the code.

1   Aspiration of one cyst, breast

    Code(s): _____

2   Simple, complete bilateral mastectomies

    Code(s): _____

3   Right modified radical mastectomy, including axillary lymph nodes without any muscles

    Code(s): _____

4   Preoperative placement of one breast wire, left breast

    Code(s): _____

5   Reconstruction of nipple/areola

    Code(s): _____

Congratulations

You made it through the entire Integumentary System subsection! The subsection is quite complicated and you have done a great job if you understand the basics of these codes. As you use them here and on the job, your knowledge will continue to grow.

CHAPTER GLOSSARY

abscess: localized collection of pus that will result in the disintegration of tissue over time

allogenic: of the same species, but genetically different

allograft: tissue graft between individuals who are not of the same genotype

allotransplantation: transplantation between individuals who are not of the same genotype

anomaly: abnormality

autogenous, autologous: from oneself

axillary nodes: lymph nodes located in the armpit

benign: not progressive or recurrent

biopsy: removal of a small piece of living tissue for diagnostic purposes

blephar(o)-: prefix meaning eyelid

conjunctiva: the lining of the eyelids and the covering of the sclera

cryosurgery: destruction of lesions using extreme cold

debridement: cleansing of or removal of dead tissue from a wound

dermis: second layer of skin, holding blood vessels, nerve endings, sweat glands, and hair follicles

destruction: killing of tissue by means of electrocautery, laser, chemicals, or other means

electrodesiccation: destruction of a lesion by the use of electric current radiated through a needle

epidermis: outer layer of skin

excision: cutting or taking away (in reference to lesion removal, it is full-thickness removal of a lesion that may include simple closure)

excisional: removal of an entire lesion for biopsy

incision and drainage: to cut and withdraw fluid

incisional: *see* incision

injection: forcing of a fluid into a vessel or cavity

lesion: abnormal or altered tissue, e.g., wound, cyst, abscess, or boil

ligation: binding or tying off, as in constricting the bloodflow of a vessel or binding fallopian tubes for sterilization

malignant: used to describe a cancerous tumor that grows worse over time

-plasty: suffix meaning technique involving molding or surgically forming

punch: use of a small hollow instrument to puncture a lesion

separate procedures: minor procedures that when done by themselves are coded as a procedure, but when performed at the same time as a major procedure are considered incidental and not coded separately

shaving: horizontal or transverse removal of dermal or epidermal lesions, without full-thickness excision

skin graft: transplantation of tissue to repair a defect

soft tissue: tissues (fascia, connective tissue, muscle, and so forth) surrounding a bone

starred procedures: procedures and services that do not include various preoperative or postoperative services

subcutaneous: tissue below the dermis, primarily fat cells that insulate the body

suture: to unite parts by stitching them together

tissue transfer: piece of skin for grafting that is still partially attached to the original blood supply and is used to cover an adjacent wound area

transplantation: grafting of tissue from one source to another

wound repair, complex: involves complicated wound closure, including revision, debridement, extensive undermining, and more than layered closure

wound repair, intermediate: requires closure of one or more subcutaneous tissues and superficial fascia, in addition to the skin closure

wound repair, simple: superficial wound repair, involving epidermis, dermis, and subcutaneous tissue, requiring only simple, one-layer suturing

CHAPTER REVIEW

CHAPTER 4, PART I, THEORY

Now is an excellent time to put all your newly learned coding skills to work by completing a Chapter Review.

1 What is the largest section of the six CPT manual sections?

_____

2 How many subsections does the Surgery section have? _____

3 The subsections in the Surgery section are usually divided according to

_____ .

4 Measurement in the CPT manual is in what system?

_____

Wound repair codes are determined by what three criteria?

5 _____

6 _____

7 _____

What are the three classifications of wound repair?

8 _____

9 _____

10 _____

11 What is the bilateral procedures modifier?

_____

List the three times when multiple procedures are coded:

12 _____

13 _____

14 _____

15 Modifier -51 indicates what?

_____

16 What is the name for the information that precedes section information?

_____

17 What is the first subsection in the Surgery section?

_____

18 If an unlisted procedure code is used, what must accompany submission of the code?

_____

19 Surgery package and surgical global fee are terms used to describe what?

_____

20 What is the five-digit code number used for documentation purposes to report nonbilled postoperative services provided to the patient under the umbrella of a surgical package?

_____

21 The major difference in destruction of lesions is whether the lesion is

_____ or _____ .

22 The division of malignant lesion excision is based on _____ and _____ .

23 What symbol in the CPT manual indicates that a procedure does not include follow-up care?

_____

24 What kind of package is developed by third-party payers and may go beyond the package described in the CPT manual?

_____

25 What two words following a procedure description alert you to the fact that you can code the procedure only if it is not done as a part of a more extensive procedure?

_____

CHAPTER 4, PART II, PRACTICAL

Code the following cases for the surgical procedures and office visits only. Do not code the radiology services or laboratory work that may be included.

26 Margaret Wilson, a 26-year-old mother of three (new patient), has routine screening mammography of both breasts. (You do not need to code the mammography.) A shadow is visualized in the right breast. The physician performs a biopsy (needle core). The biopsy indicates malignancy. The patient agrees to and has a mastectomy (simple, complete) 1 week later.

Code(s): _____

27 Shirley Peters, age 80, a new patient, presents to the office for scissors removal of 15 skin tags.

Code(s): _____

28 Removal of 180-cm^2 nevus of left cheek, autograft with split-thickness skin graft of 180 cm^2.

Code(s): _____

29 Nipple reconstruction

Code(s): _____

30 Destruction of 0.4-cm malignant lesion of the neck

Code(s): _____

31 Simple repair of a superficial wound of the genitalia; 2.4 cm

Code(s): _____

32 Adjacent tissue transfer of chin defect; 9 cm^2

Code(s): _____

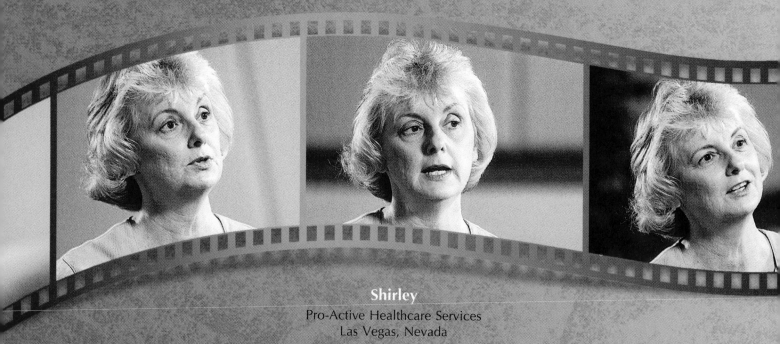

Shirley
Pro-Active Healthcare Services
Las Vegas, Nevada

chapter 5

Musculoskeletal System

LEARNING OBJECTIVES

After completing this chapter you should be able to

1 Understand and apply rules of coding fractures.

2 Differentiate among fracture treatment types.

3 Analyze cast application and strapping procedures.

4 Identify critical elements in coding incisions, wound exploration, excision, introduction, and grafts.

5 Utilize endoscopy codes.

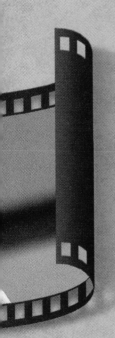

FORMAT

The Musculoskeletal System subsection is formatted by anatomic site. The subheadings in the Musculoskeletal subsection are as follows:

- General
- Head
- Neck (Soft Tissue) and Thorax
- Back and Flank
- Spine (Vertebral Column)
- Abdomen
- Shoulder
- Humerus (Upper Arm) and Elbow
- Forearm and Wrist
- Hand and Fingers
- Pelvis and Hip Joint
- Femur (Thigh Region) and Knee Joint
- Leg (Tibia and Fibula) and Ankle Joint
- Foot and Toes
- Application of Casts and Strapping
- Endoscopy/Arthroscopy

The first subheading in the subsection is General; it contains procedures that are applicable to many different anatomic sites. Other subheadings are further divided by category of procedure and usually include

- Incision
- Excision
- Introduction/Removal
- Repair/Revision/Construction
- Fracture/Dislocation
- Arthrodesis
- Amputation

Any or all of these categories of procedures may be found under each subheading.

The codes found in the Musculoskeletal System subsection are used extensively by orthopedic surgeons to describe the services they provide to restore and preserve the function of the skeletal system. There are many codes, however, that are used frequently by a wide variety of primary care and family practice physicians, such as the splinting, casting, and fracture codes. Your study of the Musculoskeletal subsection of the CPT will focus on the format of the subsection, fracture types and repair, application of casts and strapping, the General subheading, and endoscopic procedures.

CODING HIGHLIGHTS

Thorough review of the medical record will help you to identify key information necessary for coding. The following tips will help you to choose the most correct code from this subsection:

1. Identify whether the procedure is being performed on soft tissue or bone.

2. Determine whether treatment is for a traumatic injury or a medical condition.

from the trenches

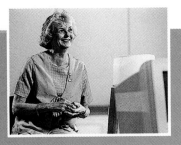

"*Read, read, read! Use your book. Highlight. Make notes. It's worth the effort in the end.*"

SHIRLEY

3. Identify the most specific anatomic site. For example, when coding vertebral procedures, it is necessary to know whether the condition was for cervical, thoracic, or lumbar vertebrae.

4. Determine whether the code description includes grafting or fixation. If grafting or fixation is not listed within the major procedure code description, each may be coded as an additional procedure.

5. Read the code carefully to determine whether it describes a procedure done on a single site (e.g., each finger). If the same procedure is performed on multiple sites (e.g., multiple fingers), you must indicate the number of units done or list the code multiple times.

Fractures

Fractures are coded by treatment—open, closed, or percutaneous. **Open repair** of a fracture is made when a surgery is performed in which the fracture is exposed by an incision made over the fracture. **Closed repair** is made when the physician repairs the fracture without opening the skin. The repair method used—open or closed—depends on the type and severity of the fracture. A simple or greenstick fracture (Fig. 5–1) may receive closed treatment, whereas a more complicated compound fracture may need open treatment so as to provide internal fixation (e.g., wires, pins, screws). Fractures are coded to the specific anatomic site and then according to whether manipulation was performed. All fractures and dislocations are coded based on the reason for the treatment. For instance, if a hip replacement (arthroplasty) is done for medical reasons such as osteoarthritis, it is coded to 27125, located under the subheading Pelvis and Hip Joint, category Repair, Revision, and/or Reconstruction. The *repair* was the reason for the treatment. If the hip replacement was performed for a fracture, it is coded 27236, located under the subheading Pelvis and Hip Joint, category Fracture and/or Dislocation. The *fracture* was the reason for the treatment.

The CPT manual more specifically defines closed, open, and percutaneous treatments as follows:

Closed treatment means that the fracture site is not surgically opened (exposed to the external environment and directly visualized). This terminology is used to describe procedures that treat fractures by three methods: (1) without manipulation, (2) with manipulation, and (3) with or without traction.

Closed treatment **without manipulation** is a procedure in which the physician immobilizes the bone with a splint, cast, or other device but without having to manipulate the fracture into alignment. Code 25500 describes a closed treatment of a radial shaft fracture without manipulation. This code is correctly used when a patient has a broken but stable radial shaft that is not displaced. The physician applies a cast and prescribes medication.

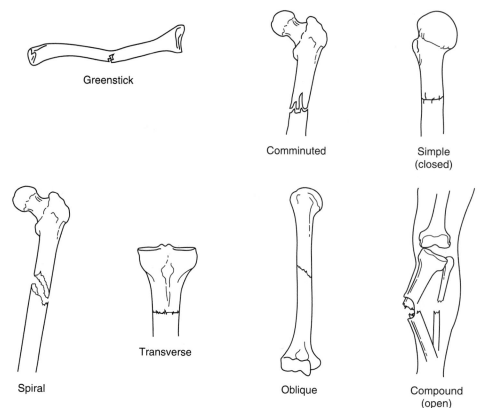

Greenstick

Comminuted

Simple
(closed)

Spiral

Transverse

Oblique

Compound
(open)

Figure 5–1 Types of fractures.

Closed treatment **with manipulation** is a procedure in which the physician has to reduce (put back in place) a fracture. Code 21320 describes a closed treatment of a nasal bone fracture with stabilization. This code is correctly used when a patient has a displaced broken nose that requires manipulation to return it to the normal position. The physician would then apply external and/or internal splints to immobilize the nose.

Open treatment is used when the fracture is surgically opened (exposed to the external environment). In this instance, the fracture (bone) is open to view and internal fixation (pins, screws, etc.) may be used.

Percutaneous skeletal fixation describes fracture treatment that is neither open nor closed. In this procedure, the fracture is not open to view, but fixation (e.g., pins) is placed across the fracture site, usually under x-ray imaging.

Other definitions are as follows:

Manipulation is a reduction, which is an attempt to maneuver the bone back into proper alignment. The physician may bend, rotate, pull, or guide the bone back into position.

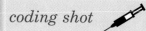

coding shot

If the physician attempts a reduction but is unable to correct the fracture successfully, you still bill for the reduction service.

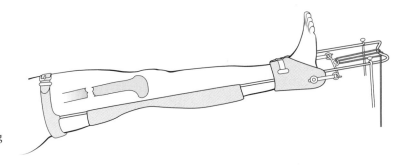

Figure 5–2 Traction is the application of a pulling force to hold a bone in alignment.

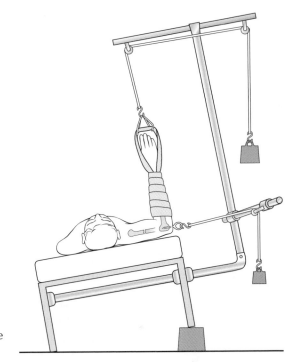

Figure 5–3 In skeletal traction, internal devices are secured in the patient bones, and traction is attached to the devices.

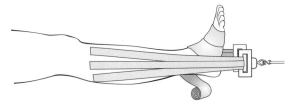

Figure 5–4 In skin traction, the traction is attached by means of strapping, wraps, or tape.

Traction is the application of pulling force to hold a bone in alignment (Fig. 5–2).

Skeletal traction is the use of internal devices, such as pins, screws, or wires, that are inserted into the bone through the skin, with ends of the pins, screws, or wires sticking out through the skin, so traction devices can be attached (Fig. 5–3).

Skin traction involves strapping, elastic wrap, or tape that is fastened to the skin or wrapped around the limb; weights attached to them apply force to the fracture (Fig. 5–4).

Dislocations

Dislocation is the displacement of a bone from its normal location, and the treatment of the dislocation injury is to return the bone to its normal

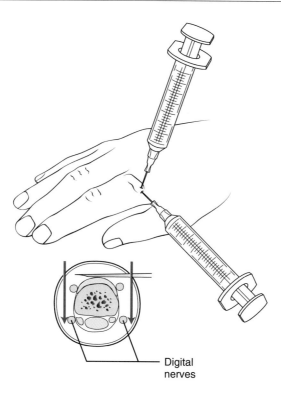

Digital
nerves

Figure 5–5   Digital nerve block.

location (anatomic alignment) by a variety of methods. For example, if a finger was dislocated and the bone did not protrude through the skin, the physician would administer a digital block (Fig. 5–5) and apply gentle traction until the finger was realigned. A splint would then be applied to keep the finger immobile for about 3 weeks. If the shoulder was dislocated, the physician might elevate the arm and rotate the humerus while applying pressure to the head of the humerus. Or the patient might lie face down on a table with the arm hanging off the edge while a weight is attached to the hand; the weight is sufficient to pull the arm back into place (Fig. 5–6). If

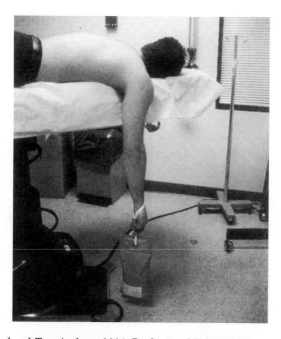

Figure 5–6   External technique for the relocation of a shoulder (Stimson technique). (From Rakel RE: Saunders Manual of Medical Practice. Philadelphia, WB Saunders, 1996, p. 817.)

external measures such as the two just described do not relocate the joint, a surgical reduction might be indicated.

EXERCISE 5-1

FRACTURES AND DISLOCATIONS

Using the CPT manual, provide the code(s) for the following:

1 Nasal bone fracture, closed treatment

   Code(s) _____

2 Uncomplicated, closed treatment of one fractured rib

   Code(s) _____

3 Interphalangeal joint dislocation, open treatment with internal fixation

   Code(s) _____

4 Open distal fibula fracture repair with internal fixation

   Code(s) _____

5 Femoral shaft fracture repair using closed treatment

   Code(s) _____

6 Percutaneous skeletal fixation of impact fracture of femoral neck

   Code(s) _____

7 Open treatment of shoulder dislocation with greater humeral tuberosity fracture

   Code(s) _____

8 Closed treatment of mandibular fracture, including interdental fixation

   Code(s) _____

9 Percutaneous skeletal fixation of a Colles-type fracture of the distal radius with manipulation and external fixation

   Code(s) _____

10 Ankle dislocation, closed treatment

   Code(s) _____

GENERAL

The first subheading in the Musculoskeletal subsection is General. As the name implies, this subheading includes a wide variety of codes.

Incisions

The first code, 20000, is for the incision of a **soft tissue abscess.** There are codes in the Integumentary System for incisions that are for skin only. What makes the 20000 code different from those in the Integumentary System is that 20000 is used when the abscess is associated with the deep tissue and possibly the bone that underlies the area of abscess. The physician would make an incision into the abscess, explore the abscess, clean the abscess, and debride it (remove dead tissue). If the underlying bone is

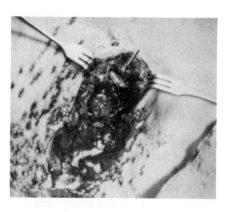

Figure 5–7 Gunshot wound requiring exploration. (From Swan KG, Swan RC: Principles of ballistics applicable to the treatment of gunshot wounds. Surg Clin North Am 71:221–239, 1991.)

affected, the physician would usually remove the affected area of the bone, irrigate the area, place a drain into the area, and pack the area. This procedure is very different from the procedures you find in the Integumentary System codes for incision of an abscess.

Wound Exploration

The Wound Exploration codes are used for traumatic wounds that result from a penetrating trauma (e.g., gunshot, knife wound). Wound Exploration codes include basic exploration and repair of the area of trauma. These codes are used specifically when the repair requires enlargement of the existing wound for exploration, cleaning, and repair. Included in the Wound Exploration codes 20100–20103 are not only the exploration and enlargement of the wound but also debridement, removal of any foreign body(s), ligation of minor blood vessels, and repair of subcutaneous tissues, muscle fascia, and muscle, as would be necessary to repair the wound (Fig. 5–7).

If the wound does not need to be enlarged, you would use a code from the Integumentary System, Skin Repair codes. If, however, the wound is more severe than a Wound Exploration code would indicate, the repair code would come from the specific repair area codes. For example, for a bullet wound to the chest that penetrated the lung, the treatment might be a thoracotomy, as illustrated in Figure 5–8, with control of the hemorrhage and repair of the tear of the lung. The thoracotomy code would come from the subsection Respiratory System under the subheading Lungs. As you can see from this example, you have to assess the extent of the procedure carefully, reading the medical record to ensure you are in the correct area so you can choose the correct service code.

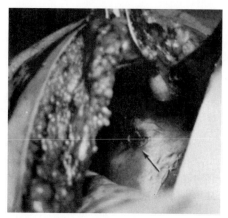

Figure 5–8 Gunshot wound requiring a thoracotomy. (From Swan KG, Swan RC: Principles of ballistics applicable to the treatment of gunshot wounds. Surg Clin North Am 71:221–239, 1991.)

Excision

The Excision category (20150–20251) contains codes for the biopsies of muscle and bone. The codes are divided based on the type of biopsy (muscle, bone), the depth of the biopsy (superficial, deep), and, in some codes, the method of obtaining the biopsy (e.g., percutaneous needle).

The procedure for a muscle or bone biopsy typically includes the administration of local anesthetic into the biopsy area, an incision into the area allowing exposure of the muscle or bone, removal of tissue for biopsy, and suturing of the area. A **percutaneous biopsy,** as represented in 20206, differs in that the area is not opened to the physician's view. A trocar (hollow needle) or needle is placed into the muscle or bone by passing the needle through the skin and into the muscle or bone and withdrawing a sample. When the percutaneous method is used to obtain a biopsy, the area does not require suturing. If the biopsy is extremely complicated, a surgeon may request the assistance of ultrasound to be able to view the biopsy area during the procedure and receive guidance as to the placement of the needle. If the ultrasonic guidance for a needle biopsy is performed by a radiologist, it is reported separately by the radiologist, using a radiology code. Also, a surgeon can use ultrasonic guidance without a radiologist. You will learn more about these radiologic services later in this text; but notice that following the percutaneous muscle biopsy code 20206, a note appears that directs you to the correct codes in the Radiology section of the CPT. This excellent directional feature will aid you as you begin to code from multiple sections of the CPT for a single case. So be certain to read all notes associated with a code.

Biopsy codes in the Excision category of the General subheading are not to be used for the excision of tumors on muscle. If the medical record indicates excision of a muscle tumor, you would have to choose a code from the correct anatomic subheading of the Musculoskeletal subsection.

Biopsy codes do not include the pathology workup that is done on the sample. You will also learn more about billing for pathology services later in this text.

Introduction and Removal

Within the Introduction and Removal category you will find a wide variety of injection, aspiration, insertion, application, removal, and adjustment codes. Because the category is within the General subheading of the Musculoskeletal subsection, the codes also have a wide application in coding for services.

Therapeutic **sinus tract injection** procedure codes are within this category. You may initially think of the nasal sinuses, but these are not the sinuses that are being injected here. The term "sinus" is referring to an abscess or cyst that is located within the body. The infection is treated by injecting an antibiotic or other substance into the sinus by way of the sinus tract (passage from the outer surface to the inner cavity). With certain sinus injections, a radiologist provides guidance to ensure the correct placement of the needle.

Removal codes located in the Introduction and Removal category are used to report the removal of foreign bodies that are lodged in muscle or bone. Recall that the Integumentary System removal codes were used for foreign bodies lodged in the skin.

Injection codes in this category are used for injections made into a tendon, ligament, or ganglion cyst (cystic tumor). An example of the use of these injection codes would be a corticosteroid injection as a ganglion cyst treatment. If more than one injection is given, use the multiple procedure modifier -51.

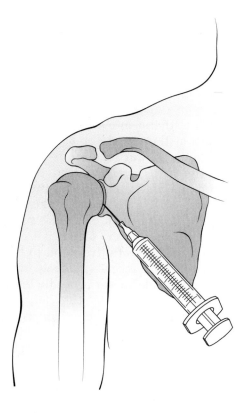

Figure 5-9   Arthrocentesis of a joint.

Arthrocentesis is injection into or aspiration of a joint (Fig. 5-9), and the codes used to report such a service are in the range of 20600-20610. This is a procedure commonly used in the treatment of joint conditions. The area over the involved joint is injected with anesthetic, a needle is inserted into the joint, and fluid is drawn out during an aspiration procedure. During an injection procedure, a drug is injected into the joint.

coding shot

The code descriptions indicate that the codes can be used for an aspiration, an injection, or both an aspiration and an injection. You would not report the performance of both an aspiration and an injection at the same session by using a multiple modifier, as that would be unbundling. You would instead report the dual service using a single code.

The arthrocentesis codes are divided according to whether the joint is small (finger, toe), intermediate (ankle, elbow), or major (shoulder, hip).

Lidocaine, marcaine, and so forth, when used as anesthetics, are not coded separately. Any injected drug such as a steroid is coded separately using a J code (drug code) from the HCPCS (CMS's Common Procedure Coding System).

Insertion of wires or pins to repair bone (20650) is a procedure often used by orthopedic physicians. The procedure is performed using a local or general anesthetic. The bone is drilled through with a power drill and pins and/or wires are placed through the holes in the bone and allowed to emerge through the skin on each side of the bone. A traction device is then attached to the pins or wires to hold the bone immobile while healing takes place. This may sound painful, but actually, the procedure is often used to alleviate pain as well as to align the bone for better healing.

coding shot

The removal of the wires or pins is included in the reimbursement for skeletal fixation; but for internal fixation removal, code separately using 20670–20680.

The **application** of many of the devices used for fixation of the bones of the body during the healing process—cranial tong, cranial halo, pelvic halo, femoral halo, caliper, stereotactic frame—is located in this category. Each of the applications includes the removal of the device, unless the device is removed by another physician (20665).

Implant removal codes are available for reporting the services of removal of buried wires, pins, rods, and so forth previously implanted by another physician or implanted by the same physician at a much earlier date. The implant removal codes are divided according to whether the implants are superficial or deep.

External fixation is the application of a device that holds a bone in place, but rather than internal fixation, the device is placed on the outside of the body and pins or wires are placed into the bone from the outside (Fig. 5–10). These wires and pins, when fastened to the bone, hold the device or system immobile. This type of fixation is commonly used with comminuted fractures that are difficult to hold in place. External fixation is used primarily in cases of limb fracture, major pelvic disruption, osteotomy, arthrodesis, bone infection, and bone lengthening.

The codes are divided according to whether the device or system is placed on one surface (uniplane) or several surfaces (multiplane). With the uni-

Figure 5–10 External fixation (Ilizarov multiplane).

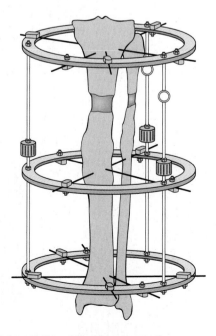

plane device, two or more pins are inserted above the fracture site and two or more pins are inserted below the fracture site. Multiplane devices are more complicated and are usually reserved for highly complex fractures.

STOP *The fixation devices codes are used in addition to the code for the treatment of the fracture, unless the application code specifically states that fracture repair is included. For example, see code 25545: "Open treatment of ulnar shaft fracture with or without internal or external fixation." Note also that the codes in the Introduction or Removal categories are for **unilateral** services, so if a procedure is bilateral you would add modifier -50.*

If the device is adjusted, the service is reported separately. Removal of external fixation devices or systems is usually accomplished under anesthesia and is coded separately from the application. However, if the removal does not require anesthesia, you would not report the service separately but would consider the removal as being bundled into the application code. If the removal was done outside the global period, some payers may reimburse it as an E/M service.

Grafts (or Implants)

Codes 20900–20938 are used to report the harvesting of bone, cartilage, fascia lata, or tissue through a incision separate from that used to implant the graft. Graft material is used in a wide variety of repair procedures. If, for example, a tibial fracture has failed to heal in 20 weeks, the surgeon may decide that the fracture requires bone grafting to achieve healing. Bone grafting is also used in cases of large defects (>6 cm). Some types of fractures commonly heal with difficulty, so after debridement and a 5- to 7-day healing period, the bone grafting procedure is performed. The grafts are obtained from the patient or a donor. Donors can be either living or deceased (a cadaver). The pieces of bone are shaped into bars or pegs and then used to repair the defect.

Fascia lata grafts are taken from the lower thigh area because the fascia is thickest in this area. Fascia is the fibrous tissue that serves as connective tissue; it is shaved off with an instrument called a stripper. The fascia lata is then used in the repair procedure. Codes for obtaining the fascia lata graft are based on whether a stripper was used to remove the fascia or whether a more complex removal procedure was required for removal of the graft material.

Tissue grafts include the obtaining of fat, dermis, paratenon, and other tissue types. **Spine surgery** codes 20930–20938 are used to report the obtaining and shaping of the tissue, whether from the patient (autograft) or from a donor (allograft). The obtaining and shaping of the spine graft material is reported in addition to reporting the implantation procedure, which is

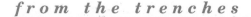

from the trenches

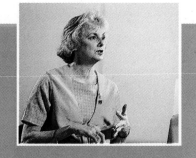

"*I heard an office manager say they didn't bill for a certain item because 'we never get paid for that.' They never used the codes!*"

SHIRLEY

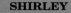

the main procedure (the definitive procedure), unless the description of the major procedure includes a graft. When reporting the obtaining of the graft and the main procedure, you do not use modifier -51, multiple procedures, as all of the codes in the category are exempt from modifier -51.

Other Procedures

Codes for monitoring muscles, microvascular bone grafts, microvascular flaps, and electronic/ultrasound stimulation are found under Other Procedures. **Monitoring of interstitial fluid pressure** (20950) is a procedure in which the physician inserts a device into the muscle to measure the pressure within the muscle. Increased pressure in the muscle indicates that the tissue is not receiving a sufficient supply of blood due to accumulation of fluid.

Bone grafts in this category are those that are performed to reconstruct the lower portion of the face. When the bone grafts are taken, the small blood vessels remain attached to the graft. The graft is then inserted and the blood vessels are attached to vessels in the area of implant, using an operating microscope. The bone grafts described by these codes are extremely complicated. The graft codes are divided based on where the bone is taken from—fibula, iliac crest, metatarsus, or another location.

Free osteocutaneous flaps are bone grafts that include the skin and tissue that overlie the bone. The skin and tissue are kept alive by the blood vessels from the bone. The surgeon then uses both the skin and tissue and the bone to reconstruct the defect, using an operating microscope. The flap procedures described by these codes are very complicated. The codes are divided based on which part of the body the flap is taken from. The grafts in the Other Procedures category differ from the grafts in the Grafts (or Implants) category; the codes in the Other Procedures category are used for grafts that include skin, blood vessels, and muscle as part of the graft.

Electric or **ultrasound stimulation** is used to promote healing. Low-voltage electricity or ultrasound is applied to the skin, and both are often used in the treatment of fractures.

The anatomic subheadings that follow the General subheading (e.g., head, neck, back, spine) contain codes divided based on the procedure, for example, incision, excision, or fracture. There are extensive notes throughout the Musculoskeletal System subsection that provide the specifics for reporting services using the codes. Many of the notes even tell you what specific anatomic areas the codes cover. For example, notes under the subheading Shoulder indicate that the areas covered are clavicle, scapula, humerus, head and neck, sternoclavicular joint, acromioclavicular joint, and shoulder joint. So be certain to read any notes carefully before using the codes.

CAUTION *As you use the codes, you will begin to know this background information, and the coding process will become faster for you. But at the beginning, reading the notes is the way to gain the knowledge that you are seeking. Now is not the time to take shortcuts.*

EXERCISE 5-2

GENERAL

Using the CPT manual, provide the codes for the following:

1 Exploration of a penetrating wound of the left leg

Code(s) _____

2 Replantation of right foot after a complete, traumatic amputation

Code(s) _____

3 Radical resection of malignant neoplasm of cheek

Code(s) _____

4 Nonoperative, electrical stimulation of nonhealing hip fracture

Code(s) _____

5 Percutaneous needle biopsy of muscle of upper arm, deep

Code(s) _____

6 Intra-articular aspiration and injection of finger joint

Code(s) _____

APPLICATION OF CASTS AND STRAPPING

Application of Casts and Strapping codes are used for subsequent treatment of fractures of the extremities, ligament sprains or tears, and overuse injuries. They may also be reported for the initial stabilization of an injury until definitive restorative treatment can be provided. Because each injury is unique, each cast is unique in terms of size and position. The cast immobilizes the fracture. Materials used to make casts are usually plaster, fiber-

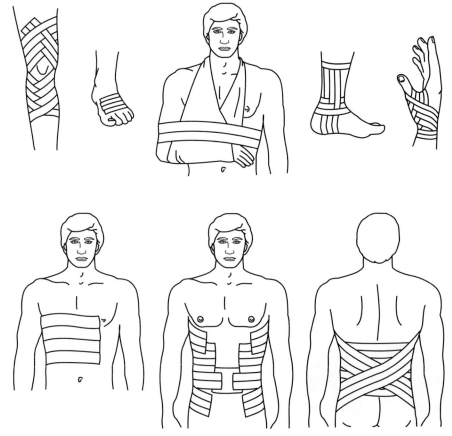

Figure 5–11 Types of strapping.

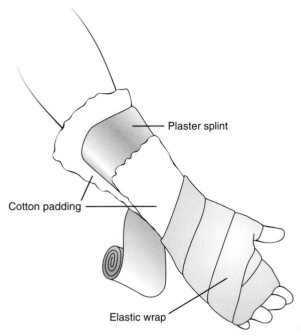

Plaster splint

Cotton padding

Elastic wrap

Figure 5–12   Splint used to immobilize a joint or bone.

glass, or thermoplastics. Each physician has a preference for the types of cast materials he or she uses. **Strapping** is the taping of a body part, as illustrated in Figure 5–11. Strapping is used to exert pressure on a body part to give it more stability; it is used in the treatment of sprains, strains, and dislocations. **Splints** are made of wood, cloth, or plastic, as illustrated in Figure 5–12, and are used to immobilize, support, or protect a body part, thereby allowing rest and healing. Both the **application** of the first cast, strapping, or splint and its later **removal** are included in each of the Application of Casts and Strapping codes.

STOP *If a cast, strapping, or splint is applied as a part of a **surgical procedure,** you do not use the codes from the Application of Casts and Strapping subheading to code for the service because the musculoskeletal surgical procedure codes include the first cast, strapping, or splint as well as its later removal. The surgery, application, and removal are all bundled into the surgical code.*

If the cast, strapping, or splint is applied as a part of a **fracture repair,** you also do not code for the service separately. The application service is bundled into all fracture repair codes, as is the removal service. If a second cast, strapping, or splint is applied within the follow-up period for either the surgical procedure or the fracture repair, you can bill for the application and the materials (99070). Most payers use A codes from HCPCS to report these services. You can bill for a separate office visit during which a second cast, strapping, or splint is applied only if the patient is provided some other, separate and significant service in addition to the application.

You can use the Application of Casts and Strapping codes only when the physician

• applies an initial cast, strapping, or splint for stabilization prior to definitive treatment.

- applies a subsequent cast, strapping, or splinting service.
- treats a sprain and does not expect to provide any additional treatment.

The subheading Application of Casts and Strapping is divided into three major categories:

- Body and Upper Extremity
- Lower Extremity
- Removal or Repair

The subcategories of Body/Upper Extremity and Lower Extremity are

- Casts
- Splints
- Strapping—Any Age

The codes in all subcategories are divided primarily according to the **location** of the cast, splint, or strapping on the body—head, hand, leg—and often on the **type**—Minerva, Velpeau, static, dynamic.

EXERCISE 5-3

APPLICATION OF CASTS AND STRAPPING

Using the CPT manual, provide the codes for the following:

1 Replacement of shoulder-to-hand (long-arm) cast

Code(s) _____

2 Initial application of a walking-type short leg cast for a sprain

Code(s) _____

3 Removal of a full leg cast by a physician who did not apply the cast

Code(s) _____

4 Strapping of a 46-year-old patient's knee

Code(s) _____

5 Replacement of a thigh-to-toes cast on the right leg of a 35-year-old female patient

Code(s) _____

ENDOSCOPY/ARTHROSCOPY

Arthroscopy is fast becoming the treatment of choice for many surgical procedures. The incisions are smaller, which decreases the risk of infection and speeds recovery time. Several small incisions are made through which lights, mirrors, and instruments are inserted. The arthroscopy codes are located separately at the end of the Musculoskeletal subsection. If multiple procedures are performed through a scope, they are reported with modifier -51. Bundled into all surgical arthroscopic procedure codes is the diagnostic arthroscopy. You must not unbundle and code a diagnostic arthroscopy and a surgical arthroscopy if both were performed during the same encounter. You also do not want to code separately for things done during a procedure that are considered a part of the procedure, such as shaving, removing, evacuating, casting, splinting, or strapping.

A note preceding the Endoscopy/Arthroscopy codes states, "When arthroscopy is performed in conjunction with arthrotomy, add modifier -51." This note indicates that if a surgeon performs an arthroscopy and during the procedure also does an arthrotomy, you can report both services. For example, a physician performs an arthroscopic shaving of the articular cartilage and also does an open capsulotomy (posterior capsular release) of the knee. Both the arthroscopic shaving (29877) and the capsulotomy (27435) would be reported, and to the least expensive procedure you would add modifier -51 (multiple procedures).

The codes in this subheading are divided according to body area—elbow, shoulder, knee—and then according to the type and extent of procedure performed. An example of type of service is as follows: code 29815 is for an arthroscopy of the shoulder for **diagnostic** purposes, whereas code 29819 is an arthroscopy of the shoulder for a **surgical** procedure. Not only are there two different codes for surgical and diagnostic arthroscopy procedures, but also the surgical procedure is significantly more expensive than the diagnostic procedure. So great care must be taken to select the code that correctly describes the services supported in the medical record.

Note the description for code 29805: "Arthroscopy, shoulder, diagnostic, with or without synovial biopsy (separate procedure)." You will find the statement "separate procedure" several times in the Endoscopy/Arthroscopy subheading because oftentimes, an arthroscopic procedure is part of a larger procedure. You cannot report the service of the arthroscopy unless it has been performed as an independent, separate procedure. Also note that the parenthetical information following the codes indicates the codes to use if the procedure was done as an open (incisional) procedure rather than as an endoscopic procedure.

EXERCISE 5-4

ENDOSCOPY/ARTHROSCOPY

Using the CPT manual, provide the codes for the following:

1   Surgical arthroscopy of ankle, which included extensive debridement

    Code(s) _____

2   Diagnostic knee arthroscopy with a synovial biopsy

    Code(s) _____

3   Diagnostic shoulder arthroscopy

    Code(s) _____

4   Arthroscopic repair of tuberosity fracture of knee with manipulation

    Code(s) _____

5   Surgical arthroscopy of ankle, including drilling and excision of tibial defect

    Code(s) _____

CHAPTER GLOSSARY

arthrodesis: surgical immobilization of a joint

arthroplasty: reshaping or reconstruction of a joint

aspiration: use of a needle and a syringe to withdraw fluid

closed treatment: fracture site that is not surgically opened and visualized

curettage: scraping of a cavity using a spoon-shaped instrument

dislocation: placement in a location other than the original location

endoscopy: inspection of body organs or cavities using a lighted scope that may be inserted through an existing opening or through a small incision

fracture: break in a bone

internal/external fixation: application of pins, wires, screws, and so on to immobilize a body part; they can be placed externally or internally

lysis: releasing

manipulation or reduction: words used interchangeably to mean the attempted restoration of a fracture or joint dislocation to its normal anatomic position

open treatment: fracture site that is surgically opened and visualized

percutaneous: through the skin

percutaneous skeletal fixation: considered neither open nor closed; the fracture is not visualized, but fixation is placed across the fracture site under x-ray imaging

traction: application of force to a limb

trocar needle: needle with a tube on the end; used to puncture and withdraw fluid from a cavity

CHAPTER REVIEW

CHAPTER 5, PART 1, THEORY

Without the use of reference material, complete the following:

1   The Musculoskeletal System subsection is formatted according to what type of sites?

_____

2   Which subspecialty would most often use the codes found in the Musculoskeletal System subsection?

_____

3   List the three types of fracture treatments and briefly describe each:

_____

_____

_____

_____

_____

4   The type of fracture treatment used by the physician depends upon the type of

_____ being repaired.

5   _____ is the application of pulling force to hold a bone in place.

6   What is the term that describes the physician's actions of bending, rotating, pulling, or guiding the bone back into place?

_____

7   What term is used to mean "put the bone back in place"? _____

8   What term describes a bone that is not in its normal location? _____

9   What term describes the cleaning of a wound?

_____

10   This is a hollow needle that is often used to withdraw samples of fluid from a joint:

_____

11   Would a biopsy code usually include the administration of any necessary anesthesia?

_____

CHAPTER 5, PART II, PRACTICAL

With the use of the CPT manual, complete the following:

12   Incision of a superficial soft tissue abscess, secondary to osteomyelitis

Code(s) _____

13 Radical resection of a malignant neoplasm of the soft tissue of the upper back

Code(s) _____

14 Closed treatment of three vertebral process fractures

Code(s) _____

15 Under general anesthesia, manipulation of a right shoulder joint fracture and application of cast

Code(s) _____

16 Lengthening of four tendons of elbow

Code(s) _____

17 Incision and drainage of bursa of elbow

Code(s) _____

18 Open treatment of a carpal scaphoid fracture with external fixation applied

Code(s) _____

19 Arthroplasty of four metacarpophalangeal joints

Code(s) _____

20 Tenotomy of two tendons

Code(s) _____

21 Amputation, lower arm, using Krukenberg procedure

Code(s) _____

22 Open treatment of radial and ulnar shaft fractures with internal fixation of both radius and ulna

Code(s) _____

23 Osteoplasty requiring shortening of both of radius and ulna

Code(s) _____

24 Fasciotomy for tennis elbow

Code(s) _____

25 Replantation of right arm, including the neck of the humerus through the elbow joint, following a complete traumatic amputation

Code(s) _____

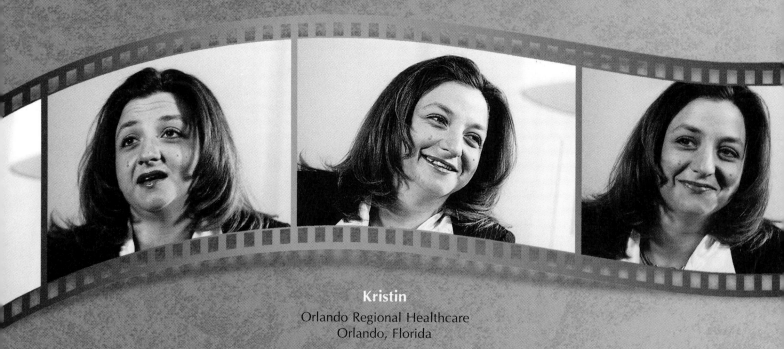

Kristin
Orlando Regional Healthcare
Orlando, Florida

chapter 6

Respiratory System

LEARNING OBJECTIVES

After completing this chapter you should be able to

1 Understand and apply rules of coding respiratory services.

2 Differentiate among codes on the basis of surgical approach.

3 Apply respiratory codes to service/procedure statements.

4 Identify the extent of endoscopic procedures.

5 Demonstrate knowledge of respiratory terminology.

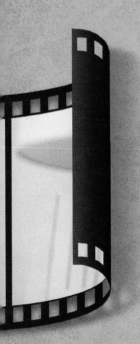

FORMAT

The Respiratory System subsection is arranged by anatomic site (e.g., nose, sinus, larynx) and then by procedure (e.g., incision, excision, introduction). Your knowledge of respiratory terminology is important (Fig. 6–1), as the coding you will learn about in the Respiratory System subsection covers the respiratory system of the entire body. In the Musculoskeletal section, the arthroscopy codes were placed at the end of the subsection, but in the Respiratory subsection, the endoscopy codes are listed throughout according to anatomic site. Fracture repair, such as of the nose or sternum, is listed in the Musculoskeletal subsection, not in the Respiratory subsection. Procedures that are performed on the throat or mouth are not located in the Respiratory System subsection, but instead are located in the Digestive System subsection.

The Respiratory subsection contains some codes that may be considered cosmetic. It is important to note the extent of the cosmetic repair indicated in the patient's medical record. The extent is important so that you do not report the same service more than once and unbundle a code. For example, under the subheading Nose and the category Repair, there is code 30420 for rhinoplasty. The rhinoplasty can be performed either through external skin incisions (open) or through intranasal incisions (closed), and both approaches can be coded to 30420. The extent of the procedure varies based on the desired outcome, but a rhinoplasty can include fracturing a deformed septum, repositioning the septum, reshaping and/or augmenting the nasal cartilage, removing fat from the area and performing a layered closure, and applying a splint or cast. If all of these components of a rhinoplasty were performed, they would all be bundled into code 30420. You have to read all of the notes and the code information carefully to ensure that each service provided to the patient is reported only once.

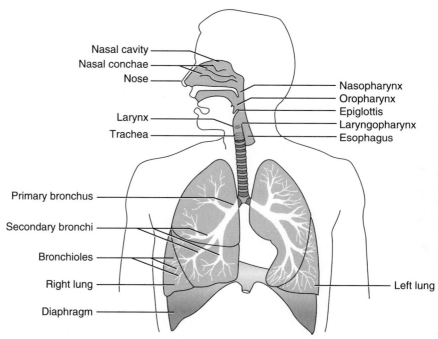

Figure 6–1   Respiratory system.

CODING HIGHLIGHTS

Endoscopy

In endoscopic procedures, a scope is placed through an existing body orifice (opening), or a small incision is made into a cavity for scope placement.

When sinus endoscopies are done, a scope is placed through the nose into the nasal cavity. Codes for sinuses are used to report unilateral (on one side) procedures except in the case of a diagnostic nasal endoscopy, which is unilateral or bilateral. Multiple procedures may be done within different sinuses (anterior and posterior sinuses, ethmoidal sinuses, sphenoidal sinuses, and frontal sinuses) during the same operative session. The CPT manual has combined into a single code some multiple sinus procedures commonly performed at the same operative session.

EXAMPLE

31276   Nasal/sinus endoscopy, surgical with frontal sinus exploration with or without removal of tissue from frontal sinus

CAUTION *Code to the* full extent *of the procedure.*

Endoscopic procedures may start at one site (such as the nose) and follow through to another site (such as the larynx or bronchial tubes). It is important to choose the code that most appropriately reflects the full extent of the procedure. For example, if a direct laryngoscopy (31515) is performed, the scope is progressed past the larynx and can include examination of the trachea. The 31515 code description states either with or without tracheoscopy. However, if it is necessary to continue the procedure to the bronchial tubes, the only code used would be 31622 (bronchoscopy). The larynx and trachea must be passed to get to the bronchial tubes and can be visualized while progressing to the farthest point (bronchial tubes).

CAUTION *Code the* correct approach *for the procedure.*

The same surgical procedure may be performed using different approaches. For example, code 32141 describes a thoracotomy with "excision-plication (removal/shortening) of bullae (blisters); with or without any pleural procedure." Code 32655 describes a surgical thoracoscopy with excision-plication of bullae, including any pleural procedures. Code 32655 describes the same procedure as 32141, except that 32655 is a procedure done through very minute incisions utilizing a thorascope, whereas code 32141 describes an open incision through the thorax, opening the full operative site to the surgeon.

Multiple endoscopic procedures may be performed through the scope during the same operative session. When this occurs, each procedure should be coded with modifier -51 (multiple procedures) placed on subsequent procedure(s). Suppose, for example, a bronchoscopy with biopsy is performed as well as a bronchoscopy with removal of a foreign body. Not only would you code a bronchoscopy, but you would also code the removal of a foreign body. The multiple procedure modifier -51 would have to be placed after the lower priced (resource-intensive) procedure.

The exception to this occurs when the CPT manual offers a code for which the description includes all the separate elements of the procedure bundled into one code.

CAUTION *Do not confuse the nasal/sinus endoscopic procedures with the intranasal procedures! Intranasal procedures may require surgical instruments' being **placed into** the nose but do not require the use of an endoscope. When an endoscope is used in a nasal/sinus procedure, use a nasal/sinus endoscopy code.*

Remember that a diagnostic endoscopy is always bundled into a surgical endoscopy. For example, if a physician began a diagnostic endoscopic nasal procedure and continued on to complete a surgical procedure, you code only for the surgical procedure. To code for both a diagnostic *and* surgical nasal endoscopy is unbundling.

When coding laryngoscopic procedure, note that the terms "indirect" and "direct" are often used. For example, see codes 31505, indirect, and 31515, direct. **Indirect** in 31505 means that the physician uses a tongue depressor to hold the tongue down and view the epiglottis (the lid that covers the larynx) with a mirror. The patient vocalizes (says "ah") and the physician can then view the vocal cords. **Direct** in 31515 means that the endoscope is passed into the larynx and the physician can look directly at the larynx through the endoscope. The patient's operative note will indicate whether the procedure was indirect or direct.

Locating Endoscopy Codes

Endoscopy codes can be located in the CPT manual index under Endoscopy and then under the anatomic subterm of the site. You can also locate an endoscopic procedure by the anatomic endoscopy title. For example, a bronchial biopsy using endoscopy would be listed under Bronchoscopy and then under the subterm Biopsy.

EXERCISE 6-1

ENDOSCOPY

Using the CPT manual, complete the following:

1 Surgical maxillary antrostomy using endoscopy

   Code(s): _____

2 Direct laryngoscopy for removal of fish bone

   Code(s): _____

3 After the airway is sufficiently anesthetized, a flexible bronchoscope is inserted through the mouth and advanced to the bronchus, where a transbronchial biopsy of the lung is obtained.

   Code(s): _____

4 Diagnostic thoracoscopy of the mediastinal space is accomplished with the use of a flexible endoscope that is inserted through a small incision on the chest.

   Code(s): _____

5 Segmental resection of the right lung using a flexible endoscope (surgical thoracoscopy)

   Code(s): _____

NOSE

Many of the codes in the Nose subheading are used by physicians who specialize in treating conditions of the nose (otorhinolaryngologist; ear, nose, and throat specialists), but there are also many codes in the subheading that are more widely used. For example, it is in the Nose subheading that you will find the codes for the following services: control of nosebleeds, incision of abscesses, removal of foreign objects from the nose (think children!), and removal of nasal cysts and lesions, all of which are commonly performed as office procedures.

Incision

Codes for incision of a nasal abscess are divided on the basis of whether the abscess is on the nasal mucosa or the septal mucosa. If a nasal abscess is approached from the outside of the nose (external approach), you would use a code from the Integumentary System subsection; but if the approach is from the inside of the nose (internal approach), you would use a code from the Respiratory System subsection. The medical record will describe the approach procedure used and the approach procedure will direct you to the correct subsection.

After the abscess has been penetrated, the physician may place a tube in the incision to ensure that the pus continues to drain from the abscess area. After the drain is removed, the abscess may be packed with gauze, with one end of the packing material left outside the surface to act as a wick, as illustrated in Figure 6–2A to C. The incision may also be closed immediately if it is felt that further drainage is not necessary. The insertion and removal of the tube and/or gauze and any required sutures and/or anesthesia are bundled into the code, so you should not report these services separately. You should report any additional supplies over and above those usually used for the procedure by using the Medicine section code for supplies, 99070, or a HCPCS code, as directed by the payer.

Excision

Within the Nose subheading, the Excision category contains a wide range of procedures that describe removal of tissue from the nose—for example, biopsy, polyp excision, and cyst excision—as well as resection of the turbinate bone.

from the trenches

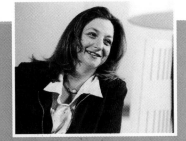

What advice would give to a new coder?
"Know your anatomy and physiology like the back of your hand. Also, practice, practice, practice . . . and always be willing to challenge yourself and learn new areas. Most important, 'not documented, not done!'"

KRISTIN

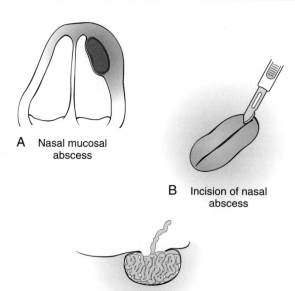

A   Nasal mucosal
abscess

B   Incision of nasal
abscess

C   Gauze packed into abscess
with end extending outside,
acting as a wick

Figure 6-2 *A,* Nasal mucosal abscess. *B,* Incision of abscess. *C,* Gauze packed into abscess with the end extending outside the abscess, acting as a wick.

The **biopsy** code (30100) is used for a biopsy that is done intranasally; but for a biopsy of the skin outside of the nose, you would use the biopsy code (11100) from the Integumentary System.

The excision of **nasal polyps** has two codes (30110 and 30115), with the difference between the codes being the extent of the excision. Code 30110 is used for a simple polyp excision that would usually be performed in the physician's office, whereas 30115 is used for a more extensive polyp excision that would usually be performed in a hospital setting.

coding shot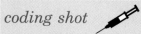

Use modifier -50 (bilateral) if the polyps are removed from both the left and right sides of the nose.

The codes for excision or destruction of **lesions** inside the nose are divided based on the approach—internal or external.

STOP *Usually, if the approach to the procedure has been external, you are referred to the Integumentary System subsection to locate the correct code; but the nasal lesion excision/destruction codes can be used for either an external or an internal approach to a lesion.*

You have to read the code descriptions carefully to ensure that you understand all of the circumstances that surround using the code, and you have to identify codes such as the lesion excision/destruction codes that are exceptions to the usual rules.

All methods of lesion destruction, including laser, are included in the Excision codes. Usually, if laser was used in the destruction of a lesion, you would be referred to a separate set of codes just for laser destruction; but with the lesion destruction codes in the Nose category, laser is included as one of the destruction methods.

coding shot

If the lesion destruction or excision is bilateral, remember to use modifier -50.

Turbinates are the bones on the outside of the nose; they are divided into three sections—inferior, middle, and superior (Fig. 6–3). Portions of or all of a turbinate bone may be removed for cosmetic reasons or because of neoplastic growth. Because third-party payers usually do not pay for cosmetic surgical procedures, you must document the noncosmetic procedures carefully to ensure appropriate reimbursement. Watch for and read the extensive notes inside the parentheses throughout this category.

Introduction

Introduction codes include injection, displacement therapy, and insertion. **Injections** into the turbinates are therapeutic injections usually used to shrink the nasal tissue to improve breathing. For example, if a patient has inflamed nasal passages due to an allergic reaction or a deviated septum, he or she may benefit from a steroid injection into the turbinates. **Displacement therapy** is a procedure in which the physician flushes saline solution into the sinuses to remove mucus or pus. The insertion of a **nasal button** is a technique used for a patient who has a hole in the septum. The physician places the button into the hole and fastens the button in place with sutures. The button is usually made of silicone or rubber. This technique is used as a method to repair the septum without surgical grafting.

Removal of a Foreign Body

A variety of objects are inserted into the various orifices (openings) of the body, and the nose is a common place into which these foreign objects are placed. The code to report an office procedure for the removal of a foreign

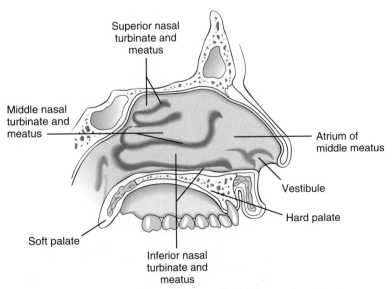

Figure 6–3 Superior, inferior, and middle nasal turbinates.

body from the nose is 30300. Codes for more extensive procedures are also available for removal of foreign objects from the nose, such as those requiring general anesthesia and a more invasive surgical procedure.

Repair

Within the Repair category you will find the plastic procedures—rhinoplasty, septoplasty, and septal dermatoplasty. **Rhinoplasty** is a procedure used to reshape the nose internally, externally, or both. The codes are divided based on the extent (minor, intermediate, major), on whether the septum was also repaired (septoplasty), and on whether the procedure was an initial or secondary procedure. **Secondary** procedures are those that are done after an initial procedure. For example, if a rhinoplasty was performed and the results were not as successful as the patient desired, the surgeon could perform a second procedure (secondary) to improve the result.

Septoplasty is rearrangement of the nasal septum. This procedure is commonly performed in a patient with a deviated septum.

CAUTION *Do not use a septoplasty code if the operative report indicates that only a resection of the turbinate(s) was performed. The resection of the turbinate(s) is reported with 30140 and is not a procedure done on the septum. The septoplasty code, 30520, is used when the nasal septum is resected. There is a note enclosed in parentheses following both codes— 30140 and 30520—that cautions you to use the correct code, which is determined by whether the turbinate or the septum was resected.*

Destruction

Destruction can be accomplished by using either cauterization or ablation. **Ablation** is removal, usually by cutting. Ablation or cauterization is used to remove excess nasal mucosa or to reduce inflammation. The destruction codes are divided according to the extent of the procedure—superficial or intramural. **Intramural** is ablation or cauterization of the deeper mucosa, as compared to **superficial** ablation or cauterization, which involves only the outer layer of mucosa.

Other Procedures

The codes for the control of nasal hemorrhage are located in the Other Procedures category and are used often. Anterior packing is packing inserted through the nose. Posterior packing is inserted through the mouth and into the back of the nose. Packing is pushing gauze into the nose to apply pressure against the side that is bleeding (Fig. 6–4). A posterior hemorrhage is more difficult to control. In the case of a posterior hemorrhage, the physician may need to place extensive packing into the nose and use extensive cauterization. A balloon may be inserted and inflated to further control bleeding (Fig. 6–5). The codes are divided according to the type and extent of control required.

coding shot

The key to correctly coding nasal hemorrhage is focusing on the type of control.

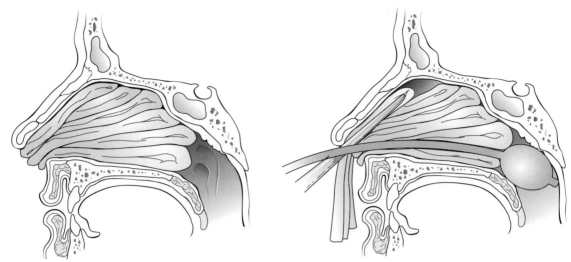

Figure 6-4 Anterior nasal packing.   **Figure 6-5** Posterior nasal packing.

There are times when neither cauterization nor packing will control a nasal hemorrhage, and ligation of the bleeding artery may be necessary. Ligation of ethmoidal arteries involves opening the upper side of the nose and locating and tying the ethmoid artery. Ligation of the internal maxillary artery is performed to gain control of nasal hemorrhage by locating and ligating the maxillary artery.

A **therapeutic fracture** of the nasal turbinate is a procedure in which the physician fractures the turbinate bone and then repositions it. The patient receives a local anesthetic. Repositioning the turbinate(s) often alleviates obstructed airflow caused by a previous fracture that has healed out of alignment and resulted in a deviation of the nose.

EXERCISE 6-2

NOSE

Using the CPT manual, complete the following:

1 Biopsy of an intranasal lesion

   Code(s): _____

2 Primary rhinoplasty including complex septal repair

   Code(s): _____

3 Anterior control of nasal hemorrhage by means of limited chemical cauterization and simple packing

   Code(s): _____

4 Septoplasty with contouring and grafting

   Code(s): _____

5 Removal of crayon from nose of 5-year-old boy, conducted as an office procedure

   Code(s): _____

ACCESSORY SINUSES

Incision

Within the Incision category are codes for services that you would not think of as being incisional. For example, the nasal sinuses can be washed (lavage) with a saline solution introduced through canula (hollow tube) to remove infection. The Incision category code 31000 describes lavage of the maxillary sinus. Lavage can be done to both the maxillary and the sphenoid sinuses (Fig. 6–6). If the lavage is of the sphenoid sinus, you use 31002 to describe the service. Both codes (31000 and 31002) are followed by an asterisk to indicate that the service includes the surgical procedure only and does not usually include any follow-up care.

> *coding shot*
>
> Use modifier -50 (bilateral) if the lavage is for both the left and right maxillary sinuses.

Many of the codes in the Incision category are for sinusotomies. A **sinusotomy** is a procedure in which the physician enlarges the passage or creates a new passage from the nasal cavity into a sinus. This procedure is performed when a patient has a chronic sinus infection; the procedure enables improved sinus drainage. The codes are divided according to the extent of the procedure.

EXERCISE
6–3

ACCESSORY SINUSES

Using the CPT manual, complete the following:

1   Lavage of the maxillary sinus, bilateral

   Code(s): _____

2   Simple frontal sinusotomy using an external approach

   Code(s): _____

3   Unilateral sinusotomy of frontal, ethmoid, and sphenoid

   Code(s): _____

4   Radical sinusotomy

   Code(s): _____

5   Total intranasal ethmoidectomy

   Code(s): _____

LARYNX

The procedures covered by the Larynx subheading include a wide range of surgical procedures, such as tracheostomy, plastic repair, and nerve destruc-

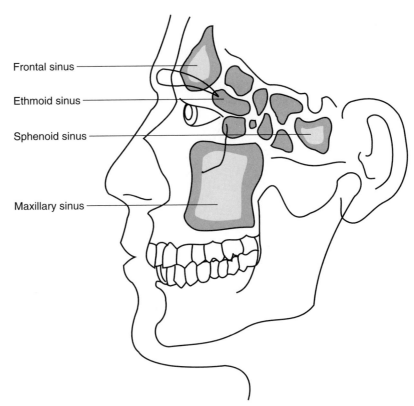

Figure 6–6   Paranasal sinuses.

tion. Make certain that you understand the terminology used in the Excision category before you code in the category.

Excision

Laryngotomy is an incision that is made over the larynx (tracheostomy) to expose the larynx to view. With the larynx exposed, the physician can remove a tumor, a laryngocele (air-filled space), or a vocal cord (cordectomy). A laryngotomy can also be performed for diagnostic purposes, without a surgical procedure's being performed.

CAUTION *Be careful not to get the codes from the Laryngotomy category confused with the tracheostomy codes located in the Trachea and Bronchi subheading, Incision category, which you will learn more about later in this chapter. The codes from the two categories differ, depending on the purpose of the procedure. The Laryngotomy category codes describe procedures in which the surgeon performs a tracheostomy for the purpose of exposing the larynx. The codes in the Trachea and Bronchi subheading Incision describe a procedure in which the surgeon performs only the tracheostomy, usually to establish airflow, and no procedure or exposure of the larynx is planned or is involved.*

Radical neck dissection, as referred to in the codes for laryngectomy, is the removal not only of the larynx but also of lymph glands and/or other surrounding tissue. Many of the codes in the Larynx subheading, Excision category, are divided according to whether radical neck dissection was or was not performed. The operative report would indicate the extent of the dissection by referring to excision of lymph nodes in a radical procedure.

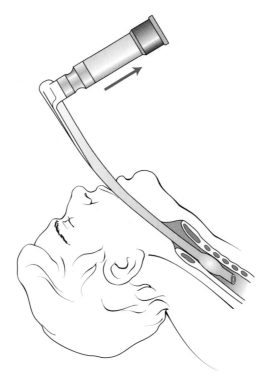

Figure 6–7   Endotracheal intubation.

Introduction

Intubation is the establishment of an airway in a patient. The intubation represented in 31500 is provided on an emergency basis at such time as the patient experiences respiratory failure or the occurrence of an inadequate airway. Figure 6–7 illustrates endotracheal intubation. The other Introduction code is for the replacement of a previously inserted tracheostomy tube.

Repair

Within the Repair category are several plastic procedures. A laryngoplasty for a **laryngeal web** is surgical procedure, usually done in two stages, for the repair of congenital webbing between the vocal cords. The surgeon removes the webbing and places a spacer between the vocal cords. At a later time, the surgeon will again expose the vocal cords, using the same tracheostomy incision made on the initial procedure, and remove the spacer.

Closed **laryngeal fracture** repair is found in the Repair category. The codes are divided according to whether the fracture required manipulation to properly align (reduce) the larynx.

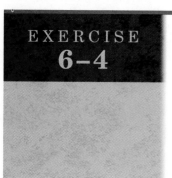

EXERCISE
6–4

LARYNX

Using the CPT manual, complete the following:

1   Diagnostic laryngotomy

Code(s): _____

2   Laryngoplasty, stage two, for repair of congenital laryngeal web, removal of spacer

Code(s): _____

3 Emergency establishment of positive airway by means of endotracheal intubation

Code(s): _____

4 Partial supraglottic laryngectomy with removal of adjacent lymph nodes and tissue

Code(s): _____

5 Pharyngolaryngectomy with radical neck dissection

Code(s): _____

TRACHEA AND BRONCHI

Procedures in the Trachea and Bronchi subheading include incisions, introductions, and repairs, in addition to the endoscopic procedures.

Incision

Tracheostomy is the major procedure in the Incision category. A tracheostomy can be planned or can be performed as an emergency procedure. A planned tracheostomy is usually done when there is a need for prolonged ventilation support, beyond the level of support that can be provided by

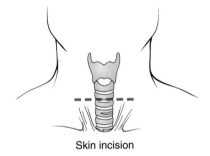

Figure 6–8   Transverse incision used in a transtracheal approach.

Skin incision

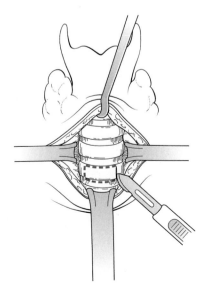

Figure 6–9   Transtracheal entry into the trachea using the transtracheal approach.

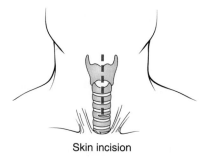

Skin incision

Figure 6–10 Vertical incision made for a cricothyroid tracheostomy.

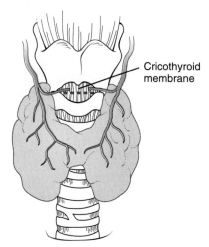

Cricothyroid membrane

Figure 6–11 Cricothyroid entry into the trachea.

endotracheal intubation, or when a patient cannot tolerate an endotracheal tube. Note that code 31603 is used for a **transtracheal** tracheostomy, and code 31605 is used for a **cricothyroid** tracheostomy. These codes represent two different approaches to establishing an airway. Figure 6–8 illustrates the transverse (across) incision used in a transtracheal approach; it is made between the cricoid cartilage and the sternal notch. Figure 6–9 illustrates entry into the trachea using the transtracheal approach. Figure 6–10 illustrates the vertical incision made for a cricothyroid tracheostomy. Figure 6–11 shows the entry into the trachea using the cricothyroid approach.

Introduction

Codes in the Introduction category are for the catheterization, instillation, injection, and aspiration of the trachea and the placement of tubes into the trachea.

A **transglottic catheterization** is one in which the physician punctures the glottis (vocal apparatus) with a needle and inserts a catheter to establish a passage. The catheter is held in place by a suture affixed to the skin and then tied to the catheter.

Some of the Introduction codes represent the instillation of **contrast material** into the larynx to improve viewing during bronchographic procedures. The contrast material is suspended in a gas that the patient inhales. The gas contains radiant energy that appears darker on the x-ray if there is an obstruction in the area, such as a tumor. Codes from the Radiology section are used in conjunction with injection of contrast material. For example, if a physician provided the service of a bronchography with contrast material injection, you would use code 31715 for the service of injecting the contrast material into the trachea, and 71040 for the supervision and interpretation of the unilateral bronchography. The injection of contrast material is not bundled into the radiology service for a bronchography, so you would have to code each part (component) of the service separately.

Repair

Repair procedures in the Trachea and Bronchi subheading include the plastic repairs, such as tracheoplasty and bronchoplasty, in addition to the excision of stenosis or of tumors, the suturing of tracheal wounds, and scar revision.

Tracheoplasty involves the surgical repair of a damaged trachea. The repair may involve reconstruction of the trachea by the use of grafts or splints formed from cartilage taken from other areas of the body or by the use of prostheses. The codes are divided according to the approach used (cervical or thoracic) and the extent and type of repair.

Bronchoplasty is the repair of the bronchus; it often involves the use of grafting repair or stents. A chest tube may be left in the area after the procedure as a drain and is not reported separately. The grafting procedure is part of the bronchoplasty code 31770.

EXERCISE 6-5

TRACHEA AND BRONCHI

Using the CPT manual, complete the following:

1 Emergency tracheostomy, cricothyroid approach

   Code(s): _____

2 Excision of a tumor of the trachea using a cervical approach

   Code(s): _____

3 Transtracheal injection for bronchography (code only the injection procedure)

   Code(s): _____

4 Planned tracheostomy in 47-year-old patient

   Code(s): _____

5 Catheterization with bronchial brush biopsy

   Code(s): _____

LUNGS AND PLEURA

The Lungs and Pleura subheading includes a wide range of codes that cover such procedures as thoracentesis, thoracostomy, and pneumonostomy, in addition to lung transplants and plastic procedures.

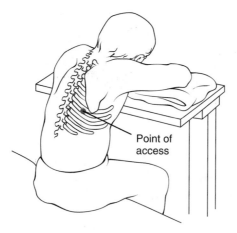

Figure 6–12 Patient in position for a thoracentesis.

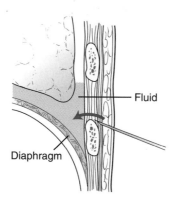

Figure 6–13 After administration of local anesthesia, a needle is inserted between the ribs, and fluid is withdrawn (thoracentesis).

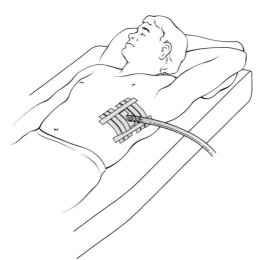

Figure 6–14 A chest tube may be inserted after thoracentesis to allow for further draining of fluid.

Incision

Thoracentesis is accomplished by having the patient sit with arms supported, as illustrated in Figure 6–12; local anesthesia is administered, a needle is inserted (Fig. 6–13) between the ribs, and fluid is withdrawn. Thoracentesis is performed to withdraw from the pleural space fluid that has accumulated as a result of a variety of conditions, such as congestive heart failure, pneumonia, tuberculosis, or carcinoma.

Thoracentesis may also be performed to insert a **chest tube** as an indwelling method of draining the accumulated fluid in the pleural space (pleural effusion), as illustrated in Figure 6–14. Local anesthesia is administered, and a small incision is made through the skin, fat, and muscle. The hole is then enlarged by using an instrument, and the tube is inserted into the pleural space. A suture is placed through the skin and tied to the tube. The tube is then secured with tape. The fluid is withdrawn by means of a suction device called a multichamber water-seal suction tube. This therapeutic procedure may be performed when the patient's pleural space contains air or gas (pneumothorax), blood (hemothorax), or a large amount of fluid (pleural effusion). These conditions can be caused by trauma, can be secondary to another disease process, or can occur spontaneously.

Thoracotomy is the procedure of making a surgical incision into the chest wall and opening the area to the view of the surgeon. This is a major surgical procedure in which the patient is under general anesthesia. The codes are divided according to the reason for the procedure, such as biopsy, control of bleeding, cyst removal, foreign body removal, and cardiac massage.

coding shot

As a part of a thoracotomy, the surgeon may insert a chest tube to allow for continued drainage of the surgical area. The placement of this tube is bundled into the surgical procedure, so you would not code separately for the placement of the tube.

Excision

The Excision category contains codes for pleurectomy, biopsy, pneumonocentesis, removal, and reconstructive lung procedures.

Pleurectomy is a procedure in which the physician opens the chest cavity to full view. With the chest open and the ribs spread apart by a rib spreader, the parietal pleura is removed. If a pleurectomy is done as part of another, more major procedure such as the removal of a lung (lobectomy), you would not report the pleurectomy separately. Note that after code 32310, pleurectomy, there is a note concerning "separate procedure," warning you not to report a separate pleurectomy if the pleurectomy was performed as a part of a more major procedure.

from the trenches

"*Good, experienced, educated coders are much in demand . . . . It seems positions are always available. Do it!*"

KRISTIN

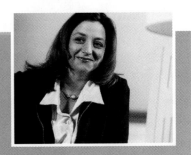

Percutaneous needle lung or mediastinum **biopsy** is often performed under radiologic guidance so that correct placement of the needle can be ensured. As with the bronchography procedure described earlier, in the discussion of the Trachea and Bronchi subheading, if radiologic guidance was used, you also use a code from the Radiology section to describe the guidance service. There is a note following code 32405 (biopsy) that directs you to the Surgery section, General subsection, code 10022, when a fine-needle aspiration is performed.

Pneumocentesis is the withdrawal of fluid from the lung by means of an aspirating needle. Air or gas in the pleural cavity is known as pneumo-thorax and is caused when the lung is traumatically ruptured or an emphy-sema bulla ruptures. Pneumothorax increases the pressure on the lung and can result in the collapse of the lung. The surgeon withdraws the fluid to allow the lung to reinflate.

The codes for the removal of the lung are based on how much of the lung is removed—segmentectomy for one segment, lobectomy for one lobe, bilo-bectomy for two lobes, total pneumonectomy for an entire lung—as well as on the extent of the procedure and the approach. If a part of the bron-chus was removed or repaired at the same time as the lobectomy or seg-mentectomy, you would indicate the service with the use of the add-on code 32501.

Surgical Collapse Therapy; Thoracoplasty

Thoracoplasty is a procedure in which a portion of the internal skeletal support is removed to treat a condition in which pus chronically collects in the chest cavity (chronic thoracic empyema). The procedure is major and requires extensive resecting of the membrane that lines the chest cavity. Gauze is left in the cavity and after several days it is removed. Note that code 32905, thoracoplasty, refers to "all stages." The subsequent stages are for the removal of the packing. Thoracoplasty procedures may also require the use of muscle grafting to close a bronchopleural fistula.

Pneumonolysis is a procedure that is performed to separate the inside of the chest cavity from the lung to permit the collapse of the lung.

Pneumothorax injection is a therapeutic procedure in which the sur-geon inserts a needle into the pleural cavity and injects air into the pleural cavity. The pressure on the lung is increased and the lung partially col-lapses. This procedure is sometimes performed to treat tuberculosis. A chest tube may be inserted into the space for further injections of air. You would not bill separately for the insertion of the chest tube, as the insertion is bundled into the procedure code.

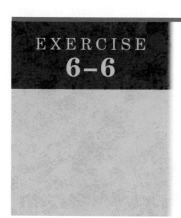

EXERCISE 6-6

LUNGS AND PLEURA

Using the CPT manual, complete the following:

1 A limited thoracotomy for lung biopsy

Code(s): _____

2 Percutaneous lung biopsy

Code(s): _____

3 Lobectomy and bronchoplasty performed at same surgical session

Code(s): _____

4 Lung resection with chest wall resection

Code(s): _____

5 Pneumonostomy with open drainage of abscess

Code(s): _____

CHAPTER GLOSSARY

ablation: removal by cutting

bilobectomy: surgical removal of two lobes of a lung

bronchoplasty: surgical repair of the bronchi

bronchoscopy: inspection of the bronchial tree using a bronchoscope

catheter: tube placed into the body to put fluid in or take fluid out

cauterization: destruction of tissue by the use of cautery

cordectomy: surgical removal of the vocal cord(s)

dermatoplasty: surgical repair of the skin

drainage: free flow or withdrawal of fluids from a wound or cavity

epiglottidectomy: excision of the covering of the larynx

intramural: within the organ wall

intubation: insertion of a tube

laryngeal web: congenital abnormality of connective tissue between the vocal cords

laryngectomy: surgical removal of the larynx

laryngo-: prefix meaning larynx

laryngoplasty: surgical repair of the larynx

laryngoscope: fiberoptic scope used to view the inside of the larynx

laryngoscopy: viewing of the larynx using a fiberoptic scope

laryngotomy: incision into the larynx

lavage: washing out of an organ

lobectomy: surgical excision of a lobe of the lung

nasal button: a synthetic circular disk used to cover a hole in the nasal septum

pharyngolaryngectomy: surgical removal of the pharynx and larynx

pleurectomy: surgical excision of the pleura

pneumonocentesis: surgical puncturing of a lung to withdraw fluid

pneumonolysis: surgical separation of the lung from the chest wall to allow the lung to collapse

pneumonostomy: surgical procedure in which the chest cavity is exposed and the lung is incised

pneumonotomy: incision of the lung

rhino-: prefix meaning nose

rhinoplasty: surgical repair of the nose

segmentectomy: surgical removal of a portion of a lung

septoplasty: surgical repair of the nasal septum

sinusotomy: surgical incision into a sinus

thoracentesis: surgical puncture of the thoracic cavity, usually using a needle, to remove fluids

thoracoplasty: surgical procedure that removes rib(s) and thereby allows the collapse of a lung

thoracoscopy: use of a lighted endoscope to view the pleural spaces and thoracic cavity or perform surgical procedures

thoracostomy: surgical incision into the chest wall and insertion of a chest tube

thoracotomy: surgical incision into the chest wall

total pneumonectomy: surgical removal of an entire lobe of a lung

tracheostomy: creation of an opening into the trachea

tracheotomy: incision into the trachea

transglottictracheoplasty: surgical repair of the vocal apparatus and trachea

transtracheal: across the trachea

CHAPTER REVIEW

CHAPTER 6, PART I, THEORY

Without the use of reference material, complete the following:

1 The Respiratory System subsection is arranged by _____ site.

2 The procedure in which a scope is placed through a small incision and into a body cavity is called a _____ .

3 When coding endoscopic procedures you must be certain to code to the fullest _____ of the procedure and to code the correct _____ for the procedure.

4 If more than one distinct procedure was performed during a endoscopic procedure, what modifier would you add to the lesser-priced service?

_____

5 What type of endoscopy is always bundled into a surgical endoscopy? _____

6 A(n) _____ laryngoscopy is performed when a physician uses a tongue depressor to hold the tongue down and view the epiglottis with a mirror.

7 A(n) _____ laryngoscopy is performed when the endoscope is passed into the larynx and the physician can look at the larynx through a scope.

8 An otorhinolaryngologist is a physician who specializes in treating conditions of the

_____ , _____ ,

and _____ .

9 When coding a nasal abscess or a nasal biopsy of the skin using the external approach, you use codes from the _____ System subsection.

10 When coding a nasal abscess or a nasal biopsy using the internal approach, you use codes from the _____ System subsection.

11 What are the three sections of turbinates?

_____ , _____ ,

and _____

12 What is the name of the therapy in which the physician flushes saline solution into the sinuses to remove mucus or pus?

_____

CHAPTER 6, PART II, PRACTICAL

With the use of the CPT manual, code the following procedures. Code only the physician services in this exercise; do not code the laboratory or radiology services.

13 A unilateral, total lung lavage
Code(s): _____

14 Performed as a separate procedure, a parietal pleurectomy
Code(s): _____

15 Resection of lung with chest wall resection
Code(s): _____

16 Removal of a crayon lodged inside nasal passage, office procedure
Code(s): _____

17 Surgical nasal endoscopy with polypectomy
Code(s): _____

18 Direct, operative laryngoscopy for removal of button lodged in 2-year-old child's larynx
Code(s): _____

19 Indirect laryngoscopy with biopsy
Code(s): _____

20 Internal approach used to drain nasal hematoma
Code(s): _____

21 External, simple, frontal sinusotomy
Code(s): _____

22 Surgical sinus endoscopy with sphenoidotomy
Code(s): _____

23 Submucous resection of nose with scoring of cartilage and contouring
Code(s): _____

24 Jack Rogers developed chest pain and difficulty breathing. He has also been coughing up thick, blood-tinged sputum. A chest radiograph shows an ill-defined mass. A diagnostic bronchoscopy is performed and a specimen of the mass is taken. The pathology report comes back positive for cancer. One week later, a lobectomy is performed.

Code(s): _____

25 James Wilson has been having difficulty breathing and has had continual sinusitis. Dr. Adams takes James to the operating room to perform a sinus endoscopy with anterior and posterior ethmoidectomy and removal of polyps.

Code(s): _____

26 Mary Bronson has a nosebleed that won't stop. She goes to the emergency department, where anterior packing is done to control the nasal hemorrhage.

Code(s): _____

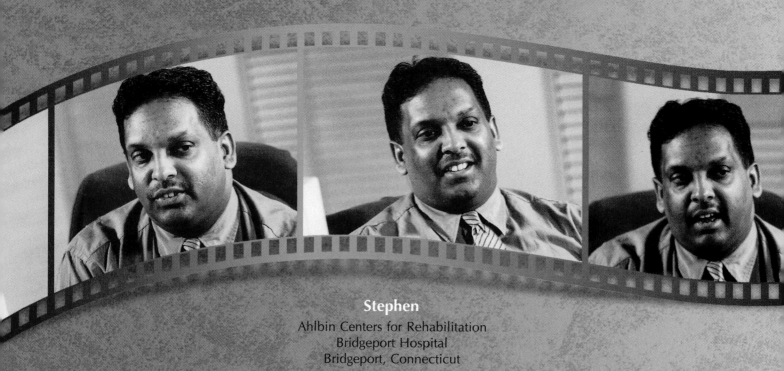

Stephen
Ahlbin Centers for Rehabilitation
Bridgeport Hospital
Bridgeport, Connecticut

chapter 7

Cardiovascular System

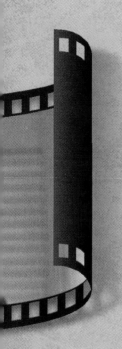

CHAPTER TOPICS

Coding Highlights

Cardiovascular Coding in the Surgery Section

Cardiovascular Coding in the Medicine Section

Cardiovascular Coding in the Radiology Section

Chapter Glossary

Chapter Review

LEARNING OBJECTIVES

After completing this chapter you should be able to

1 Code cardiovascular services using codes from three sections—Surgery, Medicine, and Radiology.

2 Apply rules of coding to cardiovascular services.

3 Differentiate among codes on the basis of surgical approach.

4 Identify selective and nonselective placement.

5 Demonstrate knowledge of coding common cardiac services.

6 Understand the various components of coding cardiovascular services.

CODING HIGHLIGHTS

Cardiology is one of the fastest growing subspecialties in medicine, and numerous modern techniques are used to diagnose and treat cardiac conditions. A **cardiologist** is an internal medicine physician who has chosen to specialize in the diagnosis and treatment of conditions of the heart. A cardiologist can further specialize in cardiovascular surgical procedures or other treatment and diagnostic specialties. In a smaller practice a cardiologist may do many of these procedures himself/herself, whereas in a larger practice a cardiologist may be more specialized and provide a more limited variety of services.

Coding from Three Sections

When you are reporting cardiology services you will often be using codes from three sections: Surgery, Medicine, and Radiology.

- The Surgery section contains the codes for cardiovascular **surgical** procedures
- The Medicine section contains codes for **nonsurgical** cardiovascular services
- The Radiology section contains **diagnostic study** codes

Figure 7–1 is a list of the section information that is most often used when reporting cardiovascular services. The confusion in coding cardiology often comes from not understanding the components (parts) of coding cardiovascular services and the various locations of these service codes in the CPT manual. To clarify cardiology coding, let's begin by reviewing the definitions of invasive, noninvasive, electrophysiology, and nuclear as they relate to cardiovascular coding.

from the trenches

What advice would you give to a new coder?
"Collect as much information as possible before announcing what the code is. Always consult a fellow coder to ensure consistency to be a reliable expert."

STEPHEN

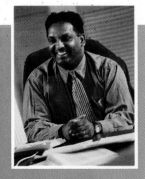

SURGERY SECTION	MEDICINE SECTION	RADIOLOGY SECTION

Cardiovascular System (33010–37799)
    Heart and Pericardium
    Arteries and Veins
	Cardiovascular System (92950–93799)
	    Therapeutic Services
	    Cardiography
	    Echocardiography
	    Cardiac Catheterization
	    Intracardiac Electrophysiological Procedures
	    Other Vascular Studies
	    Other Procedures
		Diagnostic Radiology (75552–75790)
		    Heart
		    Aorta and Arteries
		Diagnostic Ultrasound (various)
		    Ultrasonic Guidance Procedures
		Nuclear Medicine (78414–78499)
		    Cardiovascular System

Figure 7–1   A list of the section information that is most often used when reporting cardiovascular services.

Invasive

Invasive cardiology is entering the body—breaking the skin—to make a correction or for examination. An example of an invasive cardiac procedure is the removal of a tumor from the heart. The chest is opened, the ribs spread apart, the heart fully exposed to the view of the surgeon, and the tumor removed—an invasive surgical procedure. Another example is the removal of a clot from a vessel. The surgeon usually enters the body percutaneously (through the skin) by means of a catheter that is threaded to the clot's location. The clot can then be pulled out of the vein through the catheter or can be injected with a substance that dissolves it. Although an open surgical procedure was not used, the body was entered—an invasive surgical procedure. Invasive cardiology procedures are also called **interventional** procedures; some codes are located in the Surgery section and others are located in the Medicine section.

Noninvasive

Noninvasive services and procedures—not breaking the skin—are usually performed for diagnostic purposes—for example, electrocardiograms, echocardiography, and vascular studies. Performing these procedures does not require entering the body; rather, they are diagnostic tests that can be done from outside the body.

> *coding shot*
>
> To choose the correct cardiology code, first determine whether the procedure or service was invasive (interventional) or noninvasive.

Electrophysiology

Electrophysiology (EP) is the study of the electrical system of the heart and includes the study of arrhythmias. Diagnostic procedures include procedures such as recording from inside the heart by placing an electrical catheter into the heart percutaneously and taking an electrogram of the electrical activity within the heart. The code for this invasive diagnostic procedure is located in the Medicine section, Cardiology subsection.

As a treatment for abnormal electrical activity in the heart, a more invasive treatment can be performed, such as the placement of a pacemaker, cardioverter-defibrillator, or other device to regulate the rhythm of the heart. These invasive treatments are surgical procedures and the codes are located in the Surgery section, Cardiology subsection. There are also Surgery codes for operative procedures to correct electrophysiologic problems of the heart (33250–33261) when the electrical problems are corrected surgically by incision, excision, or destruction.

Nuclear

Nuclear cardiology is a diagnostic specialty that plays a very important role in modern cardiology. A physician who specializes in nuclear cardiology uses radioactive radiologic procedures to aid in the diagnosis of cardiologic conditions. For example, during angiography of the internal vessels, a nuclear cardiologist may inject a radioactive dye into the bloodstream to improve the detail of the study. The code for the angiography comes from the Radiology section, and the code for the injection procedure comes from the Surgery section.

CODING HIGHLIGHTS

Complete the following:

1 The Cardiovascular System of the Surgery section is divided into the two main subheadings of Heart/ _____ and Arteries/_____ .

2 A cardiologist is a(n) _____ medicine physician who has chosen to specialize in the diagnosis and treatment of conditions of the heart.

3 What three sections of the CPT will you often use to code cardiology services? _____ , _____ , and _____

4 What type of cardiology enters the body—breaks the skin—to make a correction or for examination? _____

5 What is the term that describes the study of the electrical system of the heart and includes the study of arrhythmias? _____

6 What type of cardiology is a diagnostic specialty in which the physician uses radioactive radiologic procedures to aid in the diagnosis of cardiology conditions? _____

Now that you are familiar with the terms "invasive," "noninvasive," "electrophysiology," and "nuclear," let's look at the three sections where you will find the components (parts) of cardiovascular coding: Surgery, Medicine, and Radiology.

CARDIOVASCULAR CODING IN THE SURGERY SECTION

The Cardiovascular System subsection of the Surgery section contains diagnostic and therapeutic procedure codes that are divided on the basis of whether the procedure was done on the heart/pericardium or on arteries/veins. It is in the Heart and Pericardium subheading that you will find codes for procedures that involve the repair of the heart and coronary vessels, such as placement of pacemakers, repair of valve disorders, and graft/bypass procedures. In the Arteries and Veins subheading you will find many of the same types of procedures, but for noncoronary (nonheart) vessels. For example, a thromboendarterectomy is the removal of a thrombus (obstruction) and a portion of the lining of an artery. When a thromboendarterectomy is performed on a coronary artery, you would use a code from the Heart and Pericardium subheading; but if the procedure was done on a noncoronary artery, you would use a code from the Arteries and Veins subheading.

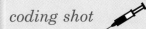

coding shot

The location of the procedure—coronary or noncoronary—is the first step in selecting the correct cardiovascular surgical code, because the CPT codes are divided on the basis of whether a procedure involved coronary or noncoronary vessels.

Heart and Pericardium

The Surgery section, Cardiovascular System subsection, Heart and Pericardium subheading contains procedures that are performed both percutaneously and through open surgical sites. There are always many revisions and additions in this subheading each year to reflect the many advances in this important health care area. Numerous notes are located throughout the subheading, and they must be read prior to coding in the subheading. Codes in the Heart and Pericardium subheading are for services provided to repair the heart (Fig. 7–2), pericardium, or coronary vessels (Fig. 7–3).

Pericardium

Pericardiocentesis is a procedure in which the surgeon withdraws fluid from the pericardial space by means of a needle that is inserted percutaneously into the space. The insertion can be done using radiologic (ultrasound) guidance—the use of which would be reported with a separate code from the Radiology section. There is a note following the pericardiocentesis codes that states: "(For radiological supervision and interpretation, use 76930)"; that is, ultrasonic guidance for pericardiocentesis, imaging supervision, and interpretation. Watch for these directional features throughout the Cardiovascular System subsection.

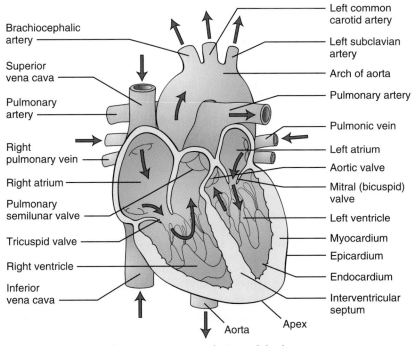

Figure 7–2   Internal view of the heart.

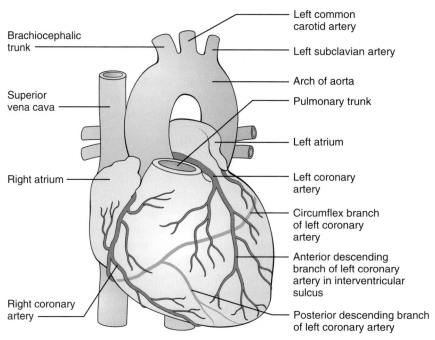

Figure 7–3   External view of the heart.

The fluid withdrawn during a pericardiocentesis is then examined for microbial agents (such as tuberculosis), neoplasia, or autoimmune diseases (such as lupus or rheumatoid arthritis). The pericardiocentesis codes are divided on the basis of whether the service was initial or subsequent.

A tube pericardiostomy uses the same procedure described earlier, but a catheter is left in the pericardium leading to the outside of the body to allow for continued drainage.

The remaining procedures in the Pericardium category are open surgical procedures for the removal of clots, foreign bodies, tumors, cysts, or a portion of the pericardium or to create a window for pericardial fluid drainage into the pleural space.

Cardiac Tumor

A procedure performed to remove a tumor of the pericardium is reported using a code from the Pericardium category, but if a tumor is removed from the heart, you would select a code from the category Cardiac Tumor. There are only two tumor-removal codes in the Cardiac Tumor category, one for a tumor that is removed from inside the heart (intracardiac) and one for a tumor that is removed from outside the heart (external). Both procedures are open surgical procedures that involve opening the chest, spreading the ribs, and excising the tumor.

Pacemaker or Pacing Cardioverter-Defibrillator

A pacemaker and a cardioverter-defibrillator are devices that are inserted into the body to electrically shock the heart into regular rhythm. When a pacemaker is inserted, a pocket is made and a generator and lead(s) are placed inside the chest (Fig. 7–4). Sometimes, only components of the pacemaker are reinserted, repaired, or replaced. You need to know three things about the service provided to correctly code the pacemaker:

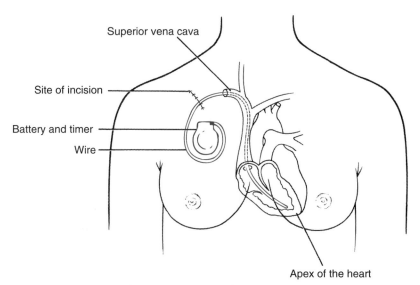

Superior vena cava

Site of incision

Battery and timer

Wire

Apex of the heart

Figure 7–4   Pacemaker insertion.

1. Where the electrode (lead) is placed: atrium, ventricle, or both
2. Whether the procedure involves initial placement, replacement, or repair of all components or separate components of the pacemaker
3. The approach used to place the pacemaker (epicardial or transvenous)

Approaches

The two approaches that can be used when inserting a pacemaker are epicardial (on the heart) and transvenous (through a vein), and the codes are divided according to the surgical approach used.

1. The **epicardial** approach involves opening the chest cavity and placing the pacemaker on the heart. A pocket is formed on the surface of the heart, and the pacemaker generator is placed into the pocket. A tunnel is made into the heart into which the wires are fed. The wires are then connected to the pacemaker generator and the chest area is closed. Codes for the epicardial process are further divided based on the approach to the chest wall that was used—thoracotomy or upper abdominal (xiphoid region).

2. The **transvenous** approach involves accessing a vein (subclavian or jugular) and inserting a needle with a wire into the vein. A fluoroscope is then passed into the heart, and the pacemaker is affixed by creating a pocket into which the pacemaker generator is placed. The fluoroscopic portion of the procedure is coded separately using a radiology code (71090) because it is not bundled into the pacemaker codes. Transvenous codes are further divided based on the area of the heart into which the pacemaker is inserted. For example, 33207 (single chamber pacemaker) is reported for transvenous placement of a pacemaker into the ventricle of the heart. If the pacemaker components were placed in both the atrium and the ventricle, 33208 (dual chamber pacemaker) is reported.

The patient record will indicate whether a pacemaker or cardioverter-defibrillator was inserted or replaced.

The same set of criteria applies to the cardioverter-defibrillator codes:

1. Revision or replacement of lead(s)
2. Replacement, repair, removal of components
3. Approach used for insertion or repair

coding shot

A change of batteries in a pacemaker or cardioverter-defibrillator is a removal of the implanted generator and the reimplantation of a new generator. Both the removal and the reimplantation are coded.

EP that was used in the diagnosis of a condition and that resulted in the insertion of a pacemaker or cardioverter-defibrillator is not included in the surgery code. If EP diagnostic services of the pacemaker system are provided, you would report services using the Medicine section codes 93731–93736.

Radiology supervision and interpretation is not included in the pacemaker implantation codes. If radiology supervision and interpretation is provided, you would report the service using the Radiology section code 71090, Insertion of pacemaker, fluoroscopy, radiography, radiological supervision and interpretation.

coding shot

If a patient with a pacemaker or other implantable device is seen by the physician within the **90-day** follow-up period for implantation but for a problem not related to the implantation, the service for the new problem can be billed. Documentation in the medical record must support the statement that the service is unrelated to the implantation. Append the unrelated E/M service code with modifier -24.

EXERCISE 7–2

PERICARDIUM, CARDIAC TUMORS, AND PACEMAKERS

Using the CPT manual, code the following:

1 Allen Jackson gets very tired walking up and down stairs. He has a hard time catching his breath and experiences instances when his heart feels as if it is beating fast. His physician has told him that he will require a pacemaker implantation. Allen goes to surgery and has a single chamber pacemaker implanted into the ventricle.

Code(s): _____

2 Five days after the pacemaker is implanted, Allen feels very dizzy and his electrocardiogram is showing some abnormalities. His physician takes him back to the operating room and discovers that the pacemaker lead is malfunctioning. The pacemaker is replaced, and Allen recovers nicely.

Code(s): _____

3 Five years later, the battery in Allen's pacemaker is found to have become depleted. He is also having some other symptoms that his physician believes necessitate not only a replacement pacemaker but also an upgrade to a dual chamber device.

Code(s): _____

4 A new patient with a chief complaint of sharp, intermittent retrosternal pain that is reduced by sitting up or leaning forward is evaluated by a cardiologist. Chest films reveal pulmonary edema with pleural effusion. The physician performs a pericardiocentesis. (Code only the procedure.)

Code(s): _____

5 Resection of an intracardiac tumor in which cardiopulmonary bypass is required

Code(s): _____

Electrophysiologic Operative Procedures

EP, as you learned earlier in this chapter, is the study of the electrical system of the heart, and most of the codes for the EP tests are in the Medicine section. The codes in the Surgery section apply to the surgical repair of a defect that causes an abnormal rhythm. Cardiopulmonary bypass is usually required during these major operative procedures, and the chest is opened to expose the heart to the full view of the surgeon. The surgeon maps the locations of the electrodes of the heart and notes the source of the arrhythmia. The source of the arrhythmia is then ablated (separated) and removed. The codes are divided on the basis of the need for cardiopulmonary bypass and the reason for the procedure (atrial fibrillation, atrial flutter, etc.).

Patient-Activated Event Recorder

A patient-activated event recorder is also known as a cardiac event recorder or a loop recorder. Codes 33282–38284 involve surgical implantation into the subcutaneous tissue in the upper left quadrant, with leads running to the outside of the body. The recorder senses the heart's rhythms, and when the patient presses a button, the device records the electrical activity. The recording can assist the physician in making a diagnosis of a hard-to-detect rhythm problem. Codes are divided on the basis of whether the device was implanted or removed.

from the trenches

Do you ever think your job is like detective work?
"Yes. Trying to decipher all of our providers' notes and medical records . . . and coming up with a code and modifier that match."

STEPHEN

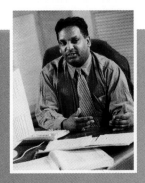

Cardiac Valves

The category Cardiac Valves has subcategory codes of aortic, mitral, tricuspid, and pulmonary valves. The procedures are about the same for each valve; some are a little more extensive than others. Code descriptions vary depending on whether a cardiopulmonary bypass (heart-lung) machine is used during the procedure. The cardiopulmonary bypass is a resource-intensive procedure that requires a heart-lung machine to assume the patient's heart and lung functions during surgery.

The procedures are located in the CPT manual index under the valve type or under what was done, such as repair or replacement. For example, the replacement of an aortic valve is located in the CPT index under "Aorta," subterm "Valve," subterm "Replacement."

EXERCISE 7-3

EP, EVENT-RECORDER, AND VALVES

Using the CPT manual, code the following:

1 Mary Black's echocardiogram and cardiac catheterization show severe mitral stenosis with regurgitation. Her physician believes that because she is symptomatic, she should have her mitral valve replaced. The mitral valve replacement includes cardiopulmonary bypass.

   Code(s): _____

2 Andrew Nelson has a loud heart murmur and, after study, is found to have severe aortic stenosis. He elects to have an aortic valve replacement. He is taken to the operating room and placed on a heart-lung machine. He then has his aortic valve replaced with a prosthetic valve.

   Code(s): _____

3 With the heart exposed through the sternum and the patient's functions supported by cardiopulmonary bypass, the right atrium is opened and the arrhythmia focuses are ablated by using electrical current. Bypass is discontinued and the atrium and sternum are closed in the usual fashion.

   Code(s): _____

4 Implantation of a patient-activated cardiac loop device with programming

   Code(s): _____

Coronary Artery Anomalies

The Coronary Artery Anomalies category contains codes to report the services of repair of the coronary artery by various methods, such as graft, ligation (tying off), and reconstruction. The codes include endarterectomy (removal of the inner lining of an artery) and angioplasty (blood vessel repair). Do not unbundle the codes and report the endarterectomy or angioplasty separately. Also, the procedures often require the use of cardiopulmonary bypass to allow the surgeon to repair the defect while the heart is without bloodflow, which makes a difference in the choice of codes.

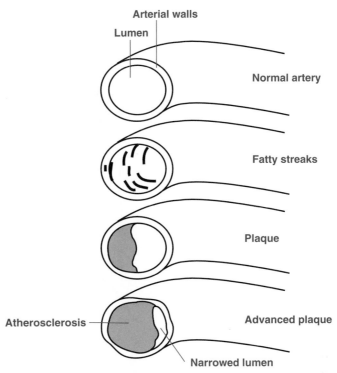

Figure 7-5   Atherosclerosis.

Coronary Artery Bypass

Arteries deliver oxygenated blood to all areas of the body, and veins return to the heart blood full of waste products. The pulmonary vessels, however, are not included in this cycle. The pulmonary vein carries oxygenated blood and the pulmonary artery carries waste products. The heart muscle is fed by coronary arteries that encircle the heart. When these arteries clog with plaque (known as arteriosclerotic coronary artery disease) (Fig. 7–5), the flow of blood lessens. Sometimes the arteries clog to the point that the heart muscle begins to perform at low levels due to lack of blood **(reversible ischemia)** or to actually die **(irreversible ischemia).** Reversible ischemia means that if the blood flow is increased to the heart muscle, the heart muscle may again begin to function at normal or near-normal levels. **Coronary artery bypass grafting** is one way to increase the flow of blood. The diseased portion of the artery is "bypassed" by attachment of a healthy vessel above and below the diseased area and allowing the healthy vessel to then become the conduit of the blood, thus bypassing the blockage (Fig. 7–6). Blockage can also be pushed to the sides of the coronary arterial walls by a procedure in which a balloon is expanded inside the artery. This procedure is known as a **percutaneous transluminal coronary angioplasty (PTCA)** (Fig. 7–7).

To correctly code coronary bypass grafts, you must know whether an artery, a vein, or both are being used as the bypass graft. You must also know how many bypass grafts are being done. There may be more than one blockage to be bypassed and, therefore, more than one graft. If only a vein is used for the graft (most often the saphenous vein from the leg is harvested and used for this purpose; see Fig. 7–6), the code reflecting the number of grafts would be chosen from the category Venous Grafting Only for Coronary Artery Bypass.

The following exercise will help you learn the differences in coding for bypass grafts using arteries, veins, or both, and for coding anomalies.

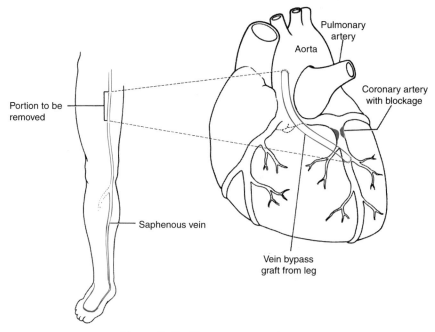

Figure 7–6   Coronary artery bypass.

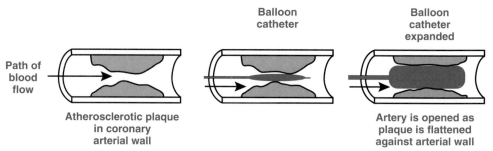

Figure 7–7   Percutaneous transluminal coronary angioplasty.

EXERCISE
7-4

CORONARY ARTERY BYPASS AND ANOMALIES

Using the CPT manual, code the following:

1 Two coronary bypass grafts using veins only

Code(s): _____

The code for Question 1 came from the category Venous Grafting Only for Coronary Artery Bypass because the bypass was accomplished using a venous graft. If the bypass was accomplished using an arterial graft, the codes in the category Arterial Grafting for Coronary Artery Bypass would be used to report the service. If both veins and arteries were used to accomplish the bypass, you would report the service by using an artery bypass code and a code from the category Combined Arterial-Venous Grafting for Coronary Bypass. Because the title of the category contains the words "arterial-venous," you might think that the codes in the category report both the artery and the vein; but this is not the case. The category codes under "arterial-venous" are used only when venous grafts have been used in addition to

arterial grafts, and they are used only in combination with the arterial graft codes.

For example, a patient has had a five-vessel coronary artery bypass graft, for which two bypasses were accomplished using internal mammary arteries and three bypasses were accomplished using veins:

2 Coronary artery bypass using two arterial grafts

    Code(s): _____

3 Coronary artery bypass using three venous grafts

    Code(s): _____

STOP *Modifier -51 would not be used with the code for the venous grafts because a note preceding the code states "list separately in addition to code for arterial graft." This means that the venous code is never used alone, but always follows an arterial code.*

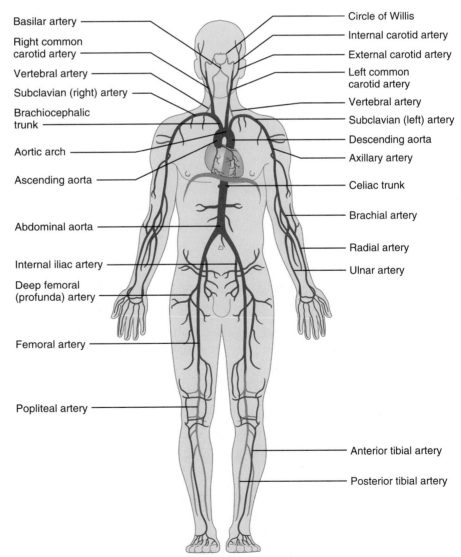

Basilar artery

Right common carotid artery

Vertebral artery

Subclavian (right) artery

Brachiocephalic trunk

Aortic arch

Ascending aorta

Abdominal aorta

Internal iliac artery

Deep femoral (profunda) artery

Femoral artery

Popliteal artery

Circle of Willis

Internal carotid artery

External carotid artery

Left common carotid artery

Vertebral artery

Subclavian (left) artery

Descending aorta

Axillary artery

Celiac trunk

Brachial artery

Radial artery

Ulnar artery

Anterior tibial artery

Posterior tibial artery

Figure 7–8 Arteries of the body.

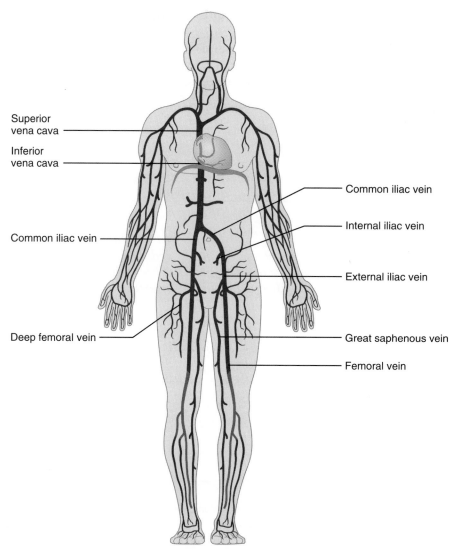

Figure 7–9 Veins of the body.

Arteries and Veins

Code groupings for arteries and veins vary according to procedures such as thrombectomies, aneurysm repairs, bypass grafting, repairs, angioplasties, arthrectomies, and all other procedures. A good book about vascular procedures will be an invaluable tool to you for coding cardiovascular services as you begin your career as a coder. Codes in the subheading Arteries and Veins refer to all arteries and veins except the coronary arteries and veins (Figs. 7–8 and 7–9).

Vascular Families—Selective or Nonselective Placement

A vascular family can be compared to a tree with branches. The tree has a main trunk from which large branches and then smaller branches grow. The same is true with vascular families. A main vessel is present, and other vessels branch off from the main vessel. Vessels that are connected in this manner are considered families.

Catheters may have to be placed in vessels for monitoring, removal of blood, injection of contrast materials, or infusion. When coding the placement of a catheter it is necessary to know where the catheter starts and where it ends up.

Catheter placement is nonselective or selective. **Nonselective catheter placement** means the catheter or needle is placed directly into an artery or vein (and not manipulated farther along) or is placed only into the aorta from any approach. **Selective catheter placement** means the catheter must be moved, manipulated, or guided into a part of the arterial system other than the aorta or the vessel punctured (that is, into the branches), generally under fluoroscopic guidance. The following codes illustrate nonselective and selective placement:

EXAMPLE

Nonselective:	36000 Introduction of needle or intracatheter, vein
Selective:	36012 Selective catheter placement, venous system; second order, or more selective, branch

Code 36000 describes the placement of a needle or catheter into a vein with no further manipulation or movement. Code 36012 describes the placement of a catheter into a vein and its manipulation or moving to a second-order vein or farther.

The first note in the Cardiovascular System subsection in the CPT manual refers to selective placement. The note appears at the beginning of the section because it is very important and applies to the entire Cardiovascular System subsection. When coding selective placement for any procedure, you report the fullest extention into one vascular family, just as you would when coding a gastrointestinal endoscopic procedure, when you code to the farthest extent of the procedure. The same is true of selective placement into a vascular family: code to the farthest extent of the placement within the vascular family.

The first order is the main artery in a vascular family, the second order is the branch off the main artery, the third order is the next branch off the second order, and so on. A vascular family can have more than one second-order, third-order, and so on, vessel, as illustrated in Figure 7–10. If the farthest extent of the placement was to the third order, only the third-order code would be reported. For example, if a catheter was placed into the first-order brachiocephalic artery and from there manipulated through the second-order artery, and finally into the third-order artery, you would report

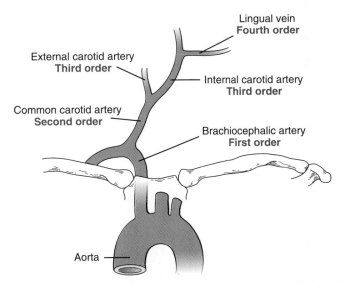

Figure 7–10 Brachiocephalic vascular family with first-, second-, third-, and fourth-order vessels.

only the third-order artery, with code 36217, which describes an initial third-order placement within the brachiocephalic family.

If the catheter placement continued from one branch of the brachiocephalic artery into another branch of the artery, you would report the additional second order, third order, and beyond using an add-on code—36218. Oftentimes, a physician will investigate not only one branch of an artery but several others. Report all subsequent catheter placement to the farthest extent of placement.

coding shot

Code to the farthest extent of the vascular family using an initial code, then code any additional services of the second order, the third order, or beyond using an add-on code.

Catheter placement codes may vary according to the vascular family into which the catheter is placed. Look at the following two codes and note the difference in vascular families:

E X A M P L E

36215   Selective catheter placement, arterial system; each first order **thoracic or brachiocephalic** branch, within a vascular family

36245   Selective catheter placement, arterial system; each first order **abdominal, pelvic, or lower extremity** artery branch, within a vascular family

Embolectomy/Thrombectomy

An **embolus** is a mass of undissolved matter that is present in blood and is transported by the blood. A **thrombus** is a blood clot that occludes, or shuts

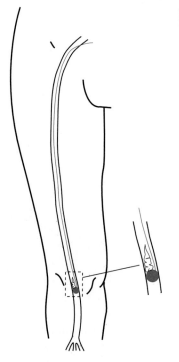

Figure 7–11   Embolectomy.

off, a vessel. When a thrombus is dislodged, it becomes an embolus. Thrombectomies or embolectomies are performed to remove the unwanted debris, or clot, from the vessel and allow unrestricted bloodflow. A thrombus or embolus may be removed by opening the vessel and scraping out the debris or by percutaneously placing a balloon within the vessel to push the material to the sides and out of the vessel (see Fig. 7–7). A catheter may also be used to draw a thrombus or embolus out of the vessel, as illustrated in Figure 7–11. Embolectomy/Thrombectomy codes begin with 34001 and are divided based on the artery or vein in which the clot or thrombus is located (e.g., radial artery, femoropopliteal vein), with the site of incision for the catheter specified (e.g., arm, leg, abdominal incision). You can locate these codes in the CPT manual index under embolectomy or thrombectomy, subdivided by arteries and veins (e.g., carotid artery, axillary vein).

When more involved procedures such as grafts are performed, inflow and outflow establishment is included in the major procedure codes. This means that if a thrombus is present and a bypass graft is performed, the removal of the thrombus is bundled into the grafting procedure if done on the same vessel. Also bundled into the aortic procedures is any sympathectomy (interruption of the sympathetic nervous system) or angiogram (radiographic view of the blood vessels).

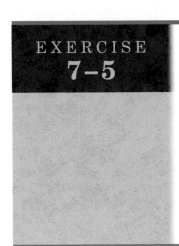

EXERCISE 7–5

EMBOLECTOMY/THROMBECTOMY

Using the CPT manual, code the following:

1 Thrombectomy of the femoropopliteal aortoiliac artery, by leg incision

   Code(s): _____

2 Embolectomy, carotid artery, by neck incision

   Code(s): _____

3 Thrombectomy of venous bypass graft

   Code(s): _____

Cardiovascular Repairs

The category Venous Reconstruction contains codes for the various repairs made to the valves of the heart, vena cava, and saphenous vein. The **valve repairs** are made by opening the site and clamping off the vessels that lead to the valve. The surgeon then tacks down excess material of the valve with sutures (plication). If there is a defect in the valve, the surgeon repairs the defect with a graft, usually harvested from elsewhere in the body. **Vein repairs** are done by locating the defective vessel, clamping the vessel off, and bypassing or grafting the defect.

The category Direct Repair of Aneurysm or Excision (Partial or Total) and Graft Insertion for Aneurysm, False Aneurysm, Ruptured Aneurysm, and Associated Occlusive Disease (35001–35162) contains **aneurysm repair** codes that are divided according to the type of aneurysm (e.g., false, ruptured) and the vessel the aneurysm is located in (subclavian artery, popliteal artery). The aneurysm, which is a sac of clotted blood, is located, and clamps are placed above and below it. The section containing the aneurysm is then removed or bypassed. The aneurysm codes often refer to a **false aneurysm,** which is an aneurysm in which the vessel is completely destroyed and the aneurysm is being contained by the tissue that surrounded the vessel.

Repair, Arteriovenous Fistula category codes (35180–35286) are used for **fistula repair** and are divided on the basis of whether the fistula (abnormal passage) is congenital, has been acquired, or is traumatic. An arteriovenous fistula occurs when blood flows between an artery and a vein. An example of an acquired arteriovenous fistula is the creation of an arteriovenous connection that is used for a hemodialysis site (Fig. 7–12). In repairing a fistula, the surgeon separates the artery and vein and then patches the area of separation with sutures or a graft.

If an **angioscopy** of the vessel or graft area is performed during a therapeutic procedure, code 35400, Angioscopy (non-coronary vessels or grafts) during therapeutic intervention, is listed in addition to the procedure code. For example, suppose the surgeon performed the repair of an arteriovenous fistula (of the neck, 35188) and then placed a scope into the artery to determine visually whether the repair was complete. Code 35188 would describe the primary therapeutic procedure of repair of the arteriovenous fistula, and code 35400 would describe the angioscopy. Note that 35400 is an add-on code and cannot be used alone, but only in conjunction with a therapeutic procedure code.

A **transluminal angioplasty** is a procedure in which a vessel is punctured and a catheter is passed into the vessel for the purposes of stretching the vessel. The category codes are divided based on the catheter being passed into the vessel by incising the skin to expose the vessel (open) or by passing the catheter through the skin (percutaneous) into the vessel. Further divisions of the codes are based on the vessel into which the catheter is placed (e.g., iliac, aortic).

A **transluminal atherectomy** is a procedure in which a vessel is punctured and a guide wire is threaded into the vessel. The surgeon then inserts a device called an atherectomy catheter into the vessel; this catheter contains a device that can destroy the materials clogging the vessel. This procedure can be done by an open or a percutaneous method, and the codes are divided on the basis of the method used and the vessel into which the catheter is passed.

Bypass Grafts, Veins

As with coronary artery bypass grafting, you must know the type of grafting material being used for vascular bypass grafts. Grafts can use vessels harvested from other areas of the body or they may be made of artificial materials. Codes are chosen on the basis of the type of graft and the specific

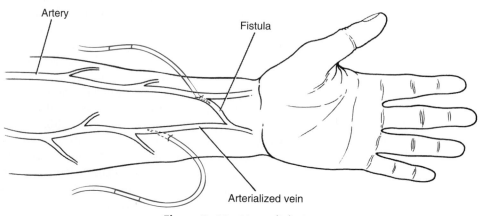

Figure 7–12   Hemodialysis.

vessel(s) that the graft is being bypassed from and to. For example, code 35506 describes a graft that is placed to bypass a portion of the subclavian artery. During this procedure the surgeon would sew a harvested vein to the side of the carotid artery and attach the other end of the vein to the subclavian artery below the damaged area, creating a bypass around the defect.

One way to locate the graft codes in the CPT manual index is to look under "Bypass Graft" and then under the subterm type (e.g., carotid, subclavian, vertebral).

Vascular Access

Some treatments are given through the blood by means of vascular access. For instance, in patients receiving hemodialysis, arteriovenous fistulas may be created for dialysis treatments (see Fig. 7–12). This means that an artificial connection is made between a vein and an artery, allowing blood to flow from the vein through the graft for dialysis (cleansing of waste products) and then be returned to the artery.

Vascular Injection Procedures

Bundled into the vascular injections are the following items:

- Local anesthesia
- Introduction of needle or catheter
- Injection of contrast media
- Pre-injection care related to procedure
- Post-injection care related to procedure

Vascular injections bundles **do not** include the following items:

- Catheter
- Drugs
- Contrast media

For items not bundled into the injection procedure, code each item separately.

STOP *Just for a moment, think about what a difference a seemingly small fact—such as what is included in the vascular injection procedures—makes in the amount received for the procedure over the course of a year! It is your responsibility as the coder to know the rules of coding to ensure appropriate reimbursement for services provided by physicians. Details are important in the business of coding!*

You will use code 99070, supplies and materials, from the Medicine section to code items such as catheters, drugs, and contrast media. There are also specific HCPCS Level II codes for many of these supply items.

As previously discussed, knowledge of the vascular families is critical in coding vascular injection procedures because the initial placement and the extent of placement are usually the characteristics that determine the codes. You now know that the initial placement of the catheter is reported first and that add-on codes report any additional services. For example, review the following initial and additional third-order placement code descriptions in the Example on page 228:

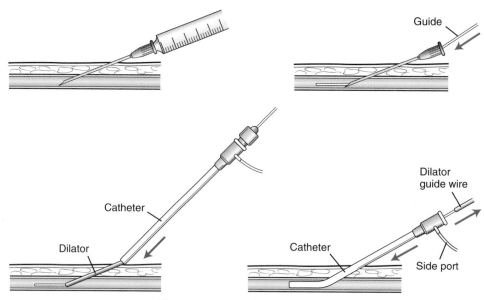

Figure 7–13   Catheter insertion.

EXAMPLE

36217   Selective catheter placement into the brachiocephalic branch, **initial** third order placement

36218   Selective catheter placement into an **additional** third order brachiocephalic branch

In the service described in 36217, the physician inserts a needle through the skin and into an artery. The needle has a guide wire attached to it, as illustrated in Figure 7–13, and when the needle is withdrawn, the guide wire is left inside the artery. The guide wire can then be manipulated into the particular artery. Once the guide wire is in the correct artery, a catheter is threaded into place over the guide wire and into the first-order brachiocephalic artery. The catheter is manipulated through the second-order artery and arrives at the third-order artery, where contrast material is injected into the artery through the catheter and an arteriography is completed.

After the completion of the service described in 36217, the physician pulls the catheter back into the artery and then manipulates the catheter into another third-order artery (36218), where contrast material is again injected into the artery through the catheter and another arteriography is completed.

EXERCISE 7–6

REPAIRS, GRAFTS, AND VASCULAR ACCESS

Using the CPT manual, code the following:

1 Bypass graft, with vein; carotid-subclavian

Code(s): _____

2 Bypass graft, with vein; femoral-popliteal

Code(s): _____

3 Bypass graft, using Gore-Tex; axillary-axillary

Code(s): _____

4 Excision, with application of a patch graft, for an aneurysm, common femoral artery

Code(s): _____

5 Selective catheter placement into the abdominal artery with manipulation into the right internal iliac artery where contrast material is injected and angiography is done. Additionally, the surgeon manipulates the catheter back to the abdominal artery and manipulates the catheter into the left internal iliac artery where contrast material is injected and angiography is completed. The catheter is withdrawn.

Code: _____ and _____

CARDIOVASCULAR CODING IN THE MEDICINE SECTION

Services in the Cardiovascular subsection of the Medicine section can be either invasive/noninvasive or diagnostic/therapeutic. The invasive treatments are not a matter of cutting open the body so the surgeon can view it, as was the case in the Cardiovascular subsection of the Surgery section, but are invasive in that there is an incision into or a puncture of the skin. The subheadings in the Cardiovascular subsection in Medicine are

- Therapeutic Services
- Cardiography
- Echocardiography
- Cardiac Catheterization
- Intracardiac Electrophysiological Procedures/Studies
- Peripheral Arterial Disease Rehabilitation
- Other Vascular Studies
- Other Procedures

Therapeutic Services

It is within the Therapeutic Services subheading that you find many commonly used cardiovascular codes, such as cardioversion, infusions, thrombolysis, placement of catheters and stents, coronary atherectomy, and angioplasty. Many of these services used to be performed as open operative procedures, but with the advent of modern techniques, many are now performed by means of percutaneous access. Division of the codes is based on **method** (balloon, blade), **location** (aorta or mitral valve), and **number** (single or multiple vessels).

Thrombolysis (92975) is a percutaneous procedure in which the physician inserts a catheter into a coronary vessel and injects contrast material into the vessel to further enhance the visualization of a blood clot. The clot is then destroyed by a drug. The Medicine section code 92975 represents the total procedure when the thrombolysis is performed in a coronary vessel. If vessels other than the coronary vessels are treated, a code from the Surgery section, Cardiovascular subsection, would be used to indicate an infusion of a thrombus (37201).

Intravascular ultrasound of the coronary vessels can be reported using the two codes 92978 and 92979, depending on the number of vessels diagnosed. A needle is inserted percutaneously into the vessel and a guide wire introduced, followed by an ultrasound probe. The probe allows a two-dimensional image of the inside of the vessel to be viewed on the ultrasound monitor. The physician can assess the vessel before and after treatment. The physician may reposition the probe to assess additional vessels, and code 92979 is used to indicate this subsequent placement. Note that both 92978 and 92979 are add-on codes and are intended to be used only in conjunction with the primary procedure. For example, intravascular ultrasound with coronary stent placement would be coded as 92980 (placement catheter) and 92978 (intravascular ultrasound).

Intracoronary stent placement using a catheter is a procedure that is performed to reinforce a coronary vessel that has collapsed or is blocked, as illustrated in Figure 7–14. The procedure requires the use of two catheters that are percutaneously inserted into the coronary vessel. The vessel is cleaned out (atherectomy) with one catheter, and the other catheter is used for the placement of a stent (support). The placement of the stent is usually accomplished with radiographic guidance. The surgeon usually reports the stent placement, and the radiologist who provides the ultrasonic guidance reports the guidance.

The codes are divided on the basis of whether more than one coronary vessel was cleared of obstruction and had a stent placed within it.

Percutaneous transluminal coronary angioplasty (PTCA), as illustrated in Figure 7–7, is described in codes 92982 and 92984. The codes are divided on the basis of whether a single vessel or multiple vessels are treated during the procedure. Add-on code 92984 (PTCA for each additional vessel) is of interest because it can be used not only with 92982 but also with other codes in the category. For example, 92984 can be used with code 92980, placement of a stent, when a stent is placed in one vessel and the PTCA is done in a different vessel. If a patient had an intracoronary stent placed in one coronary vessel, you report 92980, and if the physician also performed a PTCA on another coronary vessel, you report 92984. This is the first time

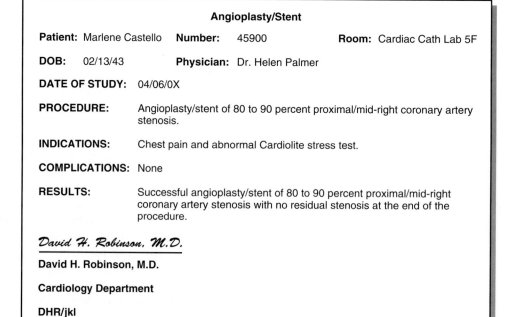

Figure 7–14 Angioplasty/Stent report.

that you have used an add-on code with a code other than the one(s) that appears directly above it in the same group of codes, so be certain to read the code descriptions for each of the codes used in the example above and pay special attention to the notes that follow 92984.

Valvuloplasty can also be performed by inserting a catheter percutaneously. The procedure opens a blocked valve by using a balloon, which is inflated to clear the blockage. The codes are divided based on the valve being repaired.

The balloon technique is also used to treat congenital heart defects such as vessels that are too narrow. A blade can also be used inside the coronary vessels or the heart. A special catheter that has a retractable blade is guided into the vessel or heart and the surgeon manipulates the blade to enlarge the area, using ultrasound or fluoroscopic guidance.

Cardiography

This category of the Cardiovascular System subsection contains frequently used codes, such as those for electrocardiograms and heart monitoring, which are certain to be used in most office practices, even if the practice does not include a cardiologist.

The Cardiography subheading is used to report diagnostic electrocardiographic procedures such as stress tests. **Stress tests** are performed to test the adequacy of the amount of oxygen getting to the heart muscle (at rest and during exercise) and thus indicate the presence or absence of heart disease. The top number on a blood pressure reading is systole (heart muscle is contracting); the bottom number is diastole (heart muscle is relaxing). The heart muscle is fed by three coronary arteries and their branches. If these arteries are clear, the amount of blood going to the muscle is adequate during rest and exercise. The heart muscle is fed only during diastole. Normal blood pressure is about 120/80 mm Hg, and the normal heart rate is about 60 beats per minute. During low blood pressure, little blood and oxygen get to the heart.

As the heart beats faster, such as during exercise, the heart rate increases and diastolic pressure time decreases, meaning that there is less time to supply blood to the heart muscle. As the heart beats faster, more oxygen is also required. With narrowing of coronary arteries and branches, too little blood may circulate to the heart muscle, supplying even less oxygen than during rest, and chest pain may result as an indication that heart muscle tissue is dying. Indications of heart disease during a stress test are chest pain and lengthening ST waves on the ECG, as illustrated in Figure 7–15.

The **Holter monitor** is similar to an **electrocardiogram (ECG)** in that leads are attached to the patient. It is portable and records the patient's ECG readings for 24 hours. Leads are attached to the chest and to a cassette machine. The monitor converts the ECG readings to sound, and the sound is converted back to an ECG reading when completed. The reading is then sped up to hundreds of times faster than normal by computers. Any reading that varies from a normal reading will be identified. The Q, R, and S waves are related to the contraction of the ventricles of the heart. The QRS waves and heartbeats can be monitored by Holter monitors. Cardiac arrhythmias can be identified using the Holter monitor process. An example of a Holter report is presented in Figure 7–16.

An **ECG** is typically conducted by attaching 12 electrodes (leads) to the patient's chest. The ECG provides a reading of the electrical currents of the heart and is a standard test conducted to detect suspected cardiac abnormalities, such as arrhythmias and conduction abnormalities. Some codes are

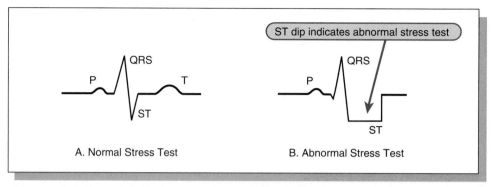

Figure 7–15 Normal and abnormal ECG results. *A,* Normal ECG reading. *B,* Abnormal ECG reading. The ST segment dips. QRS complex and T waves are related to the contraction of the ventricles. Indications of heart disease during a stress test are chest pain and lengthened ST segments.

to be used for the tracing only (the technical component), for the interpretation and report only (the professional component), or for the entire procedure of tracing and interpretation (the technical and professional components). The patient's medical record will indicate the components provided. Codes 93000–93010 are for the standard 12-lead ECG; the codes are divided on the basis of the component(s) provided.

Codes 93040–93272 are used for various ECGs and are divided according to the type of recording and the component(s) provided. Only careful reading will reveal the often slight differences between codes.

Holter Report

INDICATIONS: Patient with atrial fibrillation on Lanoxin. Patient with known cardiomyopathy.

BASELINE DATA: 84-year-old gentleman with congestive heart failure on Elavil, Vasotec, Lanoxin, and Lasix.

The patient was monitored for 24 hours.

INTERPRETATION: 1. The predominant rhythm is atrial fibrillation. The average ventricular rate is 74 beats per minute, minimal 49 beats per minute, and maximum 114 beats per minute.
2. A total of 4948 ventricular ectopic beats were detected. There were 4 forms. There were 146 couplets with 1 triplet and 5 runs of bigeminy. There were 2 runs of ventricular tachycardia, the longest for 5 beats at a rate of 150 beats per minute. There was no ventricular fibrillation.
3. There were no prolonged pauses.

CONCLUSION: 1. Predominate rhythm is atrial fibrillation with well-controlled ventricular rate.
2. There are no prolonged pauses.
3. Asymptomatic, nonsustained ventricular tachycardia.

Raymond P. Price, M.D.

Raymond P. Price, M.D.

Cardiology Department

RPP/lpm

Figure 7–16 Holter report.

Of special note is **signal-averaged electrocardiography (SAECG),** as represented in 93278. SAECG is a type of electrocardiography that can help physicians predict certain tendencies to abnormalities such as ventricular tachycardia. The signal is recorded during nine periods, each lasting 10 to 20 minutes, and the computer manipulates the data produced and predicts certain tendencies. The SAECG is a more sophisticated ECG than the standard 12-lead ECG and is used when a standard ECG is unable to demonstrate the suspected conductive abnormalities.

---

coding shot

If only the interpretation and report are done with an SAECG, report 93278-26 to indicate that only the professional component was provided.

Telephonic transmission of an electrocardiogram is made possible by a device the patient wears that records irregular rhythms. The readings from the ECG can then be sent to the physician by using a telephone to transmit the information, which is subsequently printed for the physician's review. Third-party payers usually restrict the payment of telephonic transmissions to one every 30 days. The codes 93012–93014 are divided on the basis of the component(s) the physician provides.

A **cardiovascular stress test** is a test that is used to evaluate and diagnose chest pain, to screen for heart disease, to evaluate irregular heart rhythms, and to investigate many other cardiovascular abnormalities. The patient is placed on a treadmill or a stationary bicycle and ECG leads are attached. The patient then exercises until he or she reaches maximal (220 minus age) or submaximal (85% of maximal) heart rate. During certain intervals, the physician or technician records the ECG, heart rate, and blood pressure of the patient.

The codes for stress tests (93015–93018) are divided on the basis of the components provided. The ECG is bundled into the stress test, so do not unbundle and report an ECG or any reading separately. Medication can be administered to mimic the stressing of the heart; it is used when factors are present that limit a patient's ability to exercise, such as arthritis, morbid obesity, or stroke. Stress test codes are used for both stress-induced (exercise) and pharmacologically induced (drug) studies. Medications and radiology services may be reported separately.

Echocardiography

Echocardiography is a noninvasive diagnostic method that uses ultrasonographic images to detect the presence of heart disease or valvular disease. A sliced image is used to detail the various walls of the heart. A **transducer** is placed on the outside of the chest wall, and it sends sound waves through the chest (Fig. 7–17). As the sound reflects back from each organ wall, dots are recorded, indicating the point of reflection. When the heart is in systole, it is contracting, and the dots on the recording appear farther apart. When the heart is in diastole, it is relaxing, and the dots on the recording appear closer together.

Bundled into the complete echocardiography procedures are the obtaining of the signal from the heart and great arteries by means of two-dimensional imaging and/or Doppler ultrasound, the interpretation, and the report. Mod-

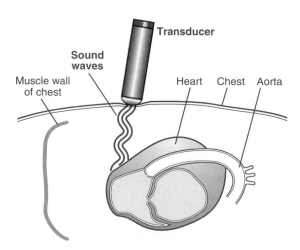

Figure 7–17 Echocardiography. A transducer is placed on the outside of the chest wall; it sends sound waves through the chest. When the heart is in systole, the heart is contracting and the dots on the echocardiogram appear farther apart. When the heart is in diastole, it is relaxing and the dots on the echocardiogram appear closer together.

ifiers -26, professional service only, and -TC, technical component, may be applied to these codes if only one component is provided. The codes are divided on the basis of whether it was a complete ECG or a follow-up/limited study, the type of ECG, and the approach used.

EXERCISE 7–7

THERAPEUTIC SERVICES, CARDIOGRAPHY, AND ECHOCARDIOGRAPHY

Using the CPT manual, code the following:

1   A physician provides CPR to a patient in cardiac arrest.

 Code(s): _____

2   Cardiovascular stress test using submaximal bicycle exercise with continuous ECG; physician was in attendance for supervision and provided the interpretation and report

 Code(s): _____

3   Percutaneous transluminal coronary balloon angioplasty of three vessels

 Code(s): _____

4   SAECG with ECG, interpretation and report only

 Code(s): _____

Cardiac Catheterization

Catheterization is an invasive diagnostic medical procedure in which the physician percutaneously inserts a catheter and manipulates the catheter into coronary vessels and/or the heart. Figure 7–18 illustrates a percutaneous method of catheterization called the Seldinger technique, after the inventor of the method. This catheterization is at the right subclavian artery. Following insertion of the fine-gauge needle, a guide wire and then a catheter are inserted. The cardiac catheter is used to measure pressure, oxygen, and blood gases, take blood samples, and measure the output of the heart. A cardiac catheterization is a study of both the circulation and the movement of the blood of the heart; the physician may inject a dye into the vessel or heart and observe the movement of the dye by means of angiogra-

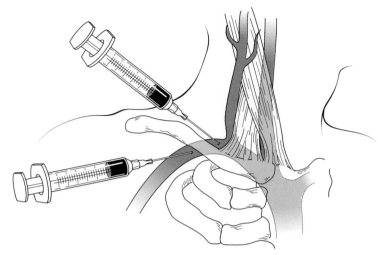

Figure 7–18   Percutaneous method of catheterization (Seldinger technique).

phy. When injection of contrast material is used to improve visualization, additional injection procedure codes (such as 93540 or 93544) must be used to specify the site of the injection.

EXAMPLE

> During a cardiac catheterization procedure, contrast medium is injected into a bypass graft and into the coronary arteries. CPT codes would be used to identify each of the areas of injection as follows:
>
> 93540   injection into the bypass graft
>
> 93545   injection into selective coronary arteries

Each of these two codes would be reported in addition to the code reflecting the type of cardiac catheterization (e.g., left and right heart catheterization, 93526). But you wouldn't be finished coding this one yet. If the cardiologist also supervises, interprets, and reports on the x-ray imaging of the angiography, codes 93555 and 93556 would be used to report the imaging services. This is a good example of component coding. Component coding requires you to examine services that were provided to the patient, identify each component, or part, of that service, identify who performed each component, and code each service provided.

Access for cardiac catheterization can be made in several locations, depending on the patient's condition and the physician's preference—for example, in the subclavian, internal jugular, femoral, external jugular, or brachial vessel.

from the trenches

What allows you to take the most pride in your career?
"Knowing our revenue per month has increased due to my consistent coding and reliability."

STEPHEN

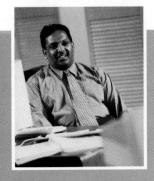

The procedure can indicate valve disorders, abnormal flow of blood, and a variety of cardiac output abnormalities. Often, a cardiac catheterization leads to a more definite treatment, such as a valvoplasty, stent placement, or angioplasty.

Bundled into the cardiac catheterization codes are the introduction, positioning, and repositioning of the catheter(s); the recording of pressures inside the heart or vessels; the taking of blood samples; rest/exercise studies; final evaluation; and final report.

There are three components in the coding of cardiac catheterization:

1. **Placement** of the catheter, using codes 93501–93533

2. **Injection** procedure, using codes 93539–93545

3. **Imaging** supervision, interpretation, and report on the injection procedure, using codes 93555–93556.

In the case of a complete cardiac catheterization, which is the usual procedure, you will find all the codes you need to fully report the service in the Medicine section, Cardiac Catheterization category. It is a good idea to make a notation of the code ranges for the three components of cardiac catheterization so you remember to look for the components when coding.

The codes in the category are not intended to be used if a catheterization was not done. For example, if a dye was injected into the vein, but it was not as a part of a cardiac catheterization, you would **not** use the injection codes from Cardiac Catheterization but instead would use codes from the Surgery section, Cardiovascular System subsection, Vascular Injection Procedures subheading, 36011–36015 or 36215–36218.

STOP *The Cardiac Catheterization injection codes are not to be used unless the injection procedure is a part of a cardiac catheterization.*

There are several codes (93561–93572) in the category that are not a part of the usual three components of the cardiac catheterization. These codes are for the **indicator dilution studies,** which are already bundled into the cardiac catheterization codes and are to be coded only when the complete cardiac catheterization procedure was **not** done. For example, if only the dye or thermal dilution study was done, without a cardiac catheterization, an indicator dilution study code would be used to report the service.

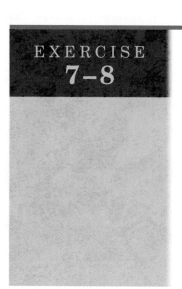

EXERCISE
7-8

CARDIAC CATHETERIZATION

Answer the following:

1 Right heart catheterization was performed by means of the introduction of a cardiac catheter into the venous system, with further manipulation into the right atrium, including injection into the right atrium of contrast material, multiple measurements, and sampling; image supervision was provided by the physician.

Code(s):

_____ Catheterization procedure

_____ Injection procedure

_____ Supervision, interpretation, and report for injection procedure

2 Retrograde left heart catheterization of left ventricle was performed, with cutdown entry into the brachiocephalic artery, and contrast medium was injected for left ventricular angiography, including supervision, interpretation, and report.

Code(s): _____

3 Indicator dilution studies when done with a cardiac catheterization are to be billed separately.

True   False

4 Bundled into the cardiac catheterization codes are the positioning and repositioning of the catheter(s).

True   False

5 Modifier -51 can be added to all codes in the Cardiac Catheterization subheading.

True   False

Intracardiac Electrophysiological Procedures

As you learned earlier in this chapter, surgical electrophysiologic procedures are those that repair the electrical system of the heart using invasive surgical procedures. In the Medicine section, the Intracardiac Electrophysiological Procedures category contains codes that are used to describe services that diagnose and treat the electrical system of the heart using less invasive procedures. Although the Medicine section procedures are invasive, they are percutaneous procedures.

Figure 7–19 illustrates the electrical conduction system of the heart, which begins with the sinoatrial node (SA), known as the heart's pacemaker. The sinoatrial node sends impulses to the atrioventricular (AV) node, which in turn passes the impulses to the bundle of His, and finally on to the Purkinje fibers to stimulate the ventricles of the heart. Lesions or diseases involving these structures along the electrical conduction pathway underlie many of the disturbances of cardiac rhythm.

To diagnose the origin of an electrophysiologic abnormality, the physician takes recordings at various sites along the pathway. The physician may also

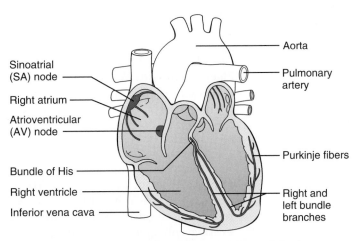

Figure 7–19 Electrical conduction system of the heart.

stimulate the heart to induce arrhythmia by means of a catheter attached to a pacing device that sends electrical impulses to various sites within the heart. A protocol (a set order) for the placement of the catheter is a **programmed stimulation.**

Pacing is the regulation of the heart rate. A cardiac pacemaker is a permanent pacer; but the pacing referred to in the EP codes is a temporary pacing done in an attempt to stabilize the beating of the heart. **Recording** is a record of the electrical activity of the heart taken by means of an ECG. Recording services are reported using codes in the range of 93600–93603, and pacing services are reported using codes in the 93610–93612 range. Combination codes that indicate both recording and pacing begin with 93619. These codes are not used as much as they used to be when EP was a new technique and readings were commonly taken at just one site. Today, more complex EP studies are usually done, including multiple pacings and recordings in combinations based on established protocols using three or more catheters. These complex services are reported with codes in the 93619–93622 range. Carefully read the notes in parentheses following several of the combination codes, as the notes indicate when the use of the combination code is appropriate and even indicate the codes that are bundled into the one combination code.

CAUTION *Most of the EP codes have many items bundled into them, so read the description of each code completely so as to avoid unbundling the services.*

A **bundle of His recording** is a reading taken inside the heart (intracardiac) at the tip of the His bundle. The physician percutaneously inserts into a vessel a special catheter that can sense electrical impulses. The catheter is advanced to the right heart. The femoral vein is the usual site of entry and fluoroscopic guidance is usually used for placement of the catheter into the heart.

Codes 93602–93603 describe a single recording based on the location—intra-arterial, right ventricle, or left ventricle. Codes 93610–93612 describe single pacing in an atrial or a ventricle location.

Code 93631 is used to report pacing and mapping done during an open surgical procedure in which the surgeon opens the chest and exposes the heart. The EP physician performs the **mapping** (locating the origin of the arrhythmia), and the surgeon then destroys the source of the arrhythmia. When reporting the services of both physicians for this procedure, use 93631 to report the mapping service and a surgery code from the range 33250–33261 to report the arrhythmia ablation. Make a notation next to the mapping code 93631 to report any surgical ablation (33250–33261) to remind yourself to code both procedures if required.

Ablation can also be performed by using a catheter with a tip that emits electric current. When the tip is placed on tissue and activated, the tissue is destroyed. Sometimes physicians destroy certain sites along the conduction pathway as a treatment for slow (bradycardia) or fast (tachycardia) heart rhythms.

Peripheral Arterial Disease Rehabilitation

Peripheral arterial disease (PAD) rehabilitation sessions last 45 to 60 minutes; these are rehabilitative physical exercises done either on a motorized treadmill or on a track to build the patient's cardiovascular endurance. An exercise physiologist or nurse supervises the sessions. If a session produces symptoms of angina or other negative symptoms, the physician reviews the information and may determine to reevaluate the patient. The physician services are reported with an additional Evaluation and Management (E/M) code.

Other Vascular Studies

If a patient has a pacemaker or defibrillator in place, periodic monitoring must occur to ensure that the device is functioning properly. Codes from the Other Vascular Studies category reflect these services. Codes are chosen according to the type of pacemaker (single or dual chamber) and whether reprogramming of an existing pacemaker or defibrillator was done.

Plethysmography (93720–93722) is a recording of the change in the size of a body part when blood passes through it and is used to determine vascular abnormalities. Respiratory function especially is assessed using total body plethysmography. There are two components in a plethysmography process—the professional component and the technical component. There are codes for the total procedure, for only the technical component of tracing, and for only the professional component of interpretation and report.

Recognize that the codes in the range 93720–93722 are only for *total* body plethysmography, in which the entire body is placed into a special chamber. There are also regional (certain parts—arm, leg, eye, etc.) recordings (plethysmography), and the codes for these regional procedures are in the 93875–93931 range. You will learn more about these regional plethysmographic procedures in the Medicine chapter because the regional studies are a diagnostic tool used in a variety of specialty areas.

Electronic analysis is an analysis of the electronic function of devices such as pacemakers and cardioverter-defibrillators after they have been implanted into a patient. The physician analyzes the devices by means of an electrocardiogram and other analyses of the device. The majority of codes in the range 93724–93744 describe a variety of electronic analytic procedures used in a variety of devices. Codes 93731–93736 describe analysis and reprogramming of single or dual chamber pacemakers, and the codes 93741–93744 describe analysis and reprogramming of cardioverter-defibrillators. Some of the pacemaker analysis codes are specifically for **telephonic analysis,** which is the analysis of a pacemaker using the telephone to transmit the information about the function of the pacemaker.

coding shot

There are no codes that specifically indicate the technical component only or the professional component only of EP, so if only the professional component was done, use modifier -26. If only the technical component was done, add the HCPCS modifier -TC.

Thermograms are visual recordings of the temperatures of the body. The variation in color on a thermogram indicates the temperature of the area. The results of a thermogram can indicate areas of vascular insufficiency.

Ambulatory blood pressure monitoring is an outpatient procedure that is done over a 24-hour period by means of a portable device worn by the patient. There is a code for the total procedure—including recording, analysis, and interpretation/report—and there are codes for each of the individual components—recording only, analysis only, and interpretation/report only.

Other Procedures

The Other Procedures codes are used for physician services that are provided for cardiac rehabilitation of outpatients, either with or without electrocardiographic monitoring.

EXERCISE 7-9

EP AND VASCULAR STUDIES

Using the CPT manual, code the following:

1 Bundle of His recording

Code(s): _____

2 Comprehensive electrophysiologic evaluation was performed, including recording and pacing of the right atrium and right ventricle. Three electrodes were repositioned. Left ventricular recordings were also made, with pacing and induction of arrhythmia.

Code(s): _____

3 Total body plethysmography, including tracing, interpretation, and report

Code(s): _____

CARDIOVASCULAR CODING IN THE RADIOLOGY SECTION

If you are employed in a clinic or office setting that has a radiology department, you will code all the components of cardiovascular services, which will often include radiology services (technical component).

Before 1992, the Radiology section of the CPT manual contained combination codes that included both the **professional** and **technical components** in one code. For example, 75659 existed to report the services of both the angiography (technical component) and the injection procedure (professional component) in a brachial angiography procedure. When the complete procedure code, 75659, was deleted, the injection procedure (professional component) was moved to the Surgery section and a code to report the technical component (angiography) remained in the Radiology section. Now, to report both the injection procedure and the angiography services (the complete procedure), you use a Surgery code to report the professional component and a Radiology code to report the technical component. The division of the technical and professional components makes it possible to specify the various parts of a procedure, which is important because some cardiologists perform both components of these cardiovascular procedures, and some cardiologists perform only the injection procedure and have a radiologist do the angiography portion of the procedure. Component coding allows for the flexibility necessary to code these various situations. Component coding also makes it easier to identify the various diagnostic tests that are used in cardiovascular conditions. For example, one cardiologist may prefer to use an ultrasonic procedure in the diagnosis of arterial stenosis and another may prefer angiography. Both procedures require the insertion of a catheter, and as such, the insertion code remains the same, but the diagnostic tools may change.

Radiology codes often contain the statement "supervision and interpretation." **Supervision** is the radiologist's overseeing of the technician who is performing the procedure or indicates that the radiologist is performing the procedure himself/herself. **Interpretation** is the summary of the findings, also known as the final report, and only the radiologist does this portion of the service. There are actually two components (parts) in a code with supervision and interpretation in the description—the professional and technical components. The technical component is the equipment and the technician who actually provides the service. The professional component is the interpretation of the results and the writing of a report about the results, as illustrated in Figure 7–20. Both components are not necessarily done by the same organization. Let's take an x-ray as an example of a service and see how you report the components.

If a clinic owns its own x-ray equipment and employs a radiologist to interpret the x-rays and write the reports, and also employs the technician who, under the supervision of the radiologist, takes the x-rays, the clinic could report the x-ray service using the appropriate radiology code, with supervision and interpretation in the description and *no modifier*. The clinic provides the total service, also known as the **global service.**

Another clinic owns the equipment and employs the technician who takes the x-ray, but then the clinic sends the x-ray out to a radiologist at another clinic who reads the x-ray and writes the report. The radiologist would report the service with the appropriate radiology code and *modifier -26* to indicate that he or she provided only the professional component of the service. The clinic that employs the technician and owns the equipment would report the same radiology code but would attach the HCPCS *modifier -TC* (technical component) to indicate that only the technical component of the service was provided by it.

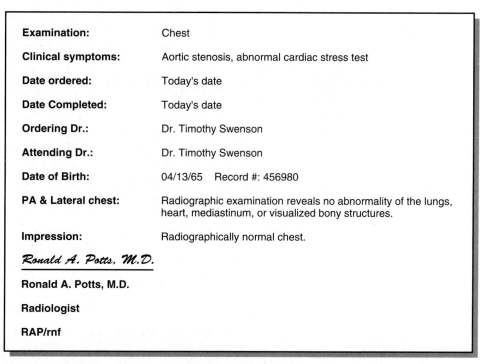

Examination:	Chest
Clinical symptoms:	Aortic stenosis, abnormal cardiac stress test
Date ordered:	Today's date
Date Completed:	Today's date
Ordering Dr.:	Dr. Timothy Swenson
Attending Dr.:	Dr. Timothy Swenson
Date of Birth:	04/13/65 Record #: 456980
PA & Lateral chest:	Radiographic examination reveals no abnormality of the lungs, heart, mediastinum, or visualized bony structures.
Impression:	Radiographically normal chest.

Ronald A. Potts, M.D.

Ronald A. Potts, M.D.

Radiologist

RAP/rnf

Figure 7–20   Final radiology report containing the radiologist's interpretation of the findings.

CAUTION *The* **professional component** *(interpreting results and writing the report) is reported using modifier -26. The* **technical component** *(technician and equipment) is reported using modifier -TC.*

A third clinic has no x-ray equipment, so the physicians in the clinic send patients to an outside radiologist who takes x-rays on equipment he or she owns, interprets the results, and writes the report. The outside radiologist would report the service using the global radiology code with *no modifier,* because both the professional component and the technical component were provided.

Contrast material is commonly used with radiology procedures to enhance the image. If the Radiology section code states "with contrast" or "with or without contrast," you will know that the injection of contrast material and the contrast material itself (the substance used for contrasting) are bundled into the code; therefore, you would not code for the contrast material or injection separately. If, however, there is no indication of contrast in the code description, and the physician used contrast, you would code both for the injection of the contrast material and for the contrast material itself. Injection of contrast is usually included in the radiology code. If guidelines state that you should code injections separately, they are coded with the appropriate code from the surgery section—for example, 47500, Injection procedure for percutaneous transhepatic cholangiography, and 74320 for the radiology portion of the service. The contrast material is reported separately using code 99070 from the Medicine section, Special Services, Procedures, and Reports subsection.

coding shot

Not all contrast material can be coded separately! Oral or rectal contrast is considered a part of the procedure and is not coded separately. Intravenous or intra-arterial injection of contrast material can be coded separately if the code description does not refer to inclusion of contrast material.

STOP *Now, don't be getting discouraged with all of these codes from all of these sections! Remember that only with repeated use of these codes can you master them. At first, it sounds so confusing that you might wonder if you can ever absorb all of this information and the variations. You can. But you must be patient with the process. To be a coder is to be able to concentrate on details and commit yourself to the process of learning the details through repeated use. Everyone starts at the same place.*

Now, let's get back to learning about component coding. Two physicians, a cardiologist and a radiologist from the same facility, perform an angiography of the brachiocephalic artery (third order) using contrast material. The coding is as follows:

- Cardiologist placing the catheter: 36217, Surgery section
- Radiologist performing the angiography: 75658, Radiology section
- Supply of the contrast material: 99070, Medicine section

Two physicians, a cardiologist and a radiologist from different facilities, perform an angiography of the brachiocephalic artery (third order) using contrast material. The coding for the cardiologist is as follows:

- Cardiologist placing the catheter: 36217, Surgery section

The coding for the radiologist is as follows:

- Radiologist performing the angiography: 75658, Radiology section
- Supply of the contrast material: 99070, Medicine section

coding shot

If the radiologist is at the same facility as the equipment, you use code 75658 (angiography). If the radiologist is hospital-based, you use code 75658-26 on the HCFA-1500 and 75658 on the UB-92.

Heart

Many of the codes that used to be in the Heart subsection of the Radiology section have been moved into the Surgery section, Cardiovascular subsection, or into the Medicine section, Cardiovascular subsection. You will see many notes in parentheses at the beginning of the Heart subheading in the Radiology section directing you to other sections of the CPT manual. For example, one note in the Radiology section indicates that code 75505, cardiac catheterization, has been deleted and that to report the service, you should use code 93555 from the Medicine section.

The remaining codes in the Heart subsection of the Radiology section are used to report cardiac magnetic resonance imaging (MRI). An **MRI** is the use of radiation to show the body in a cross-sectional view. MRI may include the use of injectable dyes (radiographic contrast) to aid in imaging. Other MRI codes are located throughout the Radiology section according to body part being imaged, but the codes in the Heart subsection are just for cardiac MRIs.

Aorta and Arteries

In Radiology, the Aorta and Arteries subsection includes codes for aortography excluding the heart—thoracic, abdominal, cervicocerebral, brachial, external carotid, carotid, vertebral, spinal, extremity, renal, visceral, adrenal pelvic, pulmonary, and internal mammary.

The codes found in the Aorta and Arteries subsection are often used in coding components of cardiovascular services.

EXERCISE 7-10

HEART, AORTA, AND ARTERIES

Using the CPT manual, code the following:

1 Code a selective catheter placement in the first-order brachiocephalic artery, with angiography, including contrast.

Code(s): _____ , _____ , and

_____

2 A cardiologist performs a selective catheter placement into the thoracic artery, first-order branch; a radiologist performs an angiographic procedure without contrast.

Code(s): _____ and _____

3 A cardiologist performs selective catheter placement into a second-order abdominal artery and also an angiography with injection of contrast.

Code(s): _____ , _____ , and

_____

4 Complete cardiac MRI with contrast

Code(s): _____

CHAPTER GLOSSARY

angioplasty: surgical or percutaneous procedure in a vessel to dilate the vessel opening; used in the treatment of atherosclerotic disease

bypass: to go around

cardiopulmonary: refers to the heart and lungs

cardiopulmonary bypass: blood bypasses the heart through a heart-lung machine during open-heart surgery

cardioverter-defibrillator: surgically placed device that directs an electric current shock to the heart to restore rhythm

component: part

electrode: lead attached to a generator that carries the electric current from the generator to the atria or ventricles

electrophysiology: the study of the electrical system of the heart, including the study of arrhythmias

embolectomy: removal of blockage (embolism) from vessels

endarterectomy: incision into an artery to remove the inner lining so as to eliminate disease or blockage

epicardial: over the heart

false aneurysm: sac of clotted blood that has completely destroyed the vessel and is being contained by the tissue that surrounds the vessel

fistula: abnormal opening from one area to another area or to the outside of the body

intracardiac: inside the heart

invasive: entering the body, breaking the skin

noninvasive: not entering the body, not breaking the skin

nuclear cardiology: diagnostic specialty that uses radiologic procedures to aid in the diagnosis of cardiologic conditions

pericardiocentesis: procedure in which a surgeon withdraws fluid from the pericardial space by means of a needle inserted percutaneously into the space

pericardium: membranous sac enclosing the heart and the ends of the great vessels

thoracostomy: surgical incision into the chest wall and insertion of a chest tube

transvenous: across a vein

CHAPTER REVIEW

CHAPTER 7, PART I, THEORY

Without the use of reference material, complete the following:

1 What are the two subheadings within the Cardiovascular System subsection?

_____ / _____ and

_____ / _____

2 The subspecialty of internal medicine that is concerned with the diagnosis and treatment of

the heart is _____ .

3 In Chapter 7 you learned about coding from which three sections of the CPT?

_____ , _____ ,

and _____

4 Procedures that break the skin for correction or examination are known as

_____

procedures.

5 Procedures that do not break the skin are

known as _____ procedures.

6 The study of the heart's electrical system is

known as _____ .

7 The use of radioactive radiologic procedures to aid in the diagnosis of cardiologic conditions

is termed _____ _____
cardiology.

8 A catheter that is inserted into an artery and manipulated to a further order is termed

_____ placement.

9 A catheter that is inserted into an artery and not manipulated to a further order is termed

_____ placement.

10 Surgical procedures in the Heart and Pericardium subheading contain procedures that are performed through both open surgical sites

and _____ .

CHAPTER 7, PART II, PRACTICAL

Code the following cases for the surgical procedures, the office visits, and the cardiology-related Radiology and Medicine section codes. Do not code the laboratory work.

11 Dennis Smith, a 42-year-old railroad employee (established patient), has a history of severe mitral stenosis with regurgitation. He is now symptomatic and his physician recommends a mitral valve replacement, to be done in 2 weeks. Dennis agrees to the surgery, and the physician does a comprehensive history and physical in preparation for surgery. The physician orders a general health panel blood workup and a urinalysis (automated). Three

weeks later, the physician performs a mitral valve replacement. Dennis recovers uneventfully and is discharged from the hospital 5 days later.
Code(s): _____

12 Thrombectomy of arterial graft
Code(s): _____

13 Direct repair of aneurysm and graft insertion for occlusive disease of the common femoral artery
Code(s): _____

14 A surgical assistant performs five venous grafts in a coronary artery bypass.
Code(s): _____

15 Open-heart repair of mitral valve with use of cardiopulmonary bypass
Code(s): _____

16 Removal of a single chamber pacing cardioverter-defibrillator pulse generator
Code(s): _____

17 Pericardiotomy for removal of clot
Code(s): _____

18 Complete repair of tetralogy of Fallot is made with closure of a ventricular septal defect, and a conduit from the pulmonary artery to the right ventricle is constructed. A pulmonary graft valve is then secured. Cardiopulmonary bypass is required.
Code(s): _____

19 Shunting from subclavian to pulmonary artery using the Blalock-Taussig operation
Code(s): _____

20 Pulmonary endarterectomy with embolectomy requiring cardiopulmonary bypass
Code(s): _____

21 Direct repair of aneurysm associated with occlusion of the vertebral artery
Code(s): _____

22 Thromboendarterectomy with patch graft of iliac artery
Code(s): _____

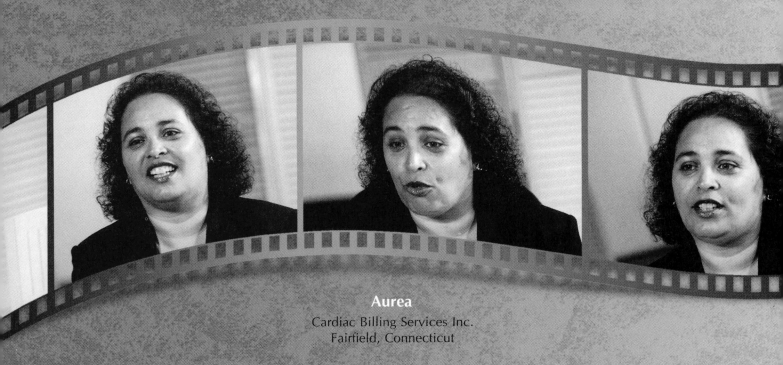

Aurea
Cardiac Billing Services Inc.
Fairfield, Connecticut

chapter 8

Female Genital System and Maternity Care and Delivery

LEARNING OBJECTIVES

After completing this chapter you should be able to

1. Code female reproductive services.

2. Apply rules of coding to female reproductive services.

3. Differentiate among codes on the basis of surgical approach.

4. Demonstrate knowledge of the coding of common female reproductive services.

5. Understand component coding in female reproductive services.

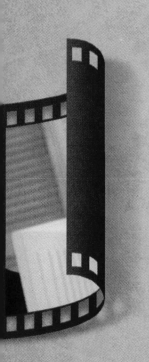

PART I: Female Genital System

FORMAT

The Female Genital System subsection is divided according to anatomic site, from the vulva up to the ovaries (Fig. 8–1). The anatomic sites are then divided on the basis of category of procedure (i.e., incision, excision, destruction). Codes for in vitro fertilization are found at the end of the subsection.

The subsection has a wide variety of codes for minor procedures that are performed in a physician's office as well as for major procedures that are performed in a hospital. It is important to read the descriptions of the codes as well as the notes to avoid unbundling in this subsection. For example, if a total abdominal hysterectomy was performed as well as a bilateral oophorectomy (removal of ovaries), only CPT code 58150 would be used. CPT code 58150 includes in the description the statement "with or without removal of ovary(s)." Bundled into the code are both the abdominal hysterectomy and the bilateral oophorectomy.

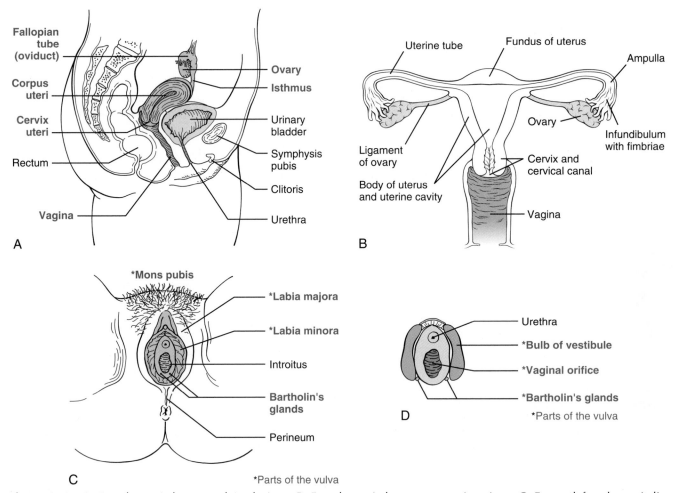

Figure 8–1 *A,* Female genital system, lateral view. *B,* Female genital system, anterior view. *C,* External female genitalia. *D,* Parts of the vulva.

CODING HIGHLIGHTS

Vulva, Perineum, and Introitus

You will see a repeated note in the Vulva, Perineum, and Introitus sub-heading indicating that the incision and drainage of Skene's gland is not coded using codes in the Female Genital System subsection but instead is coded using Surgery section, Urinary System subsection codes. That is because Skene's gland, also known as the para-urethral duct, which is a group of small mucous glands located near the lower end of the urethra, is part of the urinary system. Procedures involving Skene's gland are, therefore, always coded using Urinary System codes (53060 or 53270).

Incision

The **vulva** includes the following parts: mons pubis, labia majora, labia minora, bulb of vestibule, vaginal orifice or vestibule of the vagina, and the greater (Bartholin's gland) and lesser vestibule glands (see Fig. 8–1C and D). When the code description indicates the incision and drainage of an abscess of the vulva, the code covers an abscess of any of the anatomic areas just listed. For example, if a medical record indicates "an incision and drainage of an abscess of Bartholin's gland," you must know that Bartholin's gland is considered a part of the vulva, so the code will be located in that subheading.

Destruction

Destruction of lesions of the vulva, perineum, or introitus can be accomplished using a variety of methods—cryosurgery, electrosurgery, or chemical destruction. Destruction codes are divided on the basis of whether the destruction is simple or complex, although the code description does not define simple or complex. Complexity is based on the physician's judgment of complexity, and the complexity should be stated in the medical record

CAUTION *Destruction is not excision. Destruction is obliteration or eradication. Excision is removal. With destruction no tissue is removed, as the tissue is destroyed. There is no pathology report after a lesion has been destroyed because there is nothing for the pathologist to analyze.*

Excision

The first two codes in the Excision category are for biopsies in which the physician takes a tissue sample by removing a piece of tissue with a scalpel or punch. The area to be biopsied is anesthetized with local anesthetic before the biopsy is performed. The physician may suture the area or use clips for closure. The anesthesia and closure are included in the package of an excision code, so be careful not to unbundle. The codes are also divided on the basis of number of lesions; there is an add-on code for additional lesions beyond one. Be certain to specify the number of lesions biopsied by listing the number of units on the HCFA-1500 form in Block 24-G (refer to Fig. 4–15).

Vulvectomy is the surgical removal of a portion of the vulva. Usually a vulvectomy is performed to treat a malignant or premalignant lesion. The following definitions apply to the vulvectomy codes (56620–56640) and describe the extent and size of the vulvar area removed during the procedure.

Extent

- Simple   skin and superficial subcutaneous tissue
- Radical   skin and deep subcutaneous tissue

Size

- Partial   less than 80%
- Complete   greater than 80%

The vulvectomy codes are divided on the basis of these definitions of extent and size. The extent and size are stated in combination. For example, the term "simple partial vulvectomy" describes a *superficial subcutaneous tissue* (extent) removal of 78% (size) of the vulvar area. Bundled into the codes is usual closure, but if plastic repair is required, you would report the repair in addition to the procedure. The operative report will indicate the extent of the procedure and the closure.

The more radical procedures involving the vulva are usually performed because of a demonstrated malignancy, and more extensive removal takes place. This radical removal can include the removal of deep lymph nodes, saphenous veins, ligaments, large amounts of tissue from the lower abdomen or even from the thigh. The procedure may also be done bilaterally, so don't forget modifier -50, bilateral procedure.

Repair

The procedure codes in the Repair category describe plastic repair of the vulva, perineum, or introitus. Plastic repair of the **introitus** is surgical repair of the opening of the vagina. The extent and nature of the procedure are determined by the defect being repaired and hence vary greatly from patient to patient. **Clitoroplasty** is surgical reduction of a clitoris that has become enlarged due to an adrenal gland imbalance. **Perineoplasty** is plastic repair of the perineum, usually to provide additional support to the perineal area.

Vagina

Colpotomy is cutting into the vagina to gain access to the pelvic cavity. The procedure is performed to explore the pelvic cavity or to drain a pelvic abscess. **Colpocentesis** is incision of the vagina to gain access to the peritoneal cul-de-sac—the area between the uterus and the rectum—to explore it or to drain an abscess. If the colpocentesis is a part of a more major procedure, you do not code it separately, as it is considered to be bundled into the more major procedures. Note that the code 57020 (colpocentesis) has a star after it to designate colpocentesis as a minor procedure; it is reported only if it is the only procedure performed (separate procedure).

Destruction

As with the destruction codes for the vulva, the destruction codes for the Vagina subsection are divided on the basis of whether the destruction was

from the trenches

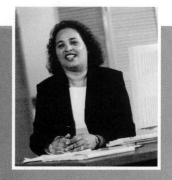

"*Coding is a challenge. You have to climb that mountain. It doesn't just come to you. You have to work at it . . . and stay current. Always read . . . books, newsletters, codes.*"

AUREA

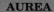

simple or extensive, in the judgment of the physician. Any method of destruction is acceptable for inclusion in these codes.

Excision

The Excision category of the Vagina subsection contains codes for reporting the services of biopsy, vaginectomy (removal of part or all of the vagina), colpocleisis (closure of the vaginal canal), and cyst/lesion removal. The vaginectomy codes are divided according to the extent of the procedure—partial or total—and the extent to which tissue and adjacent structure(s) are removed.

Introduction

The Introduction category contains codes for vaginal irrigation; insertion of a support device (pessary), diaphragm, or cervical cap (to prevent pregnancy); and packing of the vagina (for vaginal hemorrhage). The pessary and diaphragm/cervical cap are not included in these Introduction codes. The supply of these devices would be billed using code 99070, supplies, or a HCPCS code (e.g., A4561).

Repair

The Repair category is rather extensive, as the possible forms of repair of the vagina are many. A note in parentheses, "(nonobstetrical)," sometimes follows the code description in the Female Genital Systems subsection because if the procedure was performed as a part of an obstetric procedure, you would use a code from the Maternity Care and Delivery subsection.

A surgeon performs a **colporrhaphy** to strengthen an area of the wall of the vagina that is weak by pulling together the weakened vaginal area with sutures. The vaginal wall can also be reinforced with sutures placed in weakened areas. Also, excess tissue can be removed to tighten the area. The reinforcement might be performed for several reasons, but it is commonly done to prevent the bladder from protruding into the weakened vaginal wall.

In this Repair category, the codes are often divided on the basis of the approach used. For example, an abdominal approach to the repair of an enterocele (outpouching) has a different code than does a vaginal approach to the same repair; an anterior vaginal approach for the repair of a cystocele (bladder protrusion into vagina) differs from a repair in which a posterior vaginal approach was used. So, you must pay particular attention to the approach used. You will find that the approach used is noted in the operative report.

One method of vaginal repair that is *not* in the Repair category is the laparoscopic repair. Codes for repair of the vagina using a colposcope (microscope) are located in the Vagina subheading, Endoscopy category. The colposcope enables the physician to directly view changes in the vagina and cervix. For example, Figure 8–2 illustrates an endocervical polyp protruding through the external os (mouth of the cervix) as seen by the physician using a colposcope.

CAUTION *Coders need to pay close attention to the method as well as to the approach. For example, a surgeon might perform an open procedure as opposed to a laparoscopic procedure.*

Notes throughout the Repair category will often direct you to the correct code or code range in the Urinary System subsection. Often, the only difference between surgical procedures coded with Female Genital System codes and those coded with the Urinary System codes is the approach. For exam-

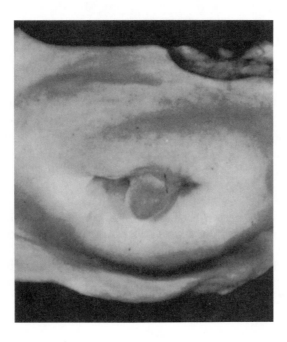

Figure 8–2 Endocervical polyp protruding through the mouth of the cervix (external os) as seen through a colposcope. (From Cotran RS, Kumar V, Robbins SL: Robbins Pathologic Basis of Disease, 5th ed. Philadelphia, WB Saunders, 1994, p. 1048.)

ple, Female Genital System code 57330 describes the closure of a vesico-vaginal fistula (abnormal channel between bladder and vagina) using a vaginal approach, whereas Urinary System code 51900 describes the same procedure using an abdominal approach. The approach method would be described in the operative report.

Manipulation

Manipulation of the vagina includes dilation (stretching), pelvic examination, and removal of foreign material. What these three different procedures have in common is that they are all performed under **general anesthesia** because a patient cannot tolerate the procedure while awake. If a local anesthetic or no anesthetic was used, you would not use a Manipulation code; instead, the service would be included in the Evaluation and Management (E/M) service. For example, if a physician removed an impacted tampon from the vagina and used no anesthetic during the procedure, only the office visit at which the removal took place would be coded.

Endoscopy

As discussed earlier in this chapter, the endoscopic procedure codes in the Endoscopy category of the Vagina subheading are for colposcopic procedures. The colposcopic procedures are often bundled into other, more major procedures. Only when colposcopic procedure is done as the only procedure or is unrelated to another procedure(s) being done is the colposcopy coded.

If a biopsy of the cervix or the endocervical canal is done, the code to report the service is 57454. The codes specifies "biopsy(s)," so whether one or multiple biopsies were taken, 57454 represents the total number. Code 57454 also indicates "and/or endocervical curettage"; therefore, you cannot unbundle the code and report the curettage (scraping) separately.

A loop electrode excision procedure is referred to as LEEP, LETZ, or cervical loop diathermy and is a new office procedure that uses heated wire (Fig. 8–3) to remove cervical tissue. The device is attached to an electric generator that heats the wire. The procedure has a lower risk level and is less expensive than other methods. A LEEP would usually be done after an abnormal Pap smear result or an abnormal examination. The cervix is

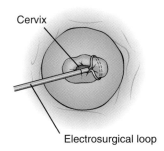

Cervix

Electrosurgical loop

Figure 8–3 The loop used in the electrosurgical excision procedure.

moistened, and the loop is positioned over the cervix and drawn across the area. The resulting slice is examined pathologically. The device is also used to cauterize the area at the end of the procedure by means of a different attachment.

Cervix Uteri

The Cervix Uteri subheading contains codes for excision, repair, and manipulation.

Excision

The codes in the Excision category often specify "(separate procedure)" because many times, the procedures are bundled into a more major procedure. For example, the excision procedure of a biopsy is often incidental to a more major surgical procedure, such as a hysterectomy, and the biopsy is not coded separately.

Codes for **conization** of the cervix are divided on the basis of the method used to obtain the tissue. In conization, a cone of tissue is removed from the cervix for a biopsy or treatment of a lesion. The laser is an often used method of conization, but the newer LEEP technology is also widely used. The LEEP device can be used for various procedures. The code for a LEEP colposcopic procedure with *cervical biopsy* in the Vagina subheading, Endoscopy category, is 57460, and the code for a LEEP colposcopic procedure with *cervical conization* is 57522; the difference is that a conization takes a deeper cut into the cervix. Be certain, when coding cervical biopsy and conization, that the information in the medical record provides sufficient detail to allow you to distinguish between a biopsy and conization. If the record is not complete enough to make the determination, obtain the information from the physician before choosing a code.

Repair

Nonobstetric cerclage repair of the cervix involves extensive suturing of the cervix to decrease the size of the opening into the vagina. **Trachelorrhaphy** is a complex cervical repair in which plastic methods are used to repair a laceration of the cervix. Both Repair codes use a vaginal approach to the procedure.

Manipulation

Dilation of the cervix is coded separately only if it is the sole procedure performed. Dilation of the cervix, like dilation of the vagina, is often bundled into a more major procedure.

Corpus Uteri

The corpus uteri is the anatomic area above the isthmus (see Fig. 8–1A) and below the opening for the fallopian tubes. The subheading contains the categories of excision, introduction, and laparoscopy/hysteroscopy procedures. Many of the procedures in the category are very complex, and some of them have several variations.

Excision

Endometrial sampling is a biopsy of the mucous lining of the uterus. The physician inserts a curet into the endocervical canal to extract tissue samples for pathologic examination. If only an endocervical sampling is taken, the biopsy is coded; but if the biopsy is done as a part of a more major procedure involving the cervix, the biopsy is considered incidental to the more major procedure and is bundled into the surgical package.

Dilation and curettage (D&C; 58120) is a diagnostic procedure that is performed when an endometrial biopsy has failed or was inconclusive, to determine the cause of abnormal bleeding, or to locate a neoplasm. Clamps are used to manipulate the cervix, a curet is inserted into the uterus, and fragments are removed from the endometrium. The tissue samples are sent to pathology for analysis. The D&C in the Corpus Uteri subheading is for nonobstetric patients only. If a D&C is performed because of postpartum hemorrhage, a code from the subsection Maternity Care and Delivery would be used to report the service.

coding shot

Many third-party payers will not reimburse for a dilation and curettage if it is performed with any other pelvic surgery because it is thought to be integral to the procedure. The CPT manual does not list a D&C as a "(separate procedure)"; therefore, you need to be familiar with reimbursement policies in your area.

Hysterectomy codes represent the majority of the codes in the Corpus Uteri subheading. A **hysterectomy** is the removal of the uterus, but in the CPT manual there are many variations of the procedure. The divisions of the hysterectomy codes are based first on the approach (abdominal or vaginal), then on the secondary procedures that were performed (removal of tubes, biopsy, bladder, etc.). You have to read the code descriptions carefully to determine what is bundled into the code. Because so many procedures are bundled into several of the codes, you also have to be careful not to unbundle and code for items already covered in the main procedure. For example, a total abdominal hysterectomy can include the removal of the ovaries and/or the fallopian tubes; therefore, billing separately for the removal of the ovaries or tubes would be undbundling.

Introduction

It is in the Introduction category that you will find the codes for some very common procedures such as the insertion and removal of an intrauterine device for birth control and for some not-so-common procedures such as artificial insemination. There are also several codes that have radiology components—your component coding skills will again be used.

Because **intrauterine device (IUD)** insertion is coded using Introduction category codes, you might think IUD removal would be in a removal category, but it is also in the Introduction category.

Don't confuse the insertion of an IUD with the placement of an implantable contraceptive such as Norplant, as described in the Integumentary subsection.

The specialized fertility procedure of **artificial insemination** and the preparation of the sperm for insemination are coded using Introduction category codes. During the insemination procedure, sperm is injected into the cervix and often, a cervical cap is inserted to keep the sperm in the cervical area. **In vitro fertilization** is a different procedure in which an egg from the female is withdrawn and fertilized with sperm in a laboratory for 2 to 3 days, then implanted into the uterus. There is an In Vitro Fertilization subheading containing codes to report these services, located at the end of the Female Genital System subsection.

Catheterization and introduction (58340) of saline or contrast material through the cervix and uterus and into the fallopian tubes (hysterosalpingography) is used by a physician to see any blockage or abnormalities of the fallopian tubes. Ultrasound can also be used for the same procedure (hysterosonography). You need to remember your component coding and code the radiology or ultrasound portion of the procedure with a code from the Radiology section. A note following 58340 in the CPT manual directs you to the correct component code. For the radiographic supervision and interpretation, the component code is 74740; for the ultrasound, the code is 76831.

The other procedure in the Introduction category that may have a radiology component is the introduction of a catheter into the fallopian tubes. The catheter is passed through the fallopian tube, and an x-ray will show where the catheter encounters an obstruction or a narrowing of the tube. A code from the Radiology section, Gynecological and Obstetrical subsection, would be used to report the radiology portion of the service.

Chromotubation is the injection of a fluid, either saline or contrast material, into the fallopian tubes during a surgical procedure to ensure that the tubes are unobstructed. This procedure, as with many in the Introduction category, is performed as a diagnostic tool in the evaluation of infertility.

Laparoscopy/Hysteroscopy

More and more procedures are being performed by using an endoscope instead of opening the area to complete view. With an endoscopic procedure, usually two or three small incisions are made through which lights, cameras, and instruments may be passed. Because endoscopic procedures are less invasive, patients are more accepting of the procedures, and recovery times and risks are reduced. Figure 8–4 illustrates a laparoscopy procedure.

The first rule of a laparoscopy or hysteroscopy is that all surgical procedures include a diagnostic procedure. You never unbundle a surgical laparo-

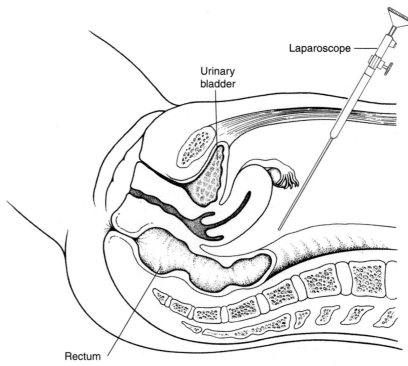

Urinary
bladder

Laparoscope

Rectum

Figure 8–4   Laparoscopy.

scopic procedure and also report a diagnostic procedure. If a procedure started out as a diagnostic laparoscopic procedure and ended up being a surgical laparoscopic procedure, still being performed through a laparoscope, you code only for the surgical laparoscopy.

CAUTION *If the laparoscopy is of the peritoneum, you use a code from the laparoscopy category of the Digestive System, Abdomen, Peritoneum, and Omentum, subheading 49320.*

The codes in the Laparoscopy/Hysteroscopy category are divided on the basis of other procedures that might have been performed during the hysteroscopy. For example, a hysteroscopy with removal of a foreign body and a hysteroscopy with ablation have different codes.

Oviduct/Ovary

The Oviduct/Ovary subheading is divided into incision, laparoscopy, excision, and repair. Fallopian tube procedures are located in this subheading.

Incision

The Incision category is where you will locate the codes for tubal ligation. **Tubal ligation** is a permanent, highly effective method of birth control. The codes are divided according to the type of ligation performed and the circumstances at the time of the ligation. The types of ligation are as follows: tying off the tube with suture material (ligation), removing a portion of the tube (transection), and blocking the tube with a clip, ring, or band (occlusion). The circumstances under which the procedure is done affect the choice of codes. For example, a procedure can be done either on one side (unilateral) or on both sides (bilateral). The procedure can be done at different times, such as during the same hospitalization period as the period of delivery, during the postpartum period, or during another surgical procedure.

CAUTION *Do not use a bilateral procedure modifier (-50) because all the code descriptions in the Incision category indicate "tube(s)" or "unilateral or bilateral." Also, do not code tubal ligations done by means of a laparoscopic procedure using the Incision category codes. There are codes for laparoscopic tubal ligation procedures in the Laparoscopy category of subheading Oviduct/Ovary.*

A ligation can be performed by taking an abdominal or a vaginal approach. If a ligation or transection of the fallopian tube(s) is done during the same operative procedure as a cesarean section or other intra-abdominal surgery, you code the ligation/transection using code 58611. Code 58611 is used only to report the tubal as a component of the more major surgical procedure but is listed in addition to the primary code.

Often at the time of an abdominal tubal ligation, lysis of adhesions is also performed. Lysis is not bundled into the ligation code. You code for the lysis of adhesions separately, using the Repair category code 58740, if so allowed by the third-party payer.

Laparoscopy

The procedures described in the Oviduct/Ovary subheading, Laparoscopy category, include only surgical laparoscopy and always include a diagnostic laparoscopy. If only a diagnostic laparoscopy was performed, you use code 49320 from the Digestive System subsection, Abdomen, Peritoneum, and Omentum category, because the scope is being passed into the abdomen for examination only. Once a definitive procedure such as a tubal ligation has begun, the examination/diagnostic laparoscopic procedure is bundled into the surgical procedure. For example, if a diagnostic laparoscopy was done and did not lead to a definitive procedure, the diagnostic laparoscopic code 49320 from the Surgery section would be submitted to describe the procedure of examining the abdomen using an endoscope. But if a diagnostic laparoscopy is done and does lead to a fulguration of the oviducts, code 58670 from the Female Genital System subsection would be used. The terminal (end or final) procedure dictates the code choice.

The laparoscopy codes are divided on the basis of the procedure performed—for example, lysis of adhesions, oophorectomy, and lesion excision.

Excision

The Excision category codes are for salpingectomy (removal of uterine tube) or salpingo-oophorectomy (removal of uterine tube and ovary). Both codes describe unilateral or bilateral procedures that are either complete or partial. An unbundling issue presents itself with the use of these codes. If either procedure is done with a more major procedure such as a hysterectomy, each is considered bundled into the more major procedure and cannot be reported separately.

Repair

Within the Repair category are codes for lysis of adhesions and various repairs to the fallopian tubes. All of the repairs are performed for the purpose of restoring fertility. Often the repairs are made through small

from the trenches

"Be open to change . . . communicate with physicians and all other clinical staff to get the information and clarification needed to code to the highest level of specificity."

AUREA

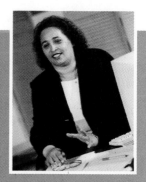

incisions above the pubic hairline, but they can also be made through a laparoscope.

Lysis of adhesions is performed in the fallopian tubes (salpingolysis) or the ovaries (ovariolysis) using a small incision to insert instrumentation and complete repairs. Lysis is a procedure that is often performed at the time of another, more major procedure and it is usually bundled into the more major procedure. If the lysis takes an extensive amount of time, you can bill for the service.

In Vitro Fertilization

In vitro fertilization means to fertilize an egg outside the body, and the codes in the In Vitro Fertilization category describe several methods that are used in modern fertility practice. Third-party payers often do not pay for the fertility treatments, and you will have to be certain that you know the policy of the payer regarding fertility treatments.

Code 58970, aspiration of the ova, is often performed with ultrasonic guidance and when it is, you use Radiology section, Ultrasonic Guidance Procedures category code 76948 to code the radiology service.

EXERCISE 8-1

FEMALE GENITAL SYSTEM

Using the CPT manual, code the following:

1 Simple destruction of one lesion of vaginal vestibule

Code(s): _____

2 Biopsy of three lesions of the vulva

Code(s): _____

3 Closure of rectovaginal fistula, abdominal approach

Code(s): _____

4 Cone biopsy (laser) of cervix with dilation and curettage

Code(s): _____

5 Unilateral salpingectomy with oophorectomy

Code(s): _____

Using the vulvectomy notes in the CPT manual, match each of the following procedures with its correct definition:

Procedure	The removal of:
6 simple _____	a. greater than 80% of the vulvar area
7 radical _____	b. skin and deep subcutaneous tissues
8 partial _____	c. skin and superficial subcutaneous tissues
9 complete _____	d. less than 80% of the vulvar area

PART II: Maternity Care and Delivery

FORMAT

The Maternity Care and Delivery subsection is divided according to type of procedure. As a general rule, the subsection progresses from antepartum procedures through delivery procedures. The guidelines are very detailed as to the services included in antepartum and delivery care, not only to facilitate coding but also to help guard against unbundling. Notes found at the beginning of this subsection describe, in depth, the services listed in obstetric care.

Abortion codes, whether for spontaneous abortion, missed abortion, or induction of abortion, are found at the end of the subsection. Abortion codes indicate treatment of a spontaneous abortion or missed abortion, including additional division on the basis of trimester and induction of abortion by method. You must be aware of the gestational age of the fetus to determine whether a delivery code or an abortion code would be appropriate.

Treatment for ectopic pregnancies is based on the site of the pregnancy, the extent of the surgery, and whether the approach was by means of laparoscopy or laparotomy.

CODING HIGHLIGHTS

Maternity and Delivery

The gestation of a fetus takes approximately 266 days; but when the **estimated date of delivery (EDD)** is calculated, 280 days are often used, counting the time from the **last menstrual period (LMP).** The gestation is divided in to three time periods, called trimesters. The trimesters are as follows:

First	LMP to week 12
Second	Weeks 13–27
Third	Weeks 28–EDD

When a maternity case is uncomplicated, the service codes normally include the antepartum care, delivery, and postpartum care in the global package. **Antepartum care** is considered to include both the initial and subsequent history and physical examinations, blood pressures, patient's weight, routine urinalysis, fetal heart tones, and monthly visits to 28 weeks of gestation, biweekly visits from gestation weeks 29 through 36, and weekly visits from week 37 to delivery when these services are provided by the same physician. If the patient is seen by the same physician for a service other than those identified as part of antepartum care, you would report that service separately. For example, if a patient in week 32 came to the office because of cold symptoms, an E/M service code would be billed.

Delivery includes admission to the hospital, which includes the admitting history and examination, management of an uncomplicated labor, and delivery that is either vaginal or by cesarean section (including any episiotomy and use of forceps). If the labor or delivery is complicated, you would report those services separately.

Included in **postpartum care** are the hospital visits and/or office visits for 6 weeks after a delivery. If the postpartum care is complicated or if services are provided to the patient during the postpartum period, but the services are not generally part of the postpartum care, you would report those services separately.

Antepartum Services

Amniocentesis is a procedure in which the physician inserts a needle into the pregnant uterus to withdraw amniotic fluid. The procedure cannot be done in the first 14 weeks of pregnancy. Usually in this procedure, ultrasound is used to guide the needle, and the Supervision and Interpretation (S&I) service is billed using a code from the Radiology section, Ultrasonic Guidance Procedures subsection, code 76946.

Several of the antepartum services require component coding in order to fully report the services provided. Attention to the code descriptions and parenthetic statements is necessary to ensure that all services are reported.

Cordocentesis is a procedure in which fetal blood is drawn. This procedure is usually done under ultrasonic guidance. As with all of the Antepartum Services codes, the purpose of the procedures is to assess the status of the fetus. These are not included in normal antepartum care and should be coded separately.

Excision

Abdominal **hysterotomy** is performed to remove a hydatidiform or an embryo. If a tubal ligation is performed at the same time as a hysterotomy, be certain to use an additional code (58611) to indicate the ligation.

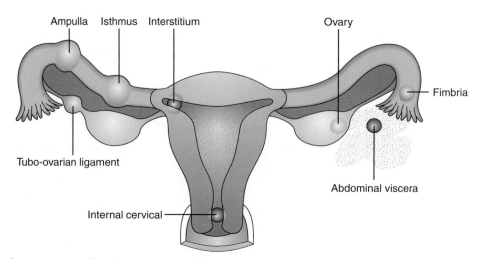

Figure 8–5 Implantation sites in ectopic pregnancy. (From Buck CJ: 2002 ICD-9-CM, and HCPCS. Philadelphia, WB Saunders, 2001, p. 730.)

An **ectopic pregnancy** is one in which the fertilized ovum has become implanted outside of the uterus, as illustrated in Figure 8–5. The surgical treatment for this condition can use either an abdominal or a vaginal approach; most often, the abdominal approach is used. If the area has not ruptured, the pregnancy is removed. If a rupture has occurred, a more extensive procedure is required. You have to know the location of the ectopic pregnancy, the extent of repair made, and the approach to the repair—vaginal, abdominal, or laparoscopic.

Postpartum curettage is performed within the first 6 weeks after delivery to remove remaining pieces of the placenta or clotted blood. Code 59160 is only for use with postpartum curettage, and if the curettage is nonobstetric, you would use 58120.

Introduction

A cervical dilator may be inserted prior to a procedure in which the cervix is to be dilated; it prepares the cervix for an abortive procedure or a delivery. The dilator initiates uterine contractions, which in turn cause cervical dilatation. Induction can be elective—at the convenience of the patient or the physician—or required, based on a medical risk factor to the mother or fetus. Physicians use a scoring system to measure the stage of the cervix ripening, as illustrated in Figure 8–6.

To induce cervical ripening, intracervical introduction of a preparation such as Prepidil gel is inserted using a catheter. The cervical ripening takes place in the delivery ward.

coding shot

You can report 59200 (cervical ripening) with an induced abortion (59840 or 59841), but not with an induced abortion by means of vaginal suppositories (59855–59857). Also, do not report an induction procedure using a code that describes a manual dilation as a part of the procedure, such as D&C.

Many third-party payers will not pay separately for an induction procedure, as it is considered to be part of the package for obstetric care. You will have to check with your payers to determine their policies regarding the induction procedure.

Score	Dilation (cm)	Effacement (%)	Station	Consistency	Cervical Position
0	Closed	0–30	−3	Firm	Posterior
1	1–2	40–50	−2	Medium	Midposition
2	3–4	60–70	−1, 0	Soft	Anterior
3	>4	>70	+1, +2	—	—

Figure 8–6   The Bishop scoring system for cervical ripening.

Repair

The obstetric repairs can be to the vulva, vagina, cervix, and uterus. All of these repairs are also located in the Female Genital subsection, but here in the Maternity Care and Delivery subsection, the codes are used only for repairs made during pregnancy. Repairs made during delivery or after pregnancy are reported using the postpartum codes, 59400–59622.

coding shot

Vaginal repairs can be reported separately only by a physician other than the attending physician. When the attending physician performs a vaginal repair such as an episiotomy, the repair is considered part of the package for obstetric care. Each third-party payer determines what is included in its own obstetric package.

Vaginal Delivery, Antepartum and Postpartum Care

The category of Vaginal Delivery, Antepartum and Postpartum Care contains codes for those times when the physician provides only part of the care. Sometimes, for example, the physician provides only the antepartum and postpartum care or only the delivery service. You must read the code descriptions carefully, as they specify which parts of the service are included in the code, so as to guard against unbundling.

CAUTION *For one to three antepartum care visits, use E/M codes to report services, not codes from Vaginal Delivery, Antepartum and Postpartum Care.*

Of special note are the codes for a patient who previously had a cesarean delivery but who, for the current delivery, is presenting for vaginal delivery. The category Delivery After Previous Cesarean Delivery is divided on the basis of the circumstances of the current delivery—previous cesarean presenting for vaginal delivery, previous cesarean and successful vaginal delivery, and previous cesarean and current delivery ending in cesarean.

from the trenches

"Coding can sometimes be frustrating . . . but look at it as an adventure or a puzzle . . . at the end you wind up with a wonderful surprise."

AUREA

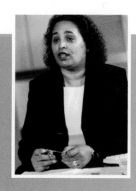

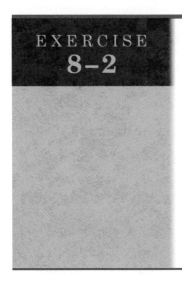

MATERNITY CARE AND DELIVERY

Using the CPT manual, code the following:

1. Laparoscopic salpingectomy of tubal ectopic pregnancy

   Code(s): _____

2. Version of breech presentation, successfully converted to cephalic presentation, with normal spontaneous delivery

   Code(s): _____

3. Thirty-year-old woman, 20 weeks' gestation, with cervical cerclage by vaginal approach

   Code(s): _____

CHAPTER GLOSSARY

abortion: termination of pregnancy

amniocentesis: percutaneous aspiration of amniotic fluid

antepartum: before childbirth

cervix uteri: rounded, cone-shaped neck of the uterus

cesarean: surgical opening through abdominal wall for delivery

chorionic villus sampling (CVS): biopsy of the outermost part of the placenta

cordocentesis: procedure to obtain a fetal blood sample; also called a percutaneous umbilical blood sampling

corpus uteri: uterus

curettage: scraping of a cavity using a spoon-shaped instrument

cystocele: herniation of the bladder into the vagina

delivery: childbirth

dilation: expansion (of the cervix)

ectopic: pregnancy outside the uterus (i.e., in the fallopian tube)

hysterectomy: surgical removal of the uterus

hysterorrhaphy: suturing of the uterus

hysteroscopy: visualization of the canal of the uterine cervix and cavity of the uterus using a scope placed through the vagina

introitus: opening or entrance to the vagina from the uterus

ligation: binding or tying off, as in constricting the bloodflow of a vessel or binding fallopian tubes for sterilization

oophor-: prefix meaning ovary

oophorectomy: surgical removal of the ovary(ies)

oviduct: fallopian tube

perineum: area between the vulva and anus; also known as the pelvic floor

postpartum: after childbirth

salpingectomy: surgical removal of the uterine tube

salping(o)-: prefix meaning tube

salpingostomy: creation of a fistula into the uterine tube

tocolysis: repression of uterine contractions

CHAPTER REVIEW

CHAPTER 8, PART I, THEORY

Without the use of reference material, complete the following:

1 The Female Genital System subsection is divided by _____ site from the vulva up to the ovaries.

2 Skene's gland procedures are reported using codes from which subsection?

_____

3 The vulva includes the following: mons _____ , labia _____ , labia _____ , bulb of _____ , vaginal orifice or vestibule, greater and lesser _____ glands.

4 Who is responsible for determining the complexity of destruction procedures?

_____

5 Destruction of a lesion is also known as excision.
True   False

6 Would you expect a pathology report to be available for a lesion that was obliterated?
Yes   No

7 The term that describes the removal of a portion of the vulva is _____ .

8 The removal of the vulvar area is reported with which two measures? _____ and _____

9 Vulvar area tissue removal that involves the skin and superficial subcutaneous tissues is termed _____ .

10 Vulvar area tissue removal that involves the skin and deep subcutaneous tissues is termed _____ .

11 Partial vulvectomy that involves less than 80% of the vulva is _____ , and that which involves more than 80% is _____ .

CHAPTER 8, PART II, PRACTICAL

Using the CPT manual, code the following:

12 Sue Lind, age 29, previously underwent excision of a vaginal cyst. The pathology report comes back positive for malignancy. Her physician recommends and performs a diagnostic laparoscopy. Evidence of further malignancy of the uterus is seen and the physician does a laparoscopically assisted vaginal hysterectomy 20 days later.
Code(s): _____

13 Diagnostic laparoscopy with fulguration of oviducts
Code(s): _____

14 Oocyte retrieval by means of a follicle puncture with radiologic assistance
Code(s): _____

15 The attending physician, who has provided Sally Fisher's obstetric care, performs a cesarean delivery and ligation of the fallopian tubes.
Code(s): _____

16 Colpopexy using an abdominal approach
Code(s): _____

17 Biopsy of three lesions of the vulva
Code(s): _____

18 Fitting and supply of a diaphragm with instructions for use
Code(s): _____

19 Extensive biopsy of mucosa of vagina, requiring closure

Code(s): _____

20 Using instrumentation, the cervical canal was dilated and examination was completed.

Code(s): _____

21 Simple incision and drainage of a valvular abscess

Code(s): _____

22 Colpocentesis

Code(s): _____

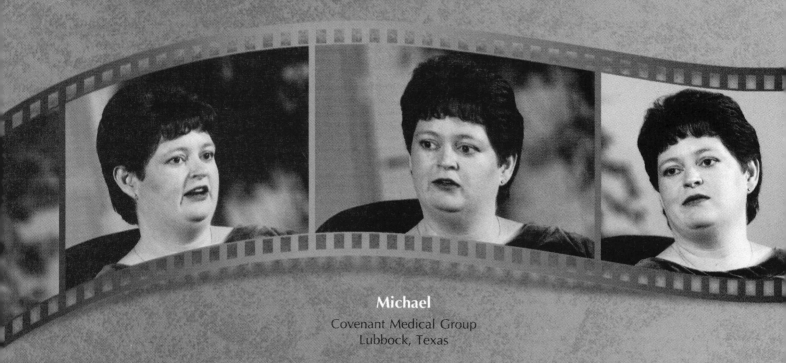

Michael
Covenant Medical Group
Lubbock, Texas

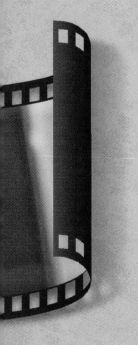

chapter 9

General Surgery I

LEARNING OBJECTIVES

After completing this chapter you should be able to

1 Code male genital, urinary, digestive, and mediastinum/diaphragm services.

2 Apply the rules of coding general surgery services.

3 Differentiate among codes on the basis of surgical approach.

4 Demonstrate knowledge of coding common general surgery services.

MALE GENITAL SYSTEM

Format

The Male Genital System subsection of the CPT manual is divided into anatomic subheadings (penis, testis, epididymis, tunica vaginalis, scrotum, vas deferens, spermatic cord, seminal vesicles, and prostate) (Fig. 9–1). The category codes are divided according to procedure. The greatest number of category codes fall under the subheading Penis because there are many repair codes in this subheading. The other subheadings are mainly for incision and excision, with only few repair codes for the remaining subheadings.

Coding Highlights

Penis Incisions and Destruction

Under the Incision category of the subheading Penis, there is an incision and drainage code (54015). Recall that under the Integumentary System section there are incision and drainage codes. The code from the Penis subheading is for a deep incision, not just an abscess of the skin. For the deep abscess described in 54015, the area is anesthetized, the abscess is opened and cleaned, and often a drain is placed to maintain adequate drainage.

Under the Destruction category of the subheading Penis there are also destruction codes for lesions of the penis. These lesion destruction codes are divided on the basis of whether the destruction is simple or extensive. Simple destruction is further divided according to the method of destruction (e.g., chemical, cryosurgery, laser). The code for extensive lesion destruction can be used no matter which method was employed.

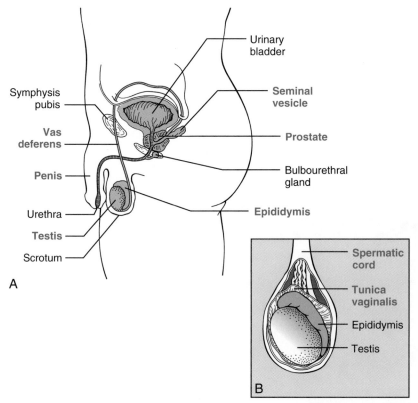

Figure 9–1   *A,* Male genital system. *B,* Scrotal contents.

EXERCISE 9-1

MALE GENITAL SYSTEM

Using the CPT manual, code the following:

1 Simple orchiectomy with insertion of prosthesis using scrotal approach

Code(s): _____

2 Epididymis exploration without biopsy

Code(s): _____

3 Aspiration of fluid sac on the testicular covering

Code(s): _____

4 Extensive electrodesiccation of a condyloma on the penis

Code(s): _____

5 Reversal of previously completed vasectomy

Code(s): _____

INTERSEX SURGERY

The Intersex Surgery subsection is located after the Male Genital Surgery subsection and contains only two codes: one for a surgical procedure to change the sex organs of a male into those of a female and one for changing the sex organs of a female into those of a male. These procedures are very specialized and are performed by physicians who have special skills and training in the procedures.

Intersex surgeries include a series of procedures that take place over an extended period of time. The procedure for changing the male genitalia into female genitalia involves removing the penis but keeping the nerves and vessels intact. These tissues are used to form a clitoris and a vagina. The urethral opening is shifted to be in the position of that of a female.

The surgical procedure for changing the female genitalia into male genitalia involves a series of procedures that uses the genitalia and surrounding skin to form a penis and testicle structures into which prostheses are inserted.

from the trenches

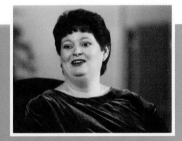

How did you decide on professional coding as a career?
"I was a nurse in a private physician's office and he needed someone to help him with coding and billing. I enjoyed it so much that I stopped nursing and have been coding ever since."

MICHAEL

URINARY SYSTEM

Format

The Urinary System subsection of the CPT manual is arranged anatomically by the subheadings of kidney, ureter, bladder, and urethra, with category codes arranged by procedure (i.e., incision, excision, introduction, repair). A wide range of terminology is used in the subsection because of the four major subheadings of the urinary system—Kidney, Ureter, Bladder, and Urethra—and each subheading has its own terminology (Fig. 9–2). The Glossary in this chapter includes many of the terms that you will encounter in the CPT manual. Always be certain you know the meaning of all the words in the code description before you assign a code.

Coding Highlights

Kidney

The first subheading in the Urinary subsection is Kidney, which contains the category Endoscopy. The endoscopy codes identify procedures (i.e., biopsy, removal, insertion, repair) for the patient who already has an established stoma. The procedure in which the stoma is created is the nephrostomy. The stoma is created by placing a catheter through the skin and into the kidney (percutaneous nephrostomy, 50395). Once a stoma has been created, the endoscopy codes can be used to indicate procedures performed using the stoma as the entry point. When coding procedures, you must

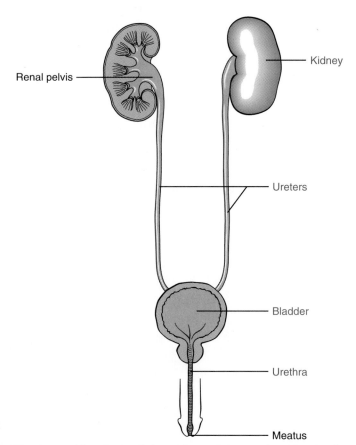

Figure 9–2 The four subheadings of the Urinary System subsection in the CPT manual are Kidney, Ureters, Bladder, and Urethra.

identify the entry method before choosing the correct code. For example, a kidney stone (calculus) can be removed by endoscopy through a stoma or surgically by opening the kidney to view and subsequently removing the stone. The codes for removal of calculus either

skin incision	50060 (nephrolithotomy)
or	
stoma	50561 (renal endoscopy)

There are Excision codes in the Kidney subheading for biopsy, nephrectomy (removal of the kidney), and removal of a cyst. The **biopsy** codes are based on the approach, either percutaneous (through the skin) or by surgical exposure of the kidney. The **nephrectomy** codes are based on the complexity and extent of the procedure (e.g., partial or total removal of the kidney, or the removal of surrounding tissues such as the bladder cuff in addition to partial or total removal of the kidney).

Introduction category codes in the Kidney subheading are for aspiration, catheters, injections for radiography, guides, and tube changes. There are extensive notes with the category codes, so you must be certain to read all notes when coding in this area.

Repair category codes include plastic surgery (pyeloplasty), suturing (nephrorrhaphy), and closure of fistula (created channels).

You will locate the kidney codes in the CPT manual index under "Kidney"; they are subtermed primarily by category (e.g., insertion, excision, repair). Another method of locating kidney codes in the CPT manual index is to look under the medical term for the procedure (e.g., nephrostomy or nephrotomy). Again, there are other index location methods; these are just a couple to help you get started locating the codes.

Ureter

The next subheading in the Urinary system subsection is Ureter. The category codes are based on procedure (i.e., incision, excision, introduction, repair, endoscopy). The endoscopy codes in this subheading are used for procedures that are performed using an established stoma (ureterostomy). The procedures conducted through the ureterostomy are similar to the types of procedures conducted through a nephrostomy (e.g., biopsy, catheterization, irrigation, instillation). Excellent medical terminology skills are essential for working within this subheading because the words can be intimidating: transureteroureterostomy, ureteroneocystostomy, ureterosigmoidostomy. Keep your medical dictionary close by to look up any words you are not absolutely sure about. You can also refer to the Glossary at the end of this chapter or at the back of the book. The time you spend now increasing the depth and breadth of your medical terminology vocabulary is an excellent investment and will greatly increase your coding accuracy.

Bladder

The Bladder subheading is next and contains category codes not only for the usual procedures, such as incision and excision, but also for urodynamics. **Urodynamics** pertains to the motion and flow of urine. Urinary tract flow can be obstructed by renal calculi, narrowing (stricture) of the ureter, cysts, and so forth. The procedures in the subheading are to be conducted by or under the direct supervision of a physician, and all the instruments, equipment, supplies, and technical assistance necessary to conduct the procedure are bundled into the codes. If the physician conducts only a portion of the service (e.g., interpretation of the results), modifier -26 (professional component) is used with the procedure code to indicate that not all the services bundled into the code were provided by the physician. For example, if a physician provides only the interpretation (-26) of a urethral pressure profile (UPP) (51772), you would report it as 51772-26.

In the Bladder subheading, there are category codes for bundled endoscopy procedures (i.e., cystoscopy, urethroscopy, cystourethroscopy). The codes contain the primary procedure of a cystourethroscopy (endoscopic procedure to view the bladder and urethra) and minor related procedures or functions performed at the same time. For example, if a cystourethroscopy is done for biopsy of the ureter with radiography, bundled into the code for the procedure (52007) are the catheterization, endoscopic procedure, and biopsy(ies). To unbundle individual components of the procedure would not be correct. If the secondary procedure(s) required significant additional time or effort, the procedure can be identified using modifier -22 (unusual procedure).

Endoscopy

Cystourethroscopy codes are found not only in the category Endoscopy—Cystoscopy, Urethroscopy, Cystourethroscopy, but also in the category Ureter and Pelvis. The Ureter and Pelvis cystourethroscopy codes include the establishment of a stent or nephrostomy, or cystourethroscopy with ureteroscopy and/or pyeloscopy (fluoroscopic examination of the renal pelvis). The notes preceding these codes indicate when modifiers should be used with the codes.

Urethra

The subheading Urethra contains codes for the usual procedures of incision, excision, and repair. There is a category called Manipulation, which has codes that are a bit different from those you encountered in the Urinary system subsection. **Manipulation** is performed on the urethra (e.g., dilation or catheterization). **Dilation** stretches, or dilates, a passage that has narrowed. The Dilation codes are based on initial or subsequent dilation of a male or female patient. The catheterization codes in the Manipulation category are for either a simple or a complicated procedure.

EXERCISE 9-2

URINARY SYSTEM

Using the CPT manual, code the following:

1 Needle aspiration of bladder

Code(s): _____

2 Endoscopy for establishment of a Gibbon ureteral stent

Code(s): _____

3 Repeat nephrolithotomy

Code(s): _____

4 Closure of a urethrostomy in a 54-year-old man

Code(s): _____

5 Second stage, Johannsen type, surgical reconstruction of the urethra

Code(s): _____

DIGESTIVE SYSTEM

Format

The format of the Digestive System subsection is divided according to anatomic site (Fig. 9–3) and procedure. Included in this subsection are codes for sites beginning with the mouth and ending with the anus.

Note that also included are those internal organs that aid in the digestive process, including the pancreas, liver, and gallbladder. This subsection includes codes for abdomen, peritoneum, omentum, and all types of hernias. Endoscopic codes can be found throughout the subsection on the basis of the anatomic site at which the particular procedure is performed.

Separate procedures are common in this subsection. Procedures such as gastrostomies and colostomies are always bundled into the major procedure unless the code specifically says to code them separately. For example, code 44141 is a colectomy (removal of part or all of the colon) with colostomy (creation of an artificial opening). Included in the description for 44141 is the establishment of the colostomy; thus, it would not be correct to report 44320, which is a separate code for the establishment of a colostomy. However, if only a colostomy was developed, it would be appropriate to code it 44320.

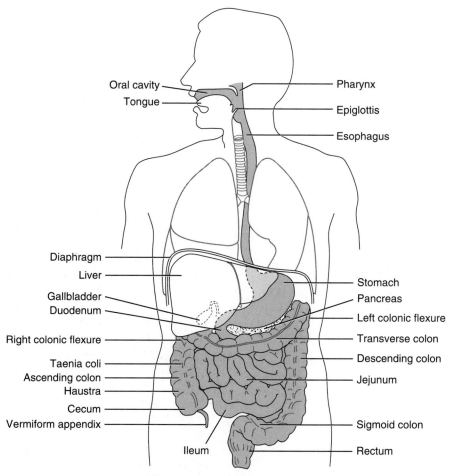

Figure 9–3   Digestive system.

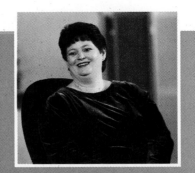

Coding Highlights

Endoscopic Procedures

Many procedures are done through endoscopes (such as the gastroscopy in Fig. 9–4). Endoscope codes are available for procedures throughout the digestive system depending on how far down (through the mouth) or up (through the anus) the scope is passed. The code selection varies according to the procedure(s) performed and includes the sites the scope passed through to accomplish the procedure. To choose the proper code, the **extent** of the procedure must be determined. For example, if a scope is passed to the esophagus only, the code would be chosen from the endoscopy codes 43200–43232. If the scoping process is continued through the esophagus to the stomach, duodenum, and/or jejunum, the code selection would be from

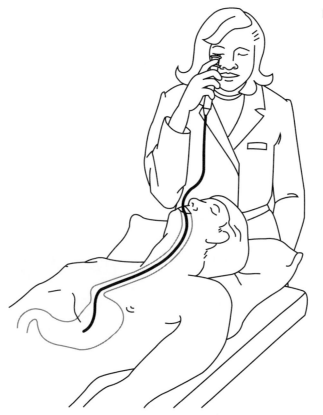

Figure 9–4   Endoscopy.

the endoscopy codes 43234–43272. Once the anatomic site of the endoscope procedure is correctly identified, the surgical procedure(s) performed would be listed. A surgical endoscopy always includes a diagnostic endoscopy, so don't unbundle and code for both. Remember to use modifier -51 if more than one procedure is performed.

---

coding shot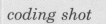

To choose the correct endoscopy code from the Digestive System subsection, choose the farthest extent to which the scope was passed.

EXERCISE 9–3

ENDOSCOPIC PROCEDURES

Using the CPT manual, code the following:

1 Esophagogastroduodenoscopy with biopsy and control of bleeding

Code(s): _____

2 Flexible sigmoidoscopy with three biopsies

Code(s): _____

3 Colonoscopy with removal of polyp by a snare

Code(s): _____

Resections

Resection of the intestine means taking out a diseased portion of the intestine and either joining the remaining ends (anastomosis) directly or developing an artificial opening (exteriorizing) through the abdominal wall. Figure 9–5 illustrates three types of anastomoses. The artificial opening (stoma) allows for the removal of body waste products (Fig. 9–6), as with the colostomy. The type of anastomosis or exteriorization depends on the medical condition of the patient and on the amount of intestine (large or small) that has to be removed. Some patients have temporary exteriorization for

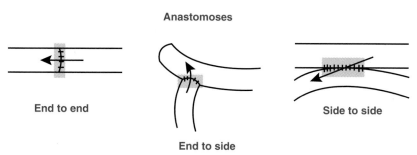

Anastomoses

End to end

End to side

Side to side

Figure 9–5   Three types of anastomoses.

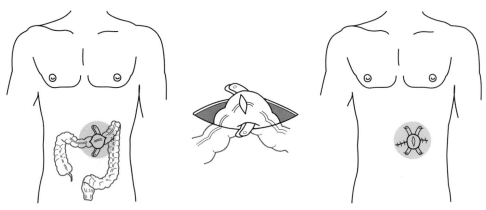

Figure 9–6   Stoma.

the length of time it takes the remaining small or large intestine to heal itself so it can perform the necessary functions. Other patients have permanent exteriorization because too much of the intestine has been removed to allow for adequate functioning. Openings to the outside of the body are named for the part of the intestine from which they are formed—colostomy is an artificial opening from the colon, ileostomy from the ileum, gastrostomy from the stomach, and so forth (Fig. 9–7). Therefore, it is critical that you identify the correct anatomic site from which the ostomy originated as well as the procedure used to establish the ostomy.

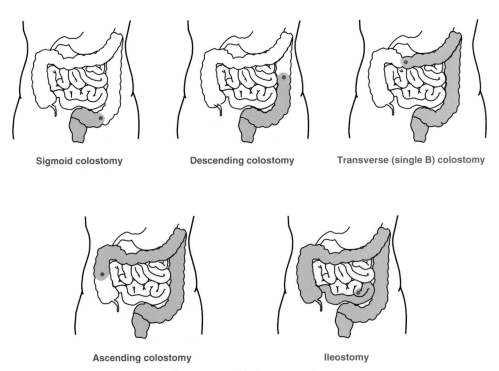

Sigmoid colostomy   Descending colostomy   Transverse (single B) colostomy

Ascending colostomy   Ileostomy

Figure 9–7   Various ostomies.

EXERCISE
9–4

RESECTIONS

Using your knowledge of medical terminology, identify what the following procedures surgically accomplish:

1 Coloproctostomy _____

2 Ileostomy _____

3 Colostomy _____

4 Enteroenterostomy _____

Using the CPT manual, code the following:

5 Partial bowel resection with colostomy

  Code(s): _____

6 Resection of small intestine, single resection, with anastomosis

  Code(s): _____

Laparotomy

A laparotomy is a surgical opening into the abdomen. Sometimes, a laparotomy is used as the approach in digestive system surgery. When it is used as a surgical approach, a laparotomy is never coded separately. An exploratory laparotomy may be done to investigate the cause of a patient's illness. If only the exploratory laparotomy is performed, it is appropriate to report it with an exploratory laparotomy code, such as 49000. However, if the exploratory procedure progresses to a more definitive surgical treatment (such as an appendectomy), only the definitive treatment (appendectomy) is reported.

Hernia

Hernia codes are listed according to type of hernia. Figure 9–8 is an illustration of an inguinal hernia that would be surgically repaired by a herniorrhaphy. The defect would be closed with sutures. Other factors in coding

Figure 9–8 Hernia.

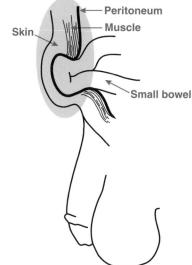

hernias are whether the hernia is **strangulated** (the blood supply is cut off) or **incarcerated** (can't be returned to the abdominal cavity); whether the repair is an initial or subsequent repair; whether the hernia is reducible (can be returned to the abdominal cavity); and the age of the patient. The hernia codes are located in the index under the main term "Hernia."

EXERCISE 9-5

MISCELLANEOUS DIGESTIVE SYSTEM CODING

Using the CPT manual, code the following:

1   Exploratory laparotomy with laparoscopic cholecystectomy

Code(s): _____

2   Cholecystotomy with exploration and removal of calculus

Code(s): _____

3   Repair of recurrent reducible incisional hernia, with implantation of a mesh graft, abdominal approach

Code(s): _____

4   Repair of an initial incarcerated inguinal hernia in a 5½-year-old

Code(s): _____

5   Biopsy of lip

Code(s): _____

MEDIASTINUM AND DIAPHRAGM

Format

The mediastinum is the area between the lungs (Fig. 9–9). The Mediastinum subheading of the Mediastinum and Diaphragm subsection of the CPT manual is divided by procedures and includes the categories of Incision, Excision, and Endoscopy. The difference between the mediastinum incision codes is the surgical approach. The approach can be either cervical (neck area) or across the thoracic area (transthoracic) or sternum. The excision codes vary based on whether a cyst or tumor was excised. Codes for the

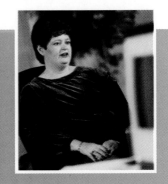

from the trenches

What is the most interesting part of your job?
"Educating the physicians and seeing them improve on their coding and documentation."

MICHAEL

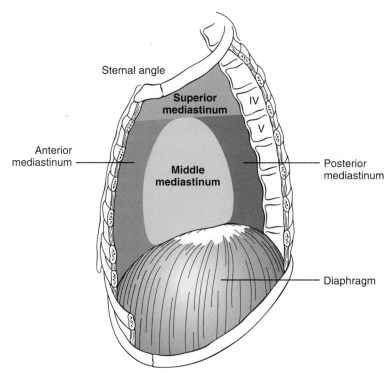

Figure 9–9 Mediastinum and diaphragm.

mediastinum procedures are usually located in the CPT manual index under "Mediastinum."

The diaphragm is the wall of muscle that separates the thoracic and abdominal cavities. The codes in the Diaphragm subheading are repair codes. Repairs are usually to a hernia or laceration. Diaphragm codes are usually located in the CPT manual index under "Diaphragm."

Coding Highlights

Mediastinum

The mediastinum incision category of codes is based on the surgical approach taken to perform the mediastinotomy. A cervical or anterior mediastinotomy is a surgical procedure in which an incision is made in the lower portion of the front of the neck for exploration, drainage, biopsy, or removal of a foreign body. Codes for removal of a foreign body are located in the Incision category. You would think removal of a foreign body would be in the Excision codes, but the Excision codes are only for cysts or tumors. The codes for Excision use a surgical approach in which the surgeon makes the operative incision just below the nipple line, pulls back the rib cage, retracts the muscles, and has exposure of the thoracic cavity. The cyst or tumor is removed and the incision closed.

Diaphragm

Other than one code for unlisted diaphragm procedures, all diaphragm codes are for repair of the diaphragm. The repairs are for lacerations or hernias, with one code for imbrication of the diaphragm. An imbrication of the diaphragm may be performed for eventration, which is when the diaphragm moves up, usually because of the paralysis of the diaphragmatic nerve (phrenic nerve). In this case the surgeon sutures the diaphragm back into place.

EXERCISE 9–6

MEDIASTINUM AND DIAPHRAGM

Using the CPT manual, code the following:

1 Repair of paraesophageal hiatus hernia, abdominal approach, with limited fundoplasty

   Code(s): _____

2 Exploratory mediastinotomy with biopsy accomplished with approach through the neck

   Code(s): _____

3 Excision of benign tumor of the mediastinum

   Code(s): _____

4 Repair of an esophageal hiatal hernia accomplished with approach across the thoracic area

   Code(s): _____

CHAPTER GLOSSARY

anastomosis: surgical connection of two tubular structures, such as two pieces of the intestine

bulbocavernosus: muscle that constricts the vagina in a female and the urethra in a male

bulbourethral gland: rounded mass of the urethra

calculus: concretion of mineral salts, also called a stone

calycoplasty: surgical reconstruction of a recess of the renal pelvis

calyx: recess of the renal pelvis

cavernosa–corpus spongiosum shunt: creation of a connection between a cavity of the penis and the urethra

cavernosa–glans penis fistulization: creation of a connection between a cavity of the penis and the glans penis, which overlaps the penis cavity

cavernosa–saphenous vein shunt: creation of a connection between the cavity of the penis and a vein

cavernosography: radiographic recording of a cavity, e.g., the pulmonary cavity or the main part of the penis

cavernosometry: measurement of the pressure in a cavity, e.g., the penis

cholangiography: radiographic recording of the bile ducts

chole-: prefix meaning bile

cholecystectomy: surgical removal of the gallbladder

cholecystoenterostomy: creation of a connection between the gallbladder and intestine

chordee: condition resulting in the penis' being bent downward

colonoscopy: fiberscopic examination of the entire colon that may include part of the terminal ileum

colostomy: artificial opening between the colon and the abdominal wall

corpora cavernosa: the two cavities of the penis

cystolithectomy: removal of a calculus (stone) from the urinary bladder

cystolithotomy: cystolithectomy

cystometrogram (CMG): measurement of the pressures and capacity of the urinary bladder

cystoplasty: surgical reconstruction of the bladder

cystorrhaphy: suture of the bladder

cystoscopy: use of a scope to view the bladder

cystostomy: surgical creation of an opening into the bladder

cystotomy: incision into the bladder

cystourethroplasty: surgical reconstruction of the bladder and urethra

cystourethroscopy: use of a scope to view the bladder and urethra

diaphragm: muscular wall that separates the thoracic and abdominal cavities

diaphragmatic hernia: hernia of the diaphragm

electrodesiccation: destruction of a lesion by the use of electric current radiated through a needle

endopyelotomy: procedure involving the bladder and ureters, including the insertion of a stent

enterocystoplasty: surgical reconstruction of the small intestine after the removal of a cyst and usually including a bowel anastomosis

epididymectomy: surgical removal of the epididymis

epididymis: tube located at the top of the testes that stores sperm

epididymovasostomy: creation of a new connection between the vas deferens and epididymis

eventration: protrusion of the bowel through the viscera of the abdomen

evisceration: pulling the viscera outside of the body through an incision

exstrophy: condition in which an organ is turned inside out

fulguration: use of electric current to destroy tissue

fundoplasty: repair of the bottom of an organ or muscle

gastro-: prefix meaning stomach

gastrointestinal: pertaining to the stomach and intestine

gastroplasty: operation on the stomach for repair or reconfiguration

gastrostomy: artificial opening between the stomach and the abdominal wall

gloss(o)-: prefix meaning tongue

hepat(o)-: prefix meaning liver

hernia: organ or tissue protruding through the wall or cavity that usually contains it

hydrocele: sac of fluid

hypospadias: congenital deformity of the urethra in which the urethral opening is on the underside of the penis rather than at the end

ileostomy: artificial opening between the ileum and the abdominal wall

imbrication: overlapping

incarcerated: regarding hernias, a constricted, irreducible hernia that may cause obstruction of an intestine

jejunostomy: artificial opening between the jejunum and the abdominal wall

Kock pouch: surgical creation of a urinary bladder from a segment of the ileum

laparoscopy: exploration of the abdomen and pelvic cavities using a scope placed through a small incision in the abdominal wall

litholapaxy: lithotripsy

lithotomy: incision into an organ or a duct for the purpose of removing a stone

lithotripsy: crushing of a gallbladder or urinary bladder stone followed by irrigation to wash the fragment out

lymphadenectomy: excision of a lymph node or nodes

marsupialization: surgical procedure that creates an exterior pouch from an internal abscess

meatotomy: surgical enlargement of the opening of the urinary meatus

mediastinoscopy: use of an endoscope inserted through a small incision to view the mediastinum

mediastinotomy: cutting into the mediastinum

mediastinum: area between the lungs that contains the heart, aorta, trachea, lymph nodes, thymus gland, esophagus, and bronchial tubes

nephrectomy, paraperitoneal: kidney transplant

nephro-: prefix meaning kidney

nephrocutaneous fistula: a channel from the kidney to the skin

nephrolithotomy: removal of a kidney stone through an incision made into the kidney

nephrorrhaphy: suturing of the kidney

nephrostolithotomy: creation of an artificial channel to the kidney

nephrostolithotomy, percutaneous: procedure to establish an artificial channel between the skin and the kidney

nephrostomy: creation of a channel into the renal pelvis of the kidney

nephrostomy, percutaneous: creation of a channel from the skin to the renal pelvis

nephrotomy: incision into the kidney

omentum: peritoneal connection between the stomach and other internal organs

orchiectomy: castration

orchiopexy: surgical procedure to release undescended testis

ostomy: artificial opening

paraesophageal hiatus hernia: hernia that is near the esophagus

pelviolithotomy: pyeloplasty

penoscrotal: referring to the penis and scrotum

perinephric cyst: cyst in the tissue around the kidney

perirenal: around the kidney

peritoneoscopy: visualization of the abdominal cavity using one scope placed through a small incision in the abdominal wall and another scope placed in the vagina

perivesical: around the bladder

perivisceral: around an organ

plethysmography: determining the changes in volume of an organ part or body

pleura: covering of the lungs and thoracic cavity

that is moistened with serous fluid to reduce friction during respiratory movements of the lungs

priapism: painful condition in which the penis is constantly erect

proctosigmoidoscopy: fiberscopic examination of the sigmoid colon and rectum

prostatotomy: incision into the prostate

pyelo-: prefix meaning renal pelvis

pyelocutaneous: from the renal pelvis to the skin

pyelolithotomy: surgical removal of a kidney stone from the renal pelvis

pyeloplasty: surgical reconstruction of the renal pelvis

pyeloscopy: viewing of the renal pelvis using a fluoroscope after injection of contrast material

pyelostolithotomy: removal of a kidney stone and establishment of a stoma

pyelostomy: surgical creation of a temporary diversion around the ureter

pyelotomy: incision into the renal pelvis

pyloroplasty: incision and repair of the pyloric channel

rectocele: herniation of the rectal wall through the posterior wall of the vagina

reducible: able to be corrected or put back into a normal position

renal pelvis: funnel-shaped sac in the kidney where urine is received

retroperitoneal: behind the sac holding the abdominal organs and viscera (peritoneum)

seminal vesicle: gland that secretes fluid into the vas deferens

sigmoidoscopy: fiberscopic examination of the entire rectum and sigmoid colon that may include a portion of the descending colon

spermatocele: cyst filled with spermatozoa

splenectomy: excision of the spleen

splenoportography: radiographic procedure to allow visualization of the splenic and portal veins of the spleen

thoracentesis: surgical puncture of the thoracic cavity, usually using a needle, to remove fluids

transabdominal: across the abdomen

transhepatic: across the liver

transthoracic: across the thorax

transureteroureterostomy: surgical connection of one ureter to the other ureter

transurethral resection, prostate: procedure performed through the urethra by means of a cystoscopy to remove part or all of the prostate

transvesical ureterolithotomy: removal of a ureter stone (calculus) through the bladder

tumescence: state of being swollen

tumor: swelling or enlargement; a spontaneous growth of tissue that forms an abnormal mass

tunica vaginalis: covering of the testes

ureterectomy: surgical removal of a ureter, either totally or partially

ureterocolon: pertaining to the ureter and colon

ureterocutaneous fistula: the channel from the ureter to the exterior skin

ureteroenterostomy: creation of a connection between the intestine and the ureter

ureterolithotomy: removal of a stone from the ureter

ureterolysis: freeing of adhesions of the ureter

ureteroneocystostomy: surgical connection of the ureter to a new site on the bladder

ureteroplasty: surgical repair of the ureter

ureteropyelography: ureter and bladder radiography

ureteropyelonephrostomy: surgical connection of the ureter to a new site on the kidney

ureteropyelostomy: ureteropyelonephrostomy

ureterosigmoidostomy: surgical connection of the ureter into the sigmoid colon

ureterotomy: incision into the ureter

ureterovisceral fistula: surgical formation of a connection between the ureter and the skin

urethrocutaneous fistula: surgically created channel from the urethra to the skin surface

urethrocystography: radiography of the bladder and urethra

urethromeatoplasty: surgical repair of the urethra and meatus

urethroplasty: surgical repair of the urethra

urethrorrhaphy: suturing of the urethra

urethroscopy: use of a scope to view the urethra

vagotomy: surgical separation of the vagus nerve

varicocele: swelling of a scrotal vein

vas deferens: tube that carries sperm from the epididymis to the urethra

vasogram: recording of the flow in the vas deferens

vasotomy: creation of an opening in the vas deferens

vasovasorrhaphy: suturing of the vas deferens

vasovasostomy: reversal of a vasectomy

vesicostomy: surgical creation of a connection of the viscera of the bladder to the skin

vesicovaginal fistula: creation of a tube between the vagina and the bladder

vesiculectomy: excision of the seminal vesicle

vesiculotomy: incision into the seminal vesicle

CHAPTER REVIEW

CHAPTER 9, PART I, THEORY

Complete the following:

1 The greatest number of category codes in the Male Genital System fall under the

_____ subheading because of the numerous repairs made to this anatomic area.

2 In what section of the CPT manual would you find a code for a superficial abscess of the

skin of the penis? _____

3 How many codes are there in the Intersex

Surgery subsection? _____

4 What is the term that pertains to the motion

and flow of urine? _____

5 What is the modifier that indicates that only the professional portion of the service was

performed? _____

6 The codes in the Digestive System subsection begin with this anatomic part,

_____ , and end with this ana-

tomic part, _____ .

7 In the Digestive System, many of the procedures performed to view the esophagus and stomach are done with this instrument.

_____

8 What type of endoscopy is always included in a surgical endoscopy and would therefore

never be reported separately? _____

9 What is the term that describes a surgical

opening into the abdomen? _____

10 When a hernia can be returned to the abdominal cavity, it is said to be _____ .

11 The difference between the mediastinum incision codes is the surgical _____ .

CHAPTER 9, PART II, PRACTICAL

Code the following cases:

12 Mary Carter, age 72, has an exploratory laparotomy with cholecystectomy through an incision.
Code(s): _____

13 Incision and drainage of deep penis abscess
Code(s): _____

14 Repair of recurrent, reducible incisional hernia
Code(s): _____

15 Extensive destruction of herpetic vesicle lesions using cryosurgery
Code(s): _____

16 Repair of an esophageal hiatal hernia using a transthoracic approach
Code(s): _____

17 Excision of full thickness of lip lesion with Abbé-Estlander flap reconstruction
Code(s): _____

18 Thoracic approach used in a diverticulectomy of hypopharynx
Code(s): _____

19 Endoscopic retrograde cholangiopancreatography (ERCP) with multiple biopsies
Code(s): _____

20 Total abdominal colectomy with ileostomy
Code(s): _____

21 Multiple biopsies of the small intestine by means of endoscopy with progression past the second portion of the duodenum
Code(s): _____

22 Proctosigmoidoscopy using rigid endoscope with collection of multiple specimens by brushing
Code(s): _____

23 Biopsy of kidney with percutaneous incision by trocar
Code(s): _____

24 Physician providing the technical and professional component of a cystography with four views
Code(s): _____

25 Drainage of abscess of Skene's gland
Code(s): _____

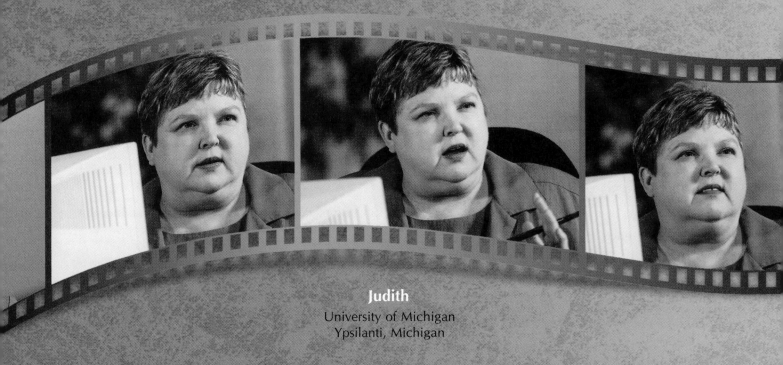

Judith
University of Michigan
Ypsilanti, Michigan

284

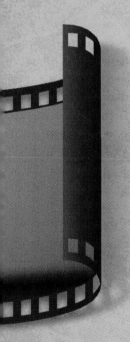

chapter 10

General Surgery II

LEARNING OBJECTIVES

After completing this chapter you should be able to

1   Code hemic/lymphatic system, endocrine system, nervous system, eye/ocular adnexa, and auditory system services.

2   Apply the rules of coding general surgery services.

3   Differentiate among codes on the basis of surgical approach.

4   Demonstrate knowledge of coding common general surgery services.

HEMIC AND LYMPHATIC SYSTEMS

Format

The Hemic and Lymphatic Systems subsection is divided into subheadings: Spleen, General, and Lymph Nodes/Lymphatic channels (Fig. 10–1). Further division is based on type of procedure (i.e., excision, incision, repair).

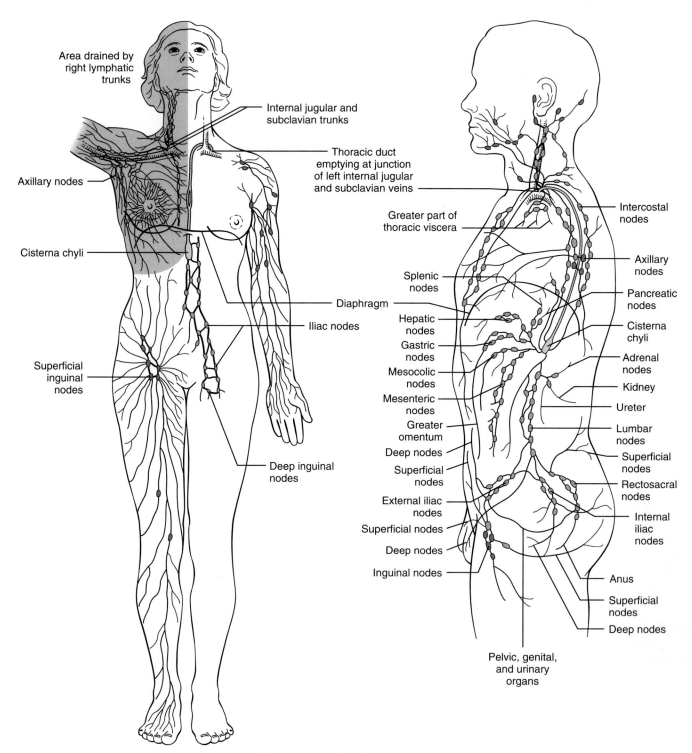

Figure 10–1 Lymphatic system.

The codes for spleen and lymph nodes are located in the CPT manual index under Spleen, General, and so forth.

Coding Highlights

Spleen

The spleen is composed of lymph tissue and is located in the left upper quadrant of the abdomen. The spleen is easily ruptured and can cause massive hemorrhage. A splenectomy is the surgical removal of the spleen; removal can be partial or total. A person can live without a spleen because the bone marrow, liver, and lymph nodes take over the work of the spleen after a total splenectomy.

Codes in the subheading Spleen are further divided into categories for excision, repair, laparoscopy, and introduction. Codes in the Excision category are based on the type of splenectomy: total, partial, or total with extensive disease. The splenectomy, total and partial, carries the designation "(separate procedure)" behind the code description. This means that if the splenectomy is an integral part of another procedure, it is bundled into the main procedure code and not reported separately. For example, if a repair of a ruptured spleen was performed and the surgeon removed a portion of the spleen as a part of the repair, you would report only the repair code (38115).

General

Bone marrow is the inner core of bones that manufactures most blood cells. Immature blood cells, called stem cells, originate in the marrow of bones. Leukemia is a malignant disease of the bone marrow in which excessive white blood cells are produced. Treatment often includes total-body irradiation or aggressive chemotherapy followed by transplantation of normal bone marrow. The bone marrow is harvested by aspiration. The immature stem cells are obtained by withdrawing blood in which the immature stem cells reside.

Allogenic bone marrow comes from a close relative, so there is a genetic similarity. **Autologous** bone marrow is collected from the patient and later transplanted or reinfused.

There are harvesting codes for the collection of bone marrow from the donor as well as codes for transplantation of bone marrow into the recipient.

Lymph Nodes

The lymphatic system is a transportation system to take fluids, proteins, and fats through the lymphatic channels and back to the bloodstream. Stations along the lymphatic system are called lymph nodes. The nodes fight disease when lymphocytes from the nodes produce antibodies. The subheading on the lymph nodes is divided on the basis of the various procedures (i.e., incision, excision, resection, and introduction).

Within the Lymph Node and Lymphatic Channels subheading are two categories of codes for lymphadenectomies that are based on whether the lymphadenectomy is limited or radical. A **limited lymphadenectomy** is the removal of the lymph nodes only; a **radical lymphadenectomy** is the removal of the lymph nodes, gland(s), and surrounding tissue. Sometimes, a limited lymphadenectomy will be bundled into a larger procedure, such as prostatectomy. If this is the case, you would not report the lymphadenectomy separately. Rather, you would report only the main procedure, such as the prostatectomy code from the Male Genital System subsection of the Surgery section.

EXERCISE 10-1

HEMIC AND LYMPHATIC SYSTEMS

Using the CPT manual, code the following:

1 Excision of an axillary cystic hygroma, which the patient record indicates involved no deep neurovascular dissection

Code(s): _____

2 Total removal of the spleen

Code(s): _____

3 Injection procedure for a radiographic view of the portal vein of the spleen

Code(s): _____

ENDOCRINE SYSTEM

Format

The endocrine system has the important job of producing and releasing hormones into the bloodstream. The endocrine glands are located throughout the body (Fig. 10–2) and regulate a wide range of body functions. (Your anatomy and physiology background is very important to you as you code.)

Coding Highlights

There are nine glands in the endocrine system, but only four are included in the Endocrine subsection of the CPT manual—thyroid, parathyroid, adrenal, and thymus. The pituitary and pineal gland procedures are in the Nervous System subsection of the CPT manual, the pancreas is in the Digestive System subsection, and the ovaries and testes are in the respective Female or Male Genital System subsections.

There are only two categories in this subsection. The first category is Thyroid Gland and the second is Parathyroid, Thymus, Adrenal Glands, and Carotid Body. **Carotid body** refers to an area adjacent to the carotid artery that can be a site of tumor excision (60600).

The CPT manual lists only one thyroid incision code and one unlisted procedure code; the remaining codes are for excisions or laparoscopy. There is also an aspiration/injection code and a biopsy code, which is under the excision category. Partial/total or subtotal/total appear in many of the descriptions; both **subtotal** and **partial** mean something *less* than the total.

from the trenches

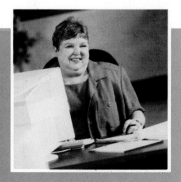

What allows you to take the most pride in your career?
"To be acknowledged as an expert in the field of primary care coding . . . . I enjoy going to work every day."

JUDITH

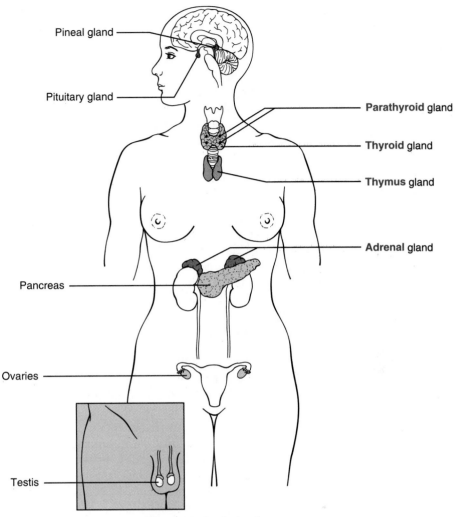

Pineal gland

Pituitary gland

Parathyroid gland

Thyroid gland

Thymus gland

Adrenal gland

Pancreas

Ovaries

Testis

Figure 10–2   Endocrine system.

<table>
<tr><td>EXERCISE
10-2</td><td>

ENDOCRINE SYSTEM

Using the CPT manual, code the following:

1 Excision of an adenoma from posterior aspect of the thyroid gland

Code(s): _____

2 Surgical removal of a thyroglossal duct cyst

Code(s): _____

3 Total removal of the thymus using the transthoracic approach, with radical mediastinal dissection

Code(s): _____

4 Removal of tumor affixed to the carotid artery

Code(s): _____

5 Partial excision of both lobes of thyroid with removal of adjacent isthmus

Code(s): _____

</td></tr>
</table>

NERVOUS SYSTEM

Format

The Nervous System subsection contains codes describing procedures done on the brain, spinal cord, nerves, and all associated parts. The subheadings are divided according to anatomic site—whether it be a part of the brain or spinal column or a type of nerve. The subheadings are further divided on the basis of type of procedure. The codes deal with both the central nervous system and the peripheral nervous system.

Two Special Considerations

Punctures, Twists, or Burr Holes

The first two categories of codes (Injection, Drainage, or Aspiration and Twist Drill, Burr Hole(s), or Trephine) deal with conditions that may require that holes or openings be made into the brain to relieve pressure, to insert monitoring devices, to place tubing, or to inject contrast material. Twist or burr holes are made through the skull to accomplish many of these procedures. Using twist or burr holes means that the skull stays intact except for the small openings (holes) that are made. Hemorrhages may also be drained through such holes.

Craniectomy/Craniotomy

Codes in the category Craniectomy or Craniotomy describe procedures that deal with actual incision of the skull with possible removal of a portion of the skull to open the operative site to the surgeon for correction of the condition. Use of these codes is determined by site and condition (e.g., evacuation of hematoma, supratentorial, subdural). Carefully review the descriptions in these codes before coding.

As in other subsections, many procedures are bundled into one code, and only by careful attention to code description can you keep from unbundling surgical procedures.

When craniectomies are performed, it is not uncommon that additional grafting must take place to repair the surgical defect caused by opening the skull. These grafting procedures would be coded separately, in addition to the major surgical procedure.

Coding Highlights

Surgery of Skull Base

The **skull base** is the area at the base of the cranium where the lobes of the brain rest. When lesions are found within the skull base, it often takes the skill of several surgeons working together to perform surgery dealing with these conditions. The operations found in the category Surgery of Skull Base are very involved, taking many hours to complete. The procedures are divided on the basis of the approach procedure, the definitive procedure, and the reconstruction/repair procedure.

The **approach procedure** is the method used to obtain exposure of the lesion (e.g., anterior cranial fossa, middle cranial fossa, posterior cranial fossa). The **definitive procedure** is what was done to the lesion (e.g., biopsy, repair, excision). If one physician did both the approach and the definitive procedures, both would be coded. For example, a neoplasm is excised at the base of the anterior cranial fossa, extradural, using an infratemporal preauricular approach to the midline skull base. This would be coded 61600 for the procedure (definitive procedure) and 61590 for the approach (approach procedure). Because two procedures were done by the same physician—61600 and 61590—the lesser procedure, the approach, would have modifier -51.

Reconstruction or repair procedures are the various repairs that will be made to the skull on closure so as to rebuild the area used for entry. This last step of reconstruction or repair is reported separately only if it is extensive.

At any given point one or more physicians may be performing distinctly different portions of the procedure. When one surgeon performs the approach procedure, another surgeon performs the definitive procedure, and another surgeon performs the reconstruction/repair procedure, each surgeon's services would be reported with the code for the specific procedure he or she individually performed. Again, if one surgeon performs more than one procedure (e.g., the approach procedure and the definitive procedure), both codes are reported, adding modifier -51 to the secondary procedure.

Aneurysms may develop in the brain, requiring surgical repair. Also present in the brain may be arteriovenous malformations, which means the arteries and veins are not in the correct anatomic position. Codes to indicate the definitive procedure or repair of these conditions are found in the category Surgery for Aneurysm, Arteriovenous Malformation, or Vascular Disease and are divided on the basis of the approach and method of procedure.

Cerebrospinal Fluid Shunts

A **shunt** can be considered a draining device that enables fluids to be drained from one area into another when the body is not able to perform this function on its own. In the case of cerebrospinal fluid (CSF) shunts, the CSF that is produced in the ventricles of the brain may not drain properly but may continue to accumulate in the brain, building pressure and causing brain damage. Drains or shunts are placed from the area of collection to a drainage area to keep the fluid level within normal ranges. For instance, code 62223 describes the creation of a shunt from the ventricle to the peritoneal space (ventriculoperitoneal). This means that the shunt starts in the ventricle of the brain and ends in the peritoneum. Codes in the CSF Shunt category describe all the various types of shunting procedures, including placement of shunting devices and their repair, replacement, and removal.

Shunt systems may also be placed to drain obstructed CSF from the spine. As in the previously described shunt procedures, codes from the category Shunt, Spinal CSF identify the creation, replacement, removal, or insertion of a shunt system.

Spine and Spinal Cord

The subheading Spine and Spinal Cord includes codes for injections, laminectomies, excisions, repairs, and shunting. You should be familiar with the terminology for parts of the spinal column, including the lamina, foramina, vertebral bodies, disks, facets, and nerve roots. The basic distinction among the codes in these ranges deals with the **condition** (a herniated intervertebral disk versus a neoplastic lesion of the spinal cord) as well as the **approach** (e.g., anterior, posterior, costovertebral).

The complexity of the procedure is determined by the condition and approach. For example, a patient with a herniated disk at L5-S1 would require less time in surgery for the removal of the disk and decompression of the nerve root than would a patient with a neoplastic growth intertwined in the same area, because removal of a piece of disk would not be as involved as separating a lesion from multiple components of the spinal column. The approaches differ in the amount of expertise and time required. Codes vary based on approach. A posterior approach means a surgical opening was formed from the back. An anterior approach means a surgical opening was formed from the front.

When coding spinal procedures, you should look for condition, approach, whether unilateral or bilateral, and whether multiple procedures were performed.

Often when a laminectomy (removal of a lamina) is performed, an arthrodesis (surgical fusion of joints) is also performed. In some cases spinal instrumentation (the use of rods, wires, and screws to create fusions) are also performed. Review the operative reports and confirm all procedures performed when coding multiple procedures.

Notes throughout the Spine and Spinal Cord subsection refer you to other code ranges for commonly performed additional procedures (e.g., arthrodesis codes are in the Musculoskeletal subsection). Remember to use the modifier -51 for multiple procedures if more than one procedure is performed.

Nerves

Nerves are our sensing devices, and they carry stimuli to and from all parts of the body. Some common procedures done on nerves include injection, destruction, decompression, and suture/repair.

Nerves can be injected with anesthetic agents to cause a temporary loss of feeling. The code is chosen according to the type of nerve being injected. Nerves may also be injected to cause destruction of the nerve and permanent loss of feeling in a specific area of the body. Persons with debilitating pain may undergo this type of procedure.

Neuroplasty is the decompression (freeing) of intact nerves (e.g., from scar tissue). If nerves receive excessive pressure from a source, such as scar

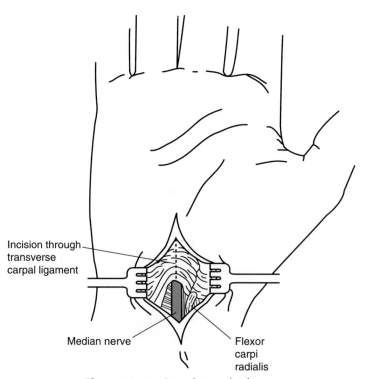

Incision through transverse carpal ligament

Median nerve

Flexor carpi radialis

Figure 10–3 Carpal tunnel release.

tissue or displacement of intervertebral disk material, severe pain may occur. Movement or freeing of nerves is reported with codes from the Neuroplasty (Exploration, Neurolysis, or Nerve Decompression) category. Perhaps the most commonly known neuroplasty procedure is a carpal tunnel release, coded to 64721, in which the median nerve and flexor tendons of the wrist are surgically released (Fig. 10–3).

Nerves can also be removed or they can be repaired (sutured). Remember, the notes found before the repair codes in the Integumentary subsection state that if repair of nerves is necessary, codes from the Nervous System are used. The codes in the Neurorraphy and the Neurorraphy with Nerve Graft categories describe nerve repairs on the basis of the specific nerve being repaired. This category also includes codes that describe grafting on the basis of the size of the graft.

EXERCISE 10-3

NERVOUS SYSTEM

Using the CPT Manual, code the following:

1 Drainage of subdural hematoma using burr holes

Code(s): _____

2 Drainage of subdural hematoma with craniectomy, supratentorial

Code(s): _____

3 Resection of neoplasm, midline skull base, extradural, using infratemporal preauricular approach to middle cranial fossa

Code(s): _____

4 Removal of complete cerebrospinal fluid shunt system, with replacement

Code(s): _____

EYE AND OCULAR ADNEXA

Format

The Eye and Ocular Adnexa subsection includes the subheadings Eyeball, Anterior Segment, Posterior Segment, Ocular Adnexa, and Conjunctiva. There are the typical incision, excision, repair, and destruction categories, but also some that are a little different. For example, the subheading Eye-

from the trenches

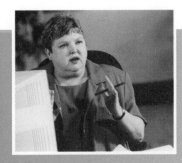

"Study hard . . . it will pay off in your career. Take every single educational opportunity you can . . . classes, mentors, publications. Also, remember 'optimization, not maximization.'"

JUDITH

ball has categories for both Removal of Eye and Removal of Foreign Bodies, although you would expect to find all removal codes in a category under one heading. Remember to use modifier -50 when the procedure is done on two eyes.

Some code groups have different codes for patients who have been operated on before. For example, in the subsection Ocular Adnexa, 67331 is used for a patient who has undergone previous eye surgery. Also, the category Prophylaxis (preventive treatment) under the subheading Posterior Segment has notes regarding the bundling in the codes. The Prophylaxis codes include all the sessions in a treatment period. The Destruction codes in this subcategory also include "one or more sessions." Be certain to read carefully so you know which elements are part of the code.

As in all sections of the CPT manual, there are directional notes throughout that will help you think about what defines a particular code. For example, code 67850 is for the "Destruction of lesion of lid margin (up to 1 cm)." Under this description is a note in parentheses: "(For Mohs' micrographic surgery, see 17304–17310)." This helpful note gives you the category of codes to refer to if the lesion destruction was done using Mohs' micrographic surgery.

Refer to Figures 10–4 through 10–7 as you prepare for coding practice.

STOP *The figures are intended as a review in preparation for coding in this interesting specialty area. Having a good medical dictionary and anatomy book available will help you to code better—when in doubt, check it out!*

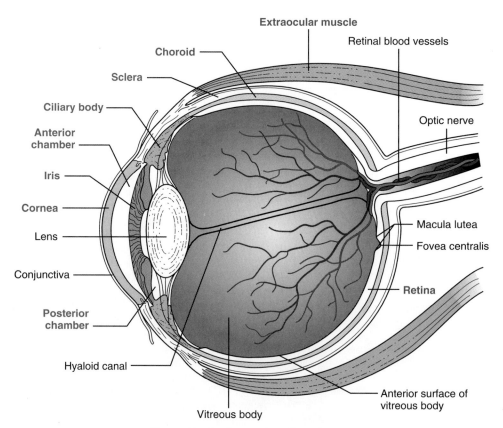

Figure 10–4 Eye and ocular adnexa.

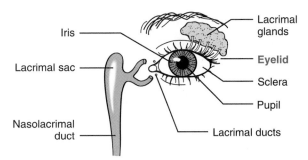

Figure 10-5   Lacrimal apparatus.

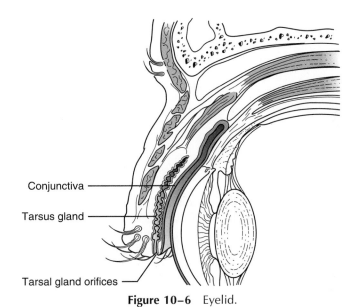

Figure 10-6   Eyelid.

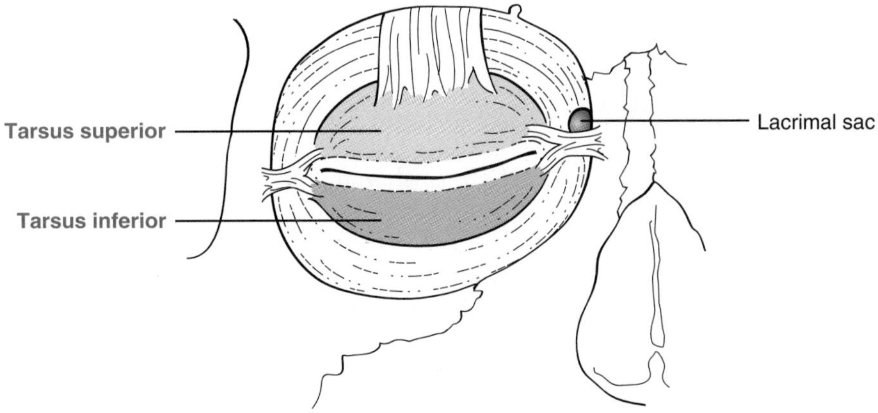

Figure 10-7   Two tarsi.

EXERCISE 10-4

EYE AND OCULAR ADNEXA

Using the CPT manual, code the following:

1 Emboli removal from anterior segment of the left eye

Code(s): _____

2 New patient strabismus surgery involving the superior oblique muscle

Code(s): _____

3 Xenon arc used in three sessions for preventive retinal detachment

Code(s): _____

4 Corneal incision for revision of earlier procedure resulting in astigmatism

Code(s): _____

5 Removal of left eye, muscles attached to implant

Code(s): _____

AUDITORY SYSTEM

Format

The Auditory System subsection is divided into the subheadings External Ear, Middle Ear, Inner Ear, and Temporal Bone/Middle Fossa Approach. The first three subheadings represent the anatomic divisions of the auditory system: external, middle, and internal ear (Fig. 10–8). The categories below each subheading include introduction, incision, excision, removal of foreign body, repair, and/or other procedures, depending on the particular subheading. The subheading Temporal Bone/Middle Fossa Approach contains codes that describe various surgical procedures in which the surgeon makes an incision in front of the ear. Using this incision, the surgeon performs a craniotomy and exposes the brain. The surgeon then repairs the nerve, removes a tumor, or otherwise repairs the area.

EXERCISE 10-5

AUDITORY SYSTEM

Using the CPT manual, code the following:

1 Labyrinthotomy with cryosurgery with multiple perfusions, transcanal

Code(s): _____

2 Bilateral insertion of eustachian tubes, using general anesthesia

Code(s): _____

3 Transcranial approach with a section of the vestibular nerve

Code(s): _____

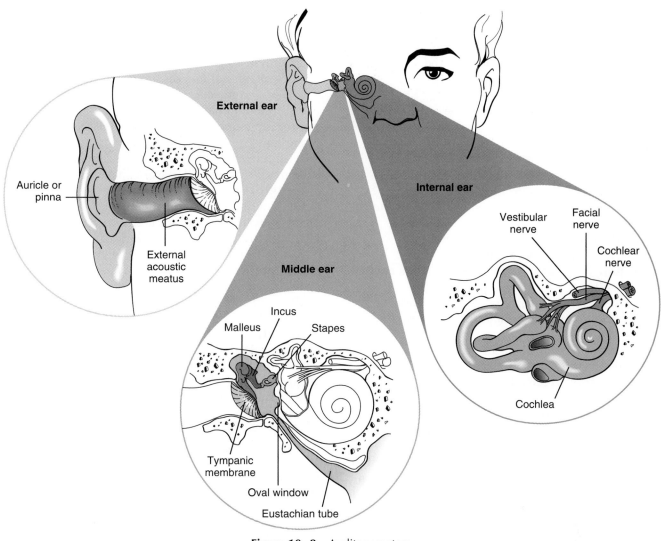

Figure 10–8   Auditory system.

4   Reconstruction of the right auditory canal, due to injury

Code(s): _____

5   Establishment of an opening on the inner wall of the inner ear, semicircular canal

Code(s): _____

CHAPTER GLOSSARY

abscess: localized collection of pus that will result in the disintegration of tissue over time

adrenal: glands, located at the top of the kidneys, that produce steroid hormones

anterior segment: those parts of the eye in the front of and including the lens, orbit, extraocular muscles, and eyelid

apicectomy: excision of a portion of the temporal bone

aspiration: use of a needle and a syringe to withdraw fluid

astigmatism: condition in which the refractive surfaces of the eye are unequal

audi-: prefix meaning hearing

aural atresia: congenital absence of the external auditory canal

autogenous, autologous: from oneself

axillary nodes: lymph nodes located in the armpit

blephar(o)-: prefix meaning eyelid

cannulation: insertion of a tube into a duct or cavity

cataract: opaque covering on or in the lens

central nervous system: brain and spinal cord

Cloquet's node: also called a gland; it is the highest of the deep groin lymph nodes

conjunctiva: the lining of the eyelids and the covering of the sclera

contralateral: affecting the opposite side

cor/o-: prefix meaning pupil

cranium: that part of the skeleton that encloses the brain

dacry/o-: prefix meaning tear or tear duct

dacryocyst/o-: prefix meaning pertaining to the lacrimal sac

enucleation: removal of an organ or organs from a body cavity

exenteration: removal of an organ all in one piece

exostosis: bony growth

fenestration: creation of a new opening in the inner wall of the middle ear

inguinofemoral: referring to the groin and thigh

isthmus: connection of two regions or structures

isthmus, thyroid: tissue connection between right and left thyroid lobes

isthmusectomy: surgical removal of the isthmus

jugular nodes: lymph nodes located next to the large vein in the neck

kerat/o-: prefix meaning cornea

keratoplasty: surgical repair of the cornea

labyrinth: inner connecting cavities, such as the internal ear

laminectomy: surgical excision of the lamina

lymph node: station along the lymphatic system

lymphadenectomy: excision of a lymph node or nodes

lymphadenitis: inflammation of a lymph node

lymphangiotomy: incision into a lymphatic vessel

mastoid-: prefix meaning posterior temporal bone

myring-: prefix meaning eardrum

ocul/o-: prefix meaning eye

ocular adnexa: orbit, extraocular muscles, and eyelid

oto-: prefix meaning ear

parathyroid: produces a hormone to mobilize calcium from the bones to the blood

peripheral nerves: 12 pairs of cranial nerves, 31 pairs of spinal nerves, and autonomic nervous system; connects peripheral receptors to the brain and spinal cord

posterior segment: those parts of the eye behind the lens

retroperitoneal: behind the sac holding the abdominal organs and viscera (peritoneum)

salping(o)-: prefix meaning tube

sclera: outer covering of the eye

shunt: divert or make an artificial passage

skull: entire skeletal framework of the head

somatic nerve: sensory or motor nerve

splenectomy: excision of the spleen

splenoportography: radiographic procedure to allow visualization of the splenic and portal veins of the spleen

stem cell: immature blood cell

stereotaxis: method of identifying a specific area or point in the brain

strabismus: extraocular muscle deviation resulting in unequal visual axes

sympathetic nerve: part of the peripheral nervous system that controls automatic body function and sympathetic nerves activated under stress

tarsorrhaphy: suturing together of the eyelids

thoracic duct: collection and distribution point for lymph, and the largest lymph vessel located in the chest

thymectomy: surgical removal of the thymus

thymus: gland that produces hormones important to the immune response

thyroglossal duct: connection between the thyroid and the pharynx

thyroid: part of the endocrine system that produces hormones that regulate metabolism

thyroidectomy: surgical removal of the thyroid

transmastoid antrostomy: called a simple mastoidectomy, it creates an opening in the mastoid for drainage

transplantation: grafting of tissue from one source to another

uveal: vascular tissue of the choroid, ciliary body, and iris

vitre/o-: prefix meaning pertaining to the vitreous body of the eye

CHAPTER REVIEW

CHAPTER 10, PART I, THEORY

Complete the following:

1 The surgical removal of the spleen is a

_____ .

2 Partial or total removal of the spleen is reported separately, even if it is a part of a more major procedure.
True   False

3 A person can live only a short time without a spleen, so every effort is made to do only a partial removal.
True   False

4 A _____ lymphadenectomy is the removal of the lymph nodes, gland(s), and surrounding tissue.

5 How many endocrine glands are included in the Endocrine subsection of the CPT manual?

_____

6 The pituitary and pineal gland procedure codes are in what subsection of the Surgery

section? _____

7 The codes for pancreatic procedures are located in what subsection of the Surgery sec-

tion? _____

8 Both subtotal and partial mean something

less than _____ .

9 Twist or _____ holes are made through the skull to accomplish procedures of the brain.

10 The _____ procedure is the method used to obtain exposure to a lesion of

the skull base, and the _____
procedure is what is done to the lesion.

11 CSF means _____ .

12 The most commonly known neuroplasty proce-

dure is a _____ release.

CHAPTER 10, PART II, PRACTICAL

Code the following cases:

13 Using a cervical approach, ligation of the thoracic duct was accomplished.
Code(s): _____

14 Surgical laparoscopy with bilateral total pelvic lymphadenectomy
Code(s): _____

15 Superficial inguinofemoral lymphadenectomy with pelvic lymphadenectomy including the external iliac, hypogastric, and obturator nodes
Code(s): _____

16 Total thyroidectomy
Code(s): _____

17 Surgical laparoscopy with partial adrenalectomy using a transabdominal approach
Code(s):_____

18 Parathyroidectomy with mediastinal exploration, sternal split approach
Code(s): _____

19 Excision of corneal lesion of right eye
Code(s): _____

20 Iridectomy with corneal section for removal of lesion from left eye
Code(s): _____

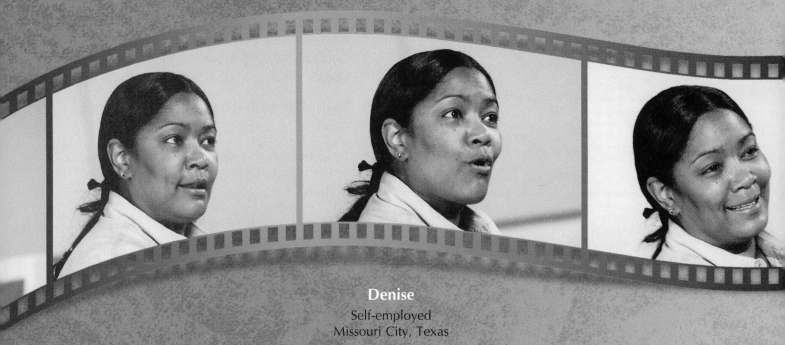

Denise
Self-employed
Missouri City, Texas

chapter 11

The Radiology Section

LEARNING OBJECTIVES

After completing this chapter you should be able to

1   Explain the format of the Radiology section.

2   Interpret the information contained in the Radiology Guidelines.

3   Demonstrate an understanding of Radiology terminology.

4   Code using Radiology codes.

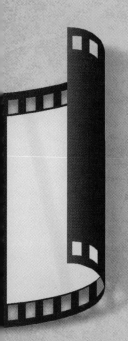

FORMAT

Radiology is the branch of medicine that uses radiant energy to diagnose and treat patients. The term originally referred to the use of x-rays to produce radiographs but is now commonly applied to all types of medical imaging. A physician who specializes in radiology is a **radiologist.** Radiologists can provide services to patients independent of or in conjunction with another physician of a different specialty. The Radiology section of the CPT manual is divided into four main subsections.

- Diagnostic Radiology
- Diagnostic Ultrasound
- Radiation Oncology
- Nuclear Medicine

RADIOLOGY TERMINOLOGY

The suffix *-graphy* means "making of a film" using a variety of methods. **Radiography** is a broad term used to indicate any number of methods used by radiologists to do diagnostic testing. The following exercise will familiarize you with some of the numerous radiographic procedures in the CPT manual.

EXERCISE 11–1

RADIOLOGY TERMINOLOGY

The following words end in "-graphy," meaning "making of a film." For example, in angiocardiography, "angio" means vessels and "cardio" means heart, so angiocardiography is the making of a film of the heart and vessels. What do the other "-graphy" words mean?

angiocardiography _____ heart and vessels _____

1   aortography _____

2   arthrography _____

3   cholangiopancreatography _____

4   cholangiography _____

5   cystography _____

6   dacryocystography _____

7   duodenography _____

8   echocardiography _____

9   encephalography _____

10   epididymography _____

11   hepatography _____

12   hysterosalpingography _____

13   laryngography _____

14 lymphangiography _____

15 myelography _____

16 pyelography _____

17 sialography _____

18 sinography _____

19 splenography _____

20 urography _____

21 venography _____

22 vesiculography _____

PROCEDURES

Here are just a few more radiographic procedures for your review:

1. **Fluoroscopy** views the inside of the body and projects it onto a television screen. Fluoroscopy provides live images and allows the study of the function of the organ (physiology) as well as the structure of the organ (anatomy).

2. **Magnetic resonance imaging (MRI)** is the use of nonionizing radiation to show the body in a cross-sectional view.

3. **Tomography** is the view of a single plane of the body by blurring out all other layers.

4. **Biometry** is the application of a statistical method to a biologic fact.

PLANES

Terminology referring to planes of the body and positioning of the body is often used in the Radiology section. A **position** is how the patient is placed during the x-ray examination, and a **projection** is the path of the x-ray beam. An example of a projection is anteroposterior, which denotes that the x-ray beam enters the patient's body at the front (anterior) and exits from the back (posterior). An example of a position is **prone,** which means the patient is lying on his or her anterior (front), but the sides of entrance and exit of the x-ray beam are not specified. Familiarity with this terminology will aid you as you review the Radiology section and begin to choose the

from the trenches

"You can do whatever you need to do . . . fall down six times, get up seven. Every person who succeeds is one who has failed and tried again."

DENISE

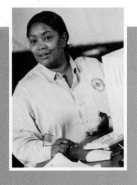

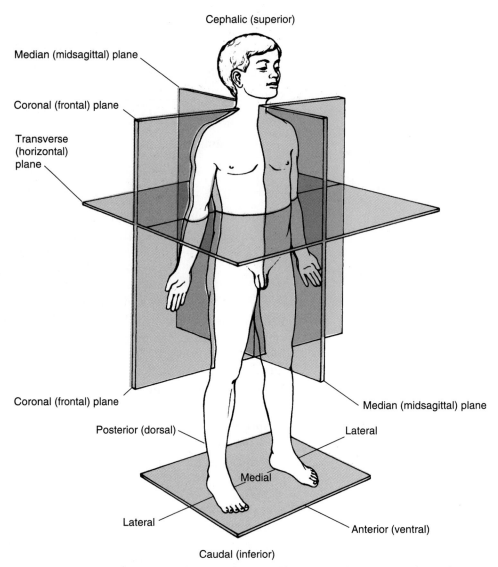

Figure 11–1   Planes of the body and terms of location and position of the body.

correct codes for physician services. Figure 11–1 illustrates the major planes and the surfaces of the body that can be accessed by positioning the body.

Figure 11–2 shows proximal and distal body references. **Proximal** and **distal** are directional body references that mean closest to (proximal) or farthest from (distal) the trunk of the body. These terms are relative, meaning they are used to describe the position of the part as compared with another part. Therefore, the term "proximal" describes a part as being closer to the body trunk than another part, and the term "distal" describes a part as being farther away from the body than another part. The knee would be described as being proximal to the ankle, and it would also be described as being distal to the thigh or hip.

Figure 11–3 illustrates the **anteroposterior (AP)** (front to back) position, in which the patient has his or her front (anterior) closest to the x-ray machine, and the x-ray travels through the patient from the front to the back. In Figure 11–4, the **posteroanterior (PA)** position, the patient has his or her back (posterior) located closest to the machine, and the beam travels through the patient from back to front.

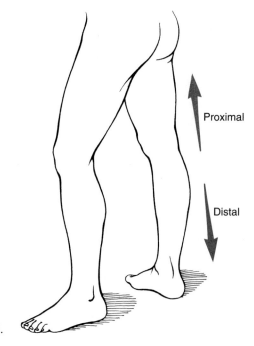

Figure 11–2   Proximal and distal.

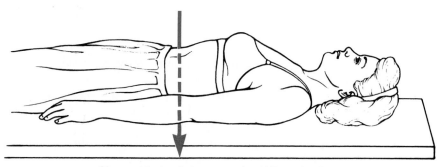

Figure 11–3   Anteroposterior (AP) projection.

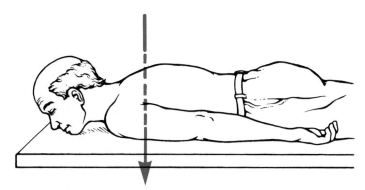

Figure 11–4   Posteroanterior (PA) projection.

Lateral positions are side positions. When the patient's right side is closest to the film, it is called *right lateral*. When the patient's left side is closest to the film, it is called *left lateral*. For example, Figure 11–5 shows a left lateral position and Figure 11–6 shows a right lateral position. The use of these various positions allows the physician to view the body from a variety of angles. Figure 11–7 shows posteroanterior and lateral positions used to view a patient's lung that contains cancer.

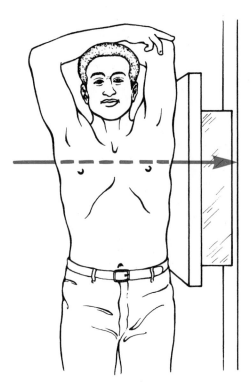

Figure 11–5 Left lateral position.

Dorsal, more commonly referred to as "supine," means lying on the back; **ventral,** more commonly referred to as "prone," means lying on the stomach; and **lateral** means lying on the **side.**

Decubitus positions are recumbent positions; the x-ray beam is placed horizontally. *Ventral decubitus* (prone) is the act of lying on the stomach (Fig. 11–8A), and *dorsal decubitus* (supine) is the act of lying on the back (Fig. 11–8B). The term "decubitus," generally shortened to "decub," has a

Figure 11–6 Right lateral position.

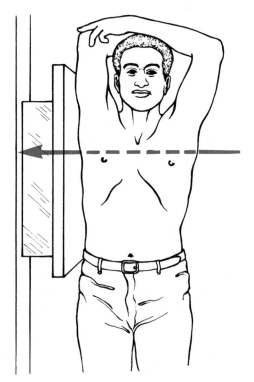

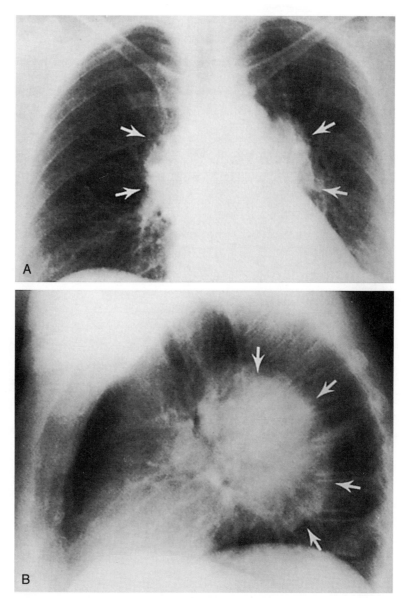

Figure 11–7 Use of posteroanterior and lateral positions to view a primary mediastinal bronchogenic carcinoma. Posteroanterior *(A)* and lateral *(B)* radiographs of this 59-year-old female smoker show a massive subcarinal mass *(arrows)* and no pulmonary mass. The subcarinal mass was surgically shown to be a large cell carcinoma of the lung. (From Woodring JH: Unusual radiographic manifestations of lung cancer. Radiol Clin North Am 28:611, 1990.)

special meaning in radiology. The simple act of lying on one's back would be referred to as lying supine, but if a horizontal x-ray beam is used, the position becomes decubitus. The type of decubitus is determined by the body surface the patient is lying on.

Recumbent means lying down. Thus, *right lateral recumbent* means the patient is lying on the right side (Fig. 11–8C), and *left lateral recumbent* means the patient is lying on the left side (Fig. 11–8D). In the ventral decubitus position, the patient is positioned prone and the x-ray beam comes into the patient from the right side and exits on the left (Fig. 11–8E).

In the *left lateral decubitus* position, the patient is lying on the left side with the beam coming from the front and passing through to the back (anteroposterior) (Fig. 11–8F).

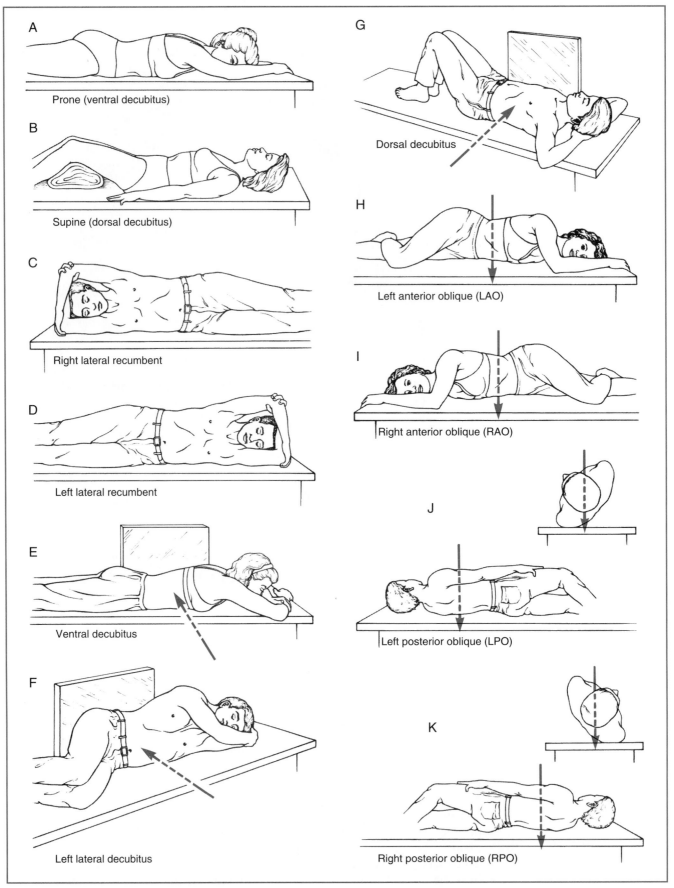

Figure 11-8 Radiographic positions. *A,* Prone (ventral decubitus). *B,* Supine (dorsal decubitus). *C,* Right lateral recumbent. *D,* Left lateral recumbent. *E,* Ventral decubitus. *F,* Left lateral decubitus. *G,* Dorsal decubitus. *H,* Left anterior oblique (LAO). *I,* Right anterior oblique (RAO). *J,* Left posterior oblique (LPO). *K,* Right posterior oblique (RPO).

When the patient is positioned on his or her back (dorsal decubitus) and the x-ray beam comes into the left side of the patient, the positioning is dorsal decubitus, but the view obtained is a right lateral (because the right side is closest to the film) (Fig. 11–8*G*).

Oblique views refer to those obtained while the body is rotated so it is not in a full anteroposterior or posteroanterior position but somewhat diagonal. Oblique views are termed according to the body surface on which the patient is lying. The *left anterior oblique (LAO)* position is depicted in Figure 11–8*H* with the patient's left side rotated forward toward the table. The patient is lying on the left anterior aspect of his or her body. The *right anterior oblique (RAO)* position has the patient on his or her right side rotated forward toward the table, as in Figure 11–8*I*.

Two more oblique views are left posterior oblique and right posterior oblique. In the *left posterior oblique (LPO)* view, the patient is rotated so that the left posterior aspect of his or her body is against the table, as in Figure 11–8*J*. The *right posterior oblique (RPO)* view has the patient on the right side rotated back, as in Figure 11–8*K*.

The last two terms that are used to describe projections are tangential and axial. **Tangential** is the patient position that allows the beam to skim the body part, which produces a profile of the structure of the body (Fig. 11–9*A*). Figure 11–9*B* illustrates the **axial** projection, which is any projection that allows the beam to pass through the body part lengthwise.

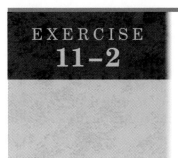

EXERCISE 11-2

PLANES

Fill in the blanks with the correct words:

1   What is the word that indicates how the patient is placed during the x-ray examination? _____

2   What is the term that indicates the path the x-ray beam travels?

_____

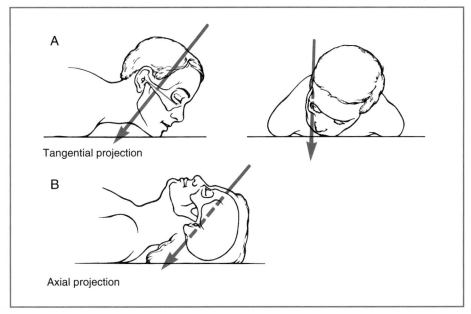

Tangential projection

Axial projection

Figure 11–9   Radiographic projections. *A,* Tangential projection. *B,* Axial projection.

What do the following abbreviations mean?

3 AP _____

4 PA _____

5 RAO _____

6 LPO _____

7 What term indicates that a patient is lying supine, or on his or her back? _____

8 What term indicates that a patient is lying prone, or on his or her stomach? _____

9 What term indicates that a patient is lying on his or her right side?

_____

10 What is the term that indicates when a patient is on his or her back and the x-ray beam comes into the right side of the patient?

_____

GUIDELINES

As with all Guidelines, the Radiology Guidelines should be read carefully before radiologic procedures or services are coded. The Guidelines contain the unique instructions used within the section and the indications for multiple procedures, separate procedures, unlisted radiology procedure codes, and applicable modifiers.

Guidelines that are used more commonly in this section than in others are those explaining the professional, technical, and global components of a procedure. These components are as follows:

1. **Professional:** describes the services of the physician, including the supervision of the taking of the x-ray film and the interpretation with report of the x-ray films
2. **Technical:** describes the services of the technologist, as well as the use of the equipment, film, and other supplies
3. **Global:** describes the combination of the professional and technical components (1 and 2)

For example, if a patient undergoes a radiology procedure in a clinic that owns its own equipment, employs its own technologist(s), and also employs the radiologist who supervises, interprets, and reports on the radiologic results, the global procedure is coded for billing. But if the radiologist is reading and interpreting films that were taken at another facility, only the professional component would be coded for physician services.

coding shot

Third-party payment is generally 40% for the professional component, 60% for the technical component, and 100% for the global service.

When only the professional component of the service is provided, the modifier -26 is placed after the CPT code. Modifier -26 alerts the third-party payer to the fact that only the professional component was provided. If, for example, an independent radiology facility takes a complete chest x-ray (71030) and sends the x-rays to an independent radiologist who reads the x-rays and writes a report of the findings in the x-rays, the coding for the independent radiologist would be

71030-26   Complete chest x-ray, four views

Professional component only

There is no CPT modifier to indicate the technical component of radiologic services. The modifier most commonly used is the HCPCS Level II modifier -TC, which stands for technical component. HCPCS codes are for use with Medicare and Medicaid claims, which you will be learning about in Chapter 12 of this text; some commercial payers may also recognize some HCPCS codes such as those for drugs and supplies. When submitting claims for radiologic services in which only the technical component was provided, use a CPT code followed by -TC. For example, if you were the coder for the independent radiology facility that took the complete chest x-ray (71030), you would code as follows:

71030-TC   Complete chest x-ray, four views

Technical component only

Supervision and Interpretation

The other coding practice most commonly used in the Radiology section is called **component** or **combination coding,** which means that a code from the Radiology section as well as a code from one of the other sections must be used to fully describe the procedure. For example, interventional radiologists may inject contrast material; place stents, catheters, or guide wires; or perform any number of procedures found throughout the CPT manual. Many times, before radiology procedures can be performed, a contrast material must be injected into the patient to make certain organs or vessels stand out more clearly on the radiographic image. When this contrast material is injected into the patient by the radiologist, a CPT code from the Surgery section must be used to indicate the injection procedure.

coding shot

Codes in the Radiology section describe only the radiology procedures, not the injections or placement of other materials necessary to do the procedure.

Suppose, for example, a voiding urethrocystography with contrast medium enhancement is performed. In this procedure, a physician injects a radioactive material into the bladder. An x-ray of the bladder (cystography) is then obtained; the x-rays show filling, voiding, and post-voiding. The injection portion of the procedure is coded with a surgery code (51600: Injection procedure for cystography or voiding urethrocystography) and the cystography is coded with a radiology code (74455: Urethrocystography, voiding, radiologic supervision and interpretation).

As a new coder, you will need to pay special attention to the information in parentheses below the codes in the Radiology section. This parenthetic material gives you information about other components of procedures. Previous editions of the CPT manual had combination codes that were used when the physician did both components of some procedures. Using the combination code replaced the use of one code from surgery and one code from radiology; but many of these combination codes have been deleted. One reason they were deleted is to allow the physicians to more specifically indicate the services provided to the patient. For example, the parenthetic phrase below code 74455 indicates that a previous combination code was deleted and directs you to code 51600 and 74455 for the complete procedure. There are many parenthetic phrases such as this throughout the Radiology section and you will want to refer to them when coding component procedures.

Odds and Ends

Many of the code descriptions state "radiologic supervision and interpretation" and alert you to component coding. When component coding, be certain that you read the parenthetic information that follows these component codes.

Some codes are divided based on the extent of the radiologic examination, such as procedures that "specify with KUB" (kidney, ureter, and bladder). You must read the radiologist's report or the details in the medical record so as to understand the extent of the procedure. Always code to the fullest extent of the procedure.

Codes are also often divided on the basis of whether contrast materials were used. The phrase "with contrast" in the CPT manual means contrast that was administered intravascularly. If the procedure indicates that contrast was administered orally or rectally, the service is coded as "without contrast."

---

coding shot

Report the supply of contrast material with Medicine section code 99070, supplies. Injection of contrast material is included in the "with contrast" radiology procedure code, unless guidelines state that a surgical code should also be used.

Radiographic procedures are located in the CPT manual index under the main term "X-ray," with subterms for the anatomic part (e.g., hand, spine).

EXERCISE 11-3

GUIDELINES

Fill in the blanks using the Radiology Guidelines of your CPT manual:

1   What procedure is one that is "performed independently of, and is not immediately related to, other services"? _____

2 If several medical services are provided in conjunction with radiologic services to a patient on the same day, what type of procedure modifier could be used?

_____

3 What are the four subsections of the Radiology section?

_____

_____

_____

_____

THE FOUR RADIOLOGY SUBSECTIONS

Diagnostic Radiology

The most standard radiographic procedures are contained in the Diagnostic Radiology subsection of the Radiology section. This subsection describes diagnostic imaging, including plain x-ray films, the use of computed axial tomography (CAT or CT) scanning, magnetic resonance imaging (MRI), magnetic resonance angiography (MRA), and angiography. CT scanning uses an x-ray beam that rotates around the patient, as illustrated in Figure 11–10. Figure 11–11 shows a right lung carcinoma in a patient and the detail that can be obtained using a CT scan. Special computer software is used with CT scanners to produce three-dimensional images, which are used to study many different internal structures. Tomography, CT scanning, and MRI may include the use of injectable dyes (radiographic contrast) to aid in imaging, and the codes are divided on the basis of whether or not contrast was used. For example, under the subheading Spine and Pelvis, the codes for CAT, MRI, and MRA are divided as follows:

    72192   Computerized axial tomography, pelvis; without contrast material

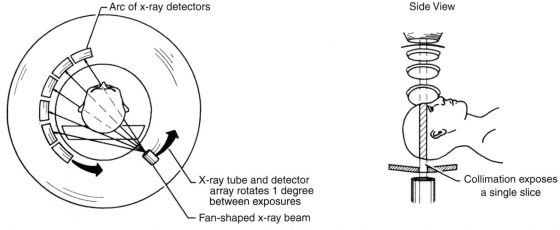

Figure 11–10 Principles of computed tomographic (CT) scanning. The x-ray tube produces a fan-shaped beam that passes through a section (slice) of the patient. This fan-shaped beam is received by a circular array of detectors at the opposite side. These detectors receive x-rays along the path through the patient's body. The detector and x-ray source rotate around the axis, producing exposures at 1-degree intervals of rotation. (From Stimac GK: Introduction to Diagnostic Imaging. Philadelphia, WB Saunders, 1992.)

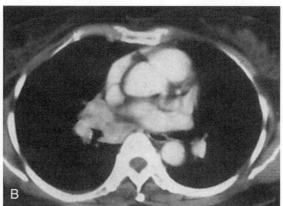

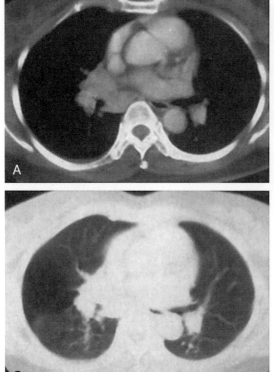

Figure 11–11   CT scans. *A,* A patient with right hilar lung carcinoma and mediastinal adenopathy showing the margins of the bones. *B,* The scan can be set to show the soft tissue. *C,* The lung organs can be shown by using additional scan settings. There is greater detail than would be obtained with conventional radiographs. (Courtesy of Bruce Porter, MD.)

72196   Magnetic resonance (e.g., proton) imaging, pelvis; with contrast material

72198   Magnetic resonance angiography, pelvis, with or without contrast material(s)

Note that there is one code for the CAT, one code for the MRI, and one code for the MRA. The codes are divided by CAT, MRI, and MRA throughout the Diagnostic Radiology subsection. So you must read the code carefully to ensure that you are using the code that represents the correct kind of imaging. Figure 11–12 is an example of a magnetic resonance image.

In **angiography,** dyes are injected into the vessels to add contrast that facilitates the visualization of vessels' lumen size and condition. The lumen is the inside layer of the vessel. Angiography is used to look for abnormalities inside the vessels. Figure 11–13 shows an angiogram of the aortic arch and brachiocephalic vessels. The radiologist studies the vessels using angiography to detect conditions such as malformations, strokes, or myocardial infarctions.

from the trenches

"Compliance starts the moment the patient calls."

DENISE

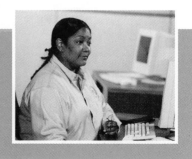

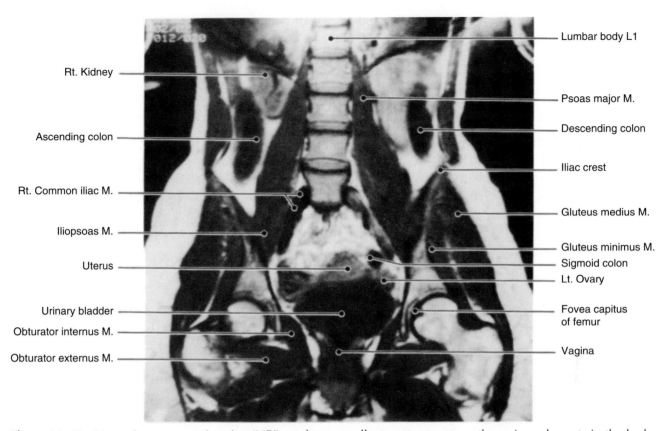

Rt. Kidney

Ascending colon

Rt. Common iliac M.

Iliopsoas M.

Uterus

Urinary bladder

Obturator internus M.

Obturator externus M.

Lumbar body L1

Psoas major M.

Descending colon

Iliac crest

Gluteus medius M.

Gluteus minimus M.
Sigmoid colon
Lt. Ovary

Fovea capitus
of femur

Vagina

Figure 11–12 Magnetic resonance imaging (MRI) produces excellent contrasts among the various elements in the body. (From Christoforidis AJ: Atlas of Axial, Sagittal, and Coronal Anatomy with CT and MRI. Philadelphia, WB Saunders, 1988.)

Mammography is the use of diagnostic radiology to detect breast tumors or other abnormal breast conditions. Three codes are used to report mammography services:

76090	Mammography, unilateral
76091	bilateral
76092	Screening mammography, bilateral (two view film study of each breast)

Figure 11–13 Angiography of the aortic arch and brachiocephalic vessels. (From Stimac GK: Introduction to Diagnostic Imaging. Philadelphia, WB Saunders, 1992.)

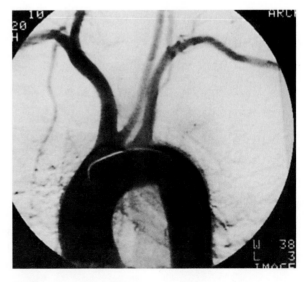

Codes 76090 and 76091 are for use when the mammography is performed to detect a tumor that is suspected. For example, a patient who upon examination has demonstrated an abnormality in a breast would appropriately have the service reported with 76090. If, however, a patient has presented for the usual screening mammography, you would report the service with 76092. Note that the description for the usual screening mammography indicates "bilateral," because screening mammography is done on both breasts.

Codes in the Diagnostic Radiology subsection are divided according to anatomic site, from the head down. Some of the codes indicate a specific number of views, such as a minimum of three views or a single view. You should pay special attention to the description in each code and understand clearly how many views are specified in the code.

---

coding shot

If fewer than the total number of views specified in the code are taken, modifier -52 would be used to indicate to the third-party payer that less of the procedure was performed than is described by the code, unless a code already exists for the smaller number of views.

EXERCISE 11-4

DIAGNOSTIC RADIOLOGY

Code the radiology portion of the procedures unless otherwise directed:

1 What is the code for a diagnostic mammography, bilateral?

Code(s): _____

2 What is the code for an unlisted diagnostic radiologic procedure?

Code(s): _____

3 What is the code for the supervision and interpretation of an aortography, thoracic, by serialography

Code(s): _____

Diagnostic Ultrasound

The second subsection in Radiology is Diagnostic Ultrasound. **Diagnostic ultrasound** is the use of high-frequency sound waves to image anatomic structures and to detect the cause of illness and disease. It is used by the physician in the diagnosis process. Ultrasound moves at different speeds through tissue, depending on the density of the tissue. Forms and outlines of organs can be identified by ultrasound as the sound waves move through or bounce back (echo) from the tissues.

There are many uses for ultrasound in medicine, such as showing a gallstone (Fig. 11–14) and showing triplets in the first trimester (Fig. 11–15). You may think that these ultrasound procedures do not produce a

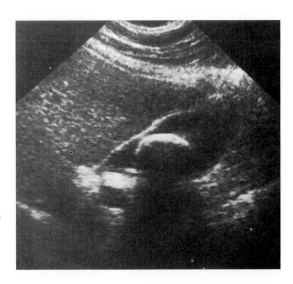

Figure 11–14 Ultrasound of the gallbladder shows the shadowing of a gallstone. (From Stimac GK: Introduction to Diagnostic Imaging. Philadelphia, WB Saunders, 1992.)

picture clear enough to be of use to the physician in the diagnosis process, but a professional trained in the interpretation of ultrasound images is able to read them clearly.

Codes for ultrasound procedures are found in three locations:

- Radiology section, Diagnostic Ultrasound subsection, 76506–76886, divided on the basis of the anatomic location of the procedure (chest, pelvis)
- Medicine section, Non-Invasive Vascular Diagnostic Studies subsection, 93875–93990, divided on the basis of the anatomic location of the procedure (cerebrovascular, extremity)
- Medicine section, Echocardiography (ultrasound of the heart and great arteries), 93303–93350

The ultrasound codes for heart and vessels are in the Medicine section; all other ultrasound codes are in the Radiology section.

An **interventional radiologist** is a physician who is skilled in both the surgical procedure and the radiology portion of an interventional radiologic service. For example, an interventional radiologist who performed a liver biopsy using CT guidance to locate the lesion would report the services by using a surgery code (47500) and a radiology code (74320). Neither code would have a modifier because the interventional radiologist provided the surgical portion of the service, reporting it with a surgery code, and provided the CT guidance service, reporting it with a code from the radiology section.

Figure 11–15 Triplets in the first trimester can be imaged on one scan. One fetus (3) is contained within its own sac with its own placenta. The other two fetuses share a placenta but are separated by a membrane. (From Benson CB, Doubilet PM: Sonography of multiple gestations. Radiol Clin North Am 28:151, 1990.)

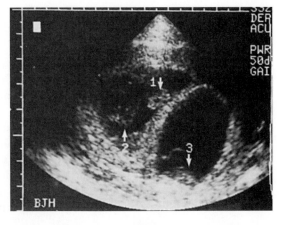

Most of the services in the Diagnostic Ultrasound subsection are located in the index of the CPT manual under the main term "Ultrasound." These terms are subdivided anatomically and by procedure, e.g., guidance or drainage.

EXERCISE 11-5

DIAGNOSTIC ULTRASOUND

In the CPT manual, Diagnostic Ultrasound is divided into subheadings.

Locate and list the subheadings:

1 _____

2 _____

3 _____

4 _____

5 _____

6 _____

7 _____

8 _____

9 _____

Modes and Scans

There are four different types of ultrasound listed in the CPT manual: A-mode, M-mode, B-scan, and real-time scan.

A-mode: one-dimensional display reflecting the time it takes the sound wave to reach a structure and reflect back. This process maps the structure's outline. "A" is for amplitude of sound return (echo).

M-mode: one-dimensional display of the movement of structures. "M" stands for motion.

B-scan: two-dimensional display of the movement of tissues and organs. "B" stands for brightness. The sound waves bounce off tissue or organs and are projected onto a black and white television screen. The strong signals display as black and the weaker signals display as lighter shades of gray. B-scan is also called gray-scale ultrasound.

Real-time scan: two-dimensional display of both the structure and the motion of tissues and organs that indicates the size, shape, and movement of the tissue or organ.

These modes and scans are used to describe the codes throughout the Diagnostic Ultrasound subsection. Codes are often divided on the basis of the scan or mode that was used. The medical record will indicate the scan or mode used.

Several codes within the subsection include the use of Doppler ultrasound. **Doppler ultrasound** is the use of sound that can be transmitted only through solids or liquids and is a specific version of ultrasonography, or ultrasound. Doppler ultrasound is named for an Austrian physicist, Johann Doppler, who discovered a relationship between sound and light waves—a relationship upon which ultrasound technology was built. Doppler ultrasound is used to measure moving objects and so is ideal for measuring bloodflow. Codes often state "with or without Doppler." Doppler ultrasound can be standard black and white or color. Color Doppler translates the standard black and white into colored images. Just imagine how much easier it is to see a leak in a vessel when the vessel is yellow and the blood is red. The code descriptions will specifically state "color-flow Doppler."

There is some component coding, but it occurs mostly under the subheading of Ultrasonic Guidance Procedures. The parenthetic information will refer you to the surgical procedure code. For example, code 76946 is for the radiologic supervision and interpretation of ultrasonic guidance for amniocentesis. The physician guides the insertion of a needle to withdraw fluid from the uterus. If the physician did both the radiologic portion of the procedure and the surgical procedure, you would code 59000 from the Surgery section and 76946 from the Radiology section.

The subheading Vascular Studies contains only parenthetic information that directs you to the Medicine section, Non-Invasive Vascular Diagnostic Studies subsection.

EXERCISE 11-6

MODES AND SCANS

Fill in the codes for the following:

1 An ultrasound of the spinal canal

   Code(s): _____

2 An ultrasound of the chest and mediastinum using B-scan

   Code(s): _____

3 A complete abdominal ultrasound in real time with image documentation

   Code(s): _____

4 A repeat uterine ultrasound in real time with image documentation of a 32-week pregnant female

   Code(s): _____

5 A fetal profile, biophysical, with nonstress testing

   Code(s): _____

Radiation Oncology

The Radiation Oncology subsection of the Radiology section deals with both professional and technical treatments utilizing radiation to destroy tumors. The subsection is divided on the basis of treatment. In this subsection, special attention must be given to reporting professional and technical components. Read all of the definitions carefully to make certain you know what the code includes. Many third-party payers have developed strict guidelines determining the number of times certain procedures are allowed within each treatment course. You should work closely with third-party payers to understand their preferred billing system.

The service codes within this subheading include codes for the initial consultation through the management of the patient throughout the course

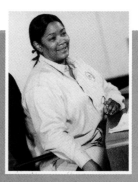

Do you ever find your job to be like detective work?

"Yes. I always feel like a detective. Most patients think that insurance companies just pay all claims. But you must have the correct information . . . this is what you search out."

DENISE

of treatment. When the initial consultation occurs, the code for the service would come from the E/M section. For example, the patient might be an inpatient when the therapeutic radiologist first sees the patient for evaluation of treatment options and before a decision for treatment is made. You would code this consultation service with an Initial Inpatient Consultation code from the E/M section.

coding shot

Normal follow-up care is included for 3 months following the completion of treatment that was reported using radiation oncology codes. You would not bill for the normal follow-up care that occurs within this 3-month period.

Clinical Treatment Planning

Clinical Treatment Planning reflects professional services by the physician. It includes interpretation of special testing, tumor localization, treatment volume determination, treatment time/dosage determination, choice of treatment modality (method), determination of number and size of treatment ports, selection of appropriate treatment devices, and any other procedures necessary to adequately develop a course of treatment. A treatment plan is set up for all patients requiring radiation therapy.

There are three types of clinical treatment plans: simple, intermediate, and complex.

Simple planning requires that there be a single treatment area of interest that is encompassed by a single port or by simple parallel opposed ports with simple or no blocking.

Intermediate planning requires that there be three or more converging ports, two separate treatment areas, multiple blocks, or special time dose constraints.

Complex planning requires that there be highly complex blocking, custom shielding blocks, tangential ports, special wedges or compensators, three or more separate treatment areas, rotational or special beam consideration, or a combination of therapeutic modalities.

Simulation

Simulation is the service of determining treatment areas and the placement of the ports for radiation treatment, but it does not include the administration of the radiation. A simulation can be performed on a simulator designated for use only in simulations in a radiation therapy treatment unit, or on a diagnostic x-ray machine. Codes are divided to indicate four levels of service:

- **Simple** simulation of a single treatment area, with either a single port or parallel opposed ports and simple or no blocking

- **Intermediate** simulation of three or more converging ports, with two separate treatment areas and multiple blocks

- **Complex** simulation of tangential ports, with three or more treatment areas, rotation or arc therapy, complex blocking, custom shielding blocks, brachytherapy source verification, hyperthermia probe verification, and any use of contrast material

- **Three-dimensional** computer-generated reconstruction of tumor volume and surrounding critical normal tissue structures based on direct CT scan and or MRI data in preparation for non-coplanar or coplanar therapy; this is a simulation that utilizes documented three-dimensional beam's-eye view volume dose displays of multiple or moving beams. Documentation of three-dimensional volume reconstruction and dose distribution is required.

Radiation oncology is a very complex area of coding. After the initial simulation and treatment plan has been established for a patient, if any change is made in the field of treatment, a new simulation billing is required. When coding for a treatment period, you will have codes for planning, simulation, the isodose plan, devices, treatment management (the number of treatments determines the number of times billed), and the radiation delivery.

The codes in Clinical Treatment Planning are located in the index of the CPT manual under the main term "Radiology" and the subterm "Therapeutic." Codes can also be located under the main term of the specific service, such as "Port Film."

EXERCISE 11-7

CLINICAL TREATMENT PLANNING

Using the CPT manual, code the following:

1 Complex therapeutic radiology simulation-aided field setting

   Code(s): _____

2 Therapeutic radiology treatment planning; simple

   Code(s): _____

Medical Radiation Physics, Dosimetry, Treatment Devices, and Special Services

Medical Radiation Physics, Dosimetry, Treatment Devices, and Special Services deals with the decision-making of the physicians as to the type of treatment (modality), dose, and development of treatment devices. It is common to have several dosimetry or device changes during a treatment course. Dosimetry is the calculation of the radiation dose and placement.

Codes in this subheading are divided mostly on the basis of the level of treatment (simple, intermediate, complex). The codes are located in the index of the CPT manual under the main term "Radiation Therapy" and the subterm of the specific service, such as dose plan or treatment.

EXERCISE 11-8

MEDICAL RADIATION, PHYSICS, DOSIMETRY, TREATMENT DEVICES, AND SPECIAL SERVICES

Using the CPT manual, code the following:

1 Design and construction of a bite block, simple

   Code(s): _____

2 Calculation of an isodose for brachytherapy, single plane, two sources, simple

   Code(s): _____

3 Teletherapy, isodose plan, to one area, simple

   Code(s): _____

Radiation Treatment Delivery

Radiation Treatment Delivery reflects the technical components only. These codes are used to bill for the actual delivery of the radiation. Radiation treatment is delivered in units called megaelectron volts (MeV). A megaelectron volt is a unit of energy. The radiation energy **delivered** by the machine is measured in megaelectron volts; the energy that is **deposited** in the patient's tissue is measured in rads (radiation-absorbed dose). The therapy dose in a cancer treatment would typically be in the thousands of rads.

To code Radiation Treatment Delivery services, you need to know the amount of radiation delivered (6–10 MeV, 11–19 MeV) and the number of

- **Areas** treated (single, two, three or more),
- **Ports** involved (single, three or more, tangential), and
- **Blocks** used (none, multiple, custom).

EXERCISE 11-9

RADIATION TREATMENT DELIVERY

Using the CPT manual, code the following:

The patient receives radiation treatment delivery:

1 To a single area at 4 MeV

   Code(s): _____

2 With superficial voltage only

   Code(s): _____

3 To four separate areas with a rotational beam at 4 MeV

Code(s): _____

4 For two separate areas, using three or more ports with multiple blocks at 5 MeV

Code(s): _____

5 For three or more separate areas using custom blocks, wedges, rotation beams, up to 5 MeV

Code(s): _____

Radiation Treatment Management

Radiation Treatment Management codes reflect the reporting of the professional component. The codes are used to bill weekly management of radiation therapy. The notes under the heading Radiation Treatment Management state that clinical management is based on five fractions or treatment sessions regardless of the time interval separating the delivery of treatment. This means these codes may be used if the patient receives a treatment at least five times within a 7-day week; it also means that if the patient receives five treatments at any time during this week (i.e., skipping a day or two between treatments), these codes may still be used.

If the patient receives five treatments and then receives an additional one or two fractions, you do not code for the additional fractions. Only if three or more fractions beyond the original five are delivered would you code using 77427 to indicate the additional treatment.

Bundled into the Radiation Treatment Management codes are the following physician services:

- Review of port films
- Review of dosimetry, dose delivery, and treatment parameters
- Review of patient treatment setup
- Examination of the patient for medical evaluation and management (e.g., assessment of the patient's response to treatment, coordination of care and treatment, review of imaging and/or lab test results).

It would be inappropriate to code these items individually. For example, the physician sees the patient in the office to evaluate the patient's response to treatment. You might think you should use an E/M code to report the office visit, but that would be incorrect because the management codes already include the office visit service.

Proton Beam Treatment Delivery

The delivery of radiation treatment using a proton beam utilizes particles that are positively charged with electricity. The use of the proton beam is an alternative delivery method for radiation in which photon (electromagnetic) radiation would traditionally be used. The Proton Beam subheading was new in the 2001 edition of the CPT manual.

The codes in the subheading are divided according to whether there was simple, intermediate, or complex delivery.

Hyperthermia

Hyperthermia is an increase in body temperature; it is used as a treatment for cancer. The heat source can be ultrasound, microwave, or another means of increasing the temperature in an area. When the temperature of an area is increased, metabolism increases, which boosts the ability of the body to eradicate cancer cells. The location of the heat source can be external (to a depth of 4 cm or less), interstitial (within the tissues), or intracavitary (inside the body). External treatment would be the application to the skin of a heat source such as ultrasound. Interstitial treatment is the insertion of a probe that delivers heat directly to the treatment area. Codes 77600–77615 are used to report external or interstitial treatment delivery.

Intracavitary treatment delivery requires the insertion of a heat-producing probe into a body orifice, such as the rectum or vagina. Code 77620 is used to report intracavitary treatment and is the only code listed under Clinical Intracavitary Hyperthermia.

EXERCISE 11-10

CLINICAL TREATMENT MANAGEMENT

Using the CPT manual, code the following management services:

1 Five radiation treatments

Code(s): _____

2 Unlisted procedure code for therapeutic radiation clinical treatment management (Submission of this unlisted procedure code would necessitate a special report and assumes that no Category III code exists for the procedure.)

Code(s): _____

Clinical Brachytherapy

Clinical **brachytherapy** is the placement of radioactive material directly into or surrounding the site of the tumor. Placement may be **intracavitary** (within a body cavity) or **interstitial** (within the tissues), and material may be placed permanently or temporarily.

The terms "source" and "ribbon" are used in the Clinical Brachytherapy codes. A **source** is a container holding a radioactive element that can be inserted directly into the body where it delivers the radiation dose over time. Sources come in various forms, such as seeds or capsules, and are placed in a cavity (intracavitary) or permanently placed within the tissue (interstitial). **Ribbons** are seeds embedded on a tape. The ribbon is cut to the desired length to control the amount of radiation the patient receives. Ribbons are inserted temporarily into the tissue.

Codes are divided on the basis of the number of sources or ribbons used in an application:

- Simple   1–4
- Intermediate   5–10
- Complex   11+

The Clinical Brachytherapy codes include the physician's work related to the patient's admission to the hospital as well as the daily hospital visits.

EXERCISE
11-11

CLINICAL BRACHYTHERAPY

Using the CPT manual, code the following:

1 A simple application of a radioactive source, intracavitary

Code(s): _____

2 A simple application of a radioactive source, interstitial

Code(s): _____

3 Surface application of a radiation source

Code(s): _____

Nuclear Medicine

Nuclear medicine deals with the placement of radionuclides within the body and the monitoring of emissions from the radioactive elements. Nuclear medicine is used not only for diagnostic studies but also for therapeutic treatment, such as treatment of thyroid conditions.

Stress tests are an example of nuclear medicine techniques. Radioactive material may be used during stress tests to monitor coronary artery blood-flow. Radioactive material adheres to red blood cells. The radioactive materials on the red blood cells allow an image of the heart to be seen and indicate areas where the blood is flowing. The radioactive materials are injected 1 minute before the end of a stress test and then again 24 hours later for a comparison study. If the bloodflow is decreased or absent, the image will show a blank area. If the coronary arteries are clear and allow blood to flow to the heart muscle, the image will show blood dispersement to all areas. If the arteries are partially blocked, the flow may be decreased but adequate during rest. During exercise, however, the necessary amount of oxygenated blood may not be adequate to keep the heart going, and that is when chest pain may occur. During a stress test, if radionuclide dispersement is absent during exercise (showing inadequate blood supply to the area during peak demand) but is present during resting periods (showing adequate flow at rest), this is called **reversible ischemia,** meaning that heart muscle death has not occurred. With intervention, arteries may be opened or bypassed to increase the supply of blood to the muscle before heart muscle death does occur. If the radionuclide is absent during rest and exercise, the ischemia is considered **irreversible,** meaning that heart muscle death has already occurred. A stress test is one of the many uses of nuclear medicine for diagnostic purposes. As you code, you will become familiar with these various diagnostic tests and how they are reported and billed.

coding shot

None of the codes in the subsection includes the radiopharmaceutical(s) used for diagnosis or therapy services. When radiopharmaceutical(s) are supplied for diagnostic purposes, you use code 78990; and when they are supplied for therapeutic purposes, you use code 79900.

There are two subheadings within the Nuclear Medicine subsection—Diagnostic and Therapeutic. The subheading Diagnostic is further divided into category codes based on system, such as the endocrine system and the cardiovascular system.

EXERCISE 11-12

NUCLEAR MEDICINE

Under which subheading in the Nuclear Medicine subsection would you look to locate codes for the following?

1 Liver _____

2 Thyroid _____

3 Spleen _____

4 Bone _____

5 Brain _____

CHAPTER GLOSSARY

A-mode: one-dimensional ultrasonic display reflecting the time it takes a sound wave to reach a structure and reflect back; maps the structure's outline

angiography: taking of x-ray films of vessels after injection of contrast material

anteroposterior: from front to back

anterior (ventral): in front of

aortography: radiographic recording of the aorta

arthrography: radiographic recording of a joint

B-scan: two-dimensional display of tissues and organs

barium enema: radiographic contrast medium—enhanced examination of the colon

bilateral: occurring on two sides

biometry: application of a statistical measure to a biologic fact

brachytherapy: therapy using radioactive sources that are placed inside the body

bronchography: radiographic recording of the lungs

caudal: same as inferior; away from the head, or the lower part of the body

cavernosography: radiographic recording of a cavity, e.g., the pulmonary cavity or the main part of the penis

cervical: pertaining to the neck or to the cervix of the uterus

cholangiography: radiographic recording of the bile ducts

cholangiopancreatography (ERCP): radiographic recording of the biliary system or pancreas

cholecystography: radiographic recording of the gallbladder

computed axial tomography (CAT or CT): procedure by which selected planes of tissue are pinpointed through computer enhancement, and images may be reconstructed by analysis of variance in absorption of the tissue

cystography: radiographic recording of the urinary bladder

dacryocystography: radiographic recording of the lacrimal sac or tear duct sac

diskography: radiographic recording of an intervertebral joint

distal: farther from the point of attachment or origin

dosimetry: scientific calculation of radiation emitted from various radioactive sources

duodenography: radiographic recording of the duodenum or first part of the small intestine

echocardiography: radiographic recording of the heart or heart walls or surrounding tissues

echoencephalography: ultrasound of the brain

echography: ultrasound procedure in which sound waves are bounced off an internal organ and the resulting image is recorded

encephalography: radiographic recording of the subarachnoid space and ventricles of the brain

epididymography: radiographic recording of the epididymis

fluoroscopy: procedure for viewing the interior of the body using x-rays and projecting the image onto a television screen

hepatography: radiographic recording of the liver

hypogastric: lowest middle abdominal area

hysterosalpingography: radiographic recording of the uterine cavity and fallopian tubes

inferior: away from the head or the lower part of the body; also known as caudal

intravenous pyelography (IVP): radiographic recording of the urinary system

laryngography: radiographic recording of the larynx

lateral: away from the midline of the body (to the side)

lymphangiography: radiographic recording of the lymphatic vessels and nodes

M-mode: one-dimensional display of movement of structures

magnetic resonance imaging (MRI): procedure that uses nonionizing radiation to view the body in a cross-sectional view

mammography: radiographic recording of the breasts

medial: toward the midline of the body

MeV: megaelectron volt

myelography: radiographic recording of the subarachnoid space of the spine

physics: scientific study of energy

posterior (dorsal): in back of

posteroanterior: from back to front

pyelography: radiographic recording of the kidneys, renal pelvis, ureters, and bladder

rad: radiation-absorbed dose, the energy deposited in patients' tissues

radiation oncology: branch of medicine concerned with the application of radiation to a tumor site for treatment (destruction) of cancerous tumors

radiograph: film on which an image is produced through exposure to x-radiation

radiologist: physician who specializes in the use of radioactive materials in the diagnosis and treatment of disease and illnesses

radiology: branch of medicine concerned with the use of radioactive substances for diagnosis and therapy

real time: two-dimensional display of both the structures and the motion of tissues and organs, with the length of time also recorded as part of the study

scan: mapping of emissions of radioactive substances after they have been introduced into the body; the density can determine normal or abnormal conditions

sialography: radiographic recording of the salivary duct and branches

sinography: radiographic recording of the sinus or sinus tract

splenography: radiographic recording of the spleen

superior: toward the head or the upper part of the body; also known as cephalic

supine: lying on the back

tomography: procedure that allows viewing of a single plane of the body by blurring out all but that particular level

transverse: horizontal

ultrasound: technique using sound waves to determine the density of the outline of tissue

unilateral: occurring on one side

uptake: absorption of a radioactive substance by body tissues; recorded for diagnostic purposes in conditions such as thyroid disease

urography: same as pyelography; radiographic recording of the kidneys, renal pelvis, ureters, and bladder

venography: radiographic recording of the veins and tributaries

vesiculography: radiographic recording of the seminal vesicles

xeroradiography: photoelectric process of radiographs

CHAPTER REVIEW

CHAPTER 11, PART I, THEORY

Without the use of the CPT manual, complete the following:

1 What is a branch of medicine that uses radiant energy to diagnose and treat patients?

_____

2 The CPT manual divides the Radiology section into subsections of Diagnostic Radiology,

_____ , _____

_____ , and Nuclear Medicine.

3 What type of procedure is "performed independently of, and is not immediately related

to, other services"?

_____

4 If several services are provided to a patient on the same day, what type of procedure modifier could be used? _____

5 The modifier used to indicate the Professional Component is _____ .

6 The two words that mean supervising the taking of the x-rays and reading/reporting the results of the films are _____ and _____ .

7 The name for the use of high-frequency sound waves in an imaging process that is used to diagnose patient illness is

_____ .

8 The Radiation Oncology section of the CPT manual is divided into subsections based on

the _____ of service provided to the patient.

9 The scientific study of energy is

_____ .

10 The scientific calculation of the radiation emitted from various radioactive sources is

_____ .

11 Radiation treatment delivery codes are based on the treatment area involved and further divided based on levels of what?

_____

12 MeV stands for _____ .

13 Radiation Treatment Management is reported in units of _____ fractions.

14 Nuclear Medicine uses these to image organs for diagnosis and treatment:

_____

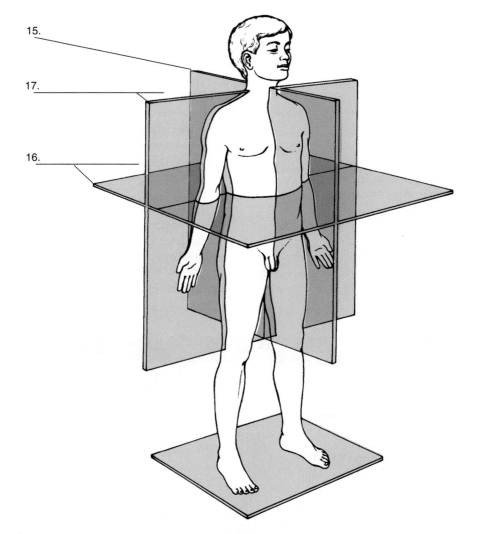

15.

17.

16.

Identify the planes of the body on the figure on the preceding page:

15 _____

16 _____

17 _____

CHAPTER 11, PART II, PRACTICAL

The coding exercise that follows uses codes from a variety of CPT sections.

Using the CPT manual, code the following:

18 An established patient is seen in the physician's office with the chief complaint of a persistent cough. Otherwise, the patient claims to be in good health. The physician collects a history, including the chief complaint and the history of the present illness. The physical examination performed focuses on the respiratory tract. The decision-making is straightforward because the physician wants to evaluate the patient for a possible case of bronchitis.

Code(s): _____

The patient is sent to the clinic's radiology department for a two-view chest x-ray study.

Code(s): _____

The radiologist sends the x-ray results to the physician, who reviews them and decides to order a consultation with a pulmonologist from another clinic. The patient sees the other clinic's pulmonologist, who performs a comprehensive history and a comprehensive examination with moderate complexity.

Code(s): _____

A fluoroscopic examination is done for transbronchial lung biopsy.

Code(s): _____

Then there is radiologic supervision and interpretation of a unilateral bronchography.

Code(s): _____

19 A new patient is seen in the office for unilateral ear pain. In the expanded problem focused history and the physical examination, the physician focuses his attention on the head, ears, nose, and throat. The physician's provisional diagnoses include otalgia and possible ear infections. The decision-making is straightforward for the physician.

Code(s): _____

The patient is sent to the clinic's radiologist for an x-ray of the ear.

Code(s): _____

The patient is then sent to the clinic's ear specialist, who inserts a ventilation tube (tympanostomy) using local anesthesia.

Code(s): _____

20 A new patient is seen in the office for a variety of complaints, but in particular a swelling and heaviness of his right leg. The physician documents the patient's complaints, collects a comprehensive history of the present illness, performs a comprehensive review of systems, and inquires about the patient's past, family, and social history. A complete multisystem physical examination is performed. The physician's working diagnosis is edema of the lower extremity, cause to be determined. Given the nature of the problem, the physician considers the decision-making process to be highly complex.

Code(s): _____

The patient is sent to radiology for a unilateral lymphangiography of one extremity.

Code(s): _____

Another physician performs the injection procedure for the lymphangiography.

Code(s): _____

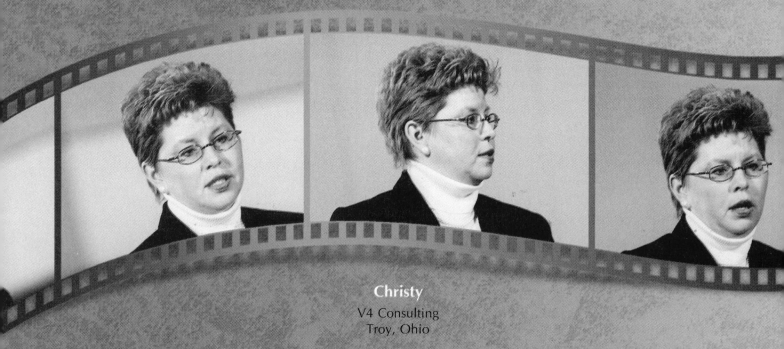

Christy
V4 Consulting
Troy, Ohio

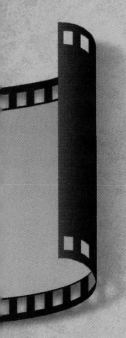

chapter 12

The Pathology/ Laboratory Section

CHAPTER TOPICS

Format

Subsections

Chapter Glossary

Chapter Review

LEARNING OBJECTIVES

After completing this chapter you should be able to

1   Explain the format of the Pathology and Laboratory terminology.

2   Interpret the information contained in the Pathology and Laboratory Guidelines.

3   Demonstrate an understanding of Pathology and Laboratory terminology.

4   Code using Pathology and Laboratory codes.

The Guidelines for the Pathology and Laboratory section indicate subsections that contain notes. Most Pathology and Laboratory subsections contain notes. Whenever notes are available, be sure to read them before assigning codes from the subsection. Specific information pertinent to subsection codes are contained in the notes.

FORMAT

The Pathology and Laboratory section of the CPT manual is formatted according to type of tests performed—automated multichannel, panels, assays, and so forth. The subsections are as follows.

- Organ or Disease Oriented Panels
- Drug Testing
- Therapeutic Drug Assays
- Evocative/Suppression Testing
- Consultations (Clinical Pathology)
- Urinalysis
- Chemistry
- Hematology and Coagulation
- Immunology
- Transfusion Medicine
- Microbiology
- Anatomic Pathology
- Cytopathology
- Cytogenetic Studies
- Surgical Pathology
- Transcutaneous Procedures
- Other Procedures

Laboratories have built-in **indicators** that allow additional tests to be performed without a written order from the physician. These standards are set by the medical facility and imply that when a certain test is found to be positive, it is assumed that the physician would want further information on the condition. For example, if a routine urinalysis is performed, a culture is performed if a **quantitative** (positive) bacteria result is found. If a culture is performed to identify the organism, a sensitivity test is performed if the bacteria is of a certain type or count, as predetermined by the medical facility to warrant the additional laboratory studies. You will code only after the tests are done. This ensures that all laboratory work will be coded. Remember that what the physician ordered may not be all the laboratory work done, depending on the facility's policy concerning further tests.

The services in the Pathology and Laboratory section include the laboratory test only. The collection of the specimen is coded separately from the analysis of the test. For example, if a patient had a technician in a clinic laboratory withdraw blood by means of a venipuncture of the finger, and the blood sample was then analyzed in the laboratory, you would code 36415 for the venipuncture, in addition to a code to report the test performed on the blood.

SUBSECTIONS

Organ or Disease Oriented Panels

The codes in the Organ or Disease Oriented Panels subsection are grouped according to the usual laboratory work ordered by a physician for the diagnosis of or screening for various diseases or conditions. Groups of tests may be performed together, depending on the situation or disease. For example, during the first obstetric visit, a mother is commonly asked to have baseline laboratory tests done to ensure that appropriate antepartum care can be given. CPT code 80055 describes an obstetric panel that would typically be used for the first obstetric visit. To code for a panel from the CPT manual, each test listed in the panel description must be performed. Additional tests are coded and billed separately. The development of panels saves the facility from having to bill for each test separately, and it is often more economical for the patient.

List each laboratory test separately unless the tests are part of a panel. If you list a panel, each test must have been done to qualify for use of the code. You cannot use modifier -52 (reduced service) with a panel. For example, if all of the tests in the obstetric panel were done except the syphilis test, you could not code 80055 (Obstetrical Panel) with modifier -52. You would instead list separately each of the tests with the corresponding CPT code.

CAUTION *Be careful when coding multiple panels on the same day for the same patient. Sometimes several panels include some of the same tests. For example, a hepatitis B surface antigen test is included in both the obstetric panel and the hepatitis panel. It would be inappropriate to code the same test twice, as it would not be performed on the same patient more than once on a single day.*

The laboratory and pathology reports in the patient record will contain the method by which the test was done. There are many different methods of performing the various tests that you will find in this subsection. For example, a urinalysis can be automated or nonautomated and can include microscopy or exclude microscopy. It is necessary to know these details if you are to choose the correct urinalysis code. If the details you need are not in the medical record, ask the laboratory staff or physician for further information.

EXERCISE 12-1

ORGAN OR DISEASE ORIENTED PANELS

Complete the following:

1 Hepatic function panel code

Code(s): _____

2 How many laboratory tests must be included in a hepatic function

panel? _____

3 Does an obstetric panel include a rubella antibody test? _____

4 Is blood typing ABO included in an obstetric panel? _____

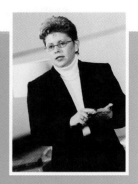

Drug Testing

Laboratory drug testing is done to identify the presence or absence of a drug. Testing that determines the presence or absence of a drug is **qualitative** (the drug is either present or not present in the specimen).

When the presence of a drug is detected in the qualitative test, a confirmation test is usually performed by using a second testing method. Code 80102 is used to describe this confirmation test. Codes from the Therapeutic Drug Assay and Chemistry subsections are used to further identify the exact amount of the drug that is present. For example, a patient who has been on a medication for a long time might need to undergo testing to determine whether the drug level is therapeutic.

The CPT manual lists the drugs most commonly tested for, although the use of the codes is not limited to the drugs listed. Modifier -51 is not used with pathology or laboratory codes; instead, each test is listed separately. For example, if a confirmation test was conducted for both alcohol and cocaine, code 80102 twice.

Therapeutic Drug Assays

Drug assays test for a specific drug and for the amount of that drug. If qualitative information is not enough, quantitative information is needed. **Quantitative** information determines not only the presence of a drug but also the exact amount present (or quantity present). Many types of drugs are listed in this subsection. If the drug is not listed, it is possible that quantitative analysis may be listed under the methodology (e.g., immunoassay, radioassay).

The drugs are listed by their generic names, not their brand names. For example, 80152 is for the generic drug amitriptyline, also sold under the brand names of Elavil and Endep. A *Physician's Desk Reference* will be helpful as you code drug testing and assays.

One location of Drug Testing codes in the index of the CPT manual is under the main term "Drug," subtermed by the reason for the tests—analysis or confirmation. Therapeutic Drug Assay subsection codes can be found under the main term "Drug Assay" and subterms of the material examined, for example, amikacin, digoxin.

EXERCISE 12-2

THERAPEUTIC DRUG TESTING AND DRUG ASSAYS

Choose the correct CPT code for the following drug tests:

1 Confirmation of cocaine (qualitative)

Code(s): _____

2 Identify the amount of digoxin in the blood (quantitative)

Code(s): _____

3 Quantitative examination of blood for amikacin

Code(s): _____

4 Examination of blood, quantitative for lithium

Code(s): _____

Evocative/Suppression Testing

Evocative/Suppression testing is done to determine measurements of the effect of evocative or suppressive agents on chemical constituents. For example, code 80400 is reported when a patient undergoes testing to determine whether adrenocorticotropic hormone is being stimulated for production in the body. The physician may suspect that the patient suffers from adrenal gland insufficiency. Note that following each of the code descriptions is a statement of the services that must have been provided for the code to be applicable. For example, the requirement to report 80400 ACTH stimulation panel is "Cortisol (82533 × 2)" or two cortisol tests as described in 82533. You will have to read the description for code 82533 to ensure it is the correct test before you can report 80400.

CAUTION *Remember that the codes from the Pathology and Laboratory section are only for the tests performed and do not reflect the complete service.*

To code the components of Evocative/Suppression Testing:
- If the physician supplied the agent, report the supply using 99070 from the Medicine section.
- If the physician administered the agent, report the infusion or injection using codes 90780–90784 from the Medicine section.
- If the test involved prolonged attendance by the physician, report the service using the appropriate E/M code.

Consultations (Clinical Pathology)

A clinical pathologist, upon request from a primary care physician, will perform a consultation to render additional medical interpretation regarding test results. For example, a primary care physician reviews lab test results and requests a clinical pathologist to review, interpret, and prepare a written report on the findings.

There are two codes under the subsection Consultations that are reserved for clinical pathology consultations. These consultations are based on whether the consultation is limited or comprehensive. A **limited consultation** is one that is done without the pathologist's reviewing the medical record of the patient, and a **comprehensive consultation** is one in which the medical record is reviewed as a part of the consultative services. When either of these consultation codes is submitted to a third-party payer, it is accompanied by a written report.

These are not the only pathology consultation codes in the Pathology and Laboratory section of the CPT manual. There are also consultation codes toward the end of the section in the Surgical Pathology subsection, codes 88321–88332. These consultation codes are used to report the services of a pathologist who reviews and gives an opinion or advice concerning pathology slides, specimens, material, or records that were prepared elsewhere or for pathology consultation during surgery.

Pathology consultations during surgery are provided to examine tissue removed from a patient during a surgical procedure. If the pathologist has not used a microscope to examine the tissue, report 88329. If a microscope has been used to examine the tissue, report 88331 or 88332, depending on the number of samples that were examined.

A **specimen** is a sample of tissue from a suspect area; a **block** is a frozen piece of a specimen; and a **section** is a slice of a frozen block. A pathologist prepares a specimen by cutting it into blocks and taking sections from the blocks. The number of sections taken depends on the judgment of the pathologist as to the number of areas of the specimen that need to be examined. The frozen section is placed (mounted) on a slide or held by other means that allow the pathologist to view the tissue under a microscope.

When one block is sectioned and examined, the service of examining that first section is reported using 88331. The second and subsequent sections of the same block are reported using 88332. If another block from another area was sectioned, the first section would be reported using 88331, and subsequent sections from the second block using 88332. You cannot use 88332 without first using 88331. Although 88332 is not marked as an add-on code (one that's used only with another code), its function is that of an add-on code as it indicates that subsequent sections were examined.

Urinalysis and Chemistry

Many types of tests are located under the Urinalysis and Chemistry subsections. Urinalysis codes are for nonspecific tests done on urine. Chemistry codes are for specific tests done on material from any source (e.g., urine, blood, breath, feces, sputum). For example, a urinalysis using a dip stick (81000–81003) would report the presence and quantity of the following constituents: bilirubin, glucose, hemoglobin, ketones, leukocytes, nitrite, pH protein, specific gravity, and urobilinogen. Any number of these constituents may be analyzed and reported using a code from the Urinalysis subsection (81000–81003). However, if the physician ordered an analysis of the urine specifically to determine the presence of urobilinogen (reduced bilirubin) and the exact amount of urobilinogen present (quantitative analysis), you would choose a code (84580) from the Chemistry subsection. The main things to remember when coding from these two subsections are

1. The identification of specific tests

2. Whether the test is automated (done by machine) or nonautomated (done manually)

3. The number of tests done

4. The identification of combination codes for similar types of tests

5. Whether the results are qualitative or quantitative

6. The methodology of testing

EXERCISE 12-3

URINALYSIS AND CHEMISTRY

Code the following:

1 An automated urinalysis without microscopy

Code(s): _____

2 Urinalysis, microscopic only

Code(s): _____

3 Albumin, serum

Code(s): _____

4 Total bilirubin

Code(s): _____

5 Gases, blood pH only

Code(s): _____

6 Sodium, urine

Code(s): _____

7 Uric acid, blood

Code(s): _____

Hematology and Coagulation

The Hematology and Coagulation subsection contains codes based on the various blood-drawing methods and tests. The method used to do the test is often what determines the code assignment. Blood counts can be manual or automated, with many variations of the tests.

There are codes within the Hematology and Coagulation subsection for bone marrow smear and smear interpretations (85060–85097). Codes to report the procurement of the bone marrow through the use of aspiration are located in the Hemic and Lymphatic Systems subsection of the Surgery section.

There are many blood coagulation tests located in the Hematology and Coagulation subsection. The codes are divided based on the particular factor being tested. Great care must be taken to ensure that the correct factor has been coded based on the information in the medical record.

Most of the tests in the Hematology and Coagulation subsection can be located in the index of the CPT manual under the name of the test, such as prothrombin time, coagulation time, or hemogram.

EXERCISE 12-4

HEMATOLOGY AND COAGULATION

Code the following:

1 Blood count by an automated hemogram (Hct, WBC, Hgb, and RBC)

   Code(s): _____

2 Blood count by an automated hemogram and platelet count with complete differential white blood cell count

   Code(s): _____

3 Blood count by a manual hemogram with a complete blood cell count

   Code(s): _____

4 Interpretation of a bone marrow smear

   Code(s): _____

As you can see, there are many variations of just one test! So read the patient record and code descriptions carefully before assigning the codes.

Immunology

Immunology codes deal with the identification of conditions of the immune system caused by the action of antibodies (e.g., hypersensitivity, allergic reactions, immunity, and alterations of body tissue).

EXERCISE 12-5

IMMUNOLOGY

Code the following:

1 ANA (antinuclear antibody) titer

   Code(s): _____

2 ASO (antistreptolysin O) screen

   Code(s): _____

3 Cold agglutinin screen

   Code(s): _____

Transfusion Medicine

The Transfusion Medicine subsection deals with tests performed on blood or blood products. Tests include screening for antibodies, Coombs testing, autologous blood collection and processing, blood typing, compatibility testing, and preparation of and treatments performed on blood and blood products.

EXERCISE 12-6

TRANSFUSION MEDICINE

Code the following:

1   ABO and Rh blood typing

    Code(s): _____

2   Irradiation of blood product, 3 units

    Code(s): _____

Microbiology

Microbiology deals with the study of microorganisms. Cultures for the identification of organisms as well as the identification of sensitivities of the organism to antibiotics (called culture and sensitivity) are found in this subsection. Culture codes must be read carefully because some codes are used to indicate screening only to detect the presence of an organism; some codes indicate the identification of specific organisms; and others indicate additional sensitivity testing to determine which antibiotic would be best for treatment of the specified bacteria. You should code all tests performed on the basis of whether they are quantitative or qualitative and/or a sensitivity study.

EXERCISE 12-7

MICROBIOLOGY

Code the following:

1   HIV-1, quantification

    Code(s): _____

2   Streptococcus, group A, using an amplified probe method

    Code(s): _____

3   Quantification of *Gardnerella vaginalis,* herpes simplex, and *Candida* species

    Code(s): _____

4   Direct probe method of mycobacteria tuberculosis, herpes simplex virus, and *Chlamydia trachomatis*

    Code(s): _____

5   Bacterial culture of urine, quantitative with colony count

    Code(s): _____

6   If code 87116 indicates that a TB organism is present, what is code 87118 used for? _____

Anatomic Pathology

Anatomic Pathology deals with examination of the body fluids or tissues in postmortem examination. Postmortem examination involves the completion of gross microscopic and limited autopsies. Codes are divided according to the extent of the examination. This subsection also contains codes for forensic examination and coroners' cases.

Cytopathology and Cytogenic Studies

The Cytopathology subsection deals with the laboratory work done to determine whether any cellular changes are present. For example, a very common cytopathology procedure is the Papanicolaou smear (Pap smear). Cytopathology may also be performed on fluids that have been aspirated from a site to identify cellular changes. Cytogenetic Studies includes tests performed for genetic and chromosomal studies.

Surgical Pathology

Surgical Pathology codes describe the evaluation of specimens to determine the pathology of disease processes. When choosing the correct code for pathology, you must identify the source of the specimen and the reason for the surgical procedure. The Surgical Pathology subsection contains codes that are divided into six levels (Levels I through VI) based on the specimen examined and the level of work required by the pathologist. Pathology testing is done on all tissue removed from the body. The surgical pathology classification level is determined by the complexity of the pathologic examination.

Level I pathology code 88300 identifies specimens that normally do not need to be viewed under a microscope for pathologic diagnosis (e.g., a tooth)—those for which the probability of disease or malignancy is minimal.

Level II pathology code 88302 deals with those tissues that are usually considered normal tissue and have been removed not because of the probability of the presence of disease or malignancy, but for some other reason (e.g., a fallopian tube for sterilization, foreskin of a newborn).

from the trenches

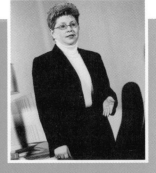

"I feel that what I do makes a difference. Physicians and hospitals look to our firm for expertise in this subject . . . . what I state and assist in preparing affects the way physicians code their charges. I must be aware of how my recommendations will change the patterns of their submissions. Therefore, I must present clear and concise coding information."

CHRISTY

Level III pathology code 88304 is assigned for specimens with a low probability of disease or malignancy. For example, a gallbladder may be neoplastic (benign or malignant), but when the gallbladder is removed for cholecystitis (inflammation of the gallbladder), it is usually inflamed from chronic disease and not because of cancerous changes.

Level IV pathology code 88305 carries a higher probability of malignancy or decision-making for disease pathology. For example, a uterus is removed because of a diagnosis of prolapse. There is a possibility that the uterus is malignant or there are other causes of disease pathology.

Level V pathology code 88307 classifies more complex pathology evaluations (e.g., examination of a uterus that was removed for reasons other than prolapse or neoplasm).

Level VI pathology code 88309 includes examination of neoplastic tissue or very involved specimens, such as a total resection of a colon.

coding shot

A specimen is defined as tissue submitted for examination. If two specimens of the same area are received and examined, each specimen is coded. For example, if two anus tags are received and each is examined, code 88304 × 2. If one anus tag is received and two different areas of the tag are examined, code 88304 only once.

The remaining codes at the end of the subsection classify specialized procedures, utilization of stains, consultations performed, preparations used, and/or instrumentation needed to complete testing.

The surgical pathology codes are located in the index under the main term "Pathology" and subterms "Surgical" and "Gross and Micro Exam."

EXERCISE 12-8

SURGICAL PATHOLOGY

Code the following using one of the six surgical pathology codes in the CPT manual:

1 The specimen is a uterus, tubes, and ovaries. The procedure was an abdominal hysterectomy for ovarian cancer.

   Code(s): _____

2 The specimen is a portion of a lung. The procedure was a left lower lobe segmental resection.

   Code(s): _____

3 The specimen is the prostate. The procedure was a transurethral resection of the prostate.

   Code(s): _____

4 What is the surgical pathology code for the pathology report in Figure 12–1?

   Code(s): _____

PATHOLOGY DEPARTMENT

Patient:	Alice C. Fisher	**Date Collected:**	02/09/0X
DOB:	12/06/37	**Date Received:**	02/09/0X
Sex	F	**Date Examined:**	02/10/0X
Record Number:	5909890	**Access Number:**	P4218
Account:	MP8352	**Surgeon:**	Dr. White

CLINICAL HISTORY: UMBILICAL HERNIA, INFLAMED

TISSUE RECEIVED: UMBILICAL HERNIA

GROSS DESCRIPTION: The specimen is labeled with the patient's name and "umbilical hernia" and consists of yellow-white fibrofatty tissue approximately 3.5 × 2 × 1 cm. Representative sections are processed in two slides.

MICROSCOPIC DIAGNOSIS: Mature adipose tissue with fibrovascular and fibrotendinous tissue with focal reactive fibrous tissue consistent with umbilical hernia.

Alberto Matusa, M.D.

Alberto Matusa, M.D.
Head, Pathology Department
Merry Brook Hospital

Figure 12–1 Pathology report.

Other Procedures

Other Procedures include miscellaneous testing on body fluids, the use of special instrumentation, and testing performed on oocyte and sperm.

CHAPTER GLOSSARY

block: frozen piece of a sample
qualitative: measuring the presence or absence of
quantitative: measuring the presence or absence of and the amount of
section: slice of a frozen block
specimen: sample of tissue or fluid
uptake: absorption of a radioactive substance by body tissues; recorded for diagnostic purposes in conditions such as thyroid disease

CHAPTER REVIEW

CHAPTER 12, PART I, THEORY

Without the use of the CPT manual, complete the following:

1 The Pathology and Laboratory section of the CPT manual is formatted according to the type of ________________ performed.

2 Laboratories have built-in ________________ that allow additional tests to be performed without the written order of the physician.

3 Codes that are grouped according to the usual laboratory work ordered by a physician for diagnosis or screening of various diseases or conditions are Organ or Disease Oriented ________________.

4 Can you use a reduced service modifier with pathology or laboratory codes?
Yes No

5 Will the medical record contain the method used to perform the test done?

Yes   No

CHAPTER 12, PART II, PRACTICAL

Answer the following:

6 The Hematology and Coagulation subsections contain codes based on the various testing methods and tests. The method used to do the test is often the code determiner. Blood cell counts can be manual or automated, with many variations of the tests. What would the code be for an automated hemogram including red blood cell count? What would the code be for an automated hemogram and platelet count with complete white blood cell count? A manual hemogram with a complete blood cell count?

Code(s): _____

Code the following three cases with the correct pathology code from the CPT manual:

7 The specimen is tonsils and adenoids. The procedure is a tonsillectomy with adenoidectomy.

Code(s): _____

8 The specimen is an appendix. The procedure is an incidental appendectomy.

Code(s): _____

9 The specimen is a tooth. The procedure is an odontectomy, gross examination only.

Code(s): _____

Code the following:

10 Western Blot of blood, with interpretation and report

Code(s): _____

11 Vitamin K analysis of blood

Code(s): _____

12 Quantitative analysis of urine for alkaloids

Code(s): _____

13 Three specimens of gastric secretions for total gastric acid

Code(s): _____

14 Blood analysis for HGH

Code(s): _____

15 Total insulin

Code(s): _____

16 LDL cholesterol using direct measurements

Code(s): _____

17 Automated hemogram (WBC, RBC, Hgb, Hct, and indices)

Code(s): _____

18 Blood smear interpretation

Code(s): _____

19 PTT of whole blood

Code(s): _____

20 Sedimentation rate, automated

Code(s): _____

21 Lee and White coagulation time

Code(s): _____

22 Clotting factor XII (Hageman factor)

Code(s): _____

23 Blood typing for paternity test, ABO, Rh, and MN

Code(s): _____

24 Culture of urine for bacteria with colony count

Code(s): _____

25 Schlichter test

Code(s): _____

26 Postmortem examination, gross only, with brain and spinal cord

Code(s): _____

27 Therapeutic drug assay for digoxin and vancomycin

Code(s): _____

28 Pathology consultation during surgery

Code(s): _____

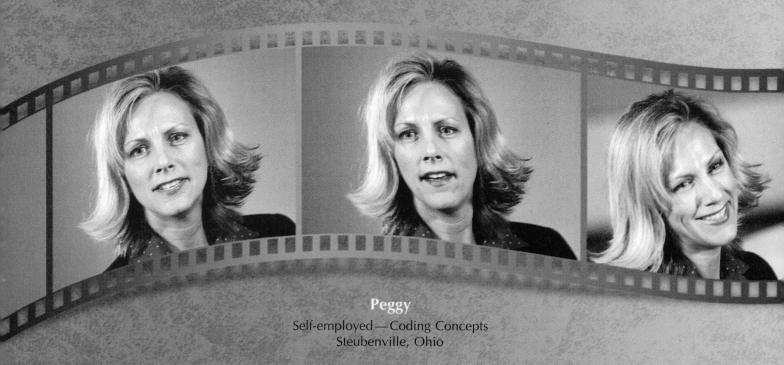

Peggy
Self-employed—Coding Concepts
Steubenville, Ohio

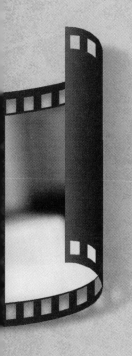

chapter 13

The Medicine Section and Level II National Codes

LEARNING OBJECTIVES

After completing this chapter you should be able to

1 Apply Medicine Guidelines when assigning codes.

2 Analyze the format of the Medicine section.

3 Apply the Medicine section codes.

4 List the major features of Level II National Codes.

5 Assign Level II National Codes and modifiers.

6 Define the terminology listed in the chapter glossary.

345

NONINVASIVE DIAGNOSTIC AND THERAPEUTIC SERVICES

The Medicine section is for coding diagnostic and therapeutic services that are generally **not invasive** (not entering a body cavity). The section begins with Guidelines applicable to all of the Medicine section codes (i.e., multiple procedures, add-on codes, separate procedures, subsection information, unlisted service/procedure, special reports, modifiers, and materials supplied by the physician).

The various subsections of Medicine contain many specific notes to be used with certain groups of codes, so be sure to read all notes that pertain to the group codes with which you are working.

Format

MEDICINE SUBSECTIONS

- Immune Globulins
- Immunization Administration for Vaccines/Toxoids
- Vaccines/Toxoids
- Therapeutic or Diagnostic Infusions (Excludes Chemotherapy)
- Therapeutic, Prophylactic, or Diagnostic Injections
- Psychiatry
- Biofeedback
- Dialysis
- Gastroenterology
- Ophthalmology
- Special Otorhinolaryngologic Services
- Cardiovascular
- Noninvasive Vascular Diagnostic Studies
- Pulmonary
- Allergy and Clinical Immunology
- Endocrinology
- Neurology and Neuromuscular Procedures
- Central Nervous System Assessments/Tests
- Health and Behavior Assessment/Interventions
- Chemotherapy Administration
- Photodynamic Therapy
- Special Dermatological Procedures
- Physical Medicine and Rehabilitation
- Medical Nutrition Therapy
- Osteopathic Manipulative Treatment
- Chiropractic Manipulative Treatment
- Special Services, Procedures, and Reports
- Qualifying Circumstances for Anesthesia
- Sedation With or Without Analgesia (Conscious Sedation)
- Other Services and Procedures
- Home Health Procedures/Services
- Home Infusion Procedures

Many specialized types of testing can be found in the Medicine section (e.g., biofeedback, audiologic function tests, electrocardiograms). Codes in

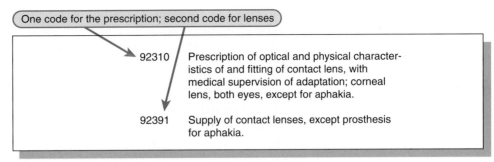

Figure 13–1   Some codes are for the supply only.

this section do not usually include the supplies used in the testing, therapy, or diagnostic treatments unless specifically stated in the code description. For example, there are codes for the prescription and fitting of an artificial eye—one code includes the supply of an artificial eye and one code does not include the supply of an artificial eye. Reading the entire code description is critical to ensure that you do not unbundle the services by billing for services already included in the code. You should code supplies, including drugs, separately unless otherwise instructed in the code information. CPT code 99070 is the supplies and materials code used to identify the supplying of drugs, trays, supplies, or materials needed to provide the service or the specific HCPCS supply code. For example, Figure 13–1 shows the code for the service of a prescription for contact lenses (92310) and the code for the supply of the contact lenses (92391). When the lenses and the prescription services are provided, both the lenses (92391) and the prescription service (92310) are billed.

Subsections

Introduction to Immunization

There are two types of immunization—active and passive. **Active immunization** is the type given when it is anticipated that the person will be in contact with the disease. Active immunization agents can be toxoids or vaccines. Toxoids are bacteria that have been made nontoxic; when injected, they produce an immune response that builds protection against a disease. Vaccines are viruses that are given in small doses and cause an immune response. **Passive immunization** doesn't cause an immune response; rather, the injected material contains a high level of antibody against a disease (e.g., rabies, hepatitis B, tetanus), called immune globulins.

The first three subsections in the Medicine section are

- Immune Globulin
- Immunization Administration for Vaccines/Toxoids
- Vaccines/Toxoids

Immune Globulins

The Immune Globulins subsection (90281–90399) is a relatively new subsection in the CPT manual. Many of the codes in the subsection were located throughout the Medicine section, but with the creation of the Immune Globulins subsection, the codes are now grouped together. The codes in this subsection identify only the immune globulin **product** and must be reported in addition to the appropriate administration code from the Therapeutic, Prophylactic, or Diagnostic Injections subsection (i.e., 90782, which is a therapeutic or diagnostic injection given subcutaneously or intramuscularly).

Codes in the Immune Globulins subsection are categorized according to the type of immune globulin (rabies, hepatitis B, etc.), the method of injection (IM, IV, SQ, etc.), and the type of dose (full dose, minidose, etc.).

Immunization Administration for Vaccines/Toxoids

The Immunization Administration subsection codes (90471–90474) are reported in conjunction with the Vaccines/Toxoids subsection codes. The codes in the Immunization Administration subsection are reported for the injection procedure. A variety of administration methods are used to deliver the vaccine/toxoid: percutaneous, intradermal, subcutaneous, intramuscular, jet injections, intranasal, and oral administration. The administration codes are divided based on the method of administration—intranasal or oral; *or* percutaneous, intradermal, subcutaneous, intramuscular, and jet injections. Report each dose administered—single or combination.

You can report multiple injections by using 90471 for the first injection and then listing 90472 for each injection after the first.

EXAMPLE

90471	Injection service for tetanus
90472	Injection service for rubella
90472	Injection service for diphtheria

Or you can report the first injection with 90471, as you would always do, and then list 90472 times the number of injections after the first one.

EXAMPLE

90471	Injection service for tetanus
90472 × 2	Injection service, rubella and diphtheria

Vaccines/Toxoids

The Vaccines/Toxoids subsection lists vaccine products given in immunizations. The subsection contains many codes for a single disease (e.g., 90703 for tetanus toxoid) as well as codes for a combination of diseases (e.g., 90701 for diphtheria, tetanus, and DPT). In many of the code descriptions, specific ages are identified. For example, 90658, influenza vaccine, specifies age 3 and above, whereas code 90657, influenza vaccine, specifies ages 6 to 35 months. The vaccines have pediatric or adult listed on the label of the vial. You must carefully review the description of the vaccine product code to determine which disease is specified. When one code is available to describe multiple products given, the combination code must be used. If each vaccine were to be listed separately when a combination code is available, it would be considered unbundling.

There are codes that describe schedules for a vaccine, such as a three-dose or four-dose schedule. For example, 90633 is a two-dose hepatitis A vaccine that is intended to be given on a two-dose schedule. Each time the vaccine is administered, 90633 is reported along with the date of the injection. A schedule is the number of doses provided and the timing of the administration. However, the doses and timing must be exactly as specified in the code; otherwise, you should use multiple codes to identify the vaccine.

from the trenches

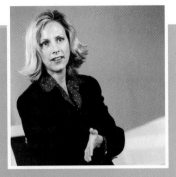

"*Coding students should be aware of the many and varied opportunities available to them. Because I am a self-employed consultant, my responsibilities vary . . . a workday may include working on coding, documentation, and reimbursement audits, writing seminars, providing educational seminars in a variety of specialties as well as fulfilling numerous other engagements in the health care setting.*"

PEGGY

coding shot

Do not use modifier -51 (multiple procedures) with the Vaccines/ Toxoid codes! List the codes multiple times or use the "times" symbol (×) and indicate the number of injections given, as described in the Immunization Administration for Vaccines/Toxoids information described earlier.

If a patient is given a vaccine in the course of an E/M service, the administration and vaccine/toxoid codes are assigned in addition to the E/M code. If the immunization is the only service that the patient receives, the immunization administration code is listed first, and then the vaccine/toxoid code is reported.

CAUTION *You do not report an E/M service if the only service provided to the patient was an injection or infusion service. Only the injection or infusion is reported. If a separate, identifiable service was provided in addition to an injection or infusion, then you can report the service using an E/M code.*

EXERCISE 13-1

IMMUNIZATION INJECTIONS

Using the CPT manual, code the following:

1   A parent takes a child to the child's physician for an oral poliomyelitis vaccine. The physician's assistant evaluates the child and administers the vaccine orally to the child.

Code(s): _____

2   The following series of vaccines is indicated as having been administered to a variety of patients; a brief history and examination are performed to assess vaccine needs and general health status. How would you code these vaccinations?

a. New patient and the only service for the visit is an injection of DTP (diphtheria, tetanus toxoid, pertussis) and oral poliovirus

Code(s): _____

b. An established patient, a 1-year-old, is brought in for a well-baby checkup (separate service) by the physician, and the following are given: DTP and injectable poliomyelitis.

Code(s): _____

c. A 64-year-old established patient comes in for an influenza virus vaccine that is administered intramuscularly by the nurse. The vaccine is the only service provided at that visit.

Code(s): _____

d. A new patient comes for an office visit at which the physician does an expanded problem focused history and physical examination (separate service) and also administers a DTP and *Haemophilus influenzae* B (Hib) vaccine.

Code(s): _____

3 A parent brings an 18-month-old infant (established patient) for a well-baby examination at which the physician administers a vaccine intramuscularly for diphtheria and tetanus toxoid (DT).

Code(s): _____

Therapeutic or Diagnostic Infusions

Therapeutic infusions are done for the purpose of healing. An **infusion** is the introducing of a liquid into the body over a long period of time, for example, fluids introduced into the vein of a patient who is dehydrated or the intravenous introduction of antibiotics into a patient with a severe infection. The physician must administer or supervise the administration of the infusion. There are only two codes in the infusion subsection, both based on the time it takes for the infusion to be completed.

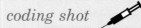

coding shot

The Therapeutic or Diagnostic Infusions codes are to be used only for the infusion service, not the substance that is infused. The drug that is infused would be reported using a HCPCS code or a CPT code.

CAUTION *Code 90780 is used to report time up to 1 hour, so a partial hour (e.g., 30 minutes) can be reported using this code.*

Therapeutic, Prophylactic, or Diagnostic Injections

Injections are the introduction of substances into the body by the use of a needle. Codes in the Therapeutic, Prophylactic, or Diagnostic Injections subsection are determined by the way the injection is introduced into the body—subcutaneous (SQ), intramuscular (IM), intravenous (IV), or intra-arterial (Fig. 13–2). Code 90782 can be used to identify any therapeutic or diagnostic injection, excluding antibiotic injections because there is a spe-

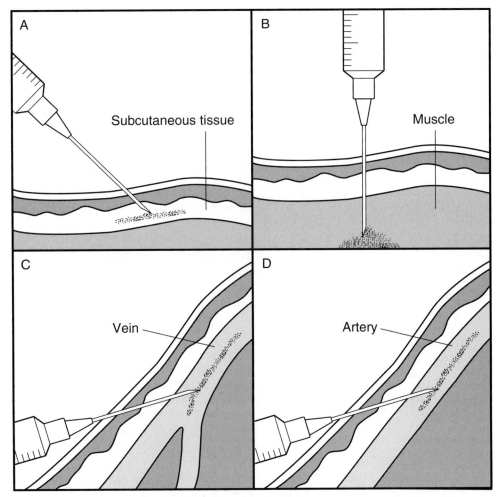

Figure 13–2   Injection methods. *A,* Subcutaneous (SQ). *B,* Intramuscular (IM). *C,* Intravenous (IV). *D,* Intra-arterial.

cific code for the injection of antibiotics—90788. When an injection is reported, specify the materials injected.

One way to locate injections in the index of the CPT manual is under the main term "Injection" and the subterm specifying the method (i.e., intravenous, intramuscular, subcutaneous).

EXERCISE 13–2

INJECTIONS

Using the CPT manual, code the following injections:

1 An established patient is seen in the office for pernicious anemia. The nurse gives the patient an injection of vitamin B_{12}.

   Code(s): _____

2 IV infusion for therapy for 1 hour

   Code(s): _____

Psychiatry

The Psychiatry subsection has a lengthy note under the heading detailing the use of psychiatric codes in conjunction with hospital and clinic E/M services. If psychiatric treatments are rendered at the same time as E/M services, both the E/M service and the psychiatric treatment should be coded. For example, if a patient is admitted to the hospital with a drug overdose secondary to depression, and the physician spends 25 minutes in supportive psychotherapy with the patient several hours after he was admitted to the hospital, services to be coded would be 99223 (Initial Hospital Care) for the E/M service provided and 90816 (Individual Medical Psychotherapy) for the psychiatric treatment. The hospital care codes include the development of orders, the review and interpretation of laboratory work or other diagnostic studies, and the review of therapy reports and other information from the medical record. When the services include not only a visit to the patient but also direction of a treatment team, an additional service code from the E/M section may be listed. You will work closely with third-party payers to determine any specific regional instructions for coding psychiatry services.

Partial hospitalization refers to a hospital setting in which the patients are in the hospital during the day and return to their homes in the evenings and on weekends. The facilities may be open only during the day, 5 days a week, although there are also facilities that are open 7 days a week. When a physician admits a patient to a partial hospital facility, the physician is responsible for preparing all of the same admission paperwork that is prepared for admission to an acute care hospital. E/M Initial Hospital Care and Subsequent Hospital Care codes (99221–99233) are used to report inpatient stays. The psychiatric services the physician provides to the patient are listed separately.

Specific descriptions dealing with services included in each of the codes appear in the Psychiatry subsection. Some codes reflect evaluation or diagnostic services, such as CPT code 90801; some reflect therapeutic procedures, such as 90804; and still others, located in the Central Nervous System Assessments/Tests, are used to report psychological testing, such as code 96100.

Time is the major billing factor in the Psychiatry subsection. Diagnostic and therapeutic time must be clearly documented in the patient record for accurate billing.

Psychiatric Diagnosis and Psychiatric Treatment are two CPT manual index locations for the psychiatric service codes.

EXERCISE 13-3

PSYCHIATRY

Using the CPT manual, code the following:

1 Individual medical psychotherapy in office for 30 minutes

   Code(s): _____

2 Psychological testing, 2 hours

   Code(s): _____

3 Psychiatric evaluation of tests, medical records, or hospital data to make appropriate diagnosis and treatment plan

   Code(s): _____

4 Initial psychiatric interview examination

   Code(s): _____

Biofeedback

Biofeedback is the process of giving a person self-information. The information can be used by patients to gain some control over their physiologic processes such as blood pressure, heart rate, or pain. Patients are trained how to use biofeedback by a professional and then continue the use of the therapy on their own. Biofeedback training is often incorporated in individual psychophysiologic therapy. When biofeedback is part of the individual psychophysiologic therapy, a code is listed for both the biofeedback training and the individual psychophysiologic therapy (90875).

Biofeedback codes are located in the CPT manual index under the main terms "Biofeedback" and "Training."

EXERCISE 13-4

BIOFEEDBACK

Using the CPT manual, code the following:

1 A 40-year-old woman has been seen by the physician for several individual psychiatric sessions as the patient attempts to give up a two-pack-a-day cigarette addiction of 15 years' duration. The patient is experiencing increased anxiety and insomnia. As a part of the last 30-minute psychiatric session, the physician teaches the patient to use biofeedback in an attempt to help her alleviate the anxiety and insomnia. The patient is instructed to use the biofeedback techniques three times a day until the next session.

Code(s): _____

2 A 52-year-old man is referred to the physician by his primary care physician for psychophysiologic therapy to regulate his blood pressure. The physician conducts a 60-minute session during which the patient is trained in the use of biofeedback.

Code(s): _____

Dialysis

Dialysis is the cleansing of the blood of waste products when it is not possible for the body to perform the cleansing function adequately on its own. Dialysis may be temporary, as in the case of a patient who has acute renal failure from which he or she recovers, or permanent, as in the case of a patient with end-stage renal disease (ESRD) who will not recover without a kidney transplant.

The Dialysis subsection of the Medicine section is divided into types of patient training in self-dialysis. The first subheading (End Stage Renal Disease Services) deals with dialysis of a permanent nature. The first four codes (90918–90921) in the category reflect all services included in treating a patient with ESRD and are listed according to patient age (e.g., younger than 2 years of age, 2–11 years of age). Dialysis services are usually billed as a monthly fee. For those cases in which a patient may be visiting the area and will not require a full month of dialysis, daily fees may be billed using the last four codes (90922–90925) in the ESRD category. Few third-party payers allow E/M codes to be billed in addition to dialysis service codes; most payers consider the dialysis codes to be bundled to include all the treatment necessary for a renal disease patient, including the E/M services.

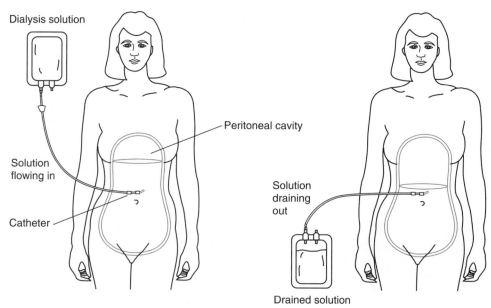

Figure 13–3 Peritoneal dialysis can be done by the patient. The dialysis solution enters the peritoneal cavity through a catheter. After the solution has remained within the patient for several hours, it is drained out through the catheter.

Hemodialysis is the routing of blood and its waste products to the outside of the body where it is filtered. After the blood is cleansed, it is returned to the body. Hemodialysis codes are billed for each day the service is provided. The codes in the hemodialysis category are based on the number of times the physician evaluates the patient during the procedure.

Peritoneal dialysis involves using the peritoneal cavity as a filter. Dialysis fluid is introduced into the cavity and left there for several hours so cleansing can take place (Fig. 13–3). The dialysis fluid is then drained from the peritoneal cavity. Peritoneal dialysis is billed on the basis of each day the service is provided. Some patients learn how to perform dialysis for themselves. Dialysis teaching codes are located under Miscellaneous Dialysis Procedures.

"Dialysis" is the main term to be referenced in the CPT manual index.

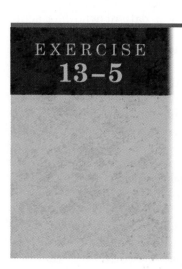

EXERCISE 13–5

DIALYSIS

Using the CPT manual, code the following dialysis services:

1 A 10-year-old patient with end-stage renal disease for a full month of services

Code(s): _____

2 Hemodialysis with a single physician evaluation

Code(s): _____

3 Peritoneal dialysis with repeated physician evaluations

Code(s): _____

Define the following subsection words or abbreviations:

4 peritoneal _____

5 hemofiltration _____

6 ESRD _____

Gastroenterology

The Gastroenterology subsection contains many types of tests and treatments that are performed on the esophagus, stomach, and intestine. Several intubation codes are listed in the Gastroenterology subsection. You must carefully review the code descriptions to determine which services are bundled into the code. For example, CPT code 91055 includes intubation, collection, and preparation of specimens. Because these three services are bundled into one code, it would be incorrect to code each service individually.

EXERCISE 13-6

GASTROENTEROLOGY

Using the CPT manual, code the following:

1 An acid reflux test of the esophagus with intraluminal pH electrode for detection of reflux

Code(s): _____

2 Insertion, positioning, and monitoring of an intestinal bleeding tube

Code(s): _____

3 Gastric intubation with washings and slide preparation for cytology

Code(s): _____

Define the following subsection words:

4 motility study _____

5 manometric studies _____

Ophthalmology

The notes found at the beginning of the Ophthalmology subsection describe the services included in the various types of ophthalmologic services. Ophthalmology is a very specialized field, and often the services provided and documented do not adequately fall into an E/M definition. Therefore, the AMA developed specialized codes that deal specifically with ophthalmology services. There are extensive subsection notes that are required reading before you code in the subsection. The notes explain the levels of service and present excellent examples to clarify the use of the codes. The general ophthalmologic services (e.g., routine yearly eye examinations) are located in the subheading General Ophthalmological Services. The codes in this subsection are based on whether the patient is a new or an established patient and on the complexity of service provided. Of special note are the

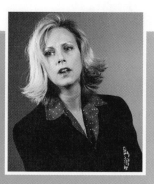

definitions of new and established patients. The definitions of the terms "new" and "established" patient are the same as those used in the E/M section. You will recall that those definitions are as follows:

New patient: one who has not received any professional service from the physician, or another physician of the same specialty who belongs to the same group practice, within the past 3 years.

Established patient: one who has received professional services from the physician, or another physician of the same specialty who belongs to the same group practice, within the past 3 years.

The subheading Special Ophthalmological Services contains **bilateral codes.** Each service in this subheading is performed on both eyes, and the codes do not require a modifier to indicate that two eyes were examined or tested. In fact, should you need to report only one eye from these codes, you would need to use modifier -52 to indicate a reduced service. It is a good idea to make a note next to the codes that are bilateral codes in the CPT manual and also to make a note of modifier -52, which you would use to reduce the service if it was performed for only one eye.

Special Ophthalmological Service codes are those services that are not normally performed in a general eye examination. Services in this group are performed for medically indicated reasons. The definitions of the codes are very comprehensive in detailing the services involved with each code.

Other codes that are found in the Ophthalmology subsection under the subheading Spectacle Services, category Supply of Materials, deal with the provision of materials to the patient (e.g., spectacles, contact lenses, or ocular prostheses). The refraction that is done to determine the lens prescription may be billed separately, depending on the policies set by third-party payers.

EXERCISE 13-7

OPHTHALMOLOGY

Using the CPT manual, code the following:

1   Established patient, comprehensive ophthalmologic examination

    Code(s): _____

2   Fitting of contact lens for treatment of a cataract, including the lens

    Code(s): _____

3 Tonography (procedure to check the intraocular pressure of the eye) with a medical diagnostic evaluation and recording of findings

Code(s): _____

4 New patient, comprehensive ophthalmologic examination

Code(s): _____

Special Otorhinolaryngologic Services

What a big word otorhinolaryngologic is! But when you take it apart it isn't so tough. "Oto" is ear, "rhino" is nose, "laryngo" is larynx, and "logy/logic" is all the knowledge about a subject—ear, nose, larynx. So all the knowledge about them is "otorhinolaryngology." The services in this subsection deal with special testing or studies for the ears, nose, and larynx. Audiology (hearing) testing is found in the Special Otorhinolaryngologic Services subsection, too. An audiology test may be performed by a physician or an audiologist trained in this area.

CAUTION *Otorhinolaryngologic diagnostic and treatment services are usually reported using codes from the E/M section. Special services are reported using these otorhinolaryngologic codes from the Medicine section. For example, a nasopharyngoscopy with endoscopy service (92511) provided during an office visit would be reported using 92511 and an office visit code from the E/M section.*

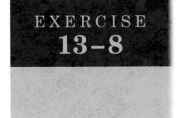

EXERCISE 13-8

SPECIAL OTORHINOLARYNGOLOGIC SERVICES

Using the CPT manual, code the following:

1 Hearing aid check in one ear (monaural: "mon" is one and "aural" is ear)

Code(s): _____

2 Screening test, pure tone, air only

Code(s): _____

3 A nasopharyngoscopy with endoscope

Code(s): _____

4 Nasal function study

Code(s): _____

Cardiovascular

The Cardiovascular subsection is discussed in Chapter 7.

Keep up the hard work; you will soon be finished with the entire CPT manual!

Noninvasive Vascular Diagnostic Studies

The codes in this subsection are used to identify procedures that are conducted to study veins and arteries other than the heart and great vessels.

These studies use the same devices as are used in heart and great-vessel echocardiography, discussed previously, except that the divisions are based on the location of the vein or artery being studied.

EXERCISE 13-9

NONINVASIVE VASCULAR DIAGNOSTIC STUDIES

Using the CPT manual, code the following:

1 A patient is referred for a single-level, bilateral venous occlusion plethysmography of the legs.

   Code(s): _____

2 A 34-year-old patient presents with a history of inability to sustain an erection. The physician uses a duplex scan to conduct a complete study of the arterial and venous flow of the penis.

   Code(s): _____

Pulmonary

Codes found in the Pulmonary subsection include codes for therapies, such as nebulizer treatments, and for diagnostic tests, such as pulmonary function tests. A nebulizer is a device that produces a spray, which is inhaled; it is used to treat patients with, for example, asthma. Pulmonary function tests are used to monitor the function of the pulmonary system; they examine the lung capacity of patients with, for example, emphysema. In most cases, several pulmonary function tests are performed together. The data are then compiled, and a diagnosis is made. Several indicators must be present from a variety of tests, and those tests must be performed many times and produce the same result each time for the results to be considered conclusive. In most cases, each type of test may be reported separately, unless it is specifically stated otherwise in the code description.

EXERCISE 13-10

PULMONARY

Using the CPT manual, code the following:

1 Pulmonary stress test, simple

   Code(s): _____

2 Vital capacity, total

   Code(s): _____

3 Bronchospasm evaluation with spirometry before and after bronchodilator treatment

   Code(s): _____

Allergy and Clinical Immunology

You are strongly encouraged to read the notes that appear at the beginning of the Allergy and Clinical Immunology subsection. The subsection is divided into several parts. The first is Allergy Testing, which describes allergy testing by various methods (percutaneous, intracutaneous, inhalation) and the type of tests (allergenic extracts, venoms, biologicals, food). The number of tests must always be specified for billing purposes because for most of these codes, payment is made per test.

The second subheading is Allergen Immunotherapy. Allergen Immunotherapy codes specify three types of services:

1. Injection only

2. Prescription and injection

3. Provision of antigen only

All the codes in Allergen Immunotherapy have specific notes that you must read to know whether the code is for injection, prescription and injection, or antigen only. For example, code 95115 covers the injection of antigen only and does not include the antigen or the prescription, but code 95120 covers the injection, antigen, and prescription. So careful reading of the descriptions is a necessity.

The professional service necessary to provide the immunotherapy is bundled into the code, so an office visit code would not usually be reported. If the physician provided another identifiable service at the time of the immunotherapy, an office visit could be reported. But for the patient who has only the injection, prescription, antigen, or any combination of these three, the codes already contain the professional service.

EXERCISE 13-11

ALLERGY AND CLINICAL IMMUNOLOGY

Using the CPT manual, code the following:

1   Direct nasal mucous membrane allergy test

    Code(s): _____

2   Percutaneous test using allergen extracts, immediate type reaction, 10 tests

    Code(s): _____

3   Single injection of allergen using extract provided by the patient

    Code(s): _____

Endocrinology

This subsection was new in the 2002 CPT manual and contains only one code used to report glucose monitoring. The monitoring is from hour 1 to hour 72 using continuous recording. The service includes the initial hook-up, calibration of the monitor, patient training, recording, and downloading of data with printout of results.

Neurology and Neuromuscular Procedures

There are codes in the Neurology and Neuromuscular Procedures subsection for sleep testing, muscle testing (electromyography), range of motion measurements, cerebral seizure monitoring, and a variety of neurologic function tests. The codes in this subsection are usually used by physicians who specialize in neurology, called neurologists. A neurologist usually is a consultant to a physician who needs the advice and input of another physician concerning a patient with suspected neurologic problems.

One of the specialized tests conducted in the neurology specialty area is sleep studies. **Sleep studies** are the monitoring of a patient's sleep for 6 or more hours. The studies include the tracing (technical component) and the physician's review, interpretation, and report (professional component). If a physician performs only the professional component, modifier -26 is used along with the CPT code.

Sleep studies are used to diagnose various sleep disorders and to measure a patient's response to therapy. An electroencephalogram (EEG) is a procedure that is used to record changes in brain waves. **Polysomnography** is the measurement of the brain waves during sleep but with the added feature of recording the various stages of sleep (i.e., excited, relaxed, drowsy, asleep, or deep sleep). During each of these stages, the rate and amplitude (height) of the brain waves are measured and compared with normal ranges. Certain neurologic conditions can be identified by the degree to which brain waves vary from normal ranges.

Parameters are what are being measured while the sleep testing is being conducted. For example, parameters include the measurement of snoring. Another parameter is blood pressure. The parameters are listed under the subheading of Sleep Testing. Be certain to read these parameters before coding in this area. The patient's record will contain the parameters, or measurements, recorded during the test. Several of the codes in the category are based on the number of parameters being measured.

To code sleep tests accurately, you must know the parameters and stages of testing. Additionally, many codes include a time component.

The electromyographic (EMG) studies use needles and electric current to stimulate nerves and record the results. Assessments of dysphasia, developmental testing, neurobehavior status, and neuropsychological test codes are also found in this subsection.

EXERCISE 13–12

NEUROLOGY AND NEUROMUSCULAR PROCEDURES

Using the notes under the the Sleep Testing subheading and the code descriptions following the notes, identify the following abbreviations:

1 NCPAP _____

2 EEG _____

3 EMG _____

4 EOG _____

Using the CPT manual, code the following:

5 Awake and drowsy EEG and photic stimulation in clinic

   Code(s): _____

6 Needle electromyography, three extremities and related paraspinal areas

   Code(s): _____

7 Range of motion measurement and report on both legs

   Code(s): _____

Central Nervous System Assessments/Tests

The Central Nervous System Assessments/Tests codes identify psychological testing, speech/language (aphasia) assessment, developmental progress assessments, and thinking/reasoning status examination (neurobehavioral). Except for the basic developmental testing, the codes are defined on a per hour basis. The results of all the tests are to be developed into a report that is included in the patient record.

EXERCISE 13-13

CENTRAL NERVOUS SYSTEM ASSESSMENTS/ TESTS

Using the CPT manual, code the following (all cases were 60 minutes in length):

1 A mother presented to the office of a psychiatrist with a 10-year-old who had been referred by the child's pediatrician for his nonconformist behavior. At the psychiatric office visit, the mother expressed great concern about the child's inability to behave as she and the child's father believed appropriate. One week later the psychiatrist conducted several developmental tests of this patient. The psychiatrist then discussed the results of the tests with the mother. Code only the developmental testing.

   Code(s): _____

2 A young executive is referred for a Minnesota Multiphasic Personality Inventory (MMPI) test by his employer. The employer requests the testing for all newly hired executives who will be working with highly sensitive government documents.

   Code(s): _____

3 A 14-year-old is seen in the office for an assessment of the child's attention span. The child is experiencing increasingly severe episodes of daydreaming. The physician conducts a clinical assessment of the child's cognitive function.

   Code(s): _____

Health and Behavior Assessment/Intervention

The codes in this subsection are not used to report preventive medicine services, nor are they used to report psychiatric treatments. Instead, these codes are used to report assessment and/or intervention for behavioral, emotional, social, psychological, or knowledge factors that are affecting the patient's health. Examples of assessments are clinical interview, behavior observation, or questionnaires. Examples of interventions are individual, group or family sessions. All services are based on 15-minute increments. These services are not performed by a physician. If these services are performed by a physician they are reported with E/M codes.

Chemotherapy Administration

Chemotherapy may be provided by several modalities. For instance, some third-party payers will pay for both an IV push and an infusion on the same day, whereas others will not. The IV push quickly puts the chemotherapy into the vein, whereas the infusion is the slower introduction of the chemotherapy into the vein. Read the patient record carefully before coding to ensure that the correct modality is identified. You must also be familiar with the coding requirements for chemotherapy of third-party payers in the area.

If a significant identifiable office visit service was provided in addition to the chemotherapy administration service, use a separate E/M code to report the service. Add modifier -25 (Significant, Separately Identifiable E/M Service by the Same Physician on the Same Day of the Procedure or Other Service) to ensure that the third-party payer is aware of the separateness of the service being reported.

If the patient is given an additional medication before or after the chemotherapy, such as an analgesic or antiemetic, you report the administration of the medication separately, using injection codes from the 90780–90788 subsection.

Chemotherapy codes are divided on the basis of method of treatment and length of time taken to complete the treatment. Pay special attention to the wording of each code in the subsection. Some codes include several hours of treatment time, whereas others specify each hour of treatment time; and unit billing or multiple coding may be necessary to accurately reflect the services provided. When reporting chemotherapy, be sure to add a code for the agent, using 96545.

coding shot

Medicare uses HCPCS code Q0081 to report chemotherapy services.

EXERCISE 13-14

CHEMOTHERAPY ADMINISTRATION

Using the CPT manual, code the following chemotherapy administrations:

1 Chemotherapy injected into the pleural cavity with thoracentesis

    Code(s): _____

2 Refilling and maintenance of a patient's portable pump

    Code(s): _____

3 Chemotherapy administered subcutaneously with local anesthesia

    Code(s): _____

4 Chemotherapy administered intravenously using the infusion technique for 50 minutes

    Code(s): _____

5 Chemotherapy injected into the central nervous system using a lumbar puncture

    Code(s): _____

from the trenches

What is the one personality trait that all coders should have?
"Patience!"

PEGGY

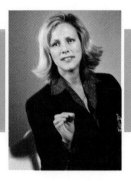

Photodynamic Therapy

The photodynamic therapy codes are used in conjunction with the codes for bronchoscopy or endoscopy. An agent is injected into the patient and remains in cancerous cells longer than in normal cells. After the agent has dissipated from the normal cells, the patient is exposed to laser light. The agent absorbs the light and the light produces oxygen, destroying the cancerous cells.

Codes for endoscopic application are divided on the basis of time—the first 30 minutes and each additional 15 minutes. External application is based on each exposure session.

Special Dermatological Procedures

The dermatology codes are usually used by a dermatologist who sees a patient in an office on a consultation basis. The dermatology codes for special procedures would typically be used in addition to the E/M consultation codes. For example, if a patient is referred by his family physician to a dermatologist for treatment of acne, the dermatologist conducts a history and examination and treats the patient with ultraviolet light (actinotherapy). The codes would be an Office or Other Outpatient Consultation code, depending on the level of service provided, *and* 96900 for the actinotherapy.

EXERCISE 13-15

SPECIAL DERMATOLOGICAL PROCEDURES

Using the CPT manual, code the following:

1 A 16-year-old patient sees a dermatologist in consultation, at which time the physician does a problem focused history and physical examination regarding the patient's acne. The physician prescribes and provides a treatment of ultraviolet light therapy.

Code(s): _____

2 Actinotherapy is provided for a 34-year-old consultative patient with severe dermatosis. The patient receives 8 hours of treatment. The physician provides a comprehensive history and physical examination with moderately complex medical decision-making.

Code(s): _____

Physical Medicine and Rehabilitation

The codes in the Physical Medicine and Rehabilitation subsection can be used by a physician or therapist. The subsection includes codes dealing with different modalities of treatments (e.g., traction, whirlpool, electrical stimulation) as well as various types of patient training (e.g., functional activities, gait training, massage). The codes are reported on the basis of time or treatment area, as stated in the description of the code. Unit coding is necessary if the time spent administering the treatment exceeds the time listed in the code. The subsection also includes other rehabilitation procedures such as shopping trips that may be arranged for residents of a Veterans' Affairs Medical Center.

EXAMPLE

Coding for patient's prosthetic training of 60 minutes would be:

97520 × 4   Prosthetic training, 60 minutes

Test and measurement codes are listed by the type of testing and the time the testing takes. The type of test would be items such as orthoses, prostheses, and musculoskeletal or functional capacity. Note the use of type and time in the following CPT code.

EXAMPLE

97750   Physical performance test or measurement (e.g., musculoskeletal, functional capacity, with written report, each 15 minutes)

Time must be noted in the documentation that is placed in the patient's medical record.

The codes in Physical Medicine and Rehabilitation are used for physical medicine and therapy as well as for other rehabilitation, for example, community/work reintegration (97537).

Active Wound Care Management

Nonphysician personnel perform the procedures described in Active Wound Care Management codes. The codes are not used with or to replace the surgical debridement represented by codes 11040–11044; a physician performs the procedures indicated by codes 11040–11044.

These wound management codes are based on selective or nonselective procedures. **Selective** debridement is that in which only the necrotic (dead) tissue is removed, without prior preparation. Prior preparation is the softening of the burn to ease the removal of necrotic tissue. Selective debridement requires more skill than nonselective debridement because selective sharp debridement involves cutting along the border between the necrotic skin and the viable tissue with scissors, a scalpel, or forceps. **Nonselective** debridement is that in which healthy tissue is removed along with necrotic tissue. The tissue is gradually loosened with water (hydrotherapy). Loosened tissue may be cut away with sharp instruments, but cutting along the border is not involved in this procedure. Nonselective debridement is usually done over several office visits.

A session usually takes approximately 30 minutes. Examples of selective and nonselective debridement can be found in the parenthetical information following each of the codes.

Medical Nutrition Therapy

These codes are used by nonphysician personnel for medical nutritional therapy assessment or intervention. If a physician provides the service, the service is reported using E/M codes or Preventive Medicine codes.

EXERCISE 13-16

PHYSICAL MEDICINE AND REHABILITATION

Using the CPT manual, code the following:

1 Application of cold packs to one area (modality)

Code(s): _____

2 Initial prosthetic training, 30 minutes

Code(s): _____

3 Physical medicine treatment procedure, gait training, 30 minutes

Code(s): _____

Osteopathic Manipulative Treatment (OMT)

Osteopathic manipulative treatment is a form of manual treatment applied by a physician to eliminate somatic (body) dysfunction and related disorders. The codes are listed according to body regions. The body regions considered are the head; cervical, thoracic, lumbar, sacral, and pelvic regions; lower extremities; upper extremities; rib cage; abdomen; and viscera. Codes are separated on the basis of the number of body regions treated. These codes are usually used by osteopathic physicians (doctors of osteopathy, D.O.).

Chiropractic Manipulative Treatment (CMT)

The Chiropractic Manipulative Treatment subsection is divided by the number of regions manipulated. For this subsection, the **spine** is divided into five regions (cervical, thoracic, lumbar, sacral, and pelvic), and the **extraspinal** regions are divided into five regions (head, lower extremities, upper extremities, rib cage, and abdomen). Chiropractic manipulation is the manipulation of the spinal column and other structures. Each of the codes in the Chiropractic Manipulative Treatment subsection has a professional assessment bundled into the code. An office visit code is used only if the patient had a significant separately identifiable service provided; otherwise, the service of the office visit is bundled into the code.

CAUTION *Use modifier -25 when reporting a separate E/M service.*

EXERCISE 13-17

MANIPULATIVE TREATMENT

Using the CPT manual, code the following:

1 Sally, a 43-year-old woman, presents with the complaint of a seizing pain in the area of her lower left hip. The physician conducts an assessment of the patient and provides an alignment to two spinal regions.

Code(s): _____

2 Lumbar manipulation (OMT), one region

Code(s): _____

Special Services, Procedures, and Reports

Special Services, Procedures, and Reports is a miscellaneous subsection that includes codes that do not fit into other sections. Codes that reflect services rendered at unusual hours of the day or on holidays, for example, are considered adjunct codes and are to be used in addition to the codes for the major service. For example, if a physician goes back to the office on a Sunday to meet an established patient and provide urgent, but not emergency, service, the correct E/M service code for the office visit would be used in addition to 99054 to indicate the unusual time at which the service was provided.

You have used 99070, supplies, from this subsection often. One of the big advantages of the HCPCS coding system is that you specifically identify the supply reported with 99070. For example, you may use 99070 to report a body sock that was given to a patient. With the HCPCS coding system, you can specify the body sock with a specific code, L0984.

The subsection also contains codes for medical testimony, the completion of complicated reports, education services, unusual travel, and supplies. Although this subsection is small, it contains codes that are used often. Take a few minutes to become familiar with the kinds of codes listed within Special Services, Procedures, and Reports and then mark the subsection for future use.

The codes for Special Services are located in the CPT manual index under the main term "Special Services."

EXERCISE 13-18

SPECIAL SERVICES, PROCEDURES, AND REPORTS

Using the CPT manual, code the following:

1 The physician is called to the emergency department on Sunday (This code is in addition to the basic service code for the services provided to the patient.)

Code(s): _____

2 Conveyance of a specimen from the physician's office to a laboratory

Code(s): _____

3 Supplies provided for an office visit exceeding those usually used

Code(s): _____

Qualifying Circumstances for Anesthesia

Anesthesia is discussed in Chapter 3.

Sedation With or Without Analgesia (Conscious Sedation)

Sedation is discussed in Chapter 3.

Other Services and Procedures

A wide variety of codes is found in this subsection of the Medicine section. For example, you will find codes for anogenital examination with a colposcope of a child in a case of suspected trauma, visual function screenings, pumping poison from the stomach, and therapeutic phlebotomy treatments. Because the codes are so varied, the way in which they are divided is also varied. For example, the code range 99190–99192 is divided on the basis of time, whereas other codes are divided according to the extent of the service.

Home Health Procedures/Services

These codes are used to report nonphysician services provided at the patient's residence. The residence may be an assisted living apartment, custodial care facility, group home, or other nontraditional residence. The codes are divided based on the reason for the service (e.g., injection, hemodialysis).

Home Infusion Procedures

The codes represent services of administration of a variety of therapies (e.g., nutrition, chemotherapy, pain management). The services are provided by nonphysician allied health professionals. Codes are divided based on the therapy and represent all services in a 24-hour period.

You did it! You made it all the way through the CPT! If there could be noise with a text, you would hear loud applause and horns blowing to celebrate all your hard work. Good job!

HISTORY OF NATIONAL LEVEL CODING

CPT coding is only one of a three-part coding system called HCPCS (pronounced hick-picks). The Centers for Medicare and Medicaid Services (CMS), formerly the Health Care Financing Administration, developed the HCFA Common Procedure Coding System in 1983. The HCPCS is a collection of codes that represent procedures, supplies, products, and services that may be provided to Medicare and Medicaid beneficiaries and to individuals enrolled in private health insurance programs.

Three Levels of Codes

HCPCS is divided into three levels or groups.

> **Level I** codes are CPT codes in the CPT manual, which was developed, maintained, and copyrighted by the AMA. The CPT is the primary coding system used in the outpatient setting to code professional services provided to patients.

> **Level II** codes (National Codes) are approved and maintained jointly by the Alpha-Numeric Workgroup, consisting of the CMS, the Health Insurance Association of America, and the Blue Cross and Blue Shield Association. Level II codes are five-position alphanumeric codes representing physician and nonphysician services that are not represented in the Level I codes.

> **Level III** codes (Local Codes) were developed by Medicare carriers for use at the local (carrier) level. These are five-position alphanumeric codes representing physician and nonphysician services that are not represented in the Level I or Level II codes.

Level II National Codes

CPT codes do not cover all services that are provided to patients. Allied health care professionals—such as dentists, orthodontists, and various technical support services, such as ambulance services—are not covered by the CPT coding system. There are also no codes in the CPT system for many of the supplies that are used in patient care (e.g., drugs, durable medical

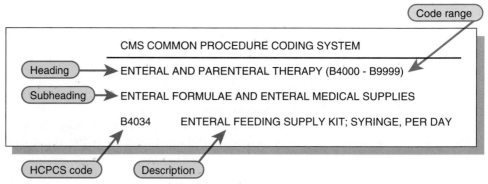

Figure 13–4 CMS Common Procedure Coding System, National Codes. (Courtesy of U.S. Department of Health and Human Services, Centers for Medicare and Medicaid Services.)

equipment, or orthoses). Use of national codes is mandatory on all Medicare and Medicaid claims submitted for payment for services of the previously listed professionals. Although the national codes were developed for use when billing for services rendered to Medicare patients, many third-party payers now require that providers use the national codes when submitting bills for non-Medicare patients too, because the system allows for continuity and specificity when billing. This uniformity also helps the effort to collect uniform health service data.

The first digit in a national code is a letter—A, B, C, D, E, G, H, J, K, L, M, P, Q, R, S, or V—which is followed by four numbers. Codes beginning with the letters K, G, and Q are for temporary assignment until a definitive decision can be made about appropriate code assignment. The K codes are temporary codes for durable medical equipment, the G codes are temporary codes for procedures and professional services, and the Q codes are temporary codes for procedures, services, and supplies. All codes and descriptions are updated annually by the CMS. The alphanumeric listing contains headings of groups of codes, as illustrated in Figure 13–4. Note that following the heading is listed the range of codes available for assignment in the category. There are also subheadings preceding the codes and the description of the codes to identify the type of codes that follow.

National codes are not used by health care facilities to code for the services provided to inpatients. Inpatient health care facilities use the diagnosis (from ICD-9-CM) as the basis of payment for their services and assign codes from ICD-9-CM, Volume 3, for inpatient procedures. The three levels of national codes are used in outpatient settings (including physician's offices) where the basis of payment is the service rendered, not the diagnosis.

General Guidelines

The HCPCS manual includes the general guidelines for use of the national codes, a list of modifiers, the codes, a Table of Drugs, and an index. We begin our study of the HCPCS manual at the index. You have to be able to locate items in the index in order to be able to identify the correct code. The main index terms include tests, services, supplies, orthoses, prostheses, medical equipment, drugs, therapies, and some medical and surgical procedures. The subterms of the index are listed under the main term to which they apply, along with the code.

EXAMPLE

Apnea monitor is found under the entry:
   Monitor
      apnea E0608

You then locate the code in the main part of the manual and read any notes that are listed with the code.

General rules for coding using the national codes are as follows:

1. Never code directly from the index. Always use both the alphanumeric listing and the index.

2. Analyze the statement or description provided that designates the item that needs a code.

3. Identify the main term in the index.

4. Check for relevant subterms under the main term. Verify the meaning of any unfamiliar abbreviations.

5. Note the code or codes found immediately after the selected main term or subterm.

6. After locating the term and the code in the index, verify the code and its full description in the alphanumeric listing to ensure the specificity of the code.

7. In most cases, for each entry a specific code is provided. In some cases, you are referred to a range of codes among which you can locate the exact code desired. You must review the entire range in the numeric listing to find the correct entry.

   If the code is a single number, locate that code number in the alphanumeric listing. Verify the code number and the description to be sure that you have selected the correct code to describe the item you are coding. You must review the alphanumeric listing to select the appropriate code number in this case.

8. In all cases, when locating an entry in the index, it is necessary to look at all descriptors under the main term and subterms in order to choose the correct entry.

CODE GROUPINGS

- A Codes — Transportation Services, including Ambulance
  Medical and Surgical Supplies
  Administrative, Miscellaneous, and Investigational
- B Codes — Enteral and Parenteral Therapy
- C Codes — Hospital Outpatient Prospective Payment System (OPPS)
- D Codes — Dental Procedures
- E Codes — Durable Medical Equipment
- G Codes — Temporary (Procedures/Professional Services)
- J Codes — Drugs Administered Other Than Oral Method
- K Codes — Temporary (Durable Medical Equipment)
- L Codes — Orthotics and Prosthetics
- M Codes — Medical Services
- P Codes — Pathology and Laboratory Services
- Q Codes — Temporary (Procedures, Services, and Supplies)
- R Codes — Diagnostic Radiology Services
- V Codes — Vision Services

Index

The index is in alphabetical order and includes main terms and subterms (Fig. 13–5). The entries in the index of the national codes may be listed under more than one main term. For example, dialysis kits can be found under the two entries "Kits" and "Dialysis," as illustrated in Figure 13–6.

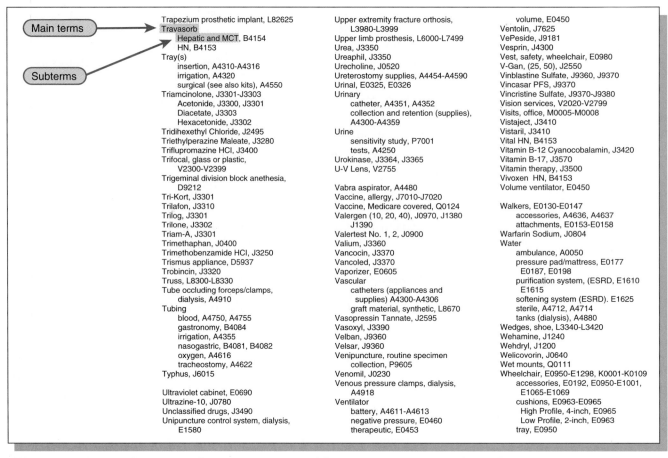

Main terms
Subterms

Trapezium prosthetic implant, L82625
Travasorb
    Hepatic and MCT, B4154
    HN, B4153
Tray(s)
    insertion, A4310-A4316
    irrigation, A4320
    surgical (see also kits), A4550
Triamcinolone, J3301-J3303
    Acetonide, J3300, J3301
    Diacetate, J3303
    Hexacetonide, J3302
Tridihexethyl Chloride, J2495
Triethylperazine Maleate, J3280
Triflupromazine HCl, J3400
Trifocal, glass or plastic,
    V2300-V2399
Trigeminal division block anethesia,
    D9212
Tri-Kort, J3301
Trilafon, J3310
Trilog, J3301
Trilone, J3302
Triam-A, J3301
Trimethaphan, J0400
Trimethobenzamide HCl, J3250
Trismus appliance, D5937
Trobincin, J3320
Truss, L8300-L8330
Tube occluding forceps/clamps,
    dialysis, A4910
Tubing
    blood, A4750, A4755
    gastronomy, B4084
    irrigation, A4355
    nasogastric, B4081, B4082
    oxygen, A4616
    tracheostomy, A4622
Typhus, J6015

Ultraviolet cabinet, E0690
Ultrazine-10, J0780
Unclassified drugs, J3490
Unipuncture control system, dialysis,
    E1580

Upper extremity fracture orthosis,
    L3980-L3999
Upper limb prosthesis, L6000-L7499
Urea, J3350
Ureaphil, J3350
Urecholine, J0520
Ureterostomy supplies, A4454-A4590
Urinal, E0325, E0326
Urinary
    catheter, A4351, A4352
    collection and retention (supplies),
        A4300-A4359
Urine
    sensitivity study, P7001
    tests, A4250
Urokinase, J3364, J3365
U-V Lens, V2755

Vabra aspirator, A4480
Vaccine, allergy, J7010-J7020
Vaccine, Medicare covered, Q0124
Valergen (10, 20, 40), J0970, J1380
    J1390
Valertest No. 1, 2, J0900
Valium, J3360
Vancocin, J3370
Vancoled, J3370
Vaporizer, E0605
Vascular
    catheters (appliances and
        supplies) A4300-A4306
    graft material, synthetic, L8670
Vasopressin Tannate, J2595
Vasoxyl, J3390
Velban, J9360
Velsar, J9360
Venipuncture, routine specimen
    collection, P9605
Venomil, J0230
Venous pressure clamps, dialysis,
    A4918
Ventilator
    battery, A4611-A4613
    negative pressure, E0460
    therapeutic, E0453

    volume, E0450
Ventolin, J7625
VePeside, J9181
Vesprin, J4300
Vest, safety, wheelchair, E0980
V-Gan, (25, 50), J2550
Vinblastine Sulfate, J9360, J9370
Vincasar PFS, J9370
Vincristine Sulfate, J9370-J9380
Vision services, V2020-V2799
Visits, office, M0005-M0008
Vistaject, J3410
Vistaril, J3410
Vital HN, B4153
Vitamin B-12 Cyanocobalamin, J3420
Vitamin B-17, J3570
Vitamin therapy, J3500
Vivoxen HN, B4153
Volume ventilator, E0450

Walkers, E0130-E0147
    accessories, A4636, A4637
    attachments, E0153-E0158
Warfarin Sodium, J0804
Water
    ambulance, A0050
    pressure pad/mattress, E0177
        E0187, E0198
    purification system, (ESRD, E1610
        E1615
    softening system (ESRD). E1625
    sterile, A4712, A4714
    tanks (dialysis), A4880
Wedges, shoe, L3340-L3420
Wehamine, J1240
Wehdryl, J1200
Welicovorin, J0640
Wet mounts, Q0111
Wheelchair, E0950-E1298, K0001-K0109
    accessories, E0192, E0950-E1001,
        E1065-E1069
    cushions, E0963-E0965
        High Profile, 4-inch, E0965
        Low Profile, 2-inch, E0963
    tray, E0950

Figure 13–5 CMS index, National Codes. (Courtesy of U.S. Department of Health and Human Services, Centers for Medicare and Medicaid Services.)

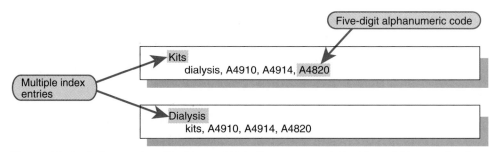

Figure 13–6 Index entries. (Courtesy of U.S. Department of Health and Human Services, Centers for Medicare and Medicaid Services.)

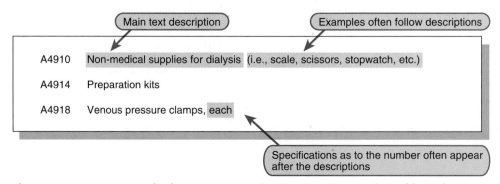

Figure 13–7 Main text display. (Courtesy of U.S. Department of Health and Human Services, Centers for Medicare and Medicaid Services.)

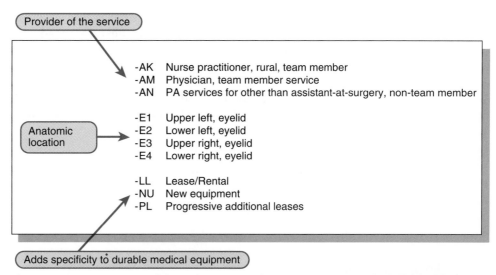

Figure 13–8 HCPCS modifiers. (Courtesy of U.S. Department of Health and Human Services, Centers for Medicare and Medicaid Services.)

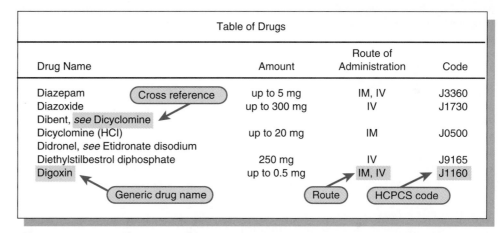

Figure 13–9 Example from Table of Drugs. (Courtesy of U.S. Department of Health and Human Services, Centers for Medicare and Medicaid Services.)

From the index, you turn to the code in the alphanumeric listing. The entries in the alphanumeric listing further explain what is included in the code. The dialysis kit code numbers are shown as they appear in the alphanumeric listing in Figure 13–7. Note that A4918 specifies "each," and A4910 lists examples of what can be considered supplies for dialysis. There are more than 50 alphabetical modifiers available for assignment to add further specificity to the five-digit national code. For example, modifiers can be used to specify the service provider, specify the anatomic site, or add specificity (Fig. 13–8). Appendix A of the CPT contains some of the Level II, HCPCS/National modifiers.

Table of Drugs

J codes are used to identify the drugs administered and the amounts or dosages given. The national codes contain a Table of Drugs (Fig. 13–9) to direct the user to the appropriate drug titles and the corresponding codes. J codes refer to drugs only by generic name. However, if a drug is known only by a brand or trade name, you will be directed to the generic name of the drug and then to the associated J code by a cross-reference system within the table. A *Physicians' Desk Reference* (PDR) is a valuable resource for the coder when using the Table of Drugs.

The Route of Administration column (see Fig. 13–9) lists the most common methods of delivering the referenced generic drug. The official definitions for Level II J codes generally describe administration other than by the oral method. Orally given drugs are not usually provided in a physician's office but are bought at a pharmacy after the visit. Therefore, with a few exceptions, orally delivered drugs are omitted from the Route of Administration column. The following abbreviations and listings are used in the Route of Administration column:

IT	Intrathecal	INH	Inhalant solution
IV	Intravenous	VAR	Various routes
IM	Intramuscular	OTH	Other routes
SC	Subcutaneous		

EXERCISE 13-19

TABLE OF DRUGS

Define the following routes of administration for drugs:

1 Intrathecal _____

_____

2 Intravenous _____

_____

3 Intramuscular _____

_____

4 Subcutaneous _____

_____

5 Inhalant solution _____

_____

CMS Common Procedure Coding System

J1120	INJECTION, ACETAZOLAMIDE SODIUM, UP TO 500 MG
J1160	INJECTION, DIGOXIN, UP TO 0.5 MG
J1165	INJECTION, PHENYTOIN SODIUM, PER 50 MG
J1170	INJECTION, HYDROMORPHONE, UP TO 4 MG
J1180	INJECTION, DYPHYLLINE, UP TO 500 MG
J1190	INJECTION, DEXRAZOXANE HYDROCHLORIDE, PER 250 MG
J1200	INJECTION, DIPHENHYDRAMINE HCL, UP TO 50 MG
J1205	INJECTION, CHLOROTHIAZIDE SODIUM, PER 500 MG

Figure 13–10 J codes. (Courtesy of U.S. Department of Health and Human Services, Centers for Medicare and Medicaid Services.)

Effective 10/XX   **DURABLE MEDICAL EQUIPMENT REGIONAL CARRIER**   **DMERC 02.01**

CERTIFICATE OF MEDICAL NECESSITY: MANUAL/MOTORIZED WHEELCHAIRS

SECTION A   CERTIFICATION: ☐ INITIAL ☐ REVISED

PATIENT NAME, ADDRESS, TELEPHONE AND HIC NO.	SUPPLIER NAME, ADDRESS, TELEPHONE, AND NSC NUMBER
(_ _ _) _ _ _ - _ _ _ _ HICN_____	(_ _ _) _ _ _ - _ _ _ _ NSC _____
PLACE OF SERVICE ____ **REPLACEMENT ITEM** ____	**HCPCS CODE(S) WARRANTY LENGTH TYPE**
NAME AND ADDRESS OF FACILITY IF APPLICABLE (SEE BACK OF FORM): _____ _____ _____ _____	

SECTION B   INFORMATION BELOW TO BE COMPLETED ONLY BY THE PHYSICIAN OR PHYSICIAN'S EMPLOYEE

DIAGNOSIS (ICD9): _____ _____ _____ _____	PT. HT. ____ (IN.) PT. WT. ____ (LBS) DOB ____/____/____
I LAST EXAMINED THIS PATIENT FOR THIS CONDITION ON: ____/____/____ PT. SEX ____ (M OR F)	DATE NEEDED INITIAL ____/____/____ REVISED ____/____/____ EST. LENGTH OF NEED: # OF MONTHS: ____ 1-99 (99 = LIFETIME)

ANSWER QUESTIONS 1-4 FOR MOTORIZED WHEELCHAIR BASE, 4, 18-22 FOR MANUAL WHEELCHAIR BASE, 4-18 FOR WHEELCHAIR OPTIONS. Use Y - Yes, N - No, or D for Does Not Apply   unless otherwise noted.

[ ] 1. Does the patient have severe weakness of the upper extremities due to a neurologic or muscular disease/condition?

[ ] 2. Is the patient unable to operate a wheelchair manually?

[ ] 3. Is the patient capable of <u>safely</u> operating the controls of a power wheelchair?

[ ] 4. Would the patient be bed or chair confined without the use of a wheelchair?

[ ] 5. Does patient have quadriplegia?

[ ] 6. Does patient have a fixed hip angle?

[ ] 7. Does patient have a trunk cast or brace that requires a reclining back feature for positioning?

[ ] 8. Does the patient have a cast or brace which prevents 90 degree flexion of the knee?

[ ] 9. Does patient have a musculoskeletal condition that prevents 90 degree flexion at the knee?

[ ] 10. Does patient have excessive extensor tone of the trunk muscles?

[ ] 11. Does patient have weak neck muscles requiring support?

[ ] 12. Does patient have weak upper body muscles, upper body instability or muscle spasticity?

[ ] 13. Does patient have use of only one hand/arm and the condition is expected to last for 6 months or more?

[ ] 14. Is there hemiplegia or uncontrolled arm movements?

[ ] 15. Does patient have a need for arm height different than that available using non-adjustable arms?

[ ] 16. Does the patient need to rest in a recumbent position two or more times during the day?

[ ] 17. Is transfer between bed and wheelchair very difficult?

____ 18. How many hours per day does the patient usually spend in the wheelchair? (round up to next hour, e.g., for 3 1/2 hours, use 4) use 1-24.

[ ] 19. Is the patient able to place his/her feet on the ground for propulsion in a standard wheelchair?

[ ] 20. Is the patient able to self-propel in a standard wheelchair?

[ ] 21. Reserved for future use.

[ ] 22. Can/does patient self-propel in a lightweight wheelchair?

I certify the medical necessity of these items for this patient. Section B of this form and any statement on my letterhead attached hereto has been completed by me, or by my employee and reviewed by me. The foregoing information is true, accurate, and complete, and I understand that any falsification, omission, or concealment of material fact may subject me to civil or criminal liability.

PHYSICIAN NAME, ADDRESS	_____ __/__/__
	PHYSICIAN'S SIGNATURE: DATE (A STAMPED SIGNATURE IS NOT ACCEPTABLE)
	☐ Attending ☐ Consulting ☐ Other ordering
	UPIN:_____
	TELEPHONE #: (_ _ _) _ _ _ - _ _ _ _

Figure 13–11 CMS Certificate of Medical Necessity. (Courtesy of U.S. Department of Health and Human Services, Centers for Medicare and Medicaid Services.)

Department of Health and Human Services
Health Care Financing Administration

Form Approved
OMB No. 0938-0534

ATTENDING PHYSICIAN'S CERTIFICATION OF MEDICAL NECESSITY FOR
HOME OXYGEN THERAPY *(Legible handwritten entries acceptable)*

Public reporting burden for this collection of information is estimated to average 15 minutes per response, including the time for reviewing instructions, searching existing data sources, gathering and maintaining the data needed, and completing and reviewing the collection of information. Send comments regarding this burden estimate or any other aspect of this collection of information, including suggestions for reducing this burden, to HCFA, P.O. Box 26684, Baltimore, MD 21207; and to the Office of Information and Regulatory Affairs, Office of Management and Budget, Washington, DC 20503.

Patient's Name, Address, and HIC No.	Supplier's Name, Address, and Identification No.

Certification: ☐ Initial ☐ Revised ☐ Renewed

INFORMATION BELOW TO BE ENTERED ONLY BY PHYSICIAN OR PHYSICIAN'S EMPLOYEE

1. Pertinent Diagnoses, ICD-9-CM Codes, and Findings - CHECK ALL THAT APPLY:

☐ Emphysema (492.8)
☐ COPD (496)
☐ Cor Pulmonale (416.9)
☐ Interstitial Disease (515)
☐ Other _____
   Specify   Code

☐ Chronic Obstructive Bronchitis (491.2)
☐ Chronic Obstructive Asthma (493.20)
☐ Congestive Heart Failure (428.0)
☐ Secondary Polycythemia (289.0)
☐ Hematocrit 57% or more Yes☐ No☐

2.A. I last examined this patient for this condition on:
___/___/___
Month   Day   Year

2.B. Home oxygen prescribed:
___/___/___
Month   Day   Year

2.C. Estimated length of need:
☐ 1-3 months ☐ 4-12 months ☐ Lifetime

3.A. Results of Most Recent Arterial Blood Gas and/or Oxygen Saturation Tests (Patient Breathing Room Air)

	PO2	02 Saturation	Date
(1) At Rest			
(2) Walking.			
(2) Sleeping.			
(3) Exercising.			
(4) Other :			

3.C. Physician/Provider Performing Test(s) *(Printed/Typed Name and Address)*:

3.B. If performed under conditions other than room air, explain:

NOTE: If PO2 Level exceeds 59 mm Hg or the arterial blood saturation exceeds 89% at rest on room air, the claim will be disallowed without compelling medical evidence. Check block ☐ If you have attached a separate statement on your letterhead of additional documentation.

4. Oxygen Flow Rate : _____ Liters per minute   ☐ Continuous (24 hrs/day)

☐ Noncontinuous (Enter hrs/day): _____ Walking _____ Sleeping _____ Exercise Program _____ Other (specify) _____

5. Oxygen Equipment Prescribed   If you have prescribed a particular form of delivery, check applicable block(s). Otherwise leave blank.

A. Supply System

(1) Stationary Source ☐ Concentrator ☐ Liquid Oxygen
   ☐ Compressed Gas ☐ Other

(2) Portable or Ambulatory Source ☐ Liquid Oxygen
   ☐ Compressed Gas
   ☐ Other _____

B. Delivery System

☐ (1) Nasal Cannula
☐ (2) 02 Conserving Device
   ☐ Pulse 02 System
   ☐ Reservoir System
   ☐ Other _____
☐ (3) Transtracheal Catheter
☐ (4) Other _____

6. If you have prescribed a portable or ambulatory system, describe activities/exercise that patient regularly pursues which require this system in the home and which cannot be met by a stationary system (e.g., amount and frequency of ambulation).

CERTIFICATION

THE PATIENT HAS APPROPRIATELY TRIED OTHER TREATMENT MEASURES WITHOUT SUCCESS. OXYGEN THERAPY AND OXYGEN EQUIPMENT AS PRESCRIBED IS MEDICALLY INDICATED AND IS REASONABLE AND NECESSARY FOR THE TREATMENT OF THIS PATIENT. THIS FORM AND ANY STATEMENT ON MY LETTERHEAD ATTACHED HERETO HAS BEEN COMPLETED BY ME, OR BY MY EMPLOYEE AND REVIEWED BY ME. THE FOREGOING INFORMATION IS TRUE, ACCURATE, AND COMPLETE, AND I UNDERSTAND THAT ANY FALSIFICATION, OMISSION, OR CONCEALMENT OF MATERIAL FACT MAY SUBJECT ME TO CIVIL OR CRIMINAL LIABILITY.

Attending Physician's Signature: *(A STAMPED SIGNATURE IS NOT ACCEPTABLE)*	Date:

Physician's Name, Address, Telephone No., and Identification No.:

Form HCFA-484 (5-90)
DMERC Region D Supplier Manual   VIII - 22

Figure 13–12 CMS Attending Physician's Certificate of Medical Necessity for Home Oxygen Therapy. (Courtesy of U.S. Department of Health and Human Services, Centers for Medicare and Medicaid Services.)

Routes of Administration of Drugs

Intravenous administration includes all methods, such as gravity infusion, injections, and timed pushes. When several routes of administration are listed, the first listing is the most common method. A "VAR" posting denotes various routes of administration and is used for drugs that are commonly administered into joints, cavities, or tissues, and as topical applications. Listings posted with "OTH" alert the coder to other administration methods, for example, suppositories or catheter injections. A dash (—) in a column signifies that no information is available for that particular listing. Figure 13–10 illustrates J code information as listed in the alphanumeric listing to which you refer after locating the drug in the Table of Drugs.

As of October 1, 2002, the J codes were to have been replaced by the National Drug Code (NDC) for reporting prescription drugs and biologicals. The NDC serves as a universal product identifier for human drugs. The NDC is maintained by the Food and Drug Administration. The unique identifiers have 11 digits—the first 5 digits represent the manufacturer, the second 4 digits identify the product, and the last two digits signify the package size. For example, NDC 00300-3612-28 identifies the manufacturer as Tap Pharmaceuticals, Inc. (00300); the drug as Lupron (3612), which is the brandname product for the generic chemical known as leuprolide acetate; and finally the package size as a single unit containing 5 milligrams of drug (28). However, the providers expressed concerns to CMS about implementation of the change to the NDC, citing insufficient time to transfer to the new system. Currently, the implementation date has not been finalized.

Durable Medical Equipment

Durable medical equipment (DME) is equipment used by a patient with a chronic disabling condition, and some equipment that is used only temporarily until the patient has healed. Claims for DME and related supplies can be paid only if the items meet the Medicare definition of covered DME and are medically necessary. The determination of medical necessity is made using documentation written by the physician. The documentation can include medical records, plans of care, discharge plans, and prescriptions or forms explicitly designed to document medical necessity. Usually these forms are referred to as Certificates of Medical Necessity (CMN) (Fig. 13–11).

Claims for other items require the use of the CMN, for example, power-operated vehicles, air-fluidized beds, decubitus care pads, seat-lift mechanisms, and paraffin baths.

Physician completion of the required medical documentation ensures that the DME items furnished to a Medicare beneficiary are those specifically needed for the unique medical condition of the patient. The CMS also requires the use of form HCFA-484 for the Attending Physician's Certification of Medical Necessity for Home Oxygen Therapy (Fig. 13–12).

National Physician Fee Schedule

Each fall, the Centers for Medicare and Medicaid Services produces the National Physician Fee Schedule, which lists all HCPCS and CPT codes along with the amount allocated for each services and the covered/noncovered status of each service. Figure 13–13 illustrates a portion of the National Physician Fee Schedule for 2002. You will learn more about CMS allocations in Chapter 16 of this text.

HCPCS	Description	Status Code	Conversion Factor
A0021	Outside state ambulance serv	I	$36.1992
A0080	Noninterest escort in non er	I	$36.1992
A0090	Interest escort in non er	I	$36.1992
A0100	Nonemergency transport taxi	I	$36.1992
A0110	Nonemergency transport bus	I	$36.1992
A0120	Noner transport mini-bus	I	$36.1992
A0130	Noner transport wheelch van	I	$36.1992
A0140	Nonemergency transport air	I	$36.1992
A0160	Noner transport case worker	I	$36.1992
A0170	Noner transport parking fees	I	$36.1992
A0180	Noner transport lodgng recip	I	$36.1992
A0190	Noner transport meals recip	I	$36.1992
A0200	Noner transport lodgng escrt	I	$36.1992
A0210	Noner transport meals escort	I	$36.1992
A0380	Basic life support mileage	X	$36.1992
A0382	Basic support routine suppls	X	$36.1992
A0384	Bls defibrillation supplies	X	$36.1992
A0390	Advanced life support mileag	X	$36.1992
A0392	Als defibrillation supplies	X	$36.1992

Figure 13–13 2002 National Physician Fee Schedule Relative Value File.

EXERCISE 13-20

NATIONAL CODES

With information provided in this chapter, complete the following:

1 HCPCS is divided into three levels. List the names of the levels, in order, and the level number:

a. _____

Level _____

b. _____

Level _____

c. _____

Level _____

2 There are three groups of codes that are used by CMS for temporary assignment until a definitive decision can be made about the correct code assignment. What are the alphabetic letters of these three groups of codes?

_____ , _____ , and _____

3 There are more than 50 modifiers in the HCPCS. Are they all numeric modifiers? _____

4 What alphabetic group of codes is used to reference drugs in the HCPCS? _____

5 The term "route of administration" generally describes the administration of drugs by methods other than _____ .

6 What group of codes is used to reference durable medical equipment in the national codes? _____

Use Figure 13–5 through Figure 13–10 to answer the following questions:

7 What is the range of codes in Figure 13–5 that is available for the coding of an allergy vaccine? _____

8 What is the modifier for each of the following (Fig. 13–8)?

a. New equipment _____

b. Lower left eyelid _____

c. The services of a physician who was a member of a team that provided service _____

9 What is the route of administration of dicyclomine (Fig. 13–9)?

_____

10 What is the amount of diazepam for code J3360 (Fig. 13–9)?

_____

11 What is the J code for an injection of diazoxide (Fig. 13–9)?

_____

12 What is the code range available for a high-profile cushion for a wheelchair (Fig. 13–5)? _____

CHAPTER GLOSSARY

actinotherapy: treatment of acne using ultraviolet rays

angiography: taking of x-ray films of vessels after injection of contrast material

anomaloscope: instrument used to test color vision

anoscopy: procedure that uses a scope to examine the anus

apexcardiography: recording of the movement of the chest wall

aphakia: absence of the lens of the eye

audiometry: hearing testing

bifocal: two focuses in eyeglasses, one usually for close work and the other for improvement of distance vision

biofeedback: process of giving a person self-information

cardioversion: electrical shock to the heart to restore normal rhythm

colonoscopy: fibroscopic examination of the entire colon that may include part of the terminal ileum

corneosclera: cornea and sclera of the eye

Doppler: ultrasonic measure of blood movement

ECG: *see* electrocardiogram

echography: ultrasound procedure in which sound waves are bounced off an internal organ and the resulting image is recorded

EEG: *see* electroencephalogram

electrocardiogram (ECG): written record of the electrical action of the heart

electrocochleography: test to measure the eighth cranial nerve (hearing test)

electroencephalogram (EEG): written record of the electrical action of the brain

electromyogram (EMG): written record of the electrical activity of the skeletal muscles

electro-oculogram (EOG): written record of the electrical activity of the eye

endomyocardial: pertaining to the inner and middle layers of the heart

ESRD: end-stage renal disease

gonioscopy: use of a scope to examine the angles of the eye

hemodialysis: cleansing of the blood outside of the body

hyposensitization: decreased sensitivity

hypothermia: low body temperature; sometimes induced during surgical procedures

immunotherapy: therapy to increase immunity

intramuscular: into a muscle

intravenous: into a vein

iontophoresis: introduction of ions into the body

ischemia: deficient blood supply due to obstruction of the circulatory system

modality: treatment method

monofocal: eyeglasses with one vision correction

MSLT: multiple sleep latency testing

myasthenia gravis: syndrome characterized by muscle weakness

nasopharyngoscopy: use of a scope to visualize the nose and pharynx

NCPAP: nasal continuous positive airway pressure

nystagmus: rapid involuntary eye movements

opacification: area that has become opaque (milky)

ophthalmodynamometry: test of the blood pressure of the eye

ophthalmology: body of knowledge regarding the eyes

optokinetic: movement of the eyes to objects moving in the visual field

orthoptic: corrective; in the correct place

percutaneous: through the skin

peritoneal: within the lining of the abdominal cavity

phlebotomy: cutting into a vein

phonocardiogram: recording of heart sounds

photochemotherapy: treatment by means of drugs that react to ultraviolet radiation or sunlight

plethysmography: determining the changes in volume of an organ part or body

pneumoplethysmography: determining the changes in the volume of the lung

proctosigmoidoscopy: fibroscopic examination of the sigmoid colon and rectum

retrograde: moving backward or against the usual direction of flow

spirometry: measurement of breathing capacity

subcutaneous: tissue below the dermis, primarily fat cells that insulate the body

thermogram: written record of temperature variation

tonography: recording of changes in intraocular pressure in response to sustained pressure on the eyeball

tonometry: measurement of pressure or tension

transcutaneous: entering by way of the skin

transesophageal echocardiogram (TEE): echocardiogram performed by placing a probe down the esophagus and sending out sound waves to obtain images of the heart and its movement

transseptal: through the septum

tympanometry: test of the inner ear using air pressure

vectorcardiogram (VCG): continuous recording of electrical direction and magnitude of the heart

CHAPTER REVIEW

CHAPTER 13, PART I, THEORY

Without the use of the CPT manual, answer the following questions:

1 There are two types of services in the Medicine section. One is diagnostic and the other is

_____ .

2 What do the following abbreviations mean?

   a. IV _____

   b. IM _____

   c. SQ _____

3 The routing of blood, including the waste products, outside of the body for cleansing is

_____ .

4 The dialysis that involves using the peritoneal cavity as a filter is known as what kind of dialysis?

_____

5 What is the name of the test that checks the intraocular pressure of the eye?

_____

6 What is the name of the scope that is used to examine color vision?

_____

7 What is the word that means the body of knowledge about the ear, nose, and larynx?

_____

8 In what subsection of the Medicine section would you find CPR, coronary atherectomies, and heart valvuloplasties? _____

_____

9 What kind of scanning uses ultrasonic technology with a display of both structure and motion with time? _____

10 What is the name of the ultrasonic documentation that records velocity mapping and imaging?

_____

11 In what Medicine subsection would you find therapies such as nebulizer treatments?

_____

12 Percutaneous, intracutaneous, and inhalation are examples of what from the Allergy subsection? _____

13 Allergenic extracts, venoms, biologicals, and food are examples of what from the Allergy subsection? _____

14 If you were looking for the code number to indicate the circumstance in which a physician sees a patient between the hours of 10 PM and 8 AM, in what subsection of the Medicine section would you find that code?

_____

CHAPTER 13, PART II, PRACTICAL

Using the CPT manual, code the following:

15 An 18-month-old established patient receives a diphtheria toxoid that is administered intramuscularly by the nurse.

Code(s): _____

16 An established patient receives a tetanus toxoid that is administered intramuscularly by the physician's assistant.

Code(s): _____

17 A DTP and an oral poliomyelitis vaccine (live) are administered to a new patient. A problem focused history and examination are done, and the medical decision-making is straightforward.

Code(s): _____

18 The physician administers an IV infusion for therapeutic purposes that takes 1 hour.

Code(s): _____

19 A patient brings his allergy medication into the office, and a single injection service is provided by the nurse.

Code(s): _____

20 A patient receives the initial 30-minute training for her prosthetic arm.

Code(s): _____

21 A patient has a bronchospasm evaluation before and after a spirometry that is administered to monitor his lung capacity.

Code(s): _____

22 Nasopharyngoscopy with endoscope

Code(s): _____

23 A 30-year-old with end-stage renal disease receives a full month of dialysis.

Code(s): _____

unit II

International Classification of Diseases, 9th Revision, Clinical Modification (ICD-9-CM)

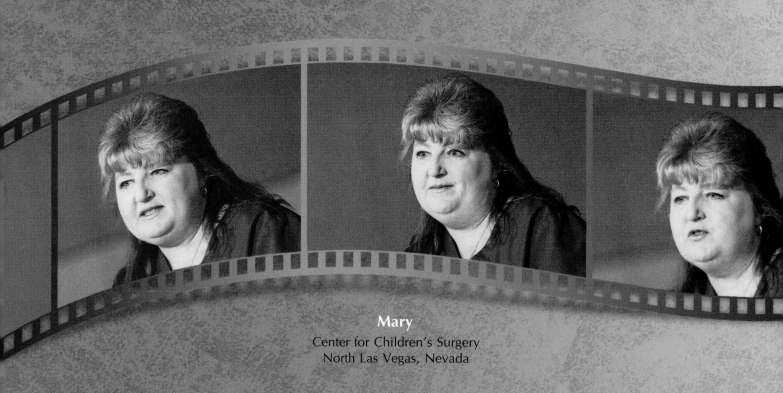

Mary
Center for Children's Surgery
North Las Vegas, Nevada

chapter 14

An Overview of the ICD-9-CM

LEARNING OBJECTIVES

After completing this chapter you should be able to

1   List the purposes of the ICD-9-CM.

2   Apply coding conventions when assigning codes.

3   Identify characteristics of Volumes 1, 2, and 3 formats.

4   Demonstrate use of ICD-9-CM.

5   Define chapter terminology.

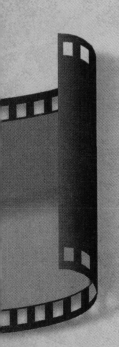

WHAT IS THE ICD-9-CM?

The International Classification of Diseases, 9th Revision, Clinical Modification (ICD-9-CM) is designed for the classification of patient morbidity (sickness) and mortality (death) information for statistical purposes and for the indexing of health records by disease and operation for data storage and retrieval.

The ICD-9-CM is based on the ICD-9—the 9th revision of the official version of the International Classification of Diseases compiled by the World Health Organization (WHO). In February 1977, a committee was convened by the National Center for Health Statistics to provide advice and counsel concerning the development of a clinical modification of the ICD-9. The ICD-9-CM is the resulting clinical modification (CM). The term "clinical" was used to emphasize the intent of the modification to serve as a tool in the area of classification of morbidity data for indexing of medical records, medical care review, ambulatory care, other medical care programs, and basic health statistics.

Through the years, the use of the ICD-9-CM (often called the ICD-9) has grown. The Medicare Catastrophic Coverage Act of 1988 (P.L. 100–330) required the submission of the appropriate ICD-9-CM diagnosis codes, with charges billed to Medicare Part B (outpatient services). The law was later repealed, but the coding requirement still stands.

Although coding was originally accomplished to provide access to medical records through retrieval for medical research, education, and administration, today codes are used to

- Facilitate payment of health services

- Evaluate patients' use of health care facilities (utilization patterns)

- Study health care costs

- Research the quality of health care

- Predict health care trends

- Plan for future health care needs

The use and results of coding are widespread and evident in our everyday lives. Many people hear the results of coding on a regular basis and don't even know it. Anytime you listen to the news and hear the newscaster refer to a specific number of AIDS cases in the United States or read a newspaper article about an epidemic of measles, you are seeing the results of ICD-9-CM coding. The ICD-9-CM is totally compatible with its parent system, ICD-9, thus meeting the need for comparability of morbidity and mortality statistics at the international level. The ICD-9-CM is a classification system for tracking morbidity and mortality. A classification system means that each condition or disease can be coded to only one code as much as possible to ensure the validity and reliability of data.

Coding must be performed correctly and consistently to produce meaningful statistics. (Refer to Figure 14–1 for the Standards of Ethical Coding.) To code accurately, it is necessary to have a working knowledge of medical terminology and to understand the guidelines, terminology, and conventions of the ICD-9-CM. Transforming verbal descriptions of diseases, injuries, conditions, and procedures into numeric designations is a complex activity and should not be undertaken without proper training. Learning to use the ICD-9-CM codes will be a valuable tool to you in any health care career.

Standards of Ethical Coding

In this era of payment based on diagnostic and procedural coding, the professional ethics of health information coding professionals continue to be challenged. A conscientious goal for coding and maintaining a quality database is accurate clinical and statistical data. The following standards of ethical coding, developed by AHIMA's Coding Policy and Strategy Committee and approved by AHIMA's Board of Directors, are offered to guide coding professionals in this process.

1. Coding professionals are expected to support the importance of accurate, complete, and consistent coding practices for the production of quality healthcare data.

2. Coding professionals in all healthcare settings should adhere to the ICD-9-CM (International Classification of Diseases, 9th Revision, Clinical Modification) coding conventions, official coding guidelines approved by the Cooperating Parties,* the CPT (Current Procedural Terminology) rules established by the American Medical Association, and any other official coding rules and guidelines established for use with mandated standard code sets. Selection and sequencing of diagnoses and procedures must meet the definitions of required data sets for applicable healthcare settings.

3. Coding professionals should use their skills, their knowledge of currently mandated coding and classification systems, and official resources to select the appropriate diagnostic and procedural codes.

4. Coding professionals should only assign and report codes that are clearly and consistently supported by physician documentation in the health record.

5. Coding professionals should consult physicians for clarification and additional documentation prior to code assignment when there is conflicting or ambiguous data in the health record.

6. Coding professionals should not change codes or the narratives of codes on the billing abstract so that meanings are misrepresented. Diagnoses or procedures should not be inappropriately included or excluded because payment or insurance policy coverage requirements will be affected. When individual payer policies conflict with official coding rules and guidelines, these policies should be obtained in writing whenever possible. Reasonable efforts should be made to educate the payer on proper coding practices in order to influence a change in the payer's policy.

7. Coding professionals, as members of the healthcare team, should assist and educate physicians and other clinicians by advocating proper documentation practices, further specificity, and resequencing or inclusion of diagnoses or procedures when needed to more accurately reflect the acuity, severity, and the occurrence of events.

8. Coding professionals should participate in the development of institutional coding policies and should ensure that coding policies complement, not conflict with, official coding rules and guidelines.

9. Coding professionals should maintain and continually enhance their coding skills, as they have a professional responsibility to stay abreast of changes in codes, coding guidelines, and regulations.

10. Coding professionals should strive for optimal payment to which the facility is legally entitled, remembering that it is unethical and illegal to maximize payment by means that contradict regulatory guidelines.

* The Official Coding Guidelines, published by the Cooperating Parties (American Hospital Association, American Health Information Management Association, Health Care Financing Administration and National Center for Health Statistics), should be followed in all facilities regardless of payment source.

Figure 14–1 Standards of Ethical Coding. (From American Health Information Management Association, 1999.)

EXERCISE 14–1

WHAT IS THE ICD-9-CM?

Using the information presented in this text, complete the following:

1 The ICD-9-CM is designed for the classification of patient

_____ or

_____ .

2 The ICD-9-CM manual is based on what text developed by the World Health Organization? _9th revision of the international classification_

3 The CM in ICD-9-CM stands for

_____ .

4 List four of the six reasons why the ICD-9-CM codes are used today.

_____

_____

_____

_____

5 The ICD-9-CM is used to translate what descriptive information into numeric codes? _____ and

_____

FORMAT AND CONVENTIONS USED IN THE ICD-9-CM

Several publishing companies produce editions of the ICD-9-CM manual. All editions are based on the official government version of the ICD-9-CM, as is this text.

Format

The ICD-9-CM manual is published in a three-volume set:

Volume 1   Diseases: Tabular List _lot of code by_
Volume 2   Diseases: Alphabetic Index
Volume 3   Procedures: Tabular List and Alphabetic Index _Hospital only procedure_

Read Vol 2 then 1

Volume 1 contains the disease and condition codes and the code descriptions (nomenclature) as well as the Supplementary Classification of Factors Influencing Health Status and Contact with Health Services (V codes) and External Causes of Injury and Poisoning (E codes). Volume 2 is the Alphabetic Index for Volume 1. Volumes 1 and 2 are used in inpatient and outpatient settings to substantiate medical services (medical necessity) by assigning diagnosis codes. Volume 3, used for coding procedures, contains codes for surgical, therapeutic, and diagnostic procedures and is used primarily by hospitals. ICD-9-CM codes are reported on the HCFA-1500 insurance claim form used in physician's offices and on the UB-92 form used in hospitals (Fig. 14–2). Private insurance carriers also require ICD-9-CM codes on forms submitted for payment for services.

There are four groups whose function it is to deal with in-depth coding principles and practices: Centers for Medicare and Medicaid Services (CMS), formerly the Health Care Financing Administration (HCFA); National Center for Health Statistics (NCHS); American Health Information Management Association (AHIMA); and American Hospital Association (AHA).

To begin the study of ICD-9-CM codes, you will be introduced to the format and content of the volumes. When the review has been completed, you will begin to practice locating codes for various diseases and illnesses using the ICD-9-CM manual, because the only way to learn to code is to practice. For now, just relax, and let's take a look at the format and content of each volume of the ICD-9-CM.

You might think that you would begin your study of the ICD-9-CM with Volume 1, the Tabular List, but you will begin with Volume 2 because this volume is the Alphabetic Index. Volume 2 is located at the beginning of the

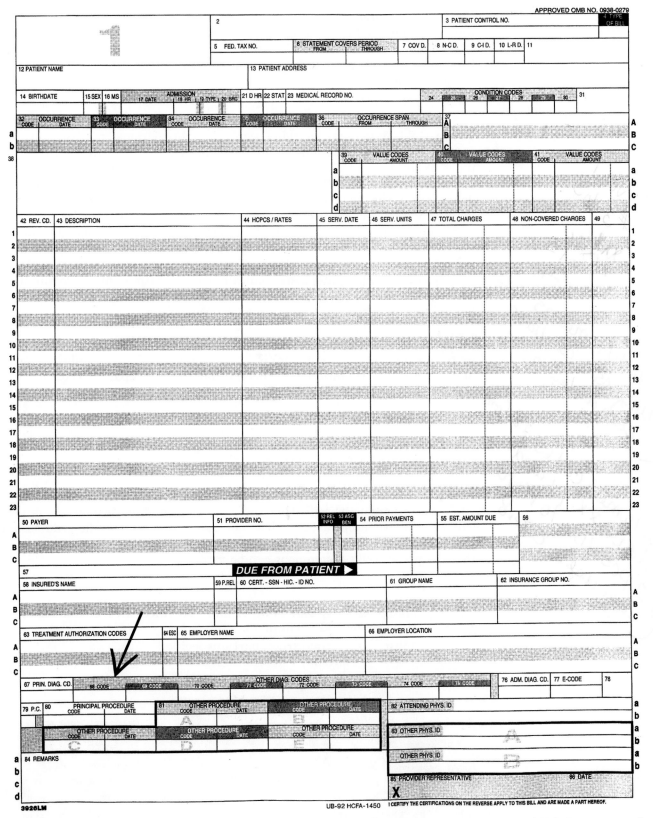

Figure 14–2   UB-92 HCFA-1450 is used by inpatient facilities for claims submissions. (Courtesy of U.S. Department of Health and Human Services, Centers for Medicare and Medicaid Services.)

ICD-9-CM manual and is followed by Volume 1. You began working with the CPT manual by learning how to locate items in the index and then moved on to the main text. We will use that same approach with the ICD-9-CM. But first, you need to know about the conventions that are used in all of the volumes.

Conventions

The ICD-9-CM manual contains symbols, abbreviations, punctuation, and notations called conventions. Some conventions are used in all three volumes of the ICD-9-CM manual, and others are used in only one or two of the volumes. The ICD-9-CM manual contains a list of the conventions and definitions to be used when assigning codes. It is important that you be familiar with the conventions as you prepare to use the ICD-9-CM codes.

Although the maintenance of the ICD-9-CM is the responsibility of the CMS, many private companies publish editions of the ICD-9-CM, and each publisher has its own conventions in addition to the standard conventions. For example, some publishers indicate that a fifth digit is required by placing a special symbol next to the code. These additional symbols are helpful to coders but are not a recognized convention.

NEC

NEC (not elsewhere classifiable) is to be used only when the information at hand specifies a condition but there is no specific separate code for that condition in the coding manual.

EXAMPLE

244.8	**Other specified acquired hypothyroidism**
	Secondary hypothyroidism NEC

NOS

NOS (not otherwise specified) is the equivalent of "unspecified." It is used when the information at hand does not permit a more specific code assignment. The coder should ask the physician for more specific information so that the proper code assignment can be made.

EXAMPLE

159	**Malignant neoplasm of other and ill-defined sites within the digestive organs and peritoneum**
159.0	**Intestinal tract, part unspecified**
	Intestine NOS

from the trenches

What advice would you give to a new coding professional?
"Listen, and read as much reference material as you can obtain."

MARY

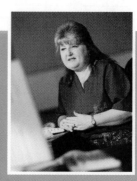

Brackets [ ]

Brackets are used to enclose synonyms, alternative wording, or explanatory phrases. They are found in the Tabular List.

EXAMPLE

426.8	**Other specified conduction disorders**
	Dissociation:
	atrioventricular [AV]
	interference
	isorhythmic
	Nonparoxysmal AV nodal tachycardia

[handwritten: Information (This is something Else it could be called tab only]

Parentheses ( )

Parentheses are used to enclose supplementary words that may be present or absent in the statement of a disease or procedure without affecting the code number to which it is assigned. Parentheses are found in both the Alphabetic Index and the Tabular List.

EXAMPLE

158	**Malignant neoplasm of retroperitoneum and peritoneum**
158.8	**Specified parts of peritoneum**
	Cul-de-sac (of Douglas)
	Mesentery

[handwritten: gives more info]

Colon :

Colons are used in the Tabular List after an incomplete term that needs one or more of the modifiers that follow in order to make it assignable to a given category.

[handwritten: could be any of these]

EXAMPLE

628	**Infertility, Female**
628.4	**Of cervical or vaginal origin**
	Infertility associated with:
	anomaly of cervical mucus
	congenital structural anomaly
	dysmucorrhea

Brace }

A brace is used to enclose a series of terms, each of which is modified by the statement appearing at the right of the brace.

EXAMPLE

473	**Chronic sinusitis**		
	Includes:	abscess	
		empyema	(chronic) of sinus
		infection	(accessory) (nasal)
		suppuration	

Lozenge □

In some versions of the ICD-9-CM, the lozenge symbol is printed in the left margin preceding the disease code to denote a four-digit number unique to the ICD-9-CM manual. The content of these codes in the ICD-9-CM is not the same as those in ICD-9. The lozenge symbol is used only in Volume 1,

Diseases: Tabular List. Coders seldom concern themselves with the differences between ICD-9-CM and ICD-9; however, these differences are important to researchers.

EXAMPLE

☐   **296.12   Manic disorder, recurrent episode, moderate**

Section Mark §

In some versions of the ICD-9-CM, the section mark in the Tabular List, Volume 1, indicates that a footnote is located at the bottom of the page.

EXAMPLE

§   **E807   Railway accident of unspecified nature**
The footnote on the page states:
§   Requires fourth digit.

Bold Type

Bold type is used for all codes and titles in the Tabular List in Volume 1.

EXAMPLE

244.8   Other specified acquired hypothyroidism
        Secondary hypothyroidism NEC

Italicized Type

Italicized type is used for all exclusion notes and to identify those codes that are not usually sequenced as the principal diagnosis. Italicized type codes cannot be assigned as a principal diagnosis because they always follow another code. Italicized codes are to be sequenced in the order specified in the Alphabetic Index, Volume 2, or according to specific coding instructions in the Tabular List, Volume 1, such as "code first . . . ."

EXAMPLE

420.0   Acute pericarditis in diseases classified elsewhere

        Code first underlying disease, as
            actinomycosis (039.8)
            amebiasis (006.8)
            nocardiosis (039.8)
            tuberculosis (017.9)
            uremia (585)

Slanted Brackets [ ] *code in Brackets would be listed second.*

Slanted brackets used in the Alphabetic Index, Volume 2, are used to enclose the manifestation of the underlying condition. When a code is listed inside the slanted brackets, you must sequence that code *after* the underlying condition code.

EXAMPLE

Diabetic retinal hemorrhage 362.01

    Hemorrhage, hemorrhagic (nontraumatic) 459.0
        retina, retinal (deep) (superficial) (vessels) 362.81
        1st diabetic 250.5 *[362.01]*

You would sequence the code 250.5X (the appropriate fifth digit would have to be included) and then 362.01 to indicate that the retinal hemorrhage was due to diabetes.

Includes

Includes notes appear in the Tabular List, Volume 1; they further define or provide examples and can apply to the chapter, section, or category. The notes at the beginning of a **chapter** apply to that entire chapter; the notes at the beginning of the **section** apply to that entire section; and the notes at the beginning of the **category** apply to that entire category. You have to refer to the beginning of the chapter or section for any Includes notes that refer to an entire chapter or section because the Includes notes are not repeated within the chapter or section. Includes notes can also be found before or after category codes.

Includes notes at the beginning of a chapter:

EXAMPLE

> ### 1. INFECTIOUS AND PARASITIC DISEASES (001–139)
>
> Note: Categories for "late effects" of infectious and parasitic diseases are to be found at 137–139.
>
> | INCLUDES | diseases generally recognized as communicable or transmissible as well as a few diseases of unknown but possibly infectious origin |
>
> | EXCLUDES | *acute respiratory infections* (460–466)
> *carrier or suspected carrier of infectious organism* (V02.0–V02.9)
> *certain localized infections*
> *influenza* (487.0–487.8) |

Includes notes at the beginning of a section:

EXAMPLE

> ### TUBERCULOSIS (010–018)
>
> | INCLUDES | infection by Mycobacterium tuberculosis (human) (bovine) |
>
> | EXCLUDES | *congenital tuberculosis* (771.2)
> *late effects of tuberculosis* (137.0–137.4) |

Includes notes at the beginning of a category (applies to the entire category):

EXAMPLE

> **006   Amebiasis**
>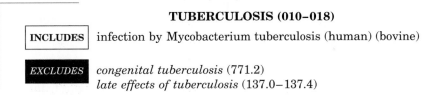
> | INCLUDES | infection due to Entamoeba histolytica |
>
> | EXCLUDES | *amebiasis due to organisms other than Entamoeba histolytica* (007.8) |
>
> **006.0   Acute amebic dysentery without mention of abscess**
> Acute amebiasis

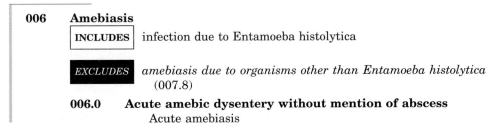

Excludes

Excludes notes appear in the Tabular List, Volume 1, and indicate terms that are to be coded elsewhere. *Excludes* notes can be located at the beginning of a chapter or section or below a category or subcategory. *Excludes* notes can be used for three reasons:

1. The condition may have to be coded elsewhere.

EXAMPLE

> **861   Injury to heart and lung**
>
>   *EXCLUDES*   *injury to blood vessels of thorax* (901.0–901.9)
>
> This *Excludes* note indicates that injuries to the blood vessels of the thorax are assigned within the codes 901.1–901.9 and are not assigned within the codes in 861.

2. The code cannot be assigned if the associated condition is present.

EXAMPLE

> **§ 463   Acute tonsillitis**
>
>   *EXCLUDES*   *streptococcal tonsillitis* (034.0)
>
> If the tonsillitis is caused by a streptococcal organism, it would be coded 034.0, not 463.

3. Additional codes may be required to fully explain the condition.

EXAMPLE

> **4. DISEASES OF BLOOD AND BLOOD-FORMING ORGANS (280–289)**
>
>   *EXCLUDES*   *Anemia complicating pregnancy or the puerperium* (648.2)
>
> This *Excludes* note tells you that you should code 648.2X (the appropriate fifth digit would have to be included) to indicate the complication of pregnancy, followed by an additional code to specify the type of anemia.

Use Additional Code

You add information (by assigning an additional code) to provide a more complete picture of the diagnosis or procedure. The use of an additional code is mandatory if supporting documentation is found in the record.

EXAMPLE

> **510   Empyema**
>
>   Use additional code to identify infectious organism (041.0–041.9)
>
> For example, if you are coding empyema due to pseudomonas, the codes would be Empyema (510.9), due to pseudomonas (041.7)

Code First Underlying Disease

The phrase "Code first underlying disease" is used in the categories in the Tabular List, Volume 1, and is not intended to indicate the principal diagnosis. In such cases, the code, title, and instructions appear in italics. The note requires that the underlying disease (etiology) be sequenced first.

EXAMPLE

> **366.4   Cataract associated with other disorders**
>
> ** *366.41   Diabetic cataract***
>
>   *Code first diabetes* (250.5)
>
> By following this convention, diabetes 250.5 is sequenced first, followed by diabetic cataract 366.41.

And and With

Although the two words "and" and "with" have similar meanings in everyday language, in ICD-9-CM terminology they have special significance and meanings. "And" means and/or, whereas "with" indicates that two conditions are included in the code.

And

EXAMPLE

474   Chronic disease of tonsils and adenoids

The code 474 is used to identify the disease as one of tonsils and/or adenoids.

With

EXAMPLE

366.4   Cataract associated with other disorders

366.41   Diabetic cataract

The code 366.4 indicates that the patient has cataracts along with another disorder, perhaps diabetes. To assign code 366.41, you have to be sure that both conditions are present.

EXERCISE 14-2

CONVENTIONS

Match the abbreviations, punctuation, symbols, and words to the correct descriptions:

1 [ ] *F*
2 NOS *G*
3 : *E, A*
4 § *I*
5 italics *H*
6 *Excludes* *L*
7 Includes *J*
8 } *E*
9 NEC *D*
10 ( ) *K*
11 [ ] *B*
12 bold type *C*

a. must be modified by an additional term to complete the code description

b. used in Volume 2 to enclose the disease manifestation codes that are to be recorded as secondary diagnoses to the diagnosis for the etiology

c. typeface used for all codes and titles in Volume 1

d. indicates the use of code assignment for "other" when a more specific code does not exist

e. encloses a series of terms that modify the statement to the right

f. encloses synonyms, alternative words, or explanatory phrases

g. equals unspecified

h. typeface used for all exclusion notes or diagnosis codes not to be used for principal diagnosis

i. footnote or section mark

j. appears under a three-digit code title to futher define or explain category content

k. encloses supplementary words that do not affect the code assignment

l. indicates terms that are to be coded elsewhere

Answer the following questions about conventions:

13 Includes and *Excludes* notes have no bearing on the code selection.
True   (False)

14 Brackets enclose synonyms, alternative wordings, or explanatory phrases.
(True)   False

VOLUME 2: ALPHABETIC INDEX

Modifiers

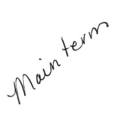

A main term in the index may be followed by a series of terms in parentheses. The presence or absence of these parenthetic terms in the diagnosis has no effect on the selection of the code listed for the main term. These are called **nonessential modifiers.**

EXAMPLE

Ileus (adynamic) (bowel) (colon) (inhibitory) (intestine) (neurogenic) (paralytic) 560.1

The nonessential modifiers are the words "(adynamic) (bowel) (colon)," and so forth. Nonessential modifiers are words that may be used to clarify the diagnosis but do not affect the code. The code for ileus is 560.1, and the code for adynamic ileus is also 560.1. The addition of the modifier "adynamic" does not affect the code assignment.

A main term may also be followed by a list of subterms that *do* have an effect on the selection of the appropriate code for a given diagnosis. These subterms are indented under the main term and offer additional specificity.

EXAMPLE

Incoordination
esophageal-pharyngeal (newborn) 787.2
muscular 781.3
papillary muscle 429.81

The term in parentheses, (newborn), is nonessential and merely supplementary. The indented subterms are essential modifiers, such as muscular or papillary muscle.

General adjectives such as "acute," "chronic," "epidemic," or "hereditary" and references to anatomic site, such as "arm," "stomach," and "uterus," will appear as main terms, but they will have a *"see"* or *"see also condition"* reference.

EXAMPLE

Hereditary—*see* condition
Uterus—*see* condition

You will now learn more about the *"see"* cross references.

Cross References

Cross references provide the coder with possible modifiers for a term or its synonyms. There are three types of cross references:

1. *see*
2. *see* also
3. *see* category

The "*see*" cross reference is an explicit direction to look elsewhere. It is used for anatomic sites and many general adjective modifiers not normally used in the Alphabetic Index. The "*see*" cross reference is also used to reference the appropriate main term under which all the information concerning a specific disease will be found.

EXAMPLE

> **Encephalomeningitis**—*see* Meningoencephalitis
>
> **Endamebiasis**—*see* Amebiasis
>
> **Kidney**—*see* condition
>
> **Leukosis**—*see* Leukemia
>
> **Lipofibroma** (M8851/0)—*see* Lipoma, by site

The "*see also*" cross reference directs you to look under another main term if all the information being searched for cannot be located under the first main term entry.

EXAMPLE

> **Laryngoplegia**—(*see also* Paralysis, vocal cord) 478.30

The "*see* category" cross reference directs you to Volume 1, Tabular List, for important information governing the use of the specific code.

EXAMPLE

> **Late**—*see also* condition
>   effect(s) (of)—*see also* condition
>   abscess
>   intracranial or intraspinal (conditions classifiable to 324)—*see* category 326

Notes

Certain main terms are followed by notes that are used to define terms and give coding instructions.

EXAMPLE

> **Amputation**
>   traumatic (complete) (partial)
>   arm 887.4
>   at or above elbow 887.2
>   complicated 887.3
>
> *Note: "Complicated" includes traumatic amputation with delayed healing, delayed treatment, foreign body, or major infection.*

Mandatory Fifth Digit

Notes are also used to list the fifth digit subclassifications for subcategories—such as the entries "Tuberculosis" or "Diabetes mellitus." Only the four-digit code is given for the individual entry, and you must refer to the note following the main term to locate the appropriate fifth digit subclassification. For example, Figure 14–3 shows the fifth digit's use when coding diabetes.

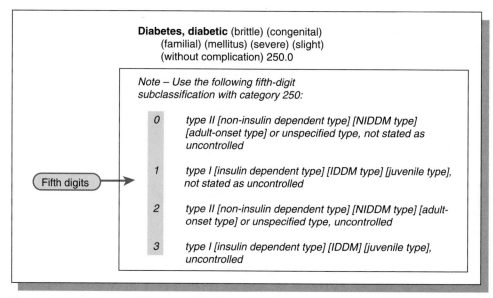

Figure 14–3   Index to Diseases, fifth digit, diabetes. (From International Classification of Diseases, 9th Revision. U.S. Department of Health and Human Services, Public Health Service, Centers for Medicare and Medicaid Services.)

Eponyms

Eponyms (diseases, procedures or syndromes named for persons) are listed both as main terms in their appropriate alphabetic sequence and under the main terms "Disease" or "Syndrome." A description of the disease or syndrome is usually included in parentheses following the eponym.

E X A M P L E

Crigler-Najjar disease or syndrome
   (congenital hyperbilirubinemia) 277.4
Disease
   Crigler-Najjar (congenital hyperbilirubinemia) 277.4
Syndrome
   Crigler-Najjar (congenital hyperbilirubinemia) 277.4

The cross reference feature will be very helpful to you as you code using the ICD-9-CM.

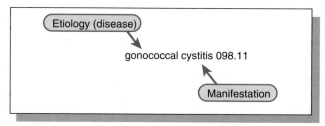

Figure 14–4   Manifestation and etiology, combination code. (From International Classification of Diseases, 9th Revision. U.S. Department of Health and Human Services, Public Health Service, Centers for Medicare and Medicaid Services.)

EXERCISE
14-3

MORE CONVENTIONS

Match the convention to the definition:

1   *see* category ___I G___
2   subterms ___B___
3   NEC ___I___
4   NOS ___E___
5   *see* ___C___
6   Notes ___D___
7   modifiers ___A___
8   *see also* ___F___
9   eponym ___H___

a. terms in parentheses or following main terms; they may or may not be essential

b. terms indented under main terms, considered essential modifiers

c. explicit direction to look elsewhere

d. follows code descriptions to define and give instructions

e. means "unspecified"

f. directs coder to look under another term if all information isn't found under the first term

g. directs coder to use Volume 1, Tabular List, for additional information

h. disease, procedure, or syndrome named for a person

i. tells the coder to use code assignment for "other" if a more specific code does not exist

Fill in the blanks in the following questions:

10   Which coding convention advises you that a more specific code is not available? _____

11   What directs you to look under another main term?

_____

Etiology and Manifestation of Disease

For certain conditions it is important to record both the etiology (cause) and the manifestation (symptom) of the disease. In many cases, the recording of the etiology and manifestation can be accomplished by using a single five-digit code. The single five-digit code is termed a **combination code.** For example, Figure 14–4 shows the etiology and manifestation combined in one code. The etiology is gonococcal, and the manifestation is cystitis; both are represented by the code 098.11.

For some conditions it is not possible to provide specific fifth digit sub-classifications that indicate both etiology and manifestation. Multiple coding is then required. In such cases the two facets of the disease—etiology and manifestation—are coded individually, as in Figure 14–5.

CAUTION *It is important to record the multiple codes in the same sequence as that used in the Alphabetic Index.*

Chapter 15 provides more information about the use of combination and multiple codes.

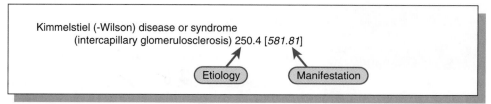

Kimmelstiel (-Wilson) disease or syndrome
(intercapillary glomerulosclerosis) 250.4 [581.81]

Etiology   Manifestation

Figure 14–5 Manifestation and etiology, multiple coding. (From International Classification of Diseases, 9th Revision. U.S. Department of Health and Human Services, Public Health Service, Centers for Medicare and Medicaid Services.)

Hypertension Table

The Hypertension Table is found in the Alphabetic Index under the main term "Hypertension." The table contains a complete list of all conditions due to or associated with hypertension. The table classifies the hypertension conditions according to malignant, benign, or unspecified. Hypertension codes will be discussed in greater detail in the hypertension guidelines in Chapter 15.

Neoplasms

Neoplasms are tumors. Two steps are needed to locate the neoplasm code in the Alphabetic Index. The first step is to locate the neoplasm by its name or

Neoplasm   **INDEX TO DISEASES**

	Malignant			Benign	Uncertain Behavior	Unspecified
	Primary	Secondary	Ca in situ			
Neoplasm, neoplastic—*continued*						
breast (connective tissue) (female) (glandular tissue) (soft parts)	174.9	198.81	233.0	217	238.3	239.3
areola	174.0	198.81	233.0	217	238.3	239.3
male	175.0	198.81	233.0	217	238.3	239.3
axillary tail	174.6	198.81	233.0	217	238.3	239.3
central portion	174.1	198.81	233.0	217	238.3	239.3
contiguous sites	174.8	—	—	—	—	—
ectopic sites	174.8	198.81	233.0	217	238.3	239.3
inner	174.8	198.81	233.0	217	238.3	239.3
lower	174.8	198.81	233.0	217	238.3	239.3
lower-inner quadrant	174.3	198.81	233.0	217	238.3	239.3
lower-outer quadrant	174.5	198.81	233.0	217	238.3	239.3
male	175.9	198.81	233.0	217	238.3	239.3
areola	175.0	198.81	233.0	217	238.3	239.3
ectopic tissue	175.9	198.81	233.0	217	238.3	239.3
nipple	175.0	198.81	233.0	217	238.3	239.3
mastectomy site (skin)	173.5	198.2	—	—	—	—
specified as breast tissue	174.8	198.81	—	—	—	—
midline	174.8	198.81	233.0	217	238.3	239.3
nipple	174.0	198.81	233.0	217	238.3	239.3

Figure 14–6 M Codes, Section 1, Index to Disease, breast. (From International Classification of Diseases, 9th Revision. U.S. Department of Health and Human Services, Public Health Service, Centers for Medicare and Medicaid Services.)

its morphology. For example, glioma, lymphoma, and adenoma are considered histologic types and are found in the Alphabetic Index. This is where hospital coders will locate the M codes to classify the morphology of the tumor. You follow the instructions in the Index to reach the proper code in the Tabular List. If you wanted to locate the correct neoplasm code for adenocarcinoma, you would find the following entry in the Index.

EXAMPLE

> **Adenocarcinoma** (M8140/3)—*see also*
>   Neoplasm, by site, malignant

This "*see also*" instruction means you are to refer to the Neoplasm Table to locate the appropriate code.

The second step is to locate the Neoplasm Table in the Alphabetic Index under "N" for neoplasm. The Neoplasm Table is organized on the basis of anatomic site. A comprehensive list of anatomic sites with subterms for greater specificity is found in this table under the main term, "Neoplasm." The table contains six columns, as indicated in Figure 14–6. For each site there are six possible code numbers; the proper code is determined by whether the neoplasm in question is malignant, and then by further specifying the malignancy as primary, secondary, or in situ (confined to the original site); benign; of uncertain behavior; or of unspecified nature. A malignant tumor is one that becomes progressively worse, and a benign tumor is one that is not malignant.

EXERCISE 14-4

NEOPLASMS

Referring to Figure 14–6, fill in the codes for the following:

1   Secondary malignant tumor of a male, breast, nipple

Code(s): _____

2   Benign neoplasm, breast, female

Code(s): _____

STOP *Morphology codes are used to supplement the appropriate ICD-9-CM neoplasm code. A complete listing of morphology codes is found in Appendix A of Volume 1, Morphology of Neoplasms, and is presented later in this chapter. M codes are optional; whether you assign these codes may depend on the particular facility's policy.*

Sections

Volume 2: Alphabetic Index serves as an index to Volume 1, Tabular List. Everything in the index is listed by condition—meaning diagnosis, signs, symptoms, and conditions such as pregnancy, admission, encounter, or complication. Volume 2: Alphabetic Index contains three sections, as illustrated in Figure 14–7.

Section 1 contains terms referring to diseases and injuries in alphabetic order.

TABLE OF CONTENTS

Volume 2

Figure 14–7   Volume 2, Table of Contents. (From International Classification of Diseases, 9th Revision. U.S. Department of Health and Human Services, Public Health Service, Centers for Medicare and Medicaid Services.)

Section 2 is the Table of Drugs and Chemicals and it includes codes for poisonings and external causes of injury by drugs or chemicals.

Section 3 is the Index to External Causes (E Codes); it is an alphabetic index of the causes of accidents and injuries.

Section 1: Index to Diseases and Injuries

Section 1 is the largest portion of the Alphabetic Index. To locate a code in the Tabular List, you must first locate the possible code in the Alphabetic Index. In the Index, main terms (conditions) are in bold type, and indented subterms (modifying words for additional specificity) are in regular type.

Main Terms and Subterms

Main terms in the Alphabetic Index are in bold type, and subterms are indented two spaces to the right.

EXAMPLE

Fracture
  styloid process
    metacarpal (closed) 815.02
      open 815.12

from the trenches

What is the one personality trait that all coders should have?
"Ethics."

                                              MARY

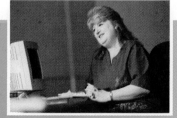

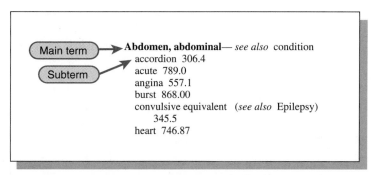

Figure 14–8 Volume 2, Format. (From International Classification of Diseases, 9th Revision. U.S. Department of Health and Human Services, Public Health Service, Centers for Medicare and Medicaid Services.)

Each term is followed by the code or codes that apply to the term (Fig. 14–8). The Alphabetic Index includes most diagnostic terms currently in use. Some types of codes may be a little difficult to find, such as those dealing with complications, late effects, and V codes.

Section 2: Table of Drugs and Chemicals

Section 2, Table of Drugs and Chemicals, contains a classification of drugs and other chemical substances associated with poisoning and external causes of adverse effects.

In Figure 14–9, the Table of Drugs and Chemicals shows that column 1 (Substance) contains the name of the drug or chemical. Column 2 (Poisoning) contains the list of poisoning codes. The remaining five columns are the E codes that are assigned to indicate how the poisoning or adverse effect occurred. Remember, E codes are never the principal diagnosis. The table headings pertaining to external causes are defined as follows:

Accident (E850–E869): instances of accidental overdose of a drug, wrong substance given or taken, drug taken inadvertently, accidents in the use of drugs and biological agents during medical and surgical procedures, and external causes of poisonings classifiable to 980–989.

Therapeutic Use (E930–E949): instances in which a correct substance properly administered in therapeutic or prophylactic dosage has been the external cause of adverse effects.

Suicide Attempt (E950–E952): instances in which self-inflicted injuries or poisonings have been involved.

Assault (E961–E962): instances in which injury or poisoning has been inflicted by another person with the intent to injure or kill.

Undetermined (E980–E982): instances in which it cannot be determined whether the poisoning or injury was intentional or accidental.

The table also contains the American Hospital Formulary Service (AHFS) List numbers, which can be used to classify new drugs not listed in the table by name. The AHFS List numbers are found in the Table of Drugs and Chemicals under the main term "Drug." The AHFS List numbers and their ICD-9-CM equivalents are also found in Appendix C of Volume 1, Tabular List.

Although certain substances are indexed with one or more subentries, the majority are listed according to one use or state (i.e., solid, liquid, or gas). It is recognized that many substances may be used in various ways, in medicine and in industry, and may cause adverse effects or poisoning whatever the state of the agent. In cases in which the reported data indicate a use or

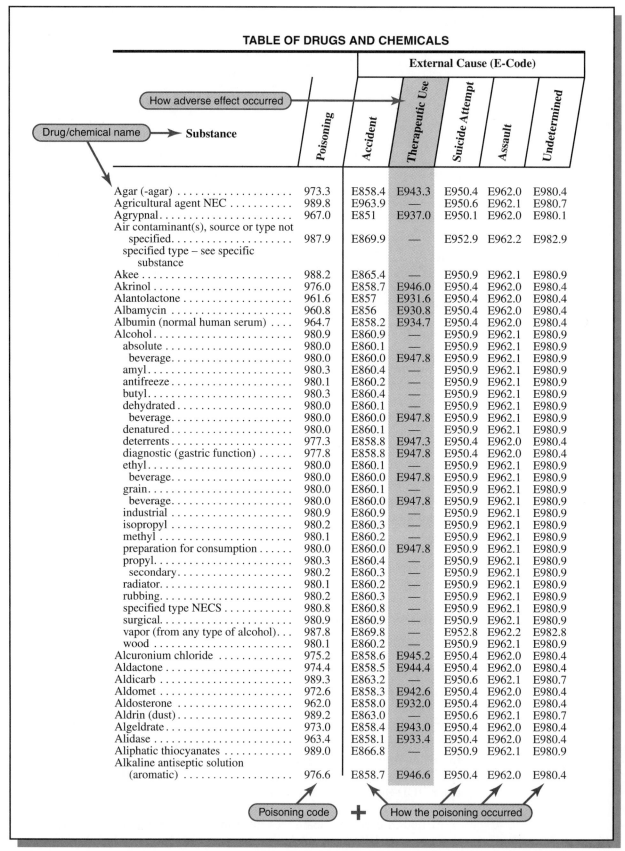

TABLE OF DRUGS AND CHEMICALS

Substance	Poisoning	Accident	Therapeutic Use	Suicide Attempt	Assault	Undetermined
Agar (-agar)	973.3	E858.4	E943.3	E950.4	E962.0	E980.4
Agricultural agent NEC	989.8	E963.9	—	E950.6	E962.1	E980.7
Agrypnal	967.0	E851	E937.0	E950.1	E962.0	E980.1
Air contaminant(s), source or type not specified	987.9	E869.9	—	E952.9	E962.2	E982.9
specified type – see specific substance						
Akee	988.2	E865.4	—	E950.9	E962.1	E980.9
Akrinol	976.0	E858.7	E946.0	E950.4	E962.0	E980.4
Alantolactone	961.6	E857	E931.6	E950.4	E962.0	E980.4
Albamycin	960.8	E856	E930.8	E950.4	E962.0	E980.4
Albumin (normal human serum)	964.7	E858.2	E934.7	E950.4	E962.0	E980.4
Alcohol	980.9	E860.9	—	E950.9	E962.1	E980.9
absolute	980.0	E860.1	—	E950.9	E962.1	E980.9
beverage	980.0	E860.0	E947.8	E950.9	E962.1	E980.9
amyl	980.3	E860.4	—	E950.9	E962.1	E980.9
antifreeze	980.1	E860.2	—	E950.9	E962.1	E980.9
butyl	980.3	E860.4	—	E950.9	E962.1	E980.9
dehydrated	980.0	E860.1	—	E950.9	E962.1	E980.9
beverage	980.0	E860.0	E947.8	E950.9	E962.1	E980.9
denatured	980.0	E860.1	—	E950.9	E962.1	E980.9
deterrents	977.3	E858.8	E947.3	E950.4	E962.0	E980.4
diagnostic (gastric function)	977.8	E858.8	E947.8	E950.4	E962.0	E980.4
ethyl	980.0	E860.1	—	E950.9	E962.1	E980.9
beverage	980.0	E860.0	E947.8	E950.9	E962.1	E980.9
grain	980.0	E860.1	—	E950.9	E962.1	E980.9
beverage	980.0	E860.0	E947.8	E950.9	E962.1	E980.9
industrial	980.9	E860.9	—	E950.9	E962.1	E980.9
isopropyl	980.2	E860.3	—	E950.9	E962.1	E980.9
methyl	980.1	E860.2	—	E950.9	E962.1	E980.9
preparation for consumption	980.0	E860.0	E947.8	E950.9	E962.1	E980.9
propyl	980.3	E860.4	—	E950.9	E962.1	E980.9
secondary	980.2	E860.3	—	E950.9	E962.1	E980.9
radiator	980.1	E860.2	—	E950.9	E962.1	E980.9
rubbing	980.2	E860.3	—	E950.9	E962.1	E980.9
specified type NECS	980.8	E860.8	—	E950.9	E962.1	E980.9
surgical	980.9	E860.9	—	E950.9	E962.1	E980.9
vapor (from any type of alcohol)	987.8	E869.8	—	E952.8	E962.2	E982.8
wood	980.1	E860.2	—	E950.9	E962.1	E980.9
Alcuronium chloride	975.2	E858.6	E945.2	E950.4	E962.0	E980.4
Aldactone	974.4	E858.5	E944.4	E950.4	E962.0	E980.4
Aldicarb	989.3	E863.2	—	E950.6	E962.1	E980.7
Aldomet	972.6	E858.3	E942.6	E950.4	E962.0	E980.4
Aldosterone	962.0	E858.0	E932.0	E950.4	E962.0	E980.4
Aldrin (dust)	989.2	E863.0	—	E950.6	E962.1	E980.7
Algeldrate	973.0	E858.4	E943.0	E950.4	E962.0	E980.4
Alidase	963.4	E858.1	E933.4	E950.4	E962.0	E980.4
Aliphatic thiocyanates	989.0	E866.8	—	E950.9	E962.1	E980.9
Alkaline antiseptic solution (aromatic)	976.6	E858.7	E946.6	E950.4	E962.0	E980.4

Figure 14–9 Section 2, Table of Drugs and Chemicals. (From International Classification of Diseases, 9th Revision. U.S. Department of Health and Human Services, Public Health Service, Centers for Medicare and Medicaid Services.)

state not in the table, or one that is clearly different from those listed, an attempt should be made to classify the substances in the category that most nearly expresses the reported facts.

<table>
<tr><td>

EXERCISE
14-5

</td><td>

TABLE OF DRUGS AND CHEMICALS

Using the ICD-9-CM manual, code the following:

1 Poisoning by the ingestion of the beverage grain alcohol

Code(s): _____

2 Undetermined poisoning by antifreeze

Code(s): _____

3 Accidental overdose due to therapeutically used akrinol

Code(s): _____

Manifestations (symptoms or signs) of poisonings and adverse effects of drugs and chemicals are found in Section 1, under the specific symptom or disease. For example, Figure 14–10 illustrates the location of the symptom Rash in Volume 2, the Alphabetic Index. If the symptom of the drug poisoning or adverse effect is a rash, the subterm "drug (internal use)" directs you to 693.0.

Turn to code 693.0 in Volume 1, Tabular List.

4 What does the description of the code state?

_____

Note the statement below the code: "Use additional E code to identify drug." In this case the condition is a rash. So when you see this statement, you know you have to identify the drug that *caused* the rash.

</td></tr>
</table>

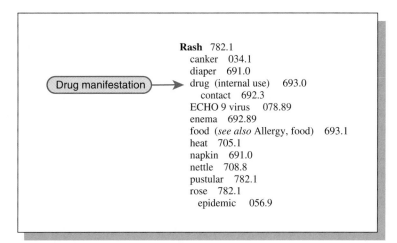

Figure 14–10 Index to Diseases, Rash. (From International Classification of Diseases, 9th Revision. U.S. Department of Health and Human Services, Public Health Service, Centers for Medicare and Medicaid Services.)

Section 3: Alphabetic Index to External Causes of Injuries and Poisonings (E Code)

Section 3: Alphabetic Index to External Causes of Injuries and Poisonings is the index for the E codes. The index classifies environmental events (tornadoes, floods), circumstances, and other conditions as the cause of injury and other adverse effects alphabetically. *E codes are never used as a principal diagnosis.* Rather, E codes are used to clarify the cause of an injury or adverse effect.

E code terms describe the circumstances under which an accident, injury, or act of violence occurred. The main terms in this section usually represent the type of accident or violence (e.g., assault, collision), with the specific agent or other circumstance listed below the main term. "Collision" in Figure 14–11 is the type of accident, and listed below collision are the circumstances of the accident.

You must be sure to read all the information under a term before choosing the code. Be sure to check for fourth digit specificity for railway accidents, motor vehicle traffic and nontraffic accidents, other road vehicle accidents, water transport accidents, and air and space transport accidents shown in the Index to External Causes section.

VOLUME 1: TABULAR LIST

Divisions

Volume 1: Tabular List is the listing of all the code numbers available for assignment, including their descriptions. When the exact word is not found in the code description in the Tabular List but the descriptive word is found in the Alphabetic Index, you must trust the code provided in the Alphabetic Index to be correct because the Index contains descriptive words that the Tabular List does not. Not listing all possible descriptive terms in the Tabular List saves space.

Anything that can happen, in the way of injury or disease, to a human body has a code number in Volume 1. Although there are certainly many things that can happen to us, the people who developed the ICD-9-CM not only included them all but organized them in a systematic way. Volume 1 is separated into two major divisions:

1. Classification of Diseases and Injuries
2. Supplementary Classification

Classification of Diseases and Injuries

The Classification of Diseases and Injuries is the main part of the ICD-9-CM, Volume 1, Tabular List; it consists of 17 chapters with codes ranging from 001 to 999. Figure 14–12 illustrates that most chapters are based on body system (e.g., nervous system [Chapter 6], respiratory system [Chapter 8], and digestive system [Chapter 9]). Some chapters are based on the cause or type of disease (e.g., infectious and parasitic diseases [Chapter 1] and neoplasms [Chapter 2]). Figure 14–13 indicates the format of each chapter.

Chapter
A chapter is the main division in the ICD-9-CM manual.

Section
A section is a group of three-digit categories that represent a group of conditions or related conditions.

Category
A three-digit category is a code that represents a single condition or disease.

INDEX TO EXTERNAL CAUSES   **Collision**

Type →

Circumstance →

Collision (accidental) — *continued*
  motor vehicle (on public highway) (traffic
    accident) — *continued*
  and — *continued*
    fallen — *continued*
      tree E815
      guard post or guard rail E815
      inter-highway divider E815
      landslide, fallen or not moving E815
        moving E909
      machinery (road) E815
      nonmotor road vehicle NEC E813
      object (any object, person, or vehicle
          off the public highway resulting
          from a noncollision motor vehicle
          nontraffic accident) E815
        off, normally not on, public
            highway resulting from a
            noncollision motor vehicle
            traffic accident E816
      pedal cycle E813
      pedestrian (conveyance) E814
      person (using pedestrian conveyance)
          E814
      post or pole (lamp) (light) (signal)
          (telephone) (utility) E815
      railway rolling stock, train, vehicle
          E810
      safety island E815
      street car E813
      traffic signal, sign, or marker
          (temporary) E815
      tree E815
      tricycle E813
      wall of cut made for road E815
    due to cataclysm — *see* categories E908,
        E909
    not on public highway, nontraffic
        accident E822
    and
      animal (carrying person, property)
          (herded) (unattended) E822
      animal-drawn vehicle E822
      another motor vehicle (moving),
          except off-road motor vehicle
          E822
        stationary E823
      avalanche, fallen, not moving
          E823
        moving E909
      landslide, fallen, not moving E823
        moving E909
      nonmotor vehicle (moving) E822
        stationary E823
      object (fallen) (normally) (fixed)
          (movable but not in motion)
          (stationary) E823
        moving, except when falling
            from, set in motion by,
            aircraft or cataclysm E822

Collision (accidental) — *continued*
  motor vehicle (on public highway) (traffic
    accident) — *continued*
  not on public highway, nontraffic
      accident — *continued*
  and — *continued*
      pedal cycle (moving) E822
        stationary E823
      pedestrian (conveyance) E822
      person (using pedestrian
          conveyance) E822
      railway rolling stock, train, vehicle
          (moving) E822
        stationary E823
      road vehicle (any) (moving) E822
        stationary E823
      tricycle (moving) E822
        stationary E823
    off-road type motor vehicle (not on public
        highway) E821
    and
      animal (being ridden) (-drawn vehicle)
          E821
      another off-road motor vehicle, except
          snow vehicle E821
      other motor vehicle, not on public
          highway E821
      other object or vehicle NEC, fixed or
          movable, not set in motion by
          aircraft, motor vehicle on
          highway, or snow vehicle, motor-
          driven E821
      pedal cycle E821
      pedestrian (conveyance) E821
      railway train E821
    on public highway — *see* Collision,
        motor vehicle
  pedal cycle E826
    and
      animal (carrying person, property)
          (herded) (unherded) E826
      animal-drawn vehicle E826
      another pedal cycle E826
      nonmotor road vehicle E826
      object (fallen) (fixed) (movable)
          (moving) not falling from or set
          in motion by aircraft, motor
          vehicle, or railway train NEC
          E826
      pedestrian (conveyance) E826
      person (using pedestrian conveyance)
          E826
      street car E826
  pedestrian(s) (conveyance) E917.9
    with fall E886.9
      in sports E886.0
    and
      crowd, human stampede (with fall)
          E917.1
      machinery — *see* Accident, machine

Figure 14–11   Section 3, Index to External Causes. (From International Classification of Diseases, 9th Revision. U.S. Department of Health and Human Services, Public Health Service, Centers for Medicare and Medicaid Services.)

TABLE OF CONTENTS

Figure 14–12 Volume 1, Diseases: Table of Contents. (From International Classification of Diseases, 9th Revision. U.S. Department of Health and Human Services, Public Health Service, Centers for Medicare and Medicaid Services.)

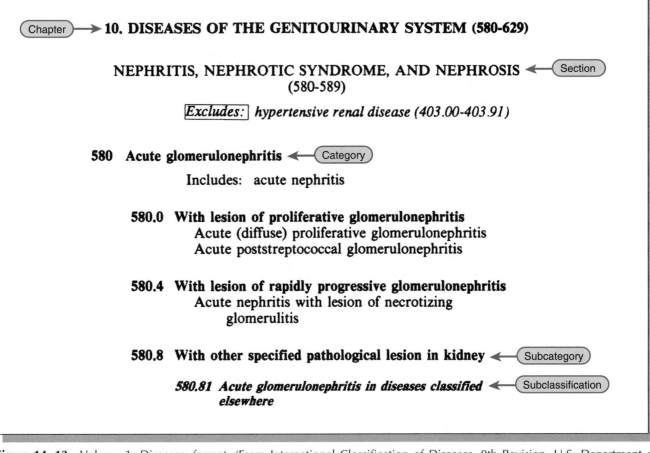

Chapter → **10. DISEASES OF THE GENITOURINARY SYSTEM (580-629)**

NEPHRITIS, NEPHROTIC SYNDROME, AND NEPHROSIS ← **Section**
(580-589)

Excludes: *hypertensive renal disease (403.00-403.91)*

580 Acute glomerulonephritis ← **Category**
         Includes: acute nephritis

580.0 With lesion of proliferative glomerulonephritis
             Acute (diffuse) proliferative glomerulonephritis
             Acute poststreptococcal glomerulonephritis

580.4 With lesion of rapidly progressive glomerulonephritis
             Acute nephritis with lesion of necrotizing
                 glomerulitis

580.8 With other specified pathological lesion in kidney ← **Subcategory**

580.81 Acute glomerulonephritis in diseases classified ← **Subclassification**
elsewhere

Figure 14–13 Volume 1, Diseases: format. (From International Classification of Diseases, 9th Revision. U.S. Department of Health and Human Services, Public Health Service, Centers for Medicare and Medicaid Services.)

Subcategory
    A four-digit subcategory code provides more information or specificity as compared to the three-digit code in terms of the cause, site, or manifestation of the condition. You must assign the fourth digit if it is available.

Subclassification
    A five-digit subclassification code adds even more information and specificity to a condition's description. You must assign the fifth digit if it is available.

EXERCISE 14-6

ICD-9-CM CHAPTER FORMAT

Using ICD-9-CM, Volume 1, Tabular List, locate the first page of Chapter 3 and answer the following questions about the chapter:

1 The name of the chapter: _____

2 The name of the first section: _____

3 The description of the first category: _____

4 The description of the first subcategory: _____

STOP *The information in this activity was important to your learning because it will enable you to communicate effectively about information in the ICD-9-CM manual using common terminology.*

Figure 14–14 illustrates the indented format used in Volume 1, Tabular List, for ease of reference.

The basic ICD-9-CM code is a three-digit code, as shown in Figure 14–15. Each code is a rubric (something under which something else is classed). Both the code number and the entry are in bold type. Diagnosis codes always contain at least three digits before the decimal point. If the diagnosis code is "1," it is written 001. Procedure codes from Volume 3 always consist of two digits, both placed before the decimal point. You can always tell a procedure code from a diagnosis code by noting the number of digits before the decimal point.

EXAMPLE

496	Diagnosis
27.54	Procedure
461.9	Diagnosis
21.1	Procedure

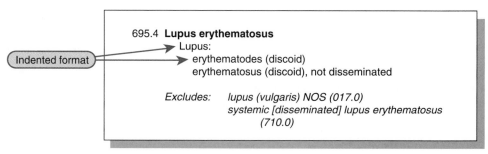

Figure 14–14 Indented format. (From International Classification of Diseases, 9th Revision. U.S. Department of Health and Human Services, Public Health Service, Centers for Medicare and Medicaid Services.)

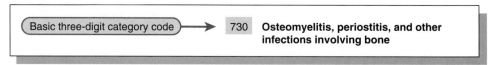

Figure 14–15 ICD-9-CM three-digit category code. (From International Classification of Diseases, 9th Revision. U.S. Department of Health and Human Services, Public Health Service, Centers for Medicare and Medicaid Services.)

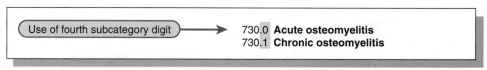

Figure 14–16 ICD-9-CM four-digit subcategory code.

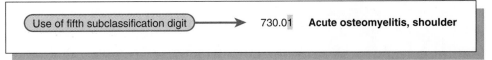

Figure 14–17   ICD-9-CM five-digit subclassification code.

Five-Digit Specificity

The addition of the fourth and fifth digits to the basic three-digit code provides greater specificity to the numeric designation of the patient's condition and reduces third-party returns. When four digits (one digit after the decimal point) are used, they are called *subcategory* codes. If five digits are used (two digits after the decimal point), they are called *subclassification* codes. Figure 14–16 shows the first three digits of the code used to identify the disease "Osteomyelitis, periostitis, and other infections involving bone"; the fourth digit provides further specificity by distinguishing between acute and chronic osteomyelitis.

Not all codes have fourth or fifth digits, but when a fourth or fifth digit is available, it must be used. It is a good idea to highlight the codes with which a fifth digit is listed. This will serve as a reminder to you to always use that fifth digit. For an example of the fifth digit: Code 730 appears with a list of fifth digits that are used to identify the location of acute osteomyelitis as

0	site unspecified
1	shoulder region
2	upper arm
3	forearm
4	hand
5	pelvic region and thigh
6	lower leg
7	ankle and foot
8	other specified sites
9	multiple sites

You indicate that acute osteomyelitis is located in the patient's shoulder by adding the fifth digit 1 to the 730.0 code (Fig. 14–17).

Remember that the goal is to be as accurate, as complete, and as specific as possible. The code(s) selected must be supported by physician documentation. If a coder notes an abnormal laboratory result, the physician should be queried before additional codes are added. Fig. 14–18 illustrates how adding the fourth and fifth digits adds specificity to the information about the patient's condition.

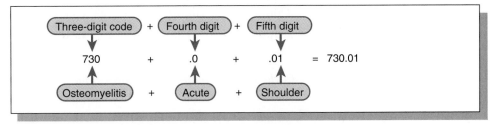

Figure 14–18   Specificity in ICD-9-CM codes.

EXERCISE 14-7

FIVE-DIGIT SPECIFICITY

Locate the first page of Chapter 13, Diseases of the Musculoskeletal System and Connective Tissues, in the ICD-9-CM manual. Notes immediately following the chapter title indicate the fifth digit subclassifications and the specific categories with which these fifth digits are used. Read the notes for Chapter 13.

The following is a part of the fifth digit subclassifications used with categories 711–712, 715–716, 718–719, and 730:

0   site unspecified

1   shoulder region
      Acromioclavicular ⎤
      Glenohumeral   ⎬ Joint(s)
      Sternoclavicular ⎦
      Clavicle
      Scapula

2   upper arm
      Elbow joint
      Humerus

The various joints of the shoulder region or the elbow joint and humerus of the upper arm are the specific anatomic terms to which the main term refers. The use of the 2 indicates the elbow joint, the humerus, and so forth. These anatomic terms serve to provide further specificity to the code selection.

Locate code 711 in the ICD-9-CM manual, then answer the following:

The patient record states: Pyogenic arthritis in lower leg.

1 What would the correct five-digit code be?

      Code(s): _____

2 Is the use of the fifth digit optional? _____

3 How is specificity added to ICD-9-CM codes?

    _____

    _____

Supplementary Classification

The Supplementary Classification in Volume 1 contains the following:

1. Supplementary Classification of Factors Influencing Health Status and Contact with Health Services (V codes)

2. Supplementary Classification of External Causes of Injury and Poisoning (E codes)

V Codes: Supplementary Classification of Factors Influencing Health Status and Contact with Health Services

V codes from the Supplementary Classification of Factors Influencing Health Status and Contact with Health Services are found under such main term references as admission, examination, history, observation, and problem. V codes are used under the following circumstances:

- When a person who is not currently sick encounters health services for some specific purpose, such as to act as a donor or receive a vaccination

- When a person with a known disease or injury presents for specific treatment of that condition—such as dialysis, chemotherapy, or cast change

- When a circumstance may influence a patient's health status

- To indicate the birth status and outcome of delivery of a newborn

The Supplementary Classification is located near the back of Volume 1, Tabular List, and contains three- or four-digit code numbers preceded by the letter V. The codes in this section are called V codes. The V codes deal with occasions in which persons who are not currently sick use health care services. This can arise mainly in two ways:

1. When a person who is currently not sick encounters the health services for some specific purpose, such as to act as donor of an organ or tissue, to receive a preventive vaccination, or to discuss a problem that is in itself not a disease or injury. Occurrences such as these will be fairly rare among hospital inpatients but will be relatively more common among outpatients at health clinics.

EXAMPLE

Code V59.4 indicates a donor of a kidney; the donor is not sick but encounters health care:

V59   Donors

    V59.4   Kidney

V59 is the category and V59.4 is the subcategory. You would first locate Donor, kidney, in the Index (Volume 2), and then verify code V59 in the V codes in the Tabular List.

EXAMPLE

A well child receives a polio vaccination:

V04   Need for prophylactic vaccination and inoculation against certain viral diseases

    V04.0   Poliomyelitis

Code V04.0 indicates a patient who is not ill but encounters health care for a polio vaccination. V04 is the category and V04.0 is the subcategory.

The Index (Volume 2) entry is vaccination, poliomyelitis. If you want to indicate that a child had been in contact with poliomyelitis, assign code V01.2, which has an Index location of Contact, poliomyelitis.

EXAMPLE

A student seeks health care to discuss a problem with school:

V62   Other psychosocial circumstances

    V62.3   Educational circumstances
        Dissatisfaction with school environment

V62 is the category code and V62.3 is the subcategory code.

Code V62.3 indicates a patient who is not ill but encounters health care for a psychosocial circumstance. Index location is Dissatisfaction with, education.

2. When some circumstance or problem is present that influences the person's health status but is not in itself a current illness or injury. For example, a family history of malignant neoplasms is significant to the patient's health care.

EXAMPLE

> **V16   Family history of malignant neoplasm**
>
> **V16.0   Gastrointestinal tract**

V16 is the category and V16.0 is the subcategory. The Index location is History, family, malignant neoplasm, gastrointestinal tract. If, however, the diagnosis was a personal history of malignant neoplasm, the Index location would be History, malignant, neoplasm, gastrointestinal tract, and the code would be V10.00.

EXAMPLE

> **V45   Other postsurgical states**
>
> **V45.01   Cardiac pacemaker**

V45 is the category, V45.0 is the subcategory, and V45.01 is the subclassification code. The Index location would be Cardiac, device, pacemaker, in situ.

EXERCISE 14-8

V CODES

Locate the V codes in the ICD-9-CM manual in Volume 2, Alphabetic Index, and then in Volume 1, Tabular List. Code the following:

1 A person who has been in contact with smallpox

Index location: _____

Code(s): _____

2 Prophylactic vaccination against smallpox

Index location: _____

Code(s): _____

3 Personal history of malignant neoplasm of the tongue

Index location: _____

Code(s): _____

E Codes: Supplementary Classification of External Causes of Injury and Poisoning

The E codes are located in Supplementary Classification of External Causes of Injury and Poisoning (E800–E999), behind the V codes in the ICD-9-CM manual. The E codes are alphanumeric designations of causes of injuries, poisonings, and adverse effects.

The E code section permits the classification of environmental events, circumstances, and conditions as the cause of injury, poisoning, and other adverse effects. With E codes, anything that can injure or have an adverse effect on a human body can be coded. The E codes can supply a code if a person is injured while pearl diving (E910.3), injured when a window on a railroad car falls on someone's head (E806.9), or hurt when pecked by a bird (E906.8). They are all in the E codes! These are rather far-fetched examples, granted, but they show how extensive and specific the codes are.

When a code from the E section is used, it is used in addition to a code from the Tabular List of the ICD-9-CM. The E code classification is used as an additional code for greater detail. Most groups of E codes have Includes or *Excludes* notes that provide further detail about using the codes in the group. Be sure to read these notes as you begin to code.

E codes have their own index. You can locate the E code index term in Volume 2, Section III, Index to External Causes of Injury, and then turn to the codes you're directed to in the E code Supplementary Classification of Volume 1.

The following information presents the E codes available in each group and an example of the type of code located in each range. The use of the fourth digit adds specificity as to who was injured in the accident. For example, if the injured person was the driver of a car involved in a motor vehicle accident, the fifth digit would be 0. If the injured person was a passenger in the vehicle, the fifth digit would be 1. E code terms are located first in the E code index in Volume 2 and then in the E code Supplementary Classification of Volume 1.

Some states have made the assignment of E codes mandatory, and the general use of E codes has increased significantly. At the beginning of Chapter 17, Injury and Poisoning (800–999), the note tells you to "Use E code(s) to identify the cause and intent of the injury or poisoning (E800–E999)."

EXERCISE 14-9

E CODES

Using the ICD-9-CM manual, locate the correct E code for each of the following in Volume 2, Alphabetic Index, and then in Volume 1, Tabular List.

1 Railway (E800–E807)
Railway accident involving derailment without antecedent collision, injuring a porter

E code index term(s): _____

Code(s): _____

2 Motor Vehicle Traffic (E810–819)
Motor vehicle traffic accident due to tire blowout; driver of the car was injured

E code index term(s): _____

Code(s): _____

3 Motor Vehicle Nontraffic (E820–E825)
Nontraffic accident of other off-road and motor vehicle, pedal cyclist injured

E code index term(s): _____

Code(s): _____

4 Other Road Vehicle (E826–E829)
Horse being ridden, rider injured, and nonmotor vehicle collision

E code index term(s): _____

Code(s): _____

5 Water Transport (E830–E838)
Accident to watercraft causing other injury, occupant of small powered boat injured due to collision

E code index term(s): _____

Code(s): _____

STOP *You are ready to move on to the appendices. There is much interesting information waiting for you in the appendices.*

THE FIVE APPENDICES IN VOLUME 1

Volume 1, Tabular List, contains five appendices:

Appendix A   Morphology of Neoplasms

Appendix B   Glossary of Mental Disorders

Appendix C   Classification of Drugs by American Hospital Formulary Service List Number and Their ICD-9-CM Equivalents

Appendix D   Classification of Industrial Accidents According to Agency

Appendix E   List of Three Digit Categories

(Note that in some commercially published ICD-9-CM texts, Appendix E or F is a listing of complications and comorbidities for the Diagnosis Related Groups.)

Appendices are included as a reference to the coder so it is possible to

- provide further information about the patient's clinical picture
- further define a diagnostic statement
- aid in classifying new drugs
- reference three-digit categories

The appendices are titled Appendix A, B, C, D, and E to indicate their positions in the back of Volume 1 of the ICD-9-CM manual.

Appendix A: Morphology of Neoplasms

The World Health Organization has published an adaptation of the International Classification of Diseases for Oncology (ICD-O). The ICD-O contains codes for the morphology of tumors. Morphology is the study of neoplasms. The morphology codes consist of five digits: the first four identify the histologic type of the neoplasm and the fifth indicates the behavior of the neoplasm.

Examples of types of neoplasm are epithelial, papillary, basal cell, and adenomas. Refer to a medical dictionary if you are not familiar with the types of neoplasms presented in Appendix A.

Examples of the behaviors of neoplasms are the terms "benign," "malignant," and "carcinoma in situ." "In situ" means the neoplasm has not spread from another site and is located in its original place.

The ICD-O one digit behavior code is as follows:

/0   Benign

/1   Uncertain whether benign or malignant
     Borderline malignancy

/2   Carcinoma in situ
        Intraepithelial
        Noninfiltrating
        Noninvasive

/3   Malignant, primary site

/6   Malignant, metastatic site
        Secondary site

/9   Malignant, uncertain whether primary or metastatic site

A primary site is the originating site of the tumor, and a secondary site is the metastatic site (spread from primary to secondary site).

Appendix B: Glossary of Mental Disorders

The psychiatric terms that appear in ICD-9-CM, Chapter 5, Mental Disorders, are listed in alphabetic order in Appendix B. Appendix B contains terminology from a variety of psychiatric sources, and the terms describe elements that are required to be present for each code to be used. Many of the terms in Appendix B appear in Chapter 5 of the ICD-9-CM manual. The Glossary of Mental Disorders is useful when a code describes a psychiatric term that you are not sure of. For example, the following shows a diagnostic code and code description.

EXAMPLE

> **309**   **Adjustment reaction**
> | INCLUDES | adjustment disorders
>   reaction (adjustment) to chronic stress

If you did not know what was meant by "Adjustment reaction," you could locate the term "Adjustment reaction" in the Glossary of Mental Disorders. You would find a complete description of the term. A portion of the description follows:

Adjustment reaction or disorder—Mild or transient disorders lasting longer than acute stress reactions which occur in individuals of any age without any apparent pre-existing mental disorder. Such disorders are often relatively circumscribed or situation-specific, are generally reversible, and usually last only a few months. They are usually closely related in time and content to

from the trenches

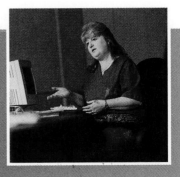

"*The sky is the limit. You can go as far in this field as you want as long as you are willing to learn.*"

MARY

stresses such as bereavement, migration, or other experiences. Reactions to major stress that last longer than a few days are also included. In children such disorders are associated with no significant distortion of development.

You will find Appendix B a helpful tool as you begin to code psychiatric conditions.

Appendix C: Drugs

This alphabetized subsection is entitled Classification of Drugs by American Hospital Formulary Service List Number and Their ICD-9-CM Equivalents. (Have you noticed how few short titles there are in the ICD-9-CM?) A division of the American Hospital Formulary Service (AHFS) regularly publishes a coded listing of drugs. These AHFS codes are as many as five digits. Each has a number, then a colon, and then up to four additional digits to provide specificity.

EXAMPLE

AHFS		ICD-9-CM
8:12.04	Antifungal Antibiotics	960.1

Note that the ICD-9-CM code and the AHFS poisoning codes mean the same thing. For example, both AHFS 8:12.04 and ICD-9-CM 960.1 are Antifungal Antibiotics.

Appendix D: Industrial Accidents

The subsection Classification of Industrial Accidents According to Agency contains three digit codes to identify occupational hazards. The subsection is divided into the following categories:

1. Machines

2. Means of Transport and Lifting Equipment

3. Other Equipment

4. Materials, Substances, and Radiation

5. Working Environments

6. Other Agencies, Not Elsewhere Classified (NEC)

7. Agencies Not Classified for Lack of Sufficient Data

The identification of occupational hazards is especially important in coding injury or death that is job-related. Statisticians analyze the data and make statements about the risks involved in various occupations based on the data collected from the forms completed by health care workers. Occupational hazard codes are not placed on the insurance or billing forms. Instead, these specialized codes are used by state and federal organizations to summarize data concerning industrial accidents.

Appendix E: Three Digit Categories

Appendix E is a list of all the three-digit codes in the ICD-9-CM, presented by each chapter. The categories are labeled 1 through 17.

EXAMPLE

> **1. INFECTIOUS AND PARASITIC DISEASES**
> **Intestinal infectious diseases (001–009)**
>
> 001   Cholera
>
> 002   Typhoid and paratyphoid fevers
>
> 003   Other salmonella infections
>
> 004   Shigellosis
>
> 005   Other food poisoning (bacterial)
>
> 006   Amebiasis
>
> 007   Other protozoal intestinal diseases
>
> 008   Intestinal infections due to other organisms
>
> 009   Ill-defined intestinal infections

Reviewing Appendix E is a good way to get a quick overview of all of the codes in the ICD-9-CM manual.

EXERCISE 14–10

THE FIVE APPENDICES IN VOLUME 1

Fill in the following:

1   In which appendix of the ICD-9-CM manual would you find the following information?

   a. Glossary of Mental Disorders _____

   b. Classification of Industrial Accidents According to Agency _____

   c. Morphology of Neoplasms _____

   d. List of Three Digit Categories _____

   e. Classification of Drugs by American Hospital Formulary Service List

   _____

2   In which appendix of the ICD-9-CM manual would you find the code to identify an injury resulting from a job-related accident involving a machine?

   _____

VOLUME 3: PROCEDURES

History

An important new development occurred with the publication of the ICD-9-CM manual—a Classification of Procedures in Medicine was added. Although some countries, notably the United States, had included classifications of surgical procedures in their adaptations of the ICD-9-CM since 1959, international agreement about classification of procedures was never reached. The classification of procedures has never been included in the ICD-9-CM manual itself but has always been a separate volume.

The WHO had recognized the growing need for a classification of procedures used in medicine and in 1971 sponsored an international working party that was convened by the American Hospital Association to coordinate the recommendations for a classification of procedures, with the primary emphasis on surgery. The International Conference for the 9th Revision of the International Classification of Diseases was convened at WHO Headquarters in Geneva in 1975. From that gathering, a proposal for a classification of procedures was submitted. The recommendations of the working party were to publish the provisional procedures classification as a supplement to the ICD-9. When the ICD-9 manual was published, a series of separate sections called fascicles (supplements) was also published. Each fascicle provides a classification of a different mode (type) of therapy (e.g., surgery, radiology, and laboratory procedures).

Subsequently, the ICD-9-CM was published in a three-volume set, including Volume 3, Procedures. Volume 3 was drawn primarily from WHO's Fascicle V, Surgical Procedures. At the same time, the codes in Volume 3 were expanded from three to four digits to allow for greater detail.

Volume 3 of the ICD-9-CM manual did not maintain compatibility with the ICD-9 as Volume 1 and 2 had done. A different approach was taken in the development of Volume 3 that was deemed more appropriate to a classification system that would deal with surgical and therapeutic procedures.

Format

Volume 3 contains two parts—the Tabular List and the Alphabetic Index. Approximately 90% of the codes in Volume 3 refer to surgical procedures (Fig. 14–19). The remaining 10% of the codes are diagnostic and therapeutic procedures, as shown in Figure 14–20. For the most part, nonsurgical procedures are segregated from surgical procedures and confined to the codes 87 to 99.

Volume 3 is not used in physicians' offices because procedures done by physicians are coded using the CPT codes. Hospitals use Volume 3 extensively to code services provided to inpatients and outpatients, including

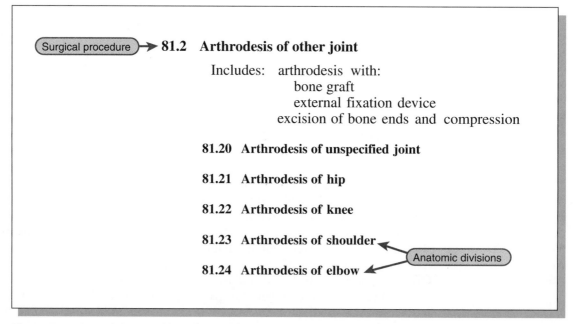

Figure 14–19 Volume 3, Surgical procedures. (From International Classification of Diseases, 9th Revision. U.S. Department of Health and Human Services, Public Health Service, Centers for Medicare and Medicaid Services.)

Therapeutic procedure → **88.4   Arteriography using contrast material**

Includes: angiography of arteries
arterial puncture for injection of
contrast material
radiography of arterres (by fluoroscopy)
retrograde arteriography

Note: The fourth-digit subclassification identifies
the site to be viewed, not the site of
injection.

Excludes: *arteriography using:*
radioisotopes or radionuclides (92.01-92.19)
ultrasound (88.71-88.79)
fluorescein angiography of eye (95.12)

88.40 Arteriography using contrast material, unspecified site

Figure 14–20   Volume 3, Therapeutic procedures. (From International Classification of Diseases, 9th Revision. U.S. Department of Health and Human Services, Public Health Service, Centers for Medicare and Medicaid Services.)

surgery, therapy, and diagnostic procedures. Hospitals use the ICD-9-CM codes to bill for facility fees (e.g., operating room, room and board, nurses, supplies). For example, a patient is admitted for a total abdominal hysterectomy. The physician would report his or her services and bill for the service of the total abdominal hysterectomy using the CPT code 58150. The hospital would report and bill for facility services for the hysterectomy procedure using the ICD-9-CM procedure code 68.4. The physician and the hospital would report the patient's diagnosis using an ICD-9-CM diagnosis code. If the patient in this example had a diagnosis of chronic endometriosis, both the physician and the hospital would indicate the patient's diagnosis and the reason for their services due to endometriosis of the uterus using the ICD-9-CM code of 617.0. However, there is an increase in the number of third-party payers that require hospitals to code surgical procedures using *both* CPT and ICD-9-CM codes.

EXERCISE 14-11

TABLE OF CONTENTS

The Table of Contents, Volume 3 (Fig. 14–21) indicates the 16 chapters in Volume 3. Note that each chapter is based on a body system, except for Chapters 13 and 16.

1   What is Chapter 13? _____

2   What is Chapter 16? _____

TABLE OF CONTENTS

Figure 14–21 Volume 3, Table of Contents. (From International Classification of Diseases, 9th Revision. U.S. Department of Health and Human Services, Public Health Service, Centers for Medicare and Medicaid Services.)

Tabular List, Volume 3

Volume 3 has abbreviations, punctuation, symbols, and words similar to those used in Volumes 1 and 2. The following are the conventions, which are the same in all volumes:

1. Abbreviations of NEC and NOS

2. Punctuation symbols brackets, parentheses, colons, and braces

3. Bold type for all codes and titles

4. Italicized type for all exclusion notes

5. Instructional notations of Includes and *Excludes*

   The term "Code also" has two purposes in Volume 3:

1. To allow the coding of each component of a procedure

2. To allow the coding of the use of special adjunctive (at the same time) procedures or equipment

These instructions are not mandatory, but they serve as a reminder to code these additional procedures if they were performed.

Using the following ICD-9-CM code as an example, let us take a closer look at the code to make sure you understand what the procedure is and how the term "Code also" is used.

EXAMPLE

> **42.6   Antesternal anastomosis of esophagus**
> Code also any synchronous:
> esophagectomy (42.40–42.42)
> gastrostomy (43.1)

You won't find the word "antesternal" in most medical dictionaries. It is at this time that your skill at taking the word apart will help you out. The prefix "ante" means before, and "sternal" refers to sternum. Anastomosis is the joining together of two openings; in this case it is an opening into the esophagus. The location of the opening into the esophagus is above the sternum, which stated in medical lingo is antesternal anastomosis of esophagus. "Synchronous" means occurring at the same time; "esophagectomy" is the removal of a part of the esophagus, and "gastrostomy" is the creation of an opening into the stomach. The statement from code 42.6 is translated into "Code also any [esophagectomy or gastrostomy] occurring at the same time." You need to know what the terminology you work with means to know what you are coding. The study of terminology is a lifelong endeavor. There are always new words to be discovered. Just remember to always look up any word you are not certain of and take the time to understand the word in the context in which it is used. If you make a practice of doing this, you will soon find that you have a very dependable medical terminology vocabulary.

An example of the second use of the instruction notation "Code also," to code the use of special adjunctive (accessory) procedures or equipment, follows.

EXAMPLE

> **39.21   Caval-pulmonary artery anastomosis**
> Code also cardiopulmonary bypass (39.61)

The "Code also" note below code 39.21 directs you to code 39.61, which is the code for extracorporeal (outside the body) circulation. Extracorporeal circulation is an auxiliary procedure performed during heart surgery.

EXERCISE 14-12

TERMINOLOGY

State the definitions of the following terms:

1 cava(l) _____

2 pulmonary _____

3 anastomosis _____

4 cardiopulmonary _____

5 extracorporeal _____

6 What is a caval-pulmonary artery anastomosis?

_____

_____

7 What does a heart-lung machine do for a patient who is having a caval-pulmonary artery anastomosis?

_____

_____

Alphabetic Index, Volume 3

The Index of Procedures is an important complement to the Tabular List of Procedures because the index contains many procedure terms that do not appear in the Tabular List of Procedures. The list of procedures included in the two-digit category code of the Tabular List of Procedures is not meant to be exhaustive; the terms serve as examples of the content of the category. The Index to Procedures, however, includes most procedure terms currently in use in North America. When the exact word is not found in the Tabular List of Procedures but is found in the Index to Procedures, you must trust that the code given in the Index to Procedures is correct.

EXAMPLE

In the Index to Procedures, you will find the entry Gastrostomy, subterm Janeway, which is a type of gastrostomy. The entry directs you to code 43.19. When you then verify the code 43.19 in the Tabular List of Procedures, you will note that code 43.19 is listed as Other gastrostomy, without mention of the term Janeway. After again checking the Index to Procedures to make certain you read the entry correctly as to the Janeway subterm, you are to trust that 43.19 is the proper code for a Janeway gastrostomy.

Never code directly from the Index to Procedures. After locating a code in the index, refer to that code in the Tabular List of Procedures for important instructions. Instructions in the form of notes suggesting the use of additional codes and exclusion notes that indicate the circumstances under

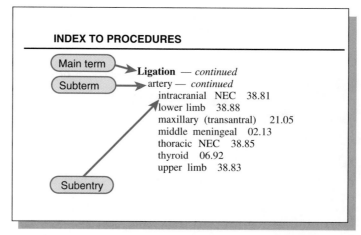

Figure 14–22 Index to procedures. (From International Classification of Diseases, 9th Revision. U.S. Department of Health and Human Services, Public Health Service, Centers for Medicare and Medicaid Services.)

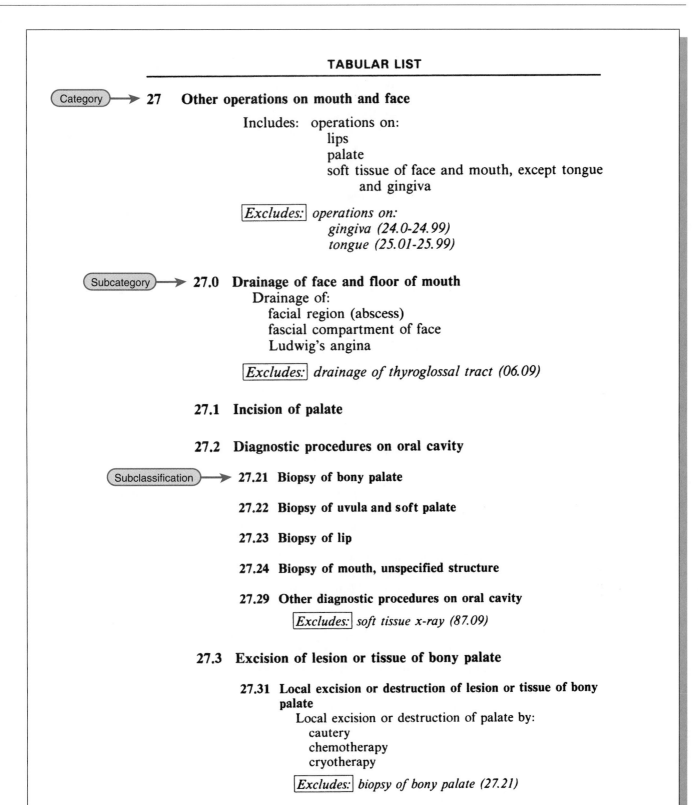

TABULAR LIST

Category → **27   Other operations on mouth and face**

Includes: operations on:
lips
palate
soft tissue of face and mouth, except tongue
and gingiva

Excludes: *operations on:*
gingiva (24.0-24.99)
tongue (25.01-25.99)

Subcategory → **27.0   Drainage of face and floor of mouth**
Drainage of:
facial region (abscess)
fascial compartment of face
Ludwig's angina

Excludes: *drainage of thyroglossal tract (06.09)*

27.1   Incision of palate

27.2   Diagnostic procedures on oral cavity

Subclassification → **27.21   Biopsy of bony palate**

27.22   Biopsy of uvula and soft palate

27.23   Biopsy of lip

27.24   Biopsy of mouth, unspecified structure

27.29   Other diagnostic procedures on oral cavity
Excludes: *soft tissue x-ray (87.09)*

27.3   Excision of lesion or tissue of bony palate

27.31   Local excision or destruction of lesion or tissue of bony palate
Local excision or destruction of palate by:
cautery
chemotherapy
cryotherapy

Excludes: *biopsy of bony palate (27.21)*

Figure 14–23   Volume 3, format. (From International Classification of Diseases, 9th Revision. U.S. Department of Health and Human Services, Public Health Service, Centers for Medicare and Medicaid Services.)

which a procedure would be coded elsewhere are found only in the Tabular List of Procedures.

The Index to Procedures is arranged primarily by procedure (Fig. 14–22) into main terms and subterms. Procedure codes are numbers only, with no alphabetic characters. The classification is based on a two-digit structure with two additional digits when necessary for additional specificity.

Figure 14–23 indicates the two-digit category codes, the three-digit subcategory codes, and the four-digit subclassification codes contained in the Tabular List of Procedures. All category codes in Volume 3, Procedures, are two-digit codes, whereas all category codes in Volume 1, Tabular List, Disease are three-digit codes.

The sequence of the Index to Procedures is letter-by-letter alphabetic order. Letter-by-letter alphabetizing ignores single spaces and hyphens and produces sequences.

EXAMPLE

> opening
>
> open reduction
>
> Upon first consideration, you would think that these two words were not in correct alphabetical order, "open" should come before "opening." The old filer's rule of "nothing comes before something" does not apply here. To alphabetize "opening" and "open reduction," you consider the beginning of the two words as "o-p-e-n"; the fifth letter in "opening" is "i" and the fifth letter in "open reduction" is "r." For alphabetizing purposes, the terms are considered as
>
> opening
>
> openreduction

Numbers, whether Arabic (1, 2, 3), Roman (I, II, III), or ordinal (first, second, third), are all placed in numeric sequence *before* alphabetic characters. Simply stated, numbers come before letters (Fig. 14–24).

The *prepositions* as, by, and with immediately follow the main term to which they refer. When multiple prepositional references are present, they are listed in alphabetic sequence.

The Index to Procedures is organized according to main terms, which are printed in bold type. Main terms usually identify the type of procedure performed, rather than the anatomic site involved.

A main term may be followed by a series of terms in parentheses. The presence or absence of these parenthetic terms in the procedure description has no effect on the selection of the code listed for the main term. These parenthetic terms are called nonessential modifiers. For example, all of the following words in parentheses are nonessential modifiers.

EXAMPLE

> **Clipping**
>   aneurysm (basilar) (carotid) (cerebellar)
>   (cerebellopontine) (communicating artery) (vertebral) 39.51

Operation
    Beck I (epicardial poudrage) 36.39
    Beck II (aorto-coronary sinus shunt) 36.39
    Beck-Jianu (permanent gastrostomy) 43.19

Figure 14–24   Numbers.

A main term may also be followed by a list of subterms (modifiers) that do have an effect on the selection of the appropriate code for a given procedure. These subterms form individual line entries and describe essential differences in site or surgical technique (e.g., see Fig. 14–25).

Terms that identify incisions are listed as main terms in the Index to Procedures. If the incision was made only for the purpose of performing further surgery, the instruction "*omit* code" is given. The incision for the surgical procedure is bundled into the surgical code and would therefore not be coded separately. Closure of a surgical wound is not coded separately unless the closure takes place during a separate operative procedure.

EXAMPLE

Arthrotomy 80.10
   as operative approach—*omit* code with
      arthrography—*see* Arthrogram
      arthroscopy—*see* Arthroscopy
      injection of drug 81.92
      removal of prothesis (*see also* Removal, prosthesis, joint structures) 80.00
   ankle 80.17
   elbow 80.12

For some operative procedures it is necessary to record the individual components of the procedure. In these instances the Index to Procedures lists both codes.

EXAMPLE

Code 57.87 describes the reconstruction of a urinary bladder, and 45.51 indicates the intestinal resection (cutting out of a portion of the intestine) necessary to create an ileal bladder.

Ileal bladder
   closed 57.87 *[45.51]*

It is important to record these codes in the same sequence as that used in the Index to Procedures.

The cross references section provides you with possible modifiers for a term or its synonyms. There are three types of cross references:

1. The term "*see*" is an explicit direction to look elsewhere. It is used with terms that do not define the type of procedure performed.

EXAMPLE

Bacterial smear—*see* Examination, microscopic

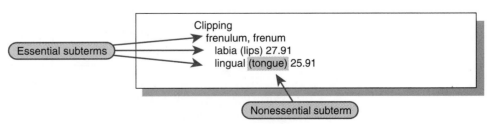

Figure 14–25 Essential and nonessential subterms. (From International Classification of Diseases, 9th Revision. U.S. Department of Health and Human Services, Public Health Service, Centers for Medicare and Medicaid Services.)

2. The term "*see also*" directs you to look under another main term because all of the information being searched for cannot be located under the first main term entry.

EXAMPLE

Immunization—*see also* Vaccination

3. The term "*see category*" directs you to the Tabular List of Procedures for further information or specific site references.

EXAMPLE

Osteolysis—*see* category 78.4

Notes are used in the Index to Procedures to list fourth digit subclassifications for those categories that use the same fourth digit. In these cases, only the three-digit code is given for the individual entry; you must refer to the note following the main term to obtain the appropriate fourth digit. For an example of a note, see Figure 14–26.

The fourth digit subclassification codes also appear in the Tabular List of Procedures with the category codes 90 and 91.

EXAMPLE

Operations named for persons (eponyms) are listed both as main terms in their appropriate alphabetic sequence and under the main term "Operation." A description of the procedure or anatomic site affected usually follows the eponym.

---

90   Microscopic examination - I

The following fourth-digit subclassification is for use with categories in section 90 to identify type of examination:

1   bacterial smear
2   culture
3   culture and sensitivity
4   parasitology
5   toxicology
6   cell block and Papanicolaou smear
7   other microscopic examination

Fourth digit also appears in the tabular list under the categories

Figure 14–26 Volume 3, Notes, Alphabetic Index. (From International Classification of Diseases, 9th Revision. U.S. Department of Health and Human Services, Public Health Service, Centers for Medicare and Medicaid Services.)

Under O:

Operation
    Thompson
        cleft lip repair 27.54
        correction of lymphedema 40.9
        quadricepsplasty 83.86
        thumb opposition with bone graft 82.69

Under T:

Thompson operation
    cleft lip repair 27.54
    correction of lymphedema 40.9
    quadricepsplasty 83.86
    thumb opposition with bone graft 82.69

EXERCISE 14-13

PROCEDURES: VOLUME 3

Code the following using Volume 3 of the ICD-9-CM manual:

1 Flexible sigmoidoscopy

Code(s): _____

2 Vasectomy

Code(s): _____

3 Closed reduction of maxillary fracture

Code(s): _____

4 Transfusion of 2 units packed cells

Code(s): _____

5 Control of epistaxis by cauterization

Code(s): _____

Congratulations

You have now completed the study of the arrangement of the information in the ICD-9-CM manual. The knowledge you have gained will be used as the foundation that will be built upon in Chapter 15. In Chapter 15 you will begin further work with the correct assignment and sequencing of ICD-9-CM codes.

CHAPTER GLOSSARY

acute: of sudden onset and short duration

benign: not progressive or recurrent

chronic: of long duration

combination code: single five-digit code used to identify etiology and manifestation of a disease

communicable disease: disease that can be transmitted from one person to another or from one species to another

etiology: study of causes of diseases

histology: study of the minute structures, composition, and function of tissues

infectious disease carrier: person who has a communicable disease

infectious disease contact: encounter with a person who has a disease that can be communicated or transmitted

malignant: used to describe a cancerous tumor that grows worse over time

manifestation: sign of a disease

morbidity: condition of being diseased or morbid

morphology: study of neoplasms

mortality: death

multiple coding: use of more than one code to identify both etiology and manifestation of a disease, as contrasted with combination coding

neoplasm: new tumor growth that can be benign or malignant

rubric: heading used as a direction or explanation as to what follows and the way in which the information is to be used. In ICD-9-CM coding, the rubric is the three-digit code that precedes the four- and five-digit codes.

secondary site: place to which a malignant tumor has spread; metastatic site

V codes: numeric designations preceded by the letter "V" used to classify persons who are not currently sick when they encounter health services

World Health Organization (WHO): group that deals with health care issues on a global basis

CHAPTER REVIEW

CHAPTER 14, PART I, THEORY

Match the appendix to the information contained in the appendix:

1   Appendix A _____

2   Appendix B _____

3   Appendix C _____

4   Appendix D _____

5   Appendix E _____

a. Industrial Accidents

b. Classification of Drugs

c. Morphology of Neoplasms

d. Three-Digit Categories

e. Mental Disorders

Circle the correct answer in each of the following:

6   The ICD-9-CM is designed to classify what two things?
a. sickness and disease
b. symptoms and illness
c. causes of morbidity and mortality
d. diagnosis and disease

7   Which of the following is *not* a stated use for the ICD-9-CM?
a. facilitate payment of health services
b. study health care costs
c. plan for future health care needs
d. evaluate appropriateness of treatment

Match the ICD-9-CM volume number to the correct name of the volume:

8   Volume 1 _____

9   Volume 2 _____

10 Volume 3 _____

a. Tabular List of Procedures and Alphabetic Index to Procedures

b. Diseases: Alphabetic Index

c. Diseases: Tabular List

Identify the format of the chapters in the ICD-9-CM Volume 1, Tabular List, in the proper sequence from first to last:

11 _____   a. subcategory

12 _____   b. chapter

13 _____   c. subclassification

14 _____   d. section

15 _____   e. category

Are the following statements about V codes true or false?

16 V codes refer primarily to persons who are not ill but use health care. _____

17 V codes do not use fourth digits. _____

18 V codes can indicate the place of birth as having been before admission or after admission.

_____

Circle the correct answer in the following:

19 The primary purpose of E codes is to
a. identify environmental events
b. designate causes of injuries and poisonings
c. both a and b
d. neither a nor b

20 Morphology is the science of
a. human anatomy
b. physiologic function
c. neoplasms
d. tissue

CHAPTER 14, PART II, PRACTICAL

Using an ICD-9-CM manual, answer the following questions:

21 What does the *Excludes* note state under category code 175? _____

_____

22 What does the Includes note state under category 444? _____

_____

23 Under category 805, which codes use the subclassification 0–8? _____

_____

24 Would code 362.72 be sequenced as the principal diagnosis? _____

_____

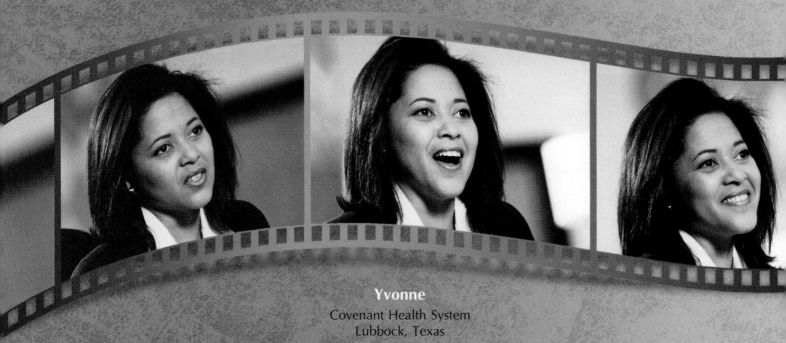

Yvonne
Covenant Health System
Lubbock, Texas

chapter 15

Using the ICD-9-CM

LEARNING OBJECTIVES

After completing this chapter you should be able to *I/P Definitive studies/testing Dx after*

1   Understand the official coding principles. *O/P*

2   Define principal and primary diagnosis.

3   Explain reporting other (additional) diagnoses.

4   Assign ICD-9-CM codes to the highest level of specificity.

5   Properly sequence ICD-9-CM codes.

6   Apply ICD-9-CM guidelines and coding conventions.

7   Apply basic coding guidelines to classifying outpatient services.

8   Recognize the major parts of ICD-10-PCS.

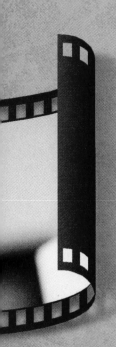

SOME GENERAL GUIDELINES

As was discussed in Chapter 14, Official Coding and Reporting Guidelines have been developed and approved for coding and reporting by the Cooperating Parties for ICD-9-CM: the American Hospital Association (AHA), American Health Information Management Association (AHIMA), Centers for Medicare and Medicaid Services (CMS), and National Center for Health Statistics (NCHS). The Central Office on ICD-9-CM of the AHA staffs guideline development activities, and the Cooperating Parties oversee the guidelines.

General Guidelines

The number that appears to the left of the coding guideline in this text is the number of the guideline as listed in the Official Coding and Reporting Guidelines published by the CMS. For the purposes of this text, the guidelines will sometimes appear out of order. For example, the two guidelines regarding burns are 8.3 and 2.11 and are presented together as you learn about sequencing burns. Appendix A of this text presents the guidelines in their entirety in numeric order.

In the examples in this text, main terms and subterms are often noted for you after the term enclosed in parentheses to help you locate the terms in the Alphabetic Index. Remember, the extensive cross-reference system in the ICD-9-CM allows you many options for locating codes in the Alphabetic Index. The examples and subsequent identification of main terms and subterms represent only one way a term can be located.

You will be practicing coding using the ICD-9-CM throughout this chapter. You need to practice using the steps that are always necessary to assign an ICD-9-CM code. If you begin your ICD-9-CM coding using these steps, you will develop good coding habits that will last throughout your career.

1. Identify the main term(s) in the diagnostic statement.
2. Locate the main term(s) in the Alphabetic Index (Volume 2) (referred to in this text as the Index).
3. Review any subterms under the main term in the Index.
4. Follow any cross-reference instructions, such as *see also*.
5. Verify the code(s) selected from the Index in the Tabular List (Volume 1) (referred to in this text as the Tabular).
6. Refer to any instructional notations in the Tabular.
7. Assign codes to the highest level of specificity. For example, if a fourth digit is available, you cannot assign only a three-digit code, and if a fifth digit is available, you cannot assign only a four-digit code.
8. Code the diagnosis until all elements are completely identified.

Each guideline is presented and is followed by examples or exercises to illustrate the rule(s).

Official Coding and Reporting Guidelines

1.1 USE OF BOTH THE ALPHABETIC INDEX AND THE TABULAR LIST

A. Use both the Alphabetic Index and the Tabular List when locating and assigning a code. Reliance on only the Alphabetic Index or the Tabular List leads to errors in code assignment and less specificity in code selection.

B. Locate each item in the Alphabetic Index and verify the code selected in the Tabular List. Read and be guided by instructional notations that appear in both the Alphabetic Index and the Tabular List.

EXAMPLES

Use of Both the Alphabetic Index and the Tabular List

Diagnosis:	Hodgkin's Disease
Index:	**Hodgkin's** (main term)
	disease (subterm) 201.9
Tabular:	**201 Hodgkin's disease** [category code]
	201.9 Hodgkin's disease, Unspecified [subcategory code]
Code:	201.9X Hodgkin's Disease [subclassification code]

Verify 201.9 in the Tabular and note that the code requires a fifth-digit assignment of 0 to 8 to indicate the disease location. You would have missed the required fifth-digit subclassification if you had used only the Index and not verified the code in the Tabular.

Diagnosis:	Stroke, due to vertebral artery occlusion
Index:	**Stroke** (main term) 436
Tabular:	**436 Acute, but ill-defined, cerebrovascular disease**

> EXCLUDES *any condition classifiable to categories 430–435*

Reading the *Excludes* note under stroke, 436, in the Tabular, you can identify that 436 can be used only if the stroke description is not classifiable to 430–435. You then must reference the occlusion portion of the diagnosis.

Index:	**Occlusion**
	artery, vertebral
Tabular:	**433 Occlusion and stenosis of precerebral arteries**
	0 without mention of cerebral infarction
	1 with cerebral infarction
	433.2 Vertebral artery
Code:	433.20 Stroke, due to vertebral artery occlusion

The diagnosis statement "fits" or is classifiable to 433.20. You would have incorrectly coded the diagnosis to 436 if you had not verified the code in the Tabular. There are no shortcuts in this process: Always check the Tabular.

Official Coding and Reporting Guidelines

1.2 LEVEL OF SPECIFICITY IN CODING

Diagnostic and procedure codes must be used at their highest level of specificity.

A. Assign three-digit codes only if there are no four-digit codes within that code category.

B. Assign four-digit codes only if there is no fifth-digit subclassification for that category.

C. Assign the five-digit subclassification code for those categories where it exists.

EXAMPLES

Level of Specificity

Three-Digit Category

Diagnosis:	Subarachnoid hemorrhage
Index:	**Hemorrhage,** subarachnoid, nontraumatic 430
Tabular:	**430 Subarachnoid hemorrhage** [category code]
Code:	430 Subarachnoid hemorrhage
Diagnosis:	AIDS
Index:	**AIDS** 042
Tabular:	**042 Human immunodeficiency virus (HIV) disease** [category code]
Code:	042 AIDS

Both of the preceding diagnostic statements are correctly assigned to three-digit category codes because there are no four-digit subcategory codes available within either code.

Four-Digit Subcategory

Diagnosis:	Crohn's disease of large intestine
Index:	**Crohn's disease** (see also Enteritis, regional) 555.9
Tabular:	**555 Regional enteritis (Includes: Crohn's disease)** [category code]
	555.1 Large intestine [subcategory code]
Code:	555.1 Crohn's disease of large intestine
Diagnosis:	Cellulitis of the upper right leg
Index:	**Cellulitis,** leg
Tabular:	**682 Other cellulitis and abscess** [category code]
	682.6 leg, except foot [subcategory code]
Code:	682.6 Cellulitis of the upper right leg

Both of the preceding diagnostic statements are correctly assigned to four-digit subcategory codes because no five-digit subclassification codes are available.

Five-Digit Subclassification

Diagnosis:	RUQ abdominal pain
Index:	**Pain,** abdominal
Tabular:	**789.0 Abdominal pain** [subcategory code]
	789.01 Right upper quadrant [subclassification code]
Code:	789.01 RUQ abdominal pain
Diagnosis:	Bilateral, congenital bowing of right femur
Index:	**Bowing**
	femur 736.89
	congenital 754.42
Tabular:	**754 Certain congenital musculoskeletal deformities** [category code]
	754.4 Congenital genu recurvatum and bowing of long bones of leg [subcategory code]
	754.42 Congenital bowing of femur [subclassification code]
Code:	754.42 Bilateral, congenital bowing of right femur

Both of the preceding diagnostic statements are correctly assigned to five-digit subclassification codes, having been carried out to the highest level of specificity available.

EXERCISE 15-1

LEVEL OF SPECIFICITY IN CODING

Identify and fill in the category, subcategory, and subclassifications of the following:

1 Diagnosis: Recurrent right inguinal hernia, with obstruction

   Index: **Hernia**

   inguinal 550.9

   Tabular: **550 Inguinal hernia** _____

   550.1 Inguinal hernia, with obstruction, without

   mention of gangrene _____

   550.11 Inguinal hernia, with obstruction, without mention of gangrene,

   unilateral _____

2 Diagnosis: Transient hypertension, 30 weeks' gestation, undelivered

   Index: **Hypertension**

   transient

   of pregnancy (soubrette) 642.3

   Tabular: **642 Hypertension complicating pregnancy, childbirth,**

   and the puerperium _____

   642.3 Transient hypertension of pregnancy _____

   642.33 Antepartum condition or

   complication _____

NEC and NOS

Official Coding and Reporting Guidelines

1.3 OTHER (NEC) AND UNSPECIFIED (NOS) CODE TITLES

Codes labeled "other specified" (NEC—not elsewhere classified) or "unspecified" (NOS—not otherwise specified) are used only when neither the diagnostic statement nor a thorough review of the medical record provides adequate information to permit assignment of a more specific code.

A. Use the code assignment for "other" or NEC when the information at hand specifies a condition but no separate code for the condition is provided.
B. Use "unspecified" (NOS) when the information at hand does not permit either a more specific or other code assignment.

When the Alphabetic Index assigns a code to a category labeled "other (NEC)" or to a category labeled "unspecified (NOS)" refer to the Tabular List and review the titles and inclusion terms in the subdivisions under that particular three-digit category (or subdivision under the four-digit code) to determine if the information at hand can be appropriately assigned to a more specific code.

EXAMPLES

> ### NEC
>
> Diagnosis: Pneumonia due to gram-negative bacteria
>
> Index: **Pneumonia**
>
>   gram-negative bacteria NEC 482.83
>
> Tabular: **482.8 Pneumonia due to other specified bacteria**
>
>   **482.83 Other gram-negative bacteria**
>
> Code: 482.83 Pneumonia due to gram-negative bacteria

Code 482.83 identifies gram-negative bacteria pneumonia that cannot be classified more specifically into the other subclassifications. The other subclassifications within 482.8 are for anaerobes, *Escherichia coli [E. coli]*, "other than gram-negative" bacteria, Legionnaire's disease, and other specified bacteria. None of these other subclassifications can be assigned to the diagnostic statement.

NEC can be used in two ways:

1. NEC directs the coder to look under other classifications if appropriate. Other subterms or *Excludes* notes may provide hints as to what the other classifications may be.
2. NEC is used when the ICD-9-CM does not have any codes that provide greater specificity.

> ### NOS
>
> Diagnosis: Bronchitis
>
> Index: **Bronchitis** 490
>
> Tabular: **490 Bronchitis, not specified as acute or chronic**
>
>   **Bronchitis NOS**
>
> Code: 490 Bronchitis

The diagnosis was not specified by the practitioner as acute or chronic; therefore, the "not otherwise specified" code 490 must be assigned. In this situation, it would be appropriate for the coder to request specificity from the practitioner.

Acute and Chronic

Official Coding and Reporting Guidelines

1.4 AND 2.3 ACUTE AND CHRONIC CONDITIONS

If the same condition is described as both acute (subacute) and chronic and separate subentries exist in the Alphabetic Index at the same indentation level, code both and sequence the acute (subacute) code first.

See Figure 15–1 for the format of acute pancreatitis and chronic pancreatitis. Both acute and chronic forms of pancreatitis are subcategorized under code 577.

EXAMPLES

> ### Acute and Chronic Conditions
>
> Diagnosis: Acute and chronic thyroiditis
>
> Index: **Thyroiditis**
>
>   acute 245.0
>
>   chronic 245.8

577.0 Acute pancreatitis

Abscess of pancreas	Pancreatitis:
Necrosis of pancreas:	NOS
acute	acute (recurrent)
infective	apoplectic
	hemorrhagic
	subacute
	suppurative

Excludes: *mumps pancreatitis (072.3)*

577.1 Chronic pancreatitis

Chronic pancreatitis:	Pancreatitis:
NOS	painless
infectious	recurrent
interstitial	relapsing

Figure 15–1 Indent level of acute and chronic. (From International Classification of Diseases, 9th Revision. U.S. Department of Health and Human Services, Public Health Service, Centers for Medicare and Medicaid Services.)

Tabular: **245 Thyroiditis**

           245.0 Acute thyroiditis

           245.8 Other and unspecified chronic thyroiditis

Sequence: 245.0, 245.8 Acute and chronic thyroiditis

Note that the acute form of thyroiditis is sequenced before the chronic form, as directed by Guideline 2.3.

Diagnosis: Acute and chronic pericarditis

Index: **Pericarditis**

        acute 420.90

        chronic 423.8

Tabular: **420 Acute pericarditis**

           420.9 Other and unspecified acute pericarditis

                420.90 Acute pericarditis, unspecified

Tabular: **423 Other diseases of pericardium**

           423.8 Other specified diseases of the pericardium

Sequence: 420.90, 423.8 Acute and chronic pericarditis

CAUTION *Note that while the Index directs you to code 423.8 for chronic pericarditis, when the Tabular is verified, there is no mention of chronic pericarditis. This is an example of a common coding situation in which you must trust the Index to have more descriptive terms than the Tabular. When the condition is both acute and chronic, and both acute and chronic are listed in the Index as separate entries and at the same indentation level, the code for* acute *is sequenced first.*

Combination Codes

Official Coding and Reporting Guidelines

1.5 COMBINATION CODE

A single code used to classify two diagnoses or a diagnosis with an associated secondary process (manifestation) or an associated complication is called a combination code. Combination codes are identified by referring to subterm entries in the Alphabetic Index and by reading the inclusion and exclusion codes in the Tabular List.

> A. Assign only the combination code when that code fully identifies the diagnostic conditions involved or when the Index so directs. Multiple coding should not be used when the classification provides a combination code that clearly identifies all of the elements documented in the diagnosis. When the combination code lacks necessary specificity in describing the manifestation or complication, an additional code may be used as a secondary code.

The following is an example of a combination code that classifies a diagnosis (hypertension) with a secondary manifestation (congestive heart failure).

EXAMPLES

Combination Codes

Diagnosis: Congestive heart failure due to hypertension

(*Note:* Beginning with this Index example, the main term will be listed first and subsequent subterm(s) will follow on the same line, separated by a comma. Index main terms and subterms will be listed on separate lines only if separate lines add to the clarity of the example.)

Index: **Failure,** heart, congestive, hypertensive 402.91

Tabular: **402 Hypertensive heart disease**

    402.9 Unspecified

      402.91 with congestive heart failure

Code: 402.91 Congestive heart failure due to hypertension

The diagnosis of congestive heart failure due to hypertension is fully described by the single code 402.91.

Another example of a diagnosis (streptococcal) and manifestation (pharyngitis—sore throat) assigned to a combination code is as follows:

Diagnosis: Streptococcal pharyngitis

Index: **Pharyngitis,** streptococcal 034.0

Tabular: **034 Streptococcal sore throat and scarlet fever**

    034.0 Streptococcal sore throat

Septic:	Streptococcal:
angina	angina
sore throat	laryngitis
	pharyngitis
	tonsillitis

The single code 034.0 fully describes the diagnosis of streptococcal pharyngitis.

Code(s):   034.0 Streptococcal pharyngitis

EXERCISE
15-2

COMBINATION CODES

Fill in the codes for the following using combination coding:

1   Pneumonia due to *Haemophilus influenzae*

  Code(s): _____

2   Candidiasis of the mouth (thrush)

  Code(s): _____

3 Enteritis due to *Clostridium difficile*

Code(s): _____

4 Hypertensive cerebrovascular disease

Code(s): _____

5 Closed fracture of the tibia and fibula

Code(s): _____

Multiple Coding

Official Coding and Reporting Guidelines

1.6 MULTIPLE CODING OF DIAGNOSES

Multiple coding is required for certain conditions not subject to the rules for combination codes.

Instructions for conditions that require multiple coding appear in the Alphabetic Index and the Tabular List:

A. Alphabetic Index: Codes for both etiology and manifestation of a disease appear following the subentry term, with the second code italicized and in slanted brackets. Assign both codes in the same sequence in which they appear in the Alphabetic Index.

B. Tabular List: Instructional terms, such as "Code first . . . ," "Use additional code for any . . . ," and "Note . . ." indicate when to use more than one code.

  1. "Code also underlying disease"—Assign the codes for both the manifestation and the underlying cause. The codes for manifestations cannot be used (designated) as principal diagnosis.

  2. "Use additional code, if desired, to identify manifestation, as . . ."— Assign also the code that identifies the manifestation such as, but not limited to, the examples listed. The codes for manifestations cannot be used (designated) as principal diagnosis.

C. Apply multiple coding instructions throughout the classification where appropriate, whether or not multiple coding directions appear in the Alphabetic Index or the Tabular List. Avoid indiscriminate multiple coding of irrelevant information such as symptoms or signs characteristic of the diagnosis.

EXAMPLES

Multiple Coding

Diagnosis: Diabetic retinopathy with type I diabetes

(*Note:* Retinopathy is the manifestation and diabetes is the etiology, or cause, of the retinopathy.)

Index: **Retinopathy,** diabetic 250.5 [362.01]

The Index subterm "diabetic" identifies the code for the etiology as 250.5 and directs you to the code for the manifestation of *[362.01]* retinopathy. The italicized code is never sequenced first as the principal diagnosis but is used to identify a manifestation.

Tabular: **250 Diabetes mellitus**

        250.5 Diabetes with ophthalmic manifestations

            Use additional code to identify manifestation

        250.51 Type I, not stated as uncontrolled

Code 250.51 is the correct code to describe the diabetes (etiology). The statement "Use additional code to identify manifestation" directs you to assign a code that identifies the manifestation (retinopathy).

Tabular: **362 Other retinal disorders**

              362.0 Diabetic retinopathy

              Code first diabetes 250.5

              362.01 Background diabetic retinopathy

Note that the *"Code first diabetes"* directs you to the etiology code.

Code: 250.51, 362.01 Diabetic retinopathy with type I diabetes

The multiple codes fully describe the diagnostic statement. The guideline directs you to place the etiology code first, followed by the manifestation code. Let's review another example of multiple coding.

Diagnosis: Staphylococcal cellulitis of the face

              (Staphylococcal infection is the etiology and cellulitis is the manifestation.)

Index: **Cellulitis,** face (any part, except eye) 682.0

Tabular: **682 Other cellulitis and abscess**

              682.0 Face

Code(s):   682.0 Cellulitis of the face

You now must identify the etiology code.

Index: **Infection,** staphylococcal NEC 041.10

Tabular: **041 Bacterial infection in conditions classified elsewhere and of unspecified site**
              Note: This category is to be used as an additional code to identify the bacterial agent in diseases classified elsewhere. This category is also used to classify bacterial infections of unspecified nature or site.

              041.1 Staphylococcus

              041.10 Staphylococcus, unspecified

Code: 682.0, 041.10 Staphylococcal cellulitis of the face

Note that it is acceptable to sequence the manifestation code first in this example because code 682.0 is not italicized in the Tabular, and the instructional notation listed under category 682 in the Tabular specifically states "Use additional code to identify organism, . . ."

EXERCISE 15–3

MULTIPLE CODING

Using multiple codes, fill in the codes for the following diagnoses:

1 Chronic prostatitis due to *Streptococcus* species

   Code(s): _____

2 Acute bronchitis due to *Pseudomonas* species

   Code(s): _____

3 Gangrene due to diabetes mellitus, type I

   Code(s): _____

4 Urinary tract infection due to *Escherichia coli*

   Code(s): _____

5 Amyloid cardiomyopathy

   Code(s): _____

Uncertain Conditions

The basis for this guideline is that the diagnostic workup and arrangements for further workup, observation, or therapies are the same whether treating the confirmed condition or ruling it out.

Because hospitals are paid a lump sum (diagnosis-related group amount) for each hospitalization, the facility resources used are averaged. In an outpatient setting, only confirmed diagnoses may be coded. Rule out, possible, or probable diagnoses are coded to the chief complaint or sign or symptom that occasioned the visit. In an outpatient setting, each visit in the process of confirming a diagnosis is coded/billed.

EXAMPLES

> *Uncertain Diagnosis*
>
> *Hospital Inpatient*
>
> Diagnosis: Probable bronchitis (code as bronchitis)
> Index: **Bronchitis** 490
> Tabular: **490 Bronchitis**
>
> *Hospital Inpatient*
>
> Diagnosis: Rule out Graves' disease (code as Graves' disease)
> Index: **Graves' Disease** 242.0
> Tabular: **242.00 Toxic diffuse goiter** (Graves' disease)
>
> *Clinic Outpatient*
>
> Diagnosis: Chest pain, rule out myocardial infarction (code as chest pain)
> Index: **Pain(s),** chest 786.50
> Tabular: **786.50 Chest pain, unspecified**
>
> *Clinic Outpatient*
>
> Diagnosis: Cough and fever, probably pneumonia (code as cough and fever)
> Index: **Cough** 786.2
> Index: **Fever** 780.6
> Tabular: **786.2 Cough**
>   **780.6 Pyrexia of unknown origin** (fever)

Impending or Threatened Condition

B. If it did not occur, reference the Alphabetic Index to determine if the condition has a subentry term for "impending" or "threatened" and also reference main term entries for Impending and for Threatened.
1. If the subterms are listed, assign the given code.
2. If the subterms are not listed, code the existing forerunner condition(s) and not the condition described as impending or threatened.

EXAMPLES

Impending or Threatened Condition

Diagnosis:	Threatened abortion
Index:	**Threatened,** abortion 640.0
Tabular:	**640 Hemorrhage in early pregnancy**
	640.0 Threatened abortion
Code:	640.03 Threatened abortion
Diagnosis:	Impending myocardial infarction
Index:	**Impending,** myocardial infarction 411.1
Tabular:	**411 Other acute and subacute forms of ischemic heart disease**
	411.1 Intermediate coronary syndrome
	Impending infarction
	Preinfarction angina
	Preinfarction syndrome
	Unstable angina
Code:	411.1 Impending myocardial infarction

If the infarction had occurred, you would have coded it as a confirmed diagnosis by coding myocardial infarction (with the appropriate fifth digit to denote the episode of care).

EXERCISE 15-4

UNCERTAIN AND IMPENDING/THREATENED CONDITION

Fill in the codes for the following:

1 Evolving stroke

Code(s): _____

2 Impending delirium tremens

Code(s): _____

3 Threatened miscarriage

Code(s): _____

4 Threatened labor

Code(s): _____

5 Impending coronary syndrome

Code(s): _____

Selection of Principal Diagnosis

Official Coding and Reporting Guidelines

The circumstances of inpatient admission always govern the selection of the principal diagnosis. The principal diagnosis is defined in the Uniform Hospital Discharge Data Set (UHDDS) as "that condition established after study to be chiefly responsible for occasioning the admission of the patient to the hospital for care."

The principal diagnosis is sequenced first. In an outpatient setting, it is important to indicate as the first diagnosis the main reason for the visit, as well as subsequent diagnoses to substantiate adjunct services (such as laboratory and radiology). In other settings, this first diagnosis is sometimes called the primary diagnosis. The terminology "principal diagnosis" only refers to the acute care setting and is used in conjunction with the DRG payment scheme.

Official Coding and Reporting Guidelines

In determining the principal diagnosis, the coding directives in the ICD-9-CM manuals, Volume I, II, and III, take precedence over all other guidelines. The importance of consistent, complete documentation in the medical record cannot be overemphasized. Without such documentation the application of all coding guidelines is a difficult, if not an impossible, task.

Symptoms, Signs, and Ill-Defined Conditions

Official Coding and Reporting Guidelines

2.1 CODES FOR SYMPTOMS, SIGNS, AND ILL-DEFINED CONDITIONS

Codes for symptoms, signs, and ill-defined conditions from Chapter 16 (Symptoms, Signs, and Ill-Defined Conditions) are not to be used as principal diagnosis when a related definitive diagnosis has been established.

EXERCISE
15-5

SYMPTOMS, SIGNS, AND ILL-DEFINED CONDITIONS

1 A 63-year-old male is admitted with chest pain. Cardiac enzyme levels are elevated and the ECG indicates an acute myocardial infarction. The principal diagnosis is acute myocardial infarction. Chest pain is not coded, because it is a symptom of the definitive diagnosis of acute myocardial infarction.

Let's code this case together.

   a. For an acute myocardial infarction, infarction is the *manifestation*. "Acute" indicates the *episode* of care and "myocardial" indicates the general *site* of the infarction.

b. Locate the term "Infarction" in the Index.

c. Under the term "Infarct, infarction" you should next locate the sub-term "myocardial." Note after "myocardium, myocardial" you find "acute. . . ." and are directed to code 410.9.

d. Now turn to 410.9 in the Tabular, Volume 1.

e. Under "410.9 Unspecified site" you are presented with a notation that a fifth digit is required.

f. Go back to the three-digit category code 410 where the fifth digits are listed. The fifth digit 0 is for an unspecified episode of care; the fifth digit 1 is for the initial episode of care; and the fifth digit 2 is for a subsequent episode of care. The myocardial infarction was diagnosed during this visit, so that would fit the initial episode of care definition in the ICD-9-CM. The correct fifth digit is 1.

g. The complete, correct code is 410.91.

Now you try one.

2   A patient is admitted to the hospital with severe flank pain and hematuria. A urinalysis is done and it is positive for *Escherichia coli*. The discharge summary states acute pyelonephritis.

a. What is the principal diagnosis? _____

b. Locate the principal diagnosis in the Index. What code does the Index direct you to locate?

Code(s): _____

c. Locate the code in the Tabular. What is the three-digit category code and the title of the category you were directed to?

Code(s) and title: _____

d. Was there mention of a lesion in the case above? _____

e. What is the correct five-digit code for this case? _____

f. Why do you think "severe flank pain and hematuria" are noted on

this patient case? _____

STOP *Wait, you're not finished with this case yet. Go back to the three-digit category code 590 and look at the entry immediately under Infections of Kidney. A note states, "Use additional code to identify organism, such as Escherichia coli [E. coli] (041.4)." You also code 041.4 to indicate the type of infection present. You have to be very careful to read all notes in the category before coding. If, in the end, you arrived at codes 590.10 and 041.4, you did a fine job.*

Codes in Brackets

Official Coding and Reporting Guidelines

2.2 CODES IN BRACKETS

Codes in brackets in the Alphabetic Index can never be sequenced as principal diagnosis. Coding directives require that the codes in brackets be sequenced in the order specified in the Alphabetic Index.

from the trenches

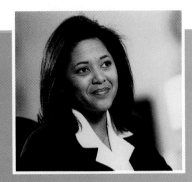

"*Many times, offices do not see the wealth of information available to them through a coding specialist. Once you are in the door, you can offer many learning opportunities to those who work with you. People want to be around knowledge and expertise.*"

YVONNE

EXERCISE 15-6

CODES IN BRACKETS

1 A patient is admitted with the diagnosis of malarial hepatitis.

a. You might not be sure whether the principal diagnosis is hepatitis or malaria.

b. Locate the term "malaria" in the Index. Under the subterm "any type, with" you will find "hepatitis 084.9 *[573.2]*." The slanted brackets alert you that *[573.2]* cannot be sequenced as the principal diagnosis.

c. Locate the term "hepatitis" and then the subterm "malarial." You again find 084.9 *[573.2]*.

d. Both Index entries direct you to the principal diagnosis of malaria. Hepatitis can be a manifestation of malaria. The slanted brackets in 084.9 *[573.2]* indicate that this hepatitis is a manifestation of the condition malaria. "Hepatitis" is the condition and "malarial" describes the hepatitis.

e. Under the four-digit code of 084.9 locate "Malarial" and then "Hepatitis." 084.9 Malaria is the principal diagnosis and *[573.2]* hepatitis is the complication, and you would record both, 084.9, 573.2.

You do the next one.

2 The patient's record states: systemic lupus erythematosus with lung involvement.

a. When you locate the term "erythematosus" in the Index, what do you find? _____

b. Locate the main term "Lupus," the subterm "erythematosus," the second subterm "systemic," and the last subterm "with lung involvement." What codes are you directed to?

Code(s): _____

c. What is the title of the three-digit category code located in the Tabular for the codes from b., above?

_____

d. What does the three-digit category code include?_____

_____

e. Under the three-digit category code you are also directed to "Use additional code to identify manifestation." Such as:

_____

That last entry tells you that you are to use *[517.8]* (lung involvement) if the principal diagnosis is in the three-digit category code 710 and further specified as "with lung involvement." This patient has lung involvement, so be alert to the use of the code in the brackets.

f. What four-digit code designates the principal diagnosis of "systemic lupus erythematosus"?

Code(s): _____

g. What are the two complete codes for this case?

Code(s): _____

Two or More Interrelated Conditions

> **Official Coding and Reporting Guidelines**
>
> **2.4 TWO OR MORE INTERRELATED CONDITIONS, EACH POTENTIALLY MEETING THE DEFINITION FOR PRINCIPAL DIAGNOSIS**
>
> When there are two or more interrelated conditions (such as a disease in the same ICD-9-CM chapter or a manifestation characteristically associated with a certain disease) potentially meeting the definition of principal diagnosis, either condition may be sequenced first, unless circumstances of the admission, the therapy provided, the Tabular List, or the Alphabetic Index indicate otherwise.

EXERCISE 15-7

TWO OR MORE INTERRELATED CONDITIONS

1 A patient is admitted with chest pain, shortness of breath, and a heart murmur. The patient undergoes a diagnostic cardiac catheterization, which shows two-vessel coronary artery disease and severe mitral (valve) stenosis. It is recommended that bypass surgery with mitral valve replacement be performed as soon as possible.

The patient has two conditions, each of which has the potential to be the principal diagnosis: mitral valve stenosis and coronary artery disease.

a. Locate stenosis in the Index: both "mitral" and "valve" indicate the type and site of the stenosis the patient has—the condition is stenosis. Under the main term "Stenosis," locate the subterm "mitral." The words in parentheses indicate the kinds of mitral stenosis, such as valve, chronic, or inactive. You are looking for valve, so the correct four-digit category code for the mitral valve stenosis is likely to be 394.0.

b. Locate coronary artery disease by locating the main term "Disease" and the subterms "artery" and "coronary." The entry you find tells you to "*see* Arteriosclerosis, coronary." Under the main term "Arteriosclerosis" and the subterm "coronary (artery)" you will be directed to code 414.00. If the Tabular validates codes 394.0 and 414.00, either code could be sequenced first because none of the information indicates one condition is more the principal diagnosis than the other.

Now you do one.

2 A patient is involved in a car accident and is admitted with an open fracture of the right humerus and an open fracture of the distal femur. Both fractures require open reduction, which means that the fracture will be repaired using an open incision into the fracture site.

a. What are the two diagnoses?

_____

Either of these diagnoses may be listed first, because both are addressed and plans are made to treat both surgically. They were equally the reason for admission to the hospital.

b. Under what main term in the Index would you look to locate both diagnoses?

_____

c. After the main term "Fracture," what would be the first subterm for the fracture of the right humerus?

_____

d. What is the word that appears in parentheses after this first subterm you just identified in c., above?

_____

Because your patient's case states "open," you know that 812.20 is not the correct code because 812.20 specifies "closed." Go farther down the list of subterms to "Fracture, humerus, open." What is the code for "open"?

Code(s): _____

e. In the Tabular, does the code you chose in the Index fit the description?

_____

You still have to locate the code for the open fracture of distal femur.

f. After looking in the Index using the main term "Fracture," what is the subterm you would locate?

_____

g. What is the word in parentheses after the first subterm?

_____

h. What is the next subterm? _____

i. What does this subterm direct you to do?

_____

j. When you take the subterm direction, what is the next subterm that you must use to get to the code?

_____

k. What is the code that you are directed to look up under "Fracture, femur, open, lower end, open"?

Code(s): _____

l. After checking the code in the Tabular, is the code correct?

_____

Two or More Diagnoses

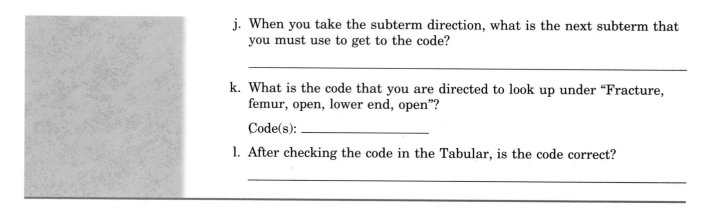

Official Coding and Reporting Guidelines

2.5 TWO OR MORE DIAGNOSES THAT EQUALLY MEET THE DEFINITION FOR PRINCIPAL DIAGNOSIS

In the usual instance when two or more diagnoses equally meet the criteria for principal diagnosis as determined by the circumstances of admission, diagnostic workup, and/or therapy provided, and the Alphabetic Index, Tabular List, or another coding guideline does not provide sequencing direction, any one of the diagnoses may be sequenced first.

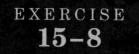

EXERCISE 15-8

TWO OR MORE DIAGNOSES

1   A patient is admitted with weakness, diarrhea of 2 days' duration, diaphoresis, and abdominal pain. The attending physician lists the diagnoses as viral gastroenteritis and dehydration. Intravenous fluids with electrolyte supplements are ordered.

a. Locate "Gastroenteritis" as the main term in the Index and then the subterm "viral." When you do this you will be directed to code 008.8 (unspecified) because the record does not specify the organism type.

b. After you have located code 008.8 in the Tabular and made sure it is the correct code, look for any notes under the three-digit category code to see if there are any fifth digits that need to be assigned.

c. The correct code is 008.8 and there are no fifth digits to be assigned. Now you need to code the other diagnosis of dehydration. It seems almost too good to be true: There is only one word in the diagnosis. "Dehydration" is the main term. Dehydration appears in the Index, and it points to only one code. Check out the code 276.5 in the Tabular.

d. The Tabular confirms that 276.5 is for dehydration or volume depletion and there is no note regarding any *Excludes* that concerns this case. There is no fifth digit with the category. The correct code is 276.5.

e. Remember, when two equally important diagnoses are indicated, it does not matter which code is sequenced first. So, the two codes for this case can be stated to be 008.8 and 276.5 *or* 276.5 and 008.8. The order of the codes may not seem too earth-shattering right now, but the order of the codes is significant. Later in this text, you will learn about how the hospital payment is made to the hospital by third-party payers based on the diagnosis codes. One of these diagnoses may be reimbursed at a higher rate than the other; therefore, selection of the principal diagnosis is critically important.

Now you have the opportunity to do the next case.

2   A patient is admitted with heavy menstrual bleeding of 2 days' duration, severe abdominal pain, and anemia due to acute blood loss. The patient is given medication intravenously to control the pain and bleeding. She also receives two units of packed cells for the anemia.

   a. What is the medical term for heavy menstrual/uterine bleeding?

   _____

   b. The medical term from the question above is the first diagnosis that you will need to locate. What code does the Index indicate and the Tabular of the text confirm as a code for the first diagnosis?

   Code(s): _____

   c. The second diagnosis is what? _____

   d. Locate the second diagnosis code and confirm your finding in the Tabular. (Hint: The subterms for the second code are "blood loss" and "acute.") What is the code?

   Code(s): _____

Comparative or Contrasting Conditions

Official Coding and Reporting Guidelines

2.6 TWO OR MORE COMPARATIVE OR CONTRASTING CONDITIONS

In those rare instances when two or more contrasting or comparative diagnoses are documented as "either/or" (or similar terminology), they are coded as if the diagnoses were confirmed, and the diagnoses are sequenced according to the circumstances of the admission. If no further determination can be made as to which diagnosis should be principal, either diagnosis may be sequenced first.

EXERCISE 15-9

COMPARATIVE OR CONTRASTING CONDITIONS

1   A patient is admitted to the hospital with chest pain, nausea, and dyspnea. The patient has a history of a prior myocardial infarction 2 years earlier. The pain is atypical. An ECG and cardiac enzyme study (creatine phosphokinase) are ordered, as well as an upper gastrointestinal series to rule out esophageal reflux. Diagnosis by the attending physician is myocardial infarction or esophageal reflux.

a. Infarction is located by the main term "Infarct, infarction" and the subterm "myocardium." In the Tabular, there is a notation of five-digit subclassifications that are used with category 410 codes. You might think that the patient was having a subsequent episode of care until you read the definitions attached to the fifth digits for initial and subsequent. "Subsequent" refers to a patient who has received care for the condition within the past 8 weeks. This patient was diagnosed and treated 2 years earlier, so this episode is considered an initial episode of care and has the fifth digit 1. The correct code is 410.91.

b. The second diagnosis is reflux, esophageal, located in the Index under the main term "Reflux" and the subterm "esophageal." You are directed to code 530.81. After checking this in the Tabular to be sure this is the correct code and has no exclusions or additions, you have the second of the two contrasting conditions, 530.81. Only further evaluation by the physician will finally determine what the principal diagnosis is; but for now, the case has been coded to the greatest specificity possible with the information available in the patient record. Either diagnosis may be selected as the principal diagnosis. You may want to consider which code would result in the higher reimbursement.

Here's a case for you to code.

2 A 75-year-old man is admitted with severe low back pain. He is known to have prostate cancer as well as severe spondylosis. Spine x-ray films and a bone scan are ordered. Differential diagnoses are compression fracture versus bone metastases from prostate cancer. (*Note:* The physician would have to be consulted to determine whether prostate cancer is "current" or "history of.")

a. What is the main term for compression fracture?

_____

b. Using "Fracture" as the main term and "compression" as the subterm, what are you directed to do?

_____

Before you continue to look up other possible subterms, you need to consider why the patient has severe low back pain. You may need to query the physician or review the record to determine whether the compression fracture was or was not due to trauma. The term **idiopathic** means of unknown cause; the term **pathologic** means due to a disease or accompanying a disease. Let us assume that the patient record substantiates a diagnosis of a fracture due to a disease (pathologic). Under Fracture locate pathologic and then the subterm "vertebrae." You are then forwarded to 733.13. Is that the correct code according to the Tabular?

c. The second diagnosis in the differential diagnoses is metastases from prostate cancer. Locating cancer in the Index you find: "*see also* Neoplasm, by site, malignant." The potential neoplasm is of the bone. "Neoplasm" is the main term and "bone" is a subterm. Secondary is the type of malignancy because the record states that this patient has had a history of prostate cancer (primary) and now has the potential to have bone (secondary) cancer. Under the "Secondary" column, what is the correct code for "Neoplasm, bone" for this patient?

Code(s): _____

An additional code would be assigned for the prostate cancer.

STOP *The difference between Guidelines 2.6 and 2.7 is the way the physician states the final diagnosis. In the Guideline 2.6 examples, symptoms are documented but the physician states "X versus Y" instead of listing the symptoms. In Guideline 2.7, the physician states the diagnosis as "symptoms due to X versus Y."*

Symptom(s) Followed by Contrasting/Comparative Diagnoses

> *Official Coding and Reporting Guidelines*
>
> **2.7 A SYMPTOM(S) FOLLOWED BY CONTRASTING/ COMPARATIVE DIAGNOSES**
>
> When a symptom(s) is followed by contrasting/comparative diagnoses, the symptom code is sequenced first. All the contrasting/comparative diagnoses should be coded as suspected conditions.

EXERCISE 15-10

SYMPTOM(S) FOLLOWED BY CONTRASTING/ COMPARATIVE DIAGNOSES

1   The patient presents with knee pain of 3 months' duration, with no known trauma, either bucket-handle tear of medial meniscus or loose body in the knee joint. The final diagnosis is knee pain due to bucket-handle tear of medial meniscus versus loose body in the knee joint.

There will be three codes for this case: one for the pain in the knee joint, one for the tear in the meniscus, and one for the loose body in the knee joint.

   a. Using "Pain, joint, knee" for the first condition, what is the correct code?

   Code(s): _____

   b. Using "Tear, meniscus, bucket handle, old," what is the correct second code?

   Code(s): _____

   c. Using "Loose, body, joint, knee," what is the correct third code?

   Code(s): _____

Observation for Suspected Conditions

> *Official Coding and Reporting Guidelines*
>
> **2.8 CODES FROM THE V71.0–V71.9 SERIES, OBSERVATION AND EVALUATION FOR SUSPECTED CONDITIONS**
>
> Codes from the V71.0–V71.9 series are assigned as principal diagnoses for encounters or admissions to evaluate the patient's condition when there is some evidence to suggest the existence of an abnormal condition or following an accident or other incident that ordinarily results in a health problem, and where no supporting evidence for the suspected condition is found and no treatment is currently required. The fact that the patient may be scheduled for continuing observation in the office/clinic setting following discharge does not limit the use of this category.

OBSERVATION FOR SUSPECTED CONDITIONS

1   The patient fell off his motorcycle when turning too sharply and hit his head on the sidewalk. The patient was wearing a helmet. The examination reveals no outwardly apparent head injury. The only injury noted on examination is abrasion of the elbow. The patient is admitted overnight to the hospital for observation to rule out head injury.

There will be two codes on this case: one for the observation of the injury (a V code) and one for the abrasion.

a.   Hospital observation is located in the Index under the main term "Observation." Listed under the main term are the reasons for observation, which you know by the word "for" in parentheses after the main term. The subterm is "accident NEC." Check the code in the Tabular. What is the V code?

Code(s): _____

b.   The second code is for the abrasion to the elbow. When you locate the term "abrasion" in the Index, you are referred to "*see also* Injury, superficial, by site." What is the code for the abrasion?

Code(s): _____

(See the cross-reference in the Tabular, and discover whether a fourth digit is needed for specificity.)

2   A patient is admitted for observation and further evaluation following an alleged rape.

a.   There is only one code for this case. What is that V code?

Code(s): _____

Original Treatment Plan Not Carried Out

Official Coding and Reporting Guidelines

2.9 ORIGINAL TREATMENT PLAN NOT CARRIED OUT

Sequence as the principal diagnosis the condition which after study occasioned the admission to the hospital, even though treatment may not have been carried out due to unforeseen circumstances.

ORIGINAL TREATMENT PLAN NOT CARRIED OUT

1   A patient is admitted to the hospital for an elective cholecystectomy. The patient has chronic cholecystitis, and gallstones were visualized on x-ray films. After admission, it is noticed that the patient has a fever, is coughing, and shows some patchy infiltrates on the chest x-ray film. Surgery is canceled because the patient may have pneumonia.

This case will have three codes: the cholecystitis with gallstones, pneumonia, and surgery not done.

a. The cholecystitis is chronic (subterm) with calculus (subterm), without mention of obstruction. What is the code?

Code(s): _____

b. What is the pneumonia code?

Code(s): _____

c. The surgery that was not done is located in the Index under "Surgery, not done because of." Why was the surgery not done?

_____

d. What is the code for the surgery not done?

Code(s): _____

No procedure code is submitted because no procedure was done.

2 A patient is admitted for elective sterilization by tubal ligation. The patient and her husband decide not to go through with the surgery, and the surgery is canceled.

a. How many codes will there be for this case and what are the main terms for each?

_____

b. What is the V code for the sterilization?

Code(s): _____

c. What is the code for the surgery not done?

Code(s): _____

TWO SPECIAL TYPES OF CODES YOU NEED TO KNOW ABOUT

There are 17 chapters in Volume 1, Tabular List, of the ICD-9-CM. Each of the chapters represents a different organ system or topic. You will review each of the chapters, but first, there are some special codes that you need to know about—V codes and late effects.

V Codes

Let's begin with the V codes. In the Tabular the V codes follow code 999.9. If you have an ICD-9-CM available, locate the V codes now. Notice that V codes have only two digits before the decimal point, and a V precedes the number. V codes can be located in the Index like any other code. Often, the most difficult thing about the V code is locating it in the Index. To help you become familiar with how to locate V codes in the Index, review the following, the most common Index terms for locating V codes:

Admission	Checking	Fitting of
Aftercare	Contraception	Follow-up
Attention to	Counseling	Health, Healthy
Boarder	Dialysis	History
Care (of)	Donor	Maintenance
Carrier	Examination	Maladjustment

Observation	Screening	Transplant
Problem	Status	Unavailability of
Procedure (surgical)	Supervision (of)	medical facilities
Prophylactic	Test	Vaccination
Replacement		

V codes are most often used in outpatient settings, that is, ambulatory care centers, physicians' offices, and outpatient departments of hospitals. There are three circumstances in which V codes are used:

1. A patient is not currently sick but receives health care services.

EXAMPLE

An elderly patient comes to the clinic for an influenza vaccination. The patient is not currently sick but receives the health care service of a vaccination.

Index: **Vaccination,** prophylactic, influenza V04.8

Tabular: **V04 Need for prophylactic vaccination and inoculation against certain viral diseases**

V04.8 Influenza

Code: V04.8 Influenza vaccination

2. A patient with a known disease or injury receives health services for specific treatment of the disease or injury.

EXAMPLE

A patient with breast cancer reports to the outpatient department of the hospital for a chemotherapy session. The patient is not currently sick but receives health care services for specific treatment of cancer.

Index: **Chemotherapy,** encounter (for) V58.1

Tabular: **V58 Other and unspecified aftercare**

V58.1 Chemotherapy

Code: V58.1 Chemotherapy treatment

The breast cancer (174.9) would also be coded, but you will learn about the details of that later in the chapter; for now, concentrate on the use of the V codes. V codes should not be mistaken for procedure codes. There is an ICD-9-CM procedure code to identify chemotherapy (99.25). Facility policy and the setting will determine the assignment of the procedure code.

3. A circumstance or problem is present and influences a patient's health status but is not in itself a current illness or injury. (In these situations the V code should be used only as a supplementary or secondary code.)

EXAMPLE

A patient who is allergic to penicillin is admitted to the hospital for treatment of pneumonia using intravenous antibiotic. The patient receives health services for the pneumonia, but the patient's allergy to penicillin is a special consideration in the treatment received.

Index: **History** (personal) of, allergy to, antibiotic agent NEC V14.1, penicillin V14.0

Tabular: **V14 Personal history of allergy to medicinal agents**

V14.0 Penicillin

Code: V14.0 History of allergy to penicillin

Additionally, the pneumonia (486) would be coded, but you are focusing only on the use of V codes right now.

EXERCISE 15-13

V CODES

Fill in the V code(s) for the following:

1   Admission for cardiac pacemaker adjustment

Code(s): _____

2   Insertion of subdermal implantable contraceptive

Code(s): _____

3   Personal history of cancer of the prostate

Code(s): _____

4   Baby in for MMR (measles, mumps, rubella) vaccination

Code(s): _____

5   Screening mammogram

Code(s): _____

6   Clinic visit for pre-employment physical examination

Code(s): _____

CAUTION *Often, the patient record states that there is a "history of" a disease: for example, "history of diabetes mellitus." This does not mean that the patient no longer has diabetes mellitus, but that the patient's medical history includes diabetes mellitus. You would not assign a V code to indicate a previous history of diabetes mellitus, but instead would assign the code for the current disease of diabetes mellitus (250.0X). If there is any question regarding the current status of the disease, check with the physician. You may also want to offer some physician education regarding the documentation of past history of diseases.*

Late Effects

Late effects codes are not assigned to a separate chapter in the Tabular. Instead, you must first identify a case as a late effect and then code it as such. You use late effects codes when the acute phase of the illness or injury has passed but a residual remains. Sometimes an acute illness or injury leaves a patient with a residual health problem that remains after the illness or injury has resolved. The residual is coded first and then the late effects code is assigned to indicate the cause of the residual. Note that the late effects code is accessed in the Index under the main term "Late." An example would be scars that remain after a severe burn.

In most instances, two codes will be assigned—one code for the residual that is being treated and one code that indicates the cause (late effect) of the residual. There is no time limit for the development of a residual. It may be evident at the time of the acute illness or it may occur months after an injury. It is also possible that a patient may develop more than one residual. For example, a patient who has had a stroke may develop right-sided hemiparesis and aphasia.

Official Coding and Reporting Guidelines

2.10 RESIDUAL CONDITION OR NATURE OF THE LATE EFFECT

The residual condition or nature of the late effect is sequenced first, followed by the late effect code for the cause of the residual condition, except in a few instances where the Alphabetic Index or Tabular List directs otherwise.

For example, a person cannot have a current hip fracture (820.8) and a late effect of hip fracture (905.3). The code is either a current injury or a condition caused by a prior injury. It cannot be both at the same time. (The only exception to this rule is in category 438, Late effects of cerebrovascular disease; this is explained in Guideline 1.7A.)

Official Coding and Reporting Guidelines

1.7 LATE EFFECT

A late effect is the residual effect (condition produced) after the acute phase of an illness or injury has terminated. There is no time limit on when a late effect code can be used. The residual may be apparent early, such as in cerebrovascular accident cases, or it may occur months or years later, such as that due to a previous injury.
   Coding of late effects requires two codes:

A. The residual condition or nature of the late effect.
B. The cause of the late effect.

The residual condition or nature of the late effect is sequenced first, followed by the cause of the late effect, except in those few instances where the code for late effect is followed by a manifestation code identified in the Tabular List and title or the late effect code has been expanded (at the fourth- and fifth-digit levels) to include the manifestation(s).
   The code for the acute phase of an illness or injury that led to the late effect is never used with a code for the cause of the late effect.

Official Coding and Reporting Guidelines

A. LATE EFFECT OF CEREBROVASCULAR DISEASE

Category 438 is used to indicate conditions classifiable to categories 430–437 as the causes of late effects (neurologic deficits), themselves classified elsewhere. These "late effects" include neurologic deficits that persist after initial onset of conditions classifiable to 430–437. The neurologic deficits caused by cerebrovascular disease may be present from the onset or may arise at any time after the onset of the condition classifiable to 430–437.
   Codes from category 438 may be assigned on a health care record with codes from 430–437 if the patient has a current CVA and deficits from an old CVA.
   Assign code V12.59 (and not a code from category 438) as an additional code for history of cerebrovascular disease when no neurologic deficits are present.

EXAMPLE

Diagnosis:	Dysphagia due to a previous cerebrovascular accident
Residual:	Dysphagia

  The dysphagia is a problem that remains following the acute illness of the cerebrovascular accident.

Cause:	Cerebrovascular accident

(This patient had a previous cerebrovascular accident.)

Terms to code:	Dysphagia [residual]
	Cerebrovascular accident [cause]

EXERCISE 15-14

RESIDUAL AND CAUSE

Write the term(s) that represent the residual and the cause of the following cases on the lines provided:

1 Scars of the face resulting from third-degree burns suffered 1 year ago

   Residual _____

   Cause _____

2 Constrictive pericarditis due to old tuberculosis infection

   Residual _____

   Cause _____

3 Residual foreign body in femur due to gunshot injury years ago

   Residual _____

   Cause _____

4 Mental retardation due to previous poliomyelitis

   Residual _____

   Cause _____

5 Leg pain resulting from old fracture of femur

   Residual _____

   Cause _____

STOP *As Guideline 1.7 indicates, you usually sequence the code for the residual condition first, followed by the late effects code. To locate the late effects codes in the ICD-9-CM, use the entry "Late Effects" in the Index. There are numerous subterms that describe the various late effects. Review and become familiar with the late effects subterms.*

If you have trouble identifying the appropriate late effects code, it may be helpful to assign the code for the acute injury or disease first; then refer to the Index for that injury or disease; and then refer to the entry "injury or condition classifiable to. . . ."

EXAMPLE

The following are the steps that you would take to correctly code the example of dysphagia due to a previous cerebrovascular accident as used in the preceding example.

Diagnosis: Dysphagia due to a previous cerebrovascular accident

Index: **Late, cerebrovascular disease with dysphagia** 438.82

EXERCISE 15-15

RESIDUAL AND CAUSE CODES

Now you identify the residual and cause terms and code the following diagnoses:

1 Traumatic arthritis following fracture of the left ankle 3 years ago

Residual _____

Code(s): _____

Cause _____

Code(s): _____

2 Aphasia due to cerebrovascular accident 6 months ago (requires one combination code)

Residual _____

Cause _____

Code: _____

3 Sensorineural deafness due to previous meningitis

Residual _____

Code(s): _____

Cause _____

Code(s): _____

CHAPTER-SPECIFIC GUIDELINES

Infectious and Parasitic Diseases

Chapter 1 in the Tabular is Infectious and Parasitic Diseases, which classifies diseases according to the etiology, or cause, of the disease. Because infectious or parasitic conditions can affect different parts of the body, the chapter contains a wide variety of codes.

In this chapter there are many instances of combination coding and multiple coding. Remember: ***Combination coding*** applies when one code fully describes the condition. ***Multiple coding*** is acceptable when it takes more than one code to fully describe the condition, so the sequencing of multiple codes may have to be considered.

from the trenches

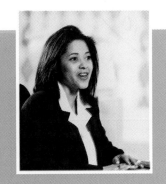

What allows you to take the most pride in your career?
"I am highly trained in what I do. When I conduct a teaching session for physicians or employees, they leave excited . . . I am proud to share my knowledge."

YVONNE

EXAMPLE

Combination Coding

Diagnosis:	Candidiasis infection of the mouth
Index:	**Candidiasis,** candidal 112.9, mouth 112.0
Tabular:	**112.0 Candidiasis of mouth**
Code:	112.0 Candidiasis infection of the mouth

The code 112.0 fully describes the diagnosis.

Multiple Coding

Diagnosis:	Urinary tract infection due to *Escherichia coli (E. coli)*
Index:	**Infection,** infected, infective, urinary (tract) NEC 599.0
Tabular:	**599.0 Urinary tract infection, site not specified**

Use additional code to identify organism, such as *Escherichia coli [E. coli]* (041.4)

Code 599.0 does not fully describe the condition. The instructions in the Tabular for code 599.0 state that you are to also code the organism causing the urinary tract infection. To locate a causative organism, you locate the main term "infection" in the Index and then the subterm of the specific organism. The urinary tract infection is sequenced first and the bacterial organism follows.

EXAMPLE

Index:	**Infection,** infected, infective, *Escherichia coli* NEC 041.4
Tabular:	**041 Bacterial infection in conditions classified elsewhere and of unspecified site**
	041.4 *Escherichia coli [E. coli]*
Codes:	599.0, 041.4 Urinary tract infection due to *Escherichia coli (E. coli)*

Multiple coding is necessary to fully describe the infection of the urinary tract and the causative organism, *E. coli.*

Human Immunodeficiency

Another important category in Chapter 1 is 042 Human Immunodeficiency Virus (HIV) Disease. Review the guidelines for HIV codes.

Know!

Official Coding and Reporting Guidelines

HUMAN IMMUNODEFICIENCY VIRUS (HIV) INFECTIONS

10.1 CODE ONLY CONFIRMED CASES OF HIV INFECTION/ILLNESS

This is an exception to Guideline 1.8, which states, "If the diagnosis documented at the time of discharge is qualified as 'probable,' 'suspect,' 'likely,' 'questionable,' 'possible,' or 'still to be ruled out,' code the condition as if it existed or was established." In this context, confirmation does not require documentation of positive serology or culture for HIV; the physician's diagnostic statement that the patient is HIV positive, or has an HIV-related illness, is sufficient.

10.2 SELECTION OF HIV CODE

042   Human Immunodeficiency Virus (HIV) Disease
        Patients with an HIV-related illness should be coded to 042, Human Immunodeficiency Virus [HIV] Disease.

V08   Asymptomatic Human Immunodeficiency Virus (HIV) Infection
        Patients with physician-documented asymptomatic HIV infections who have never had an HIV-related illness should be coded to V08, Asymptomatic Human Immunodeficiency Virus [HIV] Infection.

795.71 Nonspecific Serologic Evidence of Human Immunodeficiency Virus [HIV]
        Code 795.71, Nonspecific serologic evidence of human immunodeficiency virus [HIV] should be used for patients (including infants) with inconclusive HIV test results.

10.3 PREVIOUSLY DIAGNOSED HIV-RELATED ILLNESS

Patients with any known prior diagnosis of an HIV-related illness should be coded to 042. Once a patient has developed an HIV-related illness, the patient should always be assigned code 042 on every subsequent admission. Patients previously diagnosed with any HIV illness (042) should never be assigned with 795.71 or V08.

10.4 SEQUENCING

The sequencing of diagnoses for patients with HIV-related illnesses follows Guideline 2 for selection of principal diagnosis. That is, the circumstances of admission govern the selection of principal diagnosis, that condition established after study to be chiefly responsible for occasioning the admission of the patient to the hospital for care.

Patients who are admitted for an HIV-related illness should be assigned a minimum of two codes: first assign code 042 to identify the HIV disease and then sequence additional codes to identify the other diagnoses.

If a patient is admitted for an HIV-related condition, the principal diagnosis should be 042, followed by additional diagnosis codes for all reported HIV-related conditions.

If a patient with HIV disease is admitted for an unrelated condition (such as a traumatic injury), the code for the unrelated condition (e.g., the nature of injury code) should be the principal diagnosis. Other diagnoses would be 042 followed by additional diagnosis codes for all reported HIV-related conditions.

Whether the patient is newly diagnosed or has had previous admissions for HIV conditions (or has expired) is irrelevant to the sequencing decision.

10.5 HIV-INFECTIONS IN PREGNANCY, CHILDBIRTH, AND PUERPERIUM

During pregnancy, childbirth, or the puerperium, a patient admitted because of an HIV-related illness should receive a principal diagnosis of 647.8X, other specified infectious and parasitic diseases in the mother classifiable elsewhere, but complicating the pregnancy, childbirth, or the puerperium, followed by 042 and the code(s) for the HIV-related illness(es). This is an exception to the sequencing rule found in 10.4 above.

Patients with asymptomatic HIV infection status admitted during pregnancy, childbirth, or the puerperium should receive codes of 647.8X and V08.

10.6 ASYMPTOMATIC HIV INFECTION

V08   Asymptomatic human immunodeficiency virus (HIV) infection, is to be applied when the patient without any documentation of symptoms is listed as being HIV positive, known HIV, HIV test positive, or similar terminology. Do not use this code if the term AIDS is used or if the patient is treated for any HIV-related illness or is described as having any condition(s) resulting from his/her HIV positive status; use code 042 in these cases.

10.7 INCONCLUSIVE LABORATORY TEST FOR HIV

Patients with inconclusive HIV serology, but no definitive diagnosis or manifestations of the illness may be assigned code 795.71, inconclusive serologic test for Human Immunodeficiency Virus [HIV].

10.8 TESTING FOR HIV

If the patient is asymptomatic but wishes to know his/her HIV status, use code V73.89, Screening for other specified viral disease. Use code V69.8, Other problems related to lifestyle, as a secondary code if an asymptomatic patient is in a known high-risk group for HIV. Should a patient with signs or symptoms or illness, or a confirmed HIV-related diagnosis be tested for HIV, code the signs and symptoms or the diagnosis. An additional counseling code V65.44 may be used if counseling is provided during the encounter for the test.

When the patient returns to be informed of his/her HIV test results, use code V65.44, HIV counseling, if the results of the test are negative. If the results are positive but the patient is asymptomatic, use code V08, Asymptomatic HIV infection. If the results are positive and the patient is symptomatic, use code 042, HIV infection, with codes for the HIV-related symptoms or diagnosis. The HIV counseling code may also be used if counseling is provided for patients with positive test results.

As stated in Guideline 10.1, you do not assign 042 to a patient's record or insurance claim unless the diagnosis of HIV is a confirmed diagnosis. The assignment of the code prior to confirmation may cause the patient many unwarranted problems if the patient does not have HIV. Use extreme caution when assigning 042.

Infectious and Parasitic Diseases

Official Coding and Reporting Guidelines

7 SEPTICEMIA AND SEPTIC SHOCK

When the diagnosis of septicemia with shock or the diagnosis of general sepsis with septic shock is documented, code and list the septicemia first and report the septic shock code as a secondary condition. The septicemia code assignment should identify the type of bacteria if it is known.

Sepsis and septic shock associated with abortion, ectopic pregnancy, and molar pregnancy are classified to category codes in Chapter 11 (630–639).

Negative or inconclusive blood cultures do not preclude a diagnosis of septicemia in patients with clinical evidence of the condition.

EXERCISE 15-16

INFECTIOUS AND PARASITIC DISEASES

Code the following infectious diseases:

1 Viral gastroenteritis
Code(s): _____

2 Septicemia due to *Pseudomonas* species with septic shock
Code(s): _____

3 Acute poliomyelitis
Code(s): _____

4 Candidal vaginal infection
Code(s): _____

Neoplasms

Chapter 2 in the Tabular is similar to Chapter 1, Infectious and Parasitic Diseases, in that it classifies diseases according to the etiology, or cause, of the disease. Neoplastic conditions can affect all parts of the body. Before you learn more about what is in Chapter 2, we will quickly review some of the specific terminology.

EXERCISE 15-17

NEOPLASMS TERMINOLOGY

Match the following terms to the correct definitions:

1 neoplasm _____
2 malignant _____
3 primary _____
4 secondary _____
5 benign _____
6 in situ _____
7 uncertain behavior _____
8 unspecified nature _____
9 morphology _____

a. not progressive or recurrent

b. malignancy that is located within the original site of development

c. used to describe a cancerous tumor that grows worse over time

d. study of neoplasms

e. refers to the behavior of a neoplasm as neither malignant nor benign but having characteristics of both malignant and benign neoplasms

f. when the behavior or histology of a neoplasm is not known or not specified

g. site to which a malignant tumor has spread

h. site of origin or where the tumor originated

i. new tumor growth that can be benign or malignant

Neoplasm Codes

Locating a code for a neoplasm is a two-step process:

1. First, locate the morphology or histologic type of the neoplasm in the Index, for example, carcinoma, adenocarcinoma, sarcoma, melanoma, lymphoma, lipoma, adenoma.

2. Once you have located the morphology, review all modifiers and subterms, and then follow the instructions or verify the code listed. Most often you will be instructed to turn to the Neoplasm Table in the Index to find the code.

When you locate the morphology of the neoplasm, you can identify the "M" or morphology code. The M codes are in parentheses following the morphology. M codes are used in some inpatient settings and are optional, so facility policy would determine their usage.

M codes are alphanumeric codes and are listed in Appendix A of the ICD-9-CM code book. The alphanumeric structure of the morphology codes starts with the letter M, followed by four digits that indicate the histologic type of neoplasm, and a slash, followed by a fifth digit that indicates the behavior.

Behavior

/0 =	Benign
/1 =	Uncertain whether benign or malignant
	Borderline malignancy
/2 =	Carcinoma in situ
	Intraepithelial
	Noninfiltrating
	Noninvasive
/3 =	Malignant, primary site
/6 =	Malignant, metastatic site
	Secondary site
/9 =	Malignant, uncertain whether primary or metastatic site

EXAMPLE

> *ICD-9-CM Codes and Morphology Codes*
>
> Diagnosis: Adenocarcinoma of the upper-outer quadrant right breast with metastasis to the axillary lymph nodes.
>
> Index: **Adenocarcinoma** (M8140/3)—*see also* Neoplasm, by site, malignant
>
> Neoplasm Table: Breast, upper-outer quadrant 174.4 (primary column)
>
> Lymph, lymphatic, gland (secondary column), axilla, axillary 196.3
>
> Tabular: **174 Malignant neoplasm of female breast**
>
> **174.4 Upper-outer quadrant**
>
> **196 Secondary and unspecified malignant neoplasm of lymph nodes**
>
> **196.3 Lymph nodes of axilla and upper limb**
>
> Codes: 174.4, 196.3 Adenocarcinoma of the upper-outer quadrant right breast with metastasis to the axillary lymph nodes

But, wait, you're not finished yet. You have two M codes to assign to this diagnosis before you are finished—one for the primary adenocarcinoma and one for a secondary adenocarcinoma. Both M codes will have the same histologic type of adenocarcinoma, but the fifth digit will be different to indicate the primary and secondary behaviors.

Index:	**Adenocarcinoma** (M8140/3)—*see also* Neoplasm, by site, malignant
M code:	**primary** adenocarcinoma of the breast, M8140/**3**
M code:	**secondary** adenocarcinoma of the axillary lymph nodes, M8140/**6**
ICD-9-CM and M Codes:	174.4, M8140/3, 196.3, M8140/6 Adenocarcinoma of the upper-outer quadrant right breast with metastasis to the axillary lymph nodes

Note that the M codes are sequenced after the ICD-9-CM diagnosis code to which they refer.

Official Coding and Reporting Guidelines

2.13 NEOPLASMS

A. If the treatment is directed at the malignancy, designate the malignancy as the principal diagnosis, except when the purpose of the encounter or hospital admission is for radiotherapy session(s), V58.0, or for chemotherapy session(s), V58.1, in which instance the malignancy is coded and sequenced second.

B. When a patient is admitted for the purpose of radiotherapy or chemotherapy and develops complications, such as uncontrolled nausea and vomiting or dehydration, the principal diagnosis is Encounter for radiotherapy, V58.0, or Encounter for chemotherapy, V58.1.

C. When an episode of inpatient care involves surgical removal of a primary site or secondary site malignancy followed by adjunct chemotherapy or radiotherapy, code the malignancy as the principal diagnosis, using codes in the 140–198 series or, where appropriate in the 200–203 series.

D. When the reason for admission is to determine the extent of the malignancy, or for a procedure such as paracentesis or thoracentesis, the primary malignancy or appropriate metastatic site is designated as the principal diagnosis, even though chemotherapy or radiotherapy is administered.

E. When the primary malignancy has been previously excised or eradicated from its site and there is no adjunct treatment directed to that site and no evidence of any remaining malignancy at the primary site, use the appropriate code from the V10 series to indicate the former site of primary malignancy. Any mention of extension, invasion, or metastasis to a nearby structure or organ or to a distant site is coded as a secondary malignant neoplasm to the site and may be the principal diagnosis in the absence of the primary site.

F. When a patient is admitted because of a primary neoplasm with metastasis and treatment is directed toward the secondary site only, the secondary neoplasm is designated as the principal diagnosis even though the primary malignancy is still present.

G. Symptoms, signs, and ill-defined conditions listed in Chapter 16 characteristic of, or associated with, an existing primary or secondary site malignancy cannot be used to replace the malignancy as principal diagnosis, regardless of the number of admissions or encounters for treatment and care of the neoplasm.

H. Coding and sequencing of complications associated with the malignancy neoplasm or with the therapy thereof are subject to the following guidelines:

   1. When admission is for management of an anemia associated with the malignancy, and the treatment is only for anemia, the anemia is designated as the principal diagnosis and is followed by the appropriate code(s) for the malignancy.

2. When admission is for management of an anemia associated with chemotherapy or radiotherapy and the only treatment is for the anemia, the anemia is designated as the principal diagnosis followed by the appropriate code(s) for the malignancy.

3. When the admission is for management of dehydration due to the malignancy or the therapy, or a combination of both, and only the dehydration is being treated (intravenous rehydration), the dehydration is designated as the principal diagnosis, followed by the code(s) for the malignancy.

4. When the admission is for treatment of a complication resulting from a surgical procedure performed for the treatment of an intestinal malignancy, designate the complication as the principal diagnosis if treatment is directed at resolving the complication.

V codes are also frequently used when coding neoplasms. There are V codes present in the ICD-9-CM to indicate the history of a malignant neoplasm (V10.00–V10.9). These history codes are used to indicate a primary malignant neoplasm that is no longer present. Remember that in the V code section, you were presented with information about documenting a "history of" a disease. Be careful in determining whether the physician is indicating a past and current history of a condition or a true past history. With neoplasms there is often a true "history of" whereby the condition previously existed but is no longer present.

There are also encounter codes for chemotherapy (V58.1) and radiotherapy (V58.0). When coding an encounter for chemotherapy or radiotherapy, code the V code first, followed by the active code for the malignant neoplasm, even if that neoplasm has already been removed. As long as the neoplasm is being treated with adjunctive therapy following a surgical removal of the cancer, you can code that neoplasm as if it still exists. You would not assign a "history of" V code because the neoplasm is the reason for the treatment. Instead, the neoplasm is coded as a current or active disease.

EXERCISE 15-18

NEOPLASM CODES

1 A patient is admitted for chemotherapy for ovarian cancer.

Two codes are needed for this case: one for the encounter for chemotherapy and the other for the malignant, primary, ovarian neoplasm.

Locate in the Index and verify in the Tabular the two codes necessary to code this case.

Code(s): _____

2 A patient is admitted for radiation therapy for metastatic bone cancer. The patient had a mastectomy for breast cancer 3 years earlier.

There is a code for the admission for radiation management, which will be a V code; a code for the secondary, malignant, bone neoplasm; and a V code for the history of malignant neoplasm of the breast. What are these three codes?

Code(s): _____

3 A patient is admitted with chest pain, shortness of breath, and a history of bloody sputum. Diagnostic x-ray film shows a mass in the bronchial tube. A diagnostic bronchoscopy is performed and is positive for cancer. The pathology report states "metastatic carcinoma of bronchus, primary unknown." The patient chooses to undergo chemotherapy.

a. What is the description of the principal diagnosis? _____

b. What is the subsequent diagnosis description? _____

c. Is metastatic carcinoma of the bronchus considered a primary or secondary malignant neoplasm? _____

d. What are the diagnosis codes for this case?

Code(s): _____

4 A patient is admitted with uncontrolled nausea and vomiting after chemotherapy treatment for lung cancer.

a. How many codes would be needed to accurately reflect this case? ____

b. What is the principal diagnosis? _____

c. What is the secondary diagnosis? _____

d. What is the code for the principal diagnosis?

Code(s): _____

e. What is the code for the secondary diagnosis?

Code(s): _____

Unknown Site or Unspecified

There is an entry on the Neoplasm Table that states "unknown site or unspecified." This code, 199.1, is used to indicate either an unknown or an unspecified primary or secondary malignancy. If there is a known secondary site, a code must be assigned to the primary site or the history of a primary site. It is possible for a primary site to be unknown.

EXAMPLE

Diagnosis:	Metastatic bone cancer.

This statement indicates that the bone cancer is a secondary neoplasm, but there is no indication of the location of the primary site.

Index:	**Cancer** (M8000/3)—*see also* Neoplasm, by site, malignant
Neoplasm Table:	Bone 198.5 (secondary)
	Unknown site or unspecified 199.1 (primary)
Tabular:	**198 Secondary malignant neoplasm of other specified site**
	198.5 Bone and bone marrow
Tabular:	**199 Malignant neoplasm without specification of site**
	199.1 Other
Codes:	198.5, 199.1 Metastatic bone cancer (if the treatment is for the secondary site)
	199.1, 198.5 Metastatic bone cancer (if the treatment or diagnostic workup is for the primary site)

The sequencing of the primary and secondary neoplasms is dependent on the treatment circumstances documented in the health record. If treatment was directed toward the secondary malignancy, that code would be sequenced first. If treatment is focused on determining the site of the unknown primary malignancy, that code would be sequenced first.

EXERCISE 15-19

MORE NEOPLASMS

Practice assigning ICD-9-CM codes as well as the appropriate M codes for the following neoplasms:

1 Multiple myeloma

Code(s): _____

2 Carcinoma in situ cervix

Code(s): _____

3 Cancer of the sigmoid colon with spread to the peritoneum

Code(s): _____

4 Adenocarcinoma of the prostate with metastasis to the bone

Code(s): _____

5 Metastatic cancer to the brain; primary unknown

Code(s): _____

6 Metastatic carcinoma of the breast to the lungs; the breast carcinoma has been removed by mastectomy

Code(s): _____

Endocrine, Nutritional, and Metabolic Diseases and Immunity Disorders

Chapter 3 in the Tabular describes diseases or conditions affecting the endocrine system. The endocrine system involves glands that are located throughout the body and are responsible for secreting hormones into the bloodstream. Also included in Chapter 3 are diseases or conditions that affect nutritional and metabolic status as well as disorders of the immune system.

One of the frequently used category codes in Chapter 3 is 250 Diabetes Mellitus. When you locate diabetes in the Index, you will note that for many of the subterms, two codes are listed. The 250.X code is followed by an italicized code in brackets. This is because multiple coding is common for diabetes inasmuch as both the manifestation (symptom) and the etiology (cause—diabetes) are coded.

EXAMPLE

> Index: **Diabetes,** retinopathy, background, 250.5X *[362.01]*

There are four five-digit subclassifications for use with category 250. It is essential that you read these before assigning codes for diagnosis of diabetes mellitus (DM). The fifth digits identify the type of diabetes: 2 is type II [non−insulin-dependent type] [NIDDM type] [adult-onset type] or unspecified type, uncontrolled; and 3 is type I [insulin-dependent type] [IDDM] [juvenile type], uncontrolled. NIDDM refers to non−insulin-dependent DM and IDDM refers to insulin-dependent DM. It is possible for a type II diabetic to receive insulin, so it is best if the health care providers document the type. You should not assume that because a patient is receiving insulin that he or she is insulin-dependent. Because a type II diabetic may be receiving insulin, if there is any question regarding the type of diabetes, query the physician. In order to appropriately assign the fifth digits 2 or 3, uncontrolled diabetes, the physician must document that the patient's DM is uncontrolled or out of control. If a complication is specified (250.1–250.8), assign the appropriate fourth and fifth digits; do not use the .9 (unspecified).

EXAMPLE

Diagnosis: Diabetic iritis

Index: **Diabetes, diabetic,** iritis 250.5 *[364.42]*

The first code (250.5) indicates the etiology (diabetes) and the second code *[364.42]* indicates the manifestation (iritis). You need two codes to describe diagnosis. You will always code first the etiology and then the manifestation.

Tabular: **250.5 Diabetes with ophthalmic manifestations**

Use additional code, if desired, to identify manifestation, as:

364.4 Vascular disorders of iris and ciliary body

The Tabular also indicates that a fifth digit should be added for greater specificity.

Tabular: **364.4 Vascular disorders of iris and ciliary body**

364.42 Rubeosis iridis

Even though the 364.42 entry above does not specifically indicate iritis, you trust the code that is listed in the Index. You could also look up the main term "Iritis" in the Index and be directed to the same codes.

Index: **Iritis** 364.3, diabetic 250.5 *[364.42]*

You are directed to the same codes.

Code(s):   250.50, 364.42 Diabetic iritis

The codes must be sequenced in this order and indicate that iritis is a manifestation of the diabetes.

To code a disease or condition as a manifestation of DM, it must be stated that the disease or condition is diabetic or due to the diabetes. A cause-and-effect relationship must be evident. If you are unsure of the relationship, you must clarify this with the physician.

If a cause-and-effect relationship is not evident, the following codes would be assigned.

EXAMPLE

Diagnosis: Diabetes mellitus and iritis

Index: **Diabetes, diabetic** 250.0

Note—Use the following fifth-digit subclassification with category 250:

The Note in the Index directs you to use a fifth digit for greater specificity.

Tabular: **250.0 Diabetes mellitus without mention of complication**

Index: **Iritis** 364.3

Tabular: **364.3 Unspecified iridocyclitis**

Code(s):   250.00 Diabetes and 364.3 Iritis

Note that codes (250.00 and 364.3) are different because a cause-and-effect relationship was not established—the iritis is not a manifestation of the diabetes in this case.

EXERCISE 15-20

ENDOCRINE, NUTRITIONAL, AND METABOLIC DISEASES AND IMMUNITY DISORDERS

Fill in the codes for the following:

1 Addison's disease

Code(s): _____

2 Dehydration

Code(s): _____

3 Diabetes mellitus with hypoglycemic coma

Code(s): _____

4 Graves' disease with thyrotoxic crisis

Code(s): _____

Diseases of the Blood and Blood-Forming Organs

Chapter 4, Diseases of the Blood and Blood-Forming Organs, is a short chapter with only 10 categories. The **anemia** category is often used because anemia is the most common blood disease. Anemia is the main term under which you will find the many subterms that relate to anemia. In addition to there being numerous subterms for anemia, many of those subterms have lengthy additional subterms listed under them.

There are two anemias that are easy to confuse—anemia of chronic disease and chronic anemia. These two diagnostic statements do not have the same meaning. In anemia of chronic disease, the word "chronic" describes the nature of the disease that is the cause of the anemia, for example, Anemia due to neoplastic disease. The neoplasm is the chronic disease causing the anemia. Code anemia (285.22) and then assign the appropriate code to identify the neoplastic process. In the diagnostic statement chronic anemia, the word "chronic" describes a type of anemia. Let's see what difference these diagnostic statements make in code assignment.

EXAMPLE

Diagnosis: Anemia of chronic disease

In this diagnosis statement, you do not know what the chronic disease is.

Index: **Anemia**

The Index has a subterm (in, chronic illness, 285.29) that further directs you in the choice of the correct code.

Tabular: **285.9 Anemia of other chronic illness**

Code: **285.29** Anemia of chronic illness

Diagnosis: Chronic anemia

Index: **Anemia** 285.9, chronic simple 281.9

In this example, the Index does indicate a subterm that further directs you to chronic simple 281.9.

Tabular: **281.9 Unspecified deficiency anemia**

Code: 281.9 Chronic anemia

If there is any question about how to classify an anemia, check with the physician.

EXERCISE 15-21

DISEASES OF THE BLOOD AND BLOOD-FORMING ORGANS

Fill in the codes for the following:

1 Pernicious anemia

Code(s): _____

2 Disseminated intravascular coagulation (DIC)

Code(s): _____

3 Hemophilia

Code(s): _____

4 Acute blood-loss anemia

Code(s): _____

5 Familial polycythemia

Code(s): _____

Mental Disorders

Chapter 5 in the Tabular is Mental Disorders. The chapter includes four sections: organic psychotic conditions; other psychoses; neurotic, personality, and other nonpsychotic mental disorders; and mental retardation.

Appendix B in the ICD-9-CM is the Glossary of Mental Disorders. Your understanding of the definitions of these mental disorders is necessary to enable you to code the diagnoses accurately. When assigning codes from Chapter 5, you need to take extra care to select the appropriate code(s) and code only diagnoses that are documented in the medical record. Mental disorders can be difficult to code also because physicians are not always as specific in their diagnostic statements as might be required by the codes in this chapter. When in doubt, always check with the physician. Just one term in the medical record can make a big difference in the code(s) you use.

You should be aware that there is a V code for history of alcoholism (V11.3). Instead of using that code you use the **alcoholism** code (303.9x) with the fifth digit 3, which specifies in remission. It is rare to assign code V11.3 because the disease of alcoholism cannot be cured.

Five-Digit Subclassification

A five-digit subclassification is provided for categories 303–305 to indicate the patient's pattern of use of alcohol or drugs:

-0: unspecified

-1: continuous: Alcohol: refers to daily intake of large amounts of alcohol or regular heavy drinking on weekends or days off from work

Drugs: daily or almost daily use of drugs

-2: episodic: Alcohol: refers to alcoholic binges lasting weeks or months, followed by long periods of sobriety

Drugs: indicates short periods between drug use or use on weekends.

-3:   remission: Refers either to a complete cessation of alcohol or drug intake or to the period during which decreasing intake leading toward cessation is taking place

Another commonly encountered instance is the instruction to Use additional code to identify the associated neurological condition or Use additional code to identify cerebral atherosclerosis (437.0). Pay close attention to the instructions given in the Tabular when you see these words.

EXAMPLE

Diagnosis:	Arteriosclerotic dementia with delirium
Index:	**Dementia** 294.8, arteriosclerotic (simple type) (uncomplicated) 290.40, with, delirium 290.41
Tabular:	**290 Senile and presenile organic psychotic conditions**
	290.4 Arteriosclerotic dementia
	Use additional code to identify cerebral atherosclerosis (437.0)
	290.41 Arteriosclerotic dementia with delirium
Tabular:	**437 Other and ill-defined cerebrovascular disease**
	437.0 Cerebral atherosclerosis
Codes:	290.41, 437.0 Arteriosclerotic dementia with delirium

EXERCISE 15-22

MENTAL DISORDERS

Now you have a chance to show your skill by coding the following:

1 Alzheimer's dementia with aggressive behavior

   Code(s): _____

2 Depression with anxiety

   Code(s): _____

3 Profound mental retardation

   Code(s): _____

4 Anorexia nervosa

   Code(s): _____

5 Delirium tremens due to chronic alcoholism, continuous

   Code(s): _____

Diseases of the Nervous System and Sense Organs

Chapter 6, Diseases of the Nervous System and Sense Organs, in the Tabular describes diseases or conditions affecting the central nervous system and the peripheral nervous system. It also includes disorders and diseases of the eyes and ears.

The chapter uses some combination codes in which one code identifies both the manifestation and the etiology.

EXAMPLE

> Diagnosis: Pneumococcal meningitis
>
> This diagnostic statement means the meningitis is due to the pneumococcal bacteria.
>
> Index: **Meningitis,** pneumococcal 320.1
>
> Tabular: **320 Bacterial meningitis**
>
>   **320.1 Pneumococcal meningitis**
>
> Code: 320.1 Pneumococcal meningitis
>
> Code 320.1 includes the manifestation of meningitis and also the etiology of pneumococcal organism.

In Chapter 6, you will also find conditions that are manifestations of other diseases. These categories appear in italics in the Tabular and provide instructions to code the underlying disease process first.

EXAMPLE

> Diagnosis: Chronic iridocyclitis due to sarcoidosis
>
> Index: **Iridocyclitis** NEC 364.3, chronic, in, sarcoidosis 135 *[364.11]*
>
> Entries such as 135 *[364.11]* instruct you to code the sarcoidosis (135) first, followed by the chronic iridocyclitis (364.11). Both codes need to be verified in the Tabular.
>
> Tabular: **135 Sarcoidosis**
>
> Tabular: **364 Disorders of iris and ciliary body**
>
>   **364.11 Chronic** *iridocyclitis in diseases classified elsewhere*
>
>   Code first underlying disease, as:
>
>   sarcoidosis (135)
>
>   tuberculosis (017.3)
>
> Codes: 135, 364.11 Chronic iridocyclitis due to sarcoidosis
>
> Category 345 Epilepsy is also in Chapter 6, but the physician must specifically indicate epilepsy before the code can be assigned. If the episode was for a seizure disorder or convulsions other than epilepsy, the code would be 780.39. You should clarify any questions about the diagnosis with the physician.

EXERCISE 15–23

DISEASES OF THE NERVOUS SYSTEM AND SENSE ORGANS

Fill in the codes for the following:

1 Meningitis due to *Proteus morganii*

   Code(s): _____

2 Multiple sclerosis

   Code(s): _____

3 Acute otitis media

   Code(s): _____

4 Primary open-angle glaucoma

   Code(s): _____

5 Bell's palsy

   Code(s): _____

Diseases of the Circulatory System

Chapter 7, Diseases of the Circulatory System, in the Tabular contains diseases of heart and blood vessels.

Hypertension is probably one of the most common conditions coded in this chapter. The Hypertension Table is located in the Index, as shown in Figure 15–2. This table provides a complete listing of all conditions due to or associated with hypertension. The first column identifies the hypertensive condition, such as accelerated, antepartum, cardiovascular disease, cardiorenal, and cerebrovascular disease. The remaining three columns, entitled malignant, benign, and unspecified, constitute the subcategories of hypertensive disease.

Malignant hypertension is an accelerated, severe form of hypertension, manifested by headaches, blurred vision, dyspnea, and uremia. This type of hypertension usually causes permanent organ damage. **Benign hypertension** is a continuous, mild blood pressure elevation. **Unspecified hypertension** has not been specified as either benign or malignant.

INDEX TO DISEASES — Hypertension

	Malignant	Benign	Unspecified
Hypertension, hypertensive (arterial) (arteriolar) (crisis) (degeneration) (disease) (essential) (fluctuating) (idiopathic) (intermittent) (labile) (low renin) (orthostatic) (paroxysmal) (primary) (systemic) (uncontrolled) (vascular)	401.0	(#1) 401.1	(#3) 401.9
with heart involvement (conditions classifiable to 425.8, 428, 429.0-429.3, 429.8, 429.9 due to hypertension) (see also Hypertension, heart)	402.00	402.10	402.90
with kidney involvement — see Hypertension, cardiorenal			
renal involvement (only conditions classifiable to 585, 586, 587) (excludes conditions classifiable to 584) (see also Hypertension, kidney)	403.00	403.10	403.90
with heart involvement — see Hypertension, cardiorenal			
failure (and sclerosis) (see also Hypertension, kidney)	403.01	403.11	(#4) 403.91
sclerosis without failure (see also Hypertension, kidney)	403.00	403.10	403.90
accelerated (see also Hypertension, by type, malignant)	401.0	—	—
antepartum — see Hypertension, complicating pregnancy, childbirth, or the puerperium			
cardiorenal (disease)	404.00	404.10	404.90
with heart failure (congestive)	404.01	404.11	404.91
and renal failure	404.03	404.13	404.93
renal failure	404.02	404.12	404.92
and heart failure (congestive)	404.03	404.13	404.93
cardiovascular disease (arteriosclerotic) (sclerotic)	(#2) 402.00	402.10	402.90
with heart failure (congestive)	402.01	402.11	402.91
renal involvement (conditions classifiable to 403) (see also Hypertension, cardiorenal)	404.00	404.10	404.90
cardiovascular renal (disease) (sclerosis) (see also Hypertension, cardiorenal)	404.00	404.10	404.90

Figure 15–2 Hypertension Table, Index to Diseases. (From International Classification of Diseases, 9th Revision. U.S. Department of Health and Human Services, Public Health Service, Centers for Medicare and Medicaid Services.)

There is no defined threshold of blood pressure above which an individual is considered hypertensive. Commonly, a sustained diastolic pressure of above 90 mm Hg and a sustained systolic pressure of above 140 mm Hg constitutes hypertension.

Benign hypertension remains fairly stable over the years and is compatible with a long life, but if untreated, it is an important risk factor in coronary heart disease and cerebrovascular disease.

Malignant hypertension is commonly associated with abrupt onset and it runs a course measured in months. It causes irreversible organ damage and often ends with renal failure or cerebral hemorrhage. Usually a person with malignant hypertension complains of headaches and vision difficulties. Blood pressure of 200/140 mm Hg is common.

Hypertensive heart disease refers to the secondary effects on the heart of prolonged, sustained, systemic hypertension. The heart has to work against greatly increased resistance, and that results in high blood pressure. The primary effect is the thickening of the left ventricle, which finally results in heart failure.

There are two sections in this chapter that have instructions to Use additional code, if desired, to identify presence of hypertension (401.0–405.9). The sections are Ischemic Heart Disease (410–414) and Cerebrovascular Disease (430–438). There are also a number of guidelines that pertain to hypertension or other hypertensive disease processes.

Official Coding and Reporting Guidelines

4.1 HYPERTENSION, ESSENTIAL, OR NOS

Assign hypertension (arterial) (essential) (primary) (systemic) (NOS) to category code 401 with the appropriate fourth digit to indicate malignant (.0), benign (.1), or unspecified (.9). Do not use either .0 malignant or .1 benign unless medical record documentation supports such a designation.

4.2 HYPERTENSION WITH HEART DISEASE

Certain heart conditions (425.8, 428, 429.0–429.3, 429.8, 429.9) are assigned to a code from category 402 when a causal relationship is stated (due to hypertension) or implied (hypertensive). Use only the code from category 402. The same heart conditions (425.8, 428, 429.0–429.3, 429.8, 429.9) with hypertension, but without a stated causal relationship, are coded separately. Sequence according to the circumstances of the admission.

4.3 HYPERTENSIVE RENAL DISEASE WITH CHRONIC RENAL FAILURE

Assign codes from category 403, Hypertensive renal disease, when conditions classified to categories 585–587 are present. Unlike hypertension with heart disease, ICD-9-CM presumes a cause-and-effect relationship and classifies chronic renal failure with hypertension as hypertensive renal disease. (Acute renal failure is not included in this cause-and-effect relationship).

4.4 HYPERTENSIVE HEART AND RENAL DISEASE

Assign codes from combination category 404, Hypertensive heart and renal disease, when both hypertensive renal disease and hypertensive heart disease are stated in the diagnosis. Assume a relationship between the hypertension and the renal disease, whether or not the condition is so designated.

4.5 HYPERTENSIVE CEREBROVASCULAR DISEASE

First assign codes from 430–438, Cerebrovascular disease, then the appropriate hypertension code from categories 401–405.

4.6 HYPERTENSIVE RETINOPATHY

Two codes are necessary to identify the condition. First assign code 362.11, Hypertensive retinopathy, then the appropriate code from categories 401–405 to indicate the type of hypertension.

4.7 HYPERTENSION, SECONDARY

Two codes are required, one to identify the underlying condition and one from category 405 to identify the hypertension. Sequencing of codes is determined by the reason for admission to the hospital.

4.8 HYPERTENSION, TRANSIENT

Assign code 796.2, Elevated blood pressure reading without diagnosis of hypertension, unless patient has an established diagnosis of hypertension. Assign code 642.3X for transient hypertension of pregnancy.

4.9 HYPERTENSION, CONTROLLED

Assign appropriate code from categories 401–405. This diagnostic statement usually refers to an existing state of hypertension under control by therapy.

4.10 HYPERTENSION, UNCONTROLLED

Uncontrolled hypertension may refer to untreated hypertension or hypertension not responding to current therapeutic regimen. In either case, assign the appropriate code from categories 401–405 to designate the state and type of hypertension. Code to the type of hypertension.

Guideline 4.3 instructs you to assume that there is a cause-and-effect relationship between hypertension and renal diseases that are categorized in the range of codes 585–587. The physician might not indicate that they are related, but the coder must assume this relationship.

EXAMPLE

Diagnosis: Chronic renal failure and hypertension

There is nothing in the above diagnostic statement to indicate that the two diseases are related. Let's see how this would be coded. The guidelines instruct you to code as if there were a cause-and-effect relationship between the chronic renal failure and hypertension. Therefore, the diagnosis would be coded as hypertensive chronic renal failure.

Index: **Failure, failed,** renal 586, chronic 585, hypertensive or with hypertension (*see also* hypertension, kidney), 403.91

Tabular: **403 Hypertensive renal disease**

        403.9 Unspecified

Code 403.9 is not complete until you assign the appropriate fifth digit. You have a choice of 0 without mention of renal failure, or 1 with renal failure. Chronic renal failure is present in the diagnosis statement, so a fifth digit of 1 is assigned.

Code: 403.91 Chronic renal failure, hypertension

The code for chronic renal failure is 585; however, when you locate code 585 in the Tabular there is an *Excludes* note that states: ". . . *with any condition classifiable to 401 (403.0–403.9 with a fifth digit 1)."* Thus, chronic renal failure due to hypertension cannot be classified to code 585.

Code *410* Acute myocardial infarction (MI) requires a fifth digit assignment and includes specific instructions that must be carefully read.

A fifth digit of 1 indicates an initial episode and can be assigned to the same patient for a different admission providing treatment for the initial episode of care for the MI. A patient could be diagnosed with acute MI and be transferred to a larger facility for further investigation and care. The diagnoses at both facilities would sequence the acute MI first, and the five-digit assignment would be 1 at both facilities.

A fifth digit of 2 indicates subsequent care and is used when a patient is readmitted for testing or further care within 8 weeks of the initial episode. For example, a patient had an acute myocardial infarction and was discharged from the hospital. Four weeks later, that same patient was admitted for a cardiovascular procedure. The myocardial infarction would be coded 410.92 to indicate a subsequent episode. Note that code 412 is assigned for a healed myocardial infarction that is not showing any symptoms (asymptomatic). You would not assign a V code history of MI in this situation.

As you review the following examples, refer to Figure 15–2 for the codes highlighted for each example.

EXAMPLES

Hypertension

Diagnosis: Congestive heart failure with benign hypertension

Tabular: **428.0 Congestive heart failure**

    401.1 Hypertension, benign (indicated as 1 in Fig. 15–2)

The key word in the above diagnosis statement is "with," which indicates two conditions. Both the congestive heart failure and the benign hypertension are coded because each is a separate condition.

Diagnosis: Dilated cardiomyopathy due to malignant hypertension

Tabular: **402.00 Cardiomyopathy** (indicated as 2 in Fig. 15–2) due to:

      hypertension—See Hypertension with heart involvement malignant

In this example, the hypertension caused the cardiomyopathy. The key words here are "due to," which indicates that one condition caused the other condition.

Diagnosis: Acute renal failure with hypertension

Tabular: **584.9 Renal failure,** acute

Tabular: **401.9 Hypertension** (indicated as 3 in Fig. 15–2)

At first, you identify that you would code the hypertension separately because the word "with" is included in the diagnostic statement. Under Hypertension, renal involvement, in Figure 15–2, you will see an *Excludes* note. The note indicates that conditions classifiable to 584 (acute renal failure) are excluded from the codes for renal involvement. The condition in this example is acute renal failure, 584; therefore, you cannot assign the renal involvement hypertension codes. Codes 585–587 imply that acute renal failure is not assumed to have a cause-and-effect relationship with hypertension. Be sure to read all notes before you assign any code. Thus, the code for the hypertension in this example is 401.9, Hypertension, unspecified. When you next note the diagnosis of renal failure, you may think that only one code is to be assigned. The key term included in this diagnosis is "acute" renal failure.

Diagnosis: Hypertension with chronic renal failure

Index: **403.91 Hypertension, with renal involvement, failure** (indicated as 4 in Fig. 15–2)

Figure 15–3 shows the portion of the Hypertension Table that includes the secondary hypertension codes. **Secondary hypertension** means that the hypertension is caused by another condition.

INDEX TO DISEASES   Hypertension

	Malignant	Benign	Unspecified
Hypertension—*continued*			
pulmonary (artery) (idiopathic) (primary) (solitary)—*continued*			
with cor pulmonale (chronic)	—	—	416.0
acute.....................................	—	—	416.8
secondary...	—	—	416.8
renal (disease) (*see also* Hypertension, kidney)	403.00	403.10	403.90
renovascular NEC	405.01	405.11	405.91
secondary NEC.....................................	405.09	405.19	405.99
due to			
aldosteronism, primary...........................	405.09	405.19	405.99
brain tumor	405.09	405.19	405.99
bulbar poliomyelitis.............................	405.09	405.19	405.99
calculus			
kidney	405.09	405.19	405.99
ureter..	405.09	405.19	405.99
coarctation, aorta................................	405.09	405.19	405.99
Cushing's disease	405.09	405.19	405.99
glomerulosclerosis (*see also* Hypertension, kidney) ..	403.00	403.10	403.90
periarteritis nodosa	405.09	405.19	405.99
pheochromocytoma	405.09	405.19	405.99
polycystic kidney(s)	405.09	405.19	405.99
polycythemia	405.09	405.19	405.99
porphyria	405.09	405.19	405.99
pyelonephritis	405.09	405.19	405.99
renal (artery)			
aneurysm	405.01	405.11	405.91
anomaly	405.01	405.11	405.91
embolism	405.01	405.11	405.91
fibromuscular hyperplasia	405.01	405.11	405.91
occlusion	405.01	405.11	(#5) 405.91
stenosis	405.01	405.11	405.91
thrombosis	405.01	405.11	405.91
transient	—	—	796.2
of pregnancy	—	—	642.3

Secondary hypertension →

Figure 15–3 Secondary hypertension. (From International Classification of Diseases, 9th Revision. U.S. Department of Health and Human Services, Public Health Service, Centers for Medicare and Medicaid Services.)

EXAMPLE

Diagnosis: Secondary, benign hypertension, due to renal artery occlusion

Tabular: **405.11 Hypertension,** secondary, due to renal (artery), occlusion, benign (indicated as 5 in Fig. 15–3)

In the previous example, the renal artery occlusion caused the hypertension and so is correctly coded to category 405. You would also assign a code to the renal artery occlusion (593.81) because the renal artery occlusion is causing the secondary hypertension. Sequence the occlusion first.

EXAMPLE

Code: 593.81, 405.11 Secondary, benign hypertension, due to renal artery occlusion

The renal artery occlusion is causing the hypertension and when treated may result in the disappearance of the hypertension.

According to Guideline 4.7, the sequencing may be determined by the reason for admission to the hospital.

Official Coding and Reporting Guidelines

4.11 ELEVATED BLOOD PRESSURE

For a statement of elevated blood pressure without further specificity, assign code 796.2, Elevated blood pressure reading without diagnosis of hypertension, rather than a code from category 401.

EXERCISE 15–24

DISEASES OF THE CIRCULATORY SYSTEM

Fill in the codes for the following:

1 Congestive heart failure

Code(s): _____

2 Acute subendocardial infarction, initial episode

Code(s): _____

3 Secondary hypertension due to periarteritis nodosa

Code(s): _____

4 Cerebral infarction due to thrombosis, brain

Code(s): _____

5 Subarachnoid hemorrhage

Code(s): _____

Diseases of the Respiratory System

Chapter 8, Diseases of the Respiratory System in the Tabular includes diseases and disorders of the respiratory tract; it starts with the nasal passages and follows a path to the lungs. Note that at the beginning of Chapter 8 there is an instructional note that covers the entire chapter. The note states, "Use additional code to identify infectious organism." You should be aware that in this chapter the organism is already identified in some codes, and you would not assign an additional code to identify the specific infectious organism.

EXAMPLES

Diagnosis:	Pneumonia due to *Klebsiella pneumoniae*
Index:	**Pneumonia,** *Klebsiella pneumoniae,* 482.0
Tabular:	**482 Other bacterial pneumonia**
	482.0 Pneumonia due to *Klebsiella pneumoniae*
Code:	482.0 Pneumonia due to *Klebsiella pneumoniae*

The code 482.0 is a combination code that includes the disease process (pneumonia) with the causative organism *(Klebsiella pneumoniae)*. In this instance, you would not need to assign an additional code because the organism is identified in the code 482.0.

Diagnosis:	Acute maxillary sinusitis due to *Haemophilus influenzae*
Index:	**Sinusitis** (accessory) (nasal) (hyperplastic) (nonpurulent) (purulent) (chronic) 473.9
	acute 461.9
	maxillary 461.0
Tabular:	**461 Acute sinusitis**
	461.0 Maxillary
Index:	**Infection, infected, infective** (opportunistic), *Haemophilus influenzae* NEC 041.5
Tabular:	**041 Bacterial infection in conditions classified elsewhere and of unspecified site**
	041.5 *Haemophilus influenzae [H. influenzae]*
Codes:	461.0, 041.5 Acute maxillary sinusitis due to *Haemophilus influenzae*

The respiratory condition of chronic obstructive pulmonary disease (COPD) falls within the category 496 Chronic airway obstruction NEC. The note under code 496 indicates that this code cannot be assigned with any code from categories 491–493. The *Excludes* note under code 496 indicates that COPD specified "(as) (with) asthma (493.2)" cannot be assigned to code 496. The *Excludes* note sends you elsewhere in the ICD-9-CM.

E X A M P L E

Diagnosis:	COPD with asthma
Index:	**Asthma, asthmatic** (bronchial) (catarrh) (spasmodic) 493.9, with, chronic obstructive pulmonary disease (COPD) 493.2
Tabular:	**493 Asthma**
	493.2 Chronic obstructive asthma

This code is not complete yet because it needs a fifth digit. You have three fifth digit choices:

0 without mention of status asthmaticus

1 with status asthmaticus

2 with acute exacerbation

To code the asthma with status asthmaticus, the physician provides specific documentation of the condition. If the clinical condition is severe enough that you suspect that the patient has status asthmaticus, clarification by the physician should be sought.

Code:	493.20 COPD with asthma

EXERCISE 15-25

DISEASES OF THE RESPIRATORY SYSTEM

Fill in the codes for the following:

1 Croup

    Code(s): _____

2 Respiratory failure due to congestive heart failure

    Code(s): _____

3 COPD with chronic bronchitis

Code(s): _____

4 Influenza with acute bronchitis

Code(s): _____

5 Pneumonia due to *Haemophilus influenzae*

Code(s): _____

Diseases of the Digestive System

Chapter 9, Diseases of the Digestive System, in the Tabular describes diseases or conditions affecting the digestive system. Digestion starts when food is taken into the mouth and follows the gastrointestinal tract until it leaves the body through the anus. The categories are sequenced in a manner that follows that path, starting with disorders of the teeth.

Throughout the chapter, as in other chapters, you must pay close attention to fifth-digit assignment and carefully read the *Excludes* notes and any other instructions. Also important in the chapter is the presence of **hemorrhage** associated with the diseases. The physician may not always indicate the presence of hemorrhage, and the coder must review the record and then clarify with the physician the appropriate code assignment.

EXAMPLES

Diagnosis: Diverticulitis of the colon with hemorrhage

Index: **Diverticulitis** (acute), colon (perforated) 562.11, with hemorrhage 562.13

Note that the presence of hemorrhage makes a difference in the code assignment.

Tabular: **562 Diverticula of intestine**

        562.13 Diverticulitis of colon with hemorrhage

Code: 562.13 Diverticulitis of the colon with hemorrhage

Category **578 Gastrointestinal hemorrhage** has an *Excludes* note that is very important:

> **EXCLUDES** *that with mention of:*
> *angiodysplasia of stomach and duodenum (537.83)*
> *angiodysplasia of intestine (569.85)*
> *diverticulitis, intestine:*
>   *large (562.13)*
>   *small (562.03)*
> *diverticulosis, intestine:*
>   *large (562.12)*
>   *small (562.02)*
> *gastritis and duodenitis (535.0–535.6)*
> *ulcer:*
>   *duodenum (532.0–532.9)*
>   *gastric (531.0–531.9)*
>   *gastrojejunal (534.0–534.9)*
>   *peptic (533.0–533.9)*

If you are coding a diagnosis of gastrointestinal (GI) hemorrhage with any of the listed *Excludes* diagnoses, you are instructed to code GI hemorrhages elsewhere and not use the codes from category 578.

f r o m   t h e   t r e n c h e s

What advice would you give to a new coding professional?
"You're hard to find, and you're wanted . . . watch, learn, and code."
                                        YVONNE

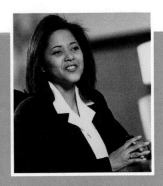

Diagnosis:	Gastrointestinal hemorrhage due to acute antral ulcer
Index:	**Ulcer, ulcerated, ulcerating, ulceration, ulcerative** 707.9, antral—*see* ulcer, stomach, stomach (eroded) (peptic) (round) 531.9, acute 531.3, with hemorrhage 531.0
Tabular:	**531 Gastric ulcer**
	531.0 Acute with hemorrhage

Code 531.0 is not a complete code. You must assign a fifth digit. There is no mention of obstruction in the diagnosis, so the fifth digit assigned would be 0, without mention of obstruction.

Index:	**Hemorrhage, hemorrhagic** (nontraumatic) 459.0
	Gastrointestinal (tract) 579.9
Tabular:	**578 Gastrointestinal hemorrhage**
	Excludes: that with mention of:
	Ulcer:
	gastric (531.0–532.9)
Code:	531.00 Gastrointestinal hemorrhage due to acute antral ulcer

CAUTION *For a hemorrhage to be coded, there does not have to be active bleeding; however, there must be documentation in the medical record that supports the fact that active bleeding has occurred.*

At this point, you discover the importance of the *Excludes* notes for 578 Gastrointestinal hemorrhage, which states that the hemorrhage is included in the ulcer code. That is one reason why it is so important to verify code assignment in the Tabular. It is only when you check the Tabular that you can know for certain about the Includes and *Excludes*, which are not listed anywhere else. So be certain to always, always check the Tabular before assigning a code.

**EXERCISE
15–26**

DISEASES OF THE DIGESTIVE SYSTEM

Fill in the codes for the following:

1   Appendicitis with peritonitis

   Code(s): _____

2   Gastrointestinal bleeding due to acute duodenal ulcer

   Code(s): _____

3 Acute and chronic cholecystitis with cholelithiasis

Code(s): _____

4 Gastroenteritis

Code(s): _____

5 Gastroesophageal reflux

Code(s): _____

Diseases of the Genitourinary System

Chapter 10, Diseases of the Genitourinary System, in the Tabular includes conditions and diseases of the male and female genital organs and urinary tract. Disorders of the breast (categories 610–611) are also included in the chapter.

Once again, when you are dealing with infections of the urinary tract or the genital organs, you are instructed to use an additional code to identify the organism.

EXAMPLE

Diagnosis:	Acute prostatitis due to *Streptococcus*
Index:	**Prostatitis** (congestive) (suppurative) 601.9
	acute 601.0
Tabular:	**601 Inflammatory diseases of prostate**
	601.1 Acute prostatitis
Index:	**Infection, infected, infective** (opportunistic)
	streptococcal NEC 041.00
Tabular:	**041 Bacterial infection in conditions classified elsewhere and of unspecified site**
	041.0 *Streptococcus*
	041.00 *Streptococcus*, unspecified
Codes:	601.1, 041.00 Acute prostatitis due to *Streptococcus*

EXERCISE
15-27

DISEASES OF THE GENITOURINARY SYSTEM

Fill in the codes for the following diagnostic statements:

1 Pelvic inflammatory disease (PID)

Code(s): _____

2 Hematuria

Code(s): _____

3 Acute and chronic pyelonephritis

Code(s): _____

4 Benign prostatic hypertrophy (BPH)

Code(s): _____

5 Fibrocystic breast disease

Code(s): _____

Complications of Pregnancy, Childbirth, and the Puerperium

Chapter 11, Complications of Pregnancy, Childbirth, and the Puerperium, of the Tabular is probably the most difficult chapter from which to code. One reason is that pregnancy and childbirth are natural functions, and physicians often overlook documentation of diagnoses that should be coded. Another reason is that there is extensive use of multiple coding in the chapter. Also, fifth digit assignment for pregnancy is often difficult to determine. There are instructions throughout this chapter that must be read thoroughly. Obstetric coding can also be difficult because you may not use this chapter as frequently as some of the other chapters, so you won't be as familiar with the special notes and coding instructions.

An ectopic pregnancy is one in which the fertilized ovum implants outside the uterus, usually in the fallopian tube. Ectopic and Molar Pregnancy (630–633) contains instructions to use an additional code from category 639 to identify any complication(s).

Category 639, Complications following abortion and ectopic and molar pregnancies, provides instructional guidelines for the use of this code. You cannot use 639, Complications, with any code from categories 634–638 because the complications are classified according to the fourth digit subcategory codes. As stated previously, you use 639, Complications, to identify any complications related to codes 630–633. You also use 639, Complications, when the complication is the reason for the medical care and the abortion, ectopic, or molar pregnancy was taken care of during a previous episode.

Complications mainly related to pregnancy (640–648) designate fifth digit subclassifications that are of special note:

0   unspecified as to episode of care or not applicable

1   delivered, with or without mention of antepartum condition

2   delivered, with mention of postpartum complication

3   antepartum condition or complication

4   postpartum condition or complication

The fifth digit 0 is used when an abortion is due to or associated with a complication included in the chapter. To use the fifth digits 1 and 2, a delivery must have occurred during that stay. The 1 is assigned to cases in which an antepartum condition has or has not been noted. The fifth digits 3 and 4 are used when no delivery has occurred during that stay or visit. The 3 is used for antepartum conditions, and the 4 for postpartum conditions. When you review the categories and subcategories throughout the chapter, you will note that many subcategories may indicate that you can use only certain fifth digits with a particular code. For example, with code 641.1, Hemorrhage from placenta previa, the only fifth digits that can be used are 0, 1, and 3. Neither 2 nor 4 can be used because placenta previa occurs before a baby is delivered.

When coding multiple diagnoses from one inpatient stay, certain combinations of fifth digits are used to classify that stay or visit. These fifth digit combinations are

1 only, or with 2; NOT with 0, 3, or 4

2 only, or with 1; NOT with 0, 3, or 4

3 only, NOT with 0, 1, 2, or 4

4 only, NOT with 0, 1, 2, or 4

Category 650, Normal delivery, cannot be used with any other code that falls within the range 630–676 because these codes refer to other than normal delivery. Code 650 is used only when all of the following are documented:

- A full-term, single liveborn infant is delivered.

- There are no antepartum or postpartum conditions classifiable to 630–676.

- The presentation is cephalic, requiring minimal assistance and without fetal manipulation or the use of instrumentation.

- An episiotomy can be performed.

Most deliveries do not fit the above criteria for a 650 Normal Delivery code assignment.

Category V27 Outcome of delivery can be assigned as an additional code to the mother's record. This is indexed under the term "Outcome."

STOP *It may be helpful to code the mother's and baby's records at the same time. Conditions documented on the birth certificate may appear on the newborn's record but may not appear on the mother's record. As always, the individual record must support the codes assigned, so additional documentation may have to be obtained from the physician.*

Official Coding and Reporting Guidelines

2.16 COMPLICATION OF PREGNANCY

When a patient is admitted because of a condition that is either a complication of pregnancy or that is complicating the pregnancy, the code for the obstetric complication is the principal diagnosis. An additional code may be assigned as needed to provide specificity.

EXAMPLE

Diagnosis: Iron deficiency anemia complicating pregnancy, antepartum

Index: **Pregnancy** (single) (uterine) (without sickness) V22.2

    complicated (by) 646.9

    anemia (conditions classifiable to 280–285) 648.2

Tabular: **648.2 Anemia**

This code is not complete because it lacks fifth digit assignment and there are instructions to Use additional code(s) to identify the condition, which means to identify the type of anemia. The code book states that you can assign fifth digits 0–4. No delivery has occurred and the condition is stated as being antepartum; therefore, the fifth digit 3 is assigned. The next step is to locate the additional code to identify the type of anemia.

EXAMPLE

Index: **Anemia** 285.9, deficiency 281.9, iron (Fe) 280.9

Tabular: **280.9 Iron deficiency anemia, unspecified**

Codes: 648.23, 280.9 Iron deficiency anemia complicating pregnancy, antepartum

The first code, 648.23, indicates that the anemia is a complication of the pregnancy, and the second code, 280.9, provides greater specificity as to the type of anemia.

Chapter 4 can be somewhat confusing at the beginning because there is an *Excludes* note that states, "anemia complicating pregnancy or the puerperium (648.2)." In Chapter 11 you are directed to "Also code the condition." This means that anemias are assumed to be complications of pregnancy and you should follow the instructions given for code 648.2. The code from the obstetric chapter would be sequenced first, followed by the anemia code.

Official Coding and Reporting Guidelines

OBSTETRICS

Introduction

These guidelines have been developed and approved by the Cooperating Parties in conjunction with the Editorial Advisory Board of Coding Clinic and the American College of Obstetricians and Gynecologists, to assist the coder in coding and reporting obstetric cases. Where feasible, previously published advice has been incorporated. Some advice in these new guidelines may supersede previous advice. The guidelines are provided for reporting purposes. Health care facilities may record additional diagnoses as needed for internal data needs.

5.1 GENERAL RULES

A. Obstetric cases require codes from Chapter 11, codes in the range 630–677, Complications of Pregnancy, Childbirth, and the Puerperium. Should the physician document that the pregnancy is incidental to the encounter, then code V22.2 should be used in place of any Chapter 11 codes. It is the physician's responsibility to state that the condition being treated is not affecting the pregnancy.

B. Chapter 11 codes have sequencing priority over codes from other chapters. Additional codes from other chapters may be used in conjunction with Chapter 11 codes to further specify conditions.

C. Chapter 11 codes are to be used only on the maternal record, never on the record of the newborn.

D. An outcome of delivery code, V27.0–V27.9, should be included on every maternal record when a delivery has occurred. These codes are not to be used on subsequent records or on the newborn record.

5.2 SELECTION OF PRINCIPAL DIAGNOSIS

A. The circumstances of the encounter govern the selection of the principal diagnosis.

B. In episodes when no delivery occurs the principal diagnosis should correspond to the principal complication of the pregnancy which necessitated the encounter. Should more than one complication exist, all of which are treated or monitored, any of the complications codes may be sequenced first.

C. When a delivery occurs, the principal diagnosis should correspond to the main circumstances or complication of the delivery. In cases of cesarean deliveries, the principal diagnosis should correspond to the reason the cesarean was performed, unless the reason for admission was unrelated to the condition resulting in the cesarean delivery.

D. For routine prenatal visits when no complications are present, codes V22.0, Supervision of normal first pregnancy, and V22.1, Supervision of other normal pregnancy, should be used as principal diagnoses. These codes should not be used in conjunction with Chapter 11 codes.

E. For prenatal outpatient visits for patients with high-risk pregnancies, a code from category V23, Supervision of high-risk pregnancy, should be used as the principal diagnosis. Secondary Chapter 11 codes may be used in conjunction with these codes if appropriate. A thorough review of any pertinent *Excludes* note is necessary to be certain that these V codes are being used properly.

5.3 CHAPTER 11 FIFTH DIGITS

A. Categories 610–648, 651–676 have required fifth digits that indicate whether the encounter is antepartum, postpartum, and whether a delivery has also occurred.
B. The fifth digits which are appropriate for each code number are listed in brackets under each code. The fifth digits for each code should all be consistent with each other. That is, should a delivery occur all of the fifth digits should indicate the delivery.

5.4 FETAL CONDITIONS AFFECTING THE MANAGEMENT OF THE MOTHER

Codes from category 655, Known or suspected fetal abnormality affecting management of the mother, and category 656, Other fetal and placental problems affecting the management of the mother, are assigned only when the fetal condition is actually responsible for modifying the management of the mother, i.e., by requiring diagnostic studies, additional observation, special care, or termination of pregnancy. The fact that the fetal condition exists does not justify assigning a code from this series to the mother's record.

5.5 NORMAL DELIVERY, 650

A. Code 650 is for use in cases when a woman is admitted for a full-term normal delivery and delivers a single, healthy infant without any complications antepartum, during the delivery, or postpartum during the delivery episode.
B. 650 may be used if the patient had complications at some point during her pregnancy but the complication is not present at the time of the admission for delivery.
C. Code 650 is always a principal diagnosis. It is not to be used if any other code from Chapter 11 is needed to describe a current complication of the antenatal delivery, or perinatal period. Additional codes from other chapters may be used with code 650 if they are not related to or are in any way complicating the pregnancy.
D. V27.0, Single liveborn, is the only outcome of delivery code appropriate for use with 650.

5.6 PROCEDURE CODES

A. In cases of cesarean delivery, the selection of the principal diagnosis should correspond to the reason the cesarean delivery was performed unless the reason for admission was unrelated to the condition resulting in the cesarean delivery.
B. A delivery procedure code should not be used for a woman who has delivered prior to admission to the hospital. Any postpartum repairs should be coded.

5.7 THE POSTPARTUM PERIOD

A. The postpartum period begins immediately after delivery and continues for 6 weeks following delivery.
B. A postpartum complication is any complication occurring within the 6 week period.
C. Chapter 11 codes may also be used to describe pregnancy related complications after the 6-week period should the physician document that a condition is pregnancy related.
D. Postpartum complications that occur during the same admission as the delivery are identified with a fifth digit of 2. Subsequent admissions for postpartum complications should be identified with a fifth digit of 4.

E. When the mother delivers outside the hospital prior to admission and is admitted for routine postpartum care and no complications are noted, code V24.0, Postpartum care and examination immediately after delivery, should be assigned as the principal diagnosis.

5.8 ABORTIONS

A. Fifth digits are required for abortion categories 634–637. Fifth digit 1, incomplete, indicates that all of the products of conception have not been expelled from the uterus. Fifth digit 2, complete, indicates that all products of conception have been expelled from the uterus prior to the episode of care.

B. A code from categories 640–648 and 651–657 may be used as additional codes with an abortion code to indicate the complication leading to the abortion. Fifth digit 3 is assigned with codes from these categories when used with an abortion code because the other fifth digits will not apply. Codes from the 660–669 series are not to be used for complications of abortion.

C. Code 639 is to be used for all complications following abortion. Code 639 cannot be assigned with codes from categories 634–638.

D. Abortion with Liveborn Fetus. When an attempted termination of pregnancy results in a liveborn fetus, assign code 644.21, Early onset of delivery, with an appropriate code from category V27, Outcome of Delivery. The procedure code for the attempted termination of pregnancy should also be assigned.

E. Retained Products of Conception Following an Abortion. Subsequent admissions for retained products of conception following a spontaneous or legally induced abortion are assigned the appropriate code from category 634, Spontaneous abortion, or legally induced abortion, with a fifth digit of 1 (incomplete). This advice is appropriate even when the patient was discharged previously with a discharge diagnosis of complete abortion.

5.9 CODE 677, LATE EFFECT OF COMPLICATION OF PREGNANCY, CHILDBIRTH, AND THE PUERPERIUM

A. Code 677, Late effect of complication of pregnancy, childbirth, and the puerperium is for use in those cases when an initial complication of a pregnancy develops a sequela requiring care or treatment at a future date.

B. This code may be used at any time after the initial postpartum period.

C. This code, like all late effect codes, is to be sequenced following the code describing the sequelae of the complication.

EXERCISE 15-28

COMPLICATIONS OF PREGNANCY, CHILDBIRTH, AND THE PUERPERIUM

Fill in the codes for the following:

1 Blighted ovum

   Code(s): _____

2 Incomplete spontaneous abortion; dilation and curettage (D&C) performed

   Code(s): _____

3 False labor of 38-week pregnancy, undelivered

   Code(s): _____

4 Vaginal delivery of liveborn single infant with fourth-degree perineal laceration; obstetric laceration repaired (Include appropriate V code for outcome of delivery.)

Code(s): _____

5 Obstructed labor due to cephalopelvic disproportion; liveborn single infant delivered by lower segment cesarean section

Code(s): _____

Diseases of the Skin and Subcutaneous Tissue

Chapter 12, Diseases of the Skin and Subcutaneous Tissue, in the Tabular describes diseases or conditions of the integumentary system. This chapter is one of the shorter chapters in the ICD-9-CM manual. When reviewing the first categories listed, such as 681, 682, and 683, you will note that multiple coding may be necessary for some conditions.

EXAMPLE

Diagnosis:	Cellulitis right small finger due to *Staphylococcus aureus*
Index:	**Cellulitis** (diffuse) (with lymphangitis) (*see also* abscess) 682.9, finger (intrathecal) (periosteal) (subcutaneous) (subcuticular) 681.00
Tabular:	**681 Cellulitis and abscess of finger and toe**
	681.0 Finger
	681.00 Cellulitis and abscess, unspecified

There is an instructional note that tells you to identify the organism when assigning code 681.00. To locate the code for the causative organism you look up the main term "infection" in the Index.

Index:	**Infection, infected, infective** (opportunistic) 136.9, staphylococcal, NEC 041.10, aureus 041.11
Tabular:	**041 Bacterial infection in conditions classified elsewhere and of unspecified site**
	041.1 *Staphylococcus*
	041.11 *Staphylococcus aureus*

The Tabular states, "Use additional code, if desired, to identify organism, such as *Staphylococcus* (041.1)." Code 041.1 must have a fifth-digit assignment before it can be assigned, and you would know this only if you verified the code in the Tabular.

Code(s):	681.00, 041.11 Cellulitis right small finger due to *Staphylococcus aureus*

The code for the organism is used as an additional code and is sequenced after the disease or condition.

DISEASES OF THE SKIN AND SUBCUTANEOUS TISSUE

Fill in the codes for the following:

1 Pruritus

Code(s): _____

2 Heat rash

Code(s): _____

3 Psoriasis

Code(s): _____

4 Decubitus ulcer coccyx

Code(s): _____

5 Dermatitis due to poison ivy

Code(s): _____

Diseases of the Musculoskeletal System and Connective Tissue

Chapter 13, Diseases of the Musculoskeletal System and Connective Tissue, in the Tabular describes diseases or conditions of the bone, joints, and muscles. It is important to refer to the note at the beginning of the chapter because that is where you will find the information on the fifth digit sub-classifications that are used for categories 711–712, 715–716, 718–719, and 730. If you turn to category 711, you will see the fifth digit subclassifications again, but not in the same detail as is found at the beginning of the chapter.

EXAMPLE

Diagnosis:	Pyogenic arthritis of the wrist
Index:	Arthritis, arthritic (acute) (chronic) (subacute) 716.9 pyogenic or pyemic 711.0
Tabular:	**711 Arthropathy associated with infections**
	711.0 Pyogenic arthritis

Code 711.0 is not a valid code because you still need to assign a fifth digit to indicate the site. When reviewing the subclassifications, you must identify whether the wrist is part of the forearm or part of the hand. You need to refer to that note at the beginning of the chapter, where you will note that fifth digit "3 forearm includes the radius, ulna and wrist joint."

Code:	711.03 Pyogenic arthritis of the wrist

Pathologic, or spontaneous, fractures are also coded in Chapter 13. A pathologic, or spontaneous, fracture is a break in a bone that occurs because of a bone disease or a change surrounding the bone tissue that makes the bone weak. For a pathologic fracture, you code the fracture and the disease process responsible for the fracture, such as osteoporosis or metastatic cancer of the bone. It is possible to have a small trauma associated with a pathologic fracture. Suppose, for example, an elderly woman with severe osteoporosis bumps her hip against the doorway and sustains a fractured hip. This would be classifiable as a pathologic fracture because a person with healthy bones would not fracture a hip as the result of a small trauma such as bumping the hip on a doorway. If there is any question about whether a fracture is pathologic or due to trauma, ask the physician what caused the fracture.

A pathologic fracture is serious because healing may be delayed by the underlying bone disease. Also, if a pathologic fracture is documented and no other disease process is indicated, review the record or clarify with the physician the underlying cause of the fracture.

EXAMPLE

Diagnosis:	Pathologic fracture of the hip due to severe osteoporosis
Index:	**Fracture** (abduction) (adduction) (avulsion) (compression) (crush) (dislocation) (oblique) (separation) (closed) 829.0 pathologic (cause unknown) 733.10 hip 733.14
Tabular:	**733.1 Pathologic fracture**
	733.14 Pathologic fracture of neck of femur
Index:	**Osteoporosis** (generalized) 733.00
Tabular:	**733.0 Osteoporosis**
	733.00 Osteoporosis, unspecified
Codes:	733.14, 733.00 Pathologic fracture of the hip due to severe osteoporosis

The instructions for category 730, Osteomyelitis, periostitis, and other infections involving bone, direct you to identify any organism as an additional code. It is easy to miss the instructions when they are stuck between an *Excludes* note and the list of fifth digit subclassifications. Highlight these instructions in your ICD-9-CM until you become familiar with their use when coding in this area.

EXERCISE 15–30

DISEASES OF THE MUSCULOSKELETAL SYSTEM AND CONNECTIVE TISSUE

Fill in the codes for the following:

1 Rheumatoid arthritis

   Code(s): _____

2 Pain in the neck

   Code(s): _____

3 Recurrent dislocation right shoulder

   Code(s): _____

4 Systemic lupus erythematosus with lung involvement

   Code(s): _____

5 Spontaneous fracture left humerus due to metastatic bone cancer; history of cancer of the breast previously excised

   Code(s): _____

Congenital Anomalies and Certain Conditions Originating in the Perinatal Period

Chapters 14 and 15, Congenital Anomalies and Certain Conditions Originating in the Perinatal Period, in the Tabular describe congenital anomalies and conditions that originate in the perinatal period. An **anomaly** is an abnormality of a structure or organ. **Congenital** means that it is an abnormality that one was born with. Some anomalies are noticeable and so are discovered at birth. In cases of other anomalies, it may be a number of months or even years before they are discovered. If there is any question about whether a condition is acquired or congenital, you can review the record or clarify the case with the physician.

The **perinatal period** extends through the 28 days following birth. Codes from this chapter can still be used beyond that time frame, but as the chapter title indicates, the condition must have originated during the perinatal period.

Official Coding and Reporting Guidelines

6 NEWBORN GUIDELINES

Definition

The newborn period is defined as beginning at birth and lasting through the 28th day following birth.

The following guidelines are provided for reporting purposes. Hospitals may record other diagnoses as needed for internal data use.

General Rule

All clinically significant conditions noted on routine newborn examination should be coded. A condition is clinically significant if it requires

- clinical evaluation
- therapeutic treatment
- diagnostic procedures
- extended length of hospital stay
- increased nursing care and/or monitoring
- has implications for future health care needs

Note: The newborn guidelines listed previously are the same as the general coding guidelines for other diagnoses, except for the final item regarding implications for future health care needs. Whether a condition is clinically significant can be determined only by the physician.

6.1 USE OF CODES V30–V39

When coding the birth of an infant, assign a code from categories V30–V39, according to the type of birth. A code from this series is assigned as a principal diagnosis, and assigned only once to a newborn at the time of birth.

6.2 NEWBORN TRANSFERS

If the newborn is transferred to another institution, the V30 series is not used.

6.3 USE OF CATEGORY V29

A. Assign a code from V29, Observation and evaluation of newborns and infants for suspected conditions not found, to identify those instances when a healthy newborn is evaluated for a suspected condition that is determined after study not to be present. Do not use a code from category V29 when the patient has identified signs or symptoms of a suspected problem; in such case, code the sign or symptom.

B. A V29 code is to be used as a secondary code after the V30, Outcome of delivery, code. It may also be assigned as a principal code for readmissions or encounters when the V30 code no longer applies. It is for use only for healthy newborns and infants for which no condition after study is found to be present.

6.4 MATERNAL CAUSES OF PERINATAL MORBIDITY

Codes from categories 760–763, Maternal causes of perinatal morbidity and mortality, are assigned only when the maternal condition has actually affected the fetus or newborn. The fact that the mother has an associated medical condition or experiences some complication of pregnancy, labor, or delivery does not justify the routine assignment of codes from these categories to the newborn record.

6.5 CONGENITAL ANOMALIES

Assign an appropriate code from categories 740–759, Congenital Anomalies, when a specific abnormality is diagnosed for an infant. Such abnormalities may occur as a set of symptoms or multiple malformations. A code should be assigned for each presenting manifestation of the syndrome if the syndrome is not specifically indexed in ICD-9-CM.

6.6 CODING OF OTHER (ADDITIONAL) DIAGNOSES

A. Assign codes for conditions that require treatment or further investigation, prolong the length of stay, or require resource utilization.
B. Assign codes for conditions that have been specified by the physician as having implications for future health care needs. Note: This guideline should not be used for adult patients.
C. Assign a code for Newborn conditions originating in the perinatal period (categories 760–779), as well as complications arising during the current episode of care classified in other chapters, only if the diagnoses have been documented by the responsible physician at the time of transfer or discharge as having affected the fetus or newborn.
D. Insignificant conditions or signs or symptoms that resolve without treatment are not coded.

6.7 PREMATURITY AND FETAL GROWTH RETARDATION

Codes from categories 764 and 765 should not be assigned based solely on recorded birthweight or estimated gestational age, but upon the attending physician's clinical assessment of maturity of infant.

Note: Since physicians may utilize different criteria in determining prematurity, do not code the diagnosis of prematurity unless the physician documents this condition.

As Guideline 6.1 states, code the birth from categories V30–V39. This code is used only once on the birth record because it indicates the type of birth. If the baby is transferred to another facility, a code from categories V30–39 would not be assigned.

On the baby's birth record the appropriate V code is sequenced first as the principal diagnosis. If any other conditions or congenital anomalies are documented, they are coded as secondary diagnoses.

EXAMPLE

Diagnosis:	Newborn male delivered in the hospital by cesarean section and with Down's syndrome
Index:	**Newborn** (infant) (liveborn), single, born in hospital (without mention of cesarean delivery or section) V30.00; with cesarean delivery or section V30.01
Tabular:	**V30 Single liveborn**

You are instructed to check the fourth and fifth digits. The code is not complete until you have coded it to the fifth digit subclassification. In this case, the code would be V30.01, as indicated in the Index.

Index:	**Syndrome**—*see also* disease, Down's (mongolism) 758.0
Tabular:	**758 Chromosomal anomalies**
	758.0 Down's syndrome
Codes:	V30.01, 758.0 Newborn male delivered by cesarean section in the hospital; Down's syndrome

In the preceding example, if that baby was transferred to a second facility for treatment of the Down's syndrome there would be no V code to identify the delivery. The V code can be used only once, as the principal diagnosis at the birthing facility. The principal diagnosis code would be Down's syndrome (758.0) at the second facility.

You have to be careful about assigning codes from the 760–763 categories, Maternal Causes of Perinatal Morbidity and Mortality. Many times the mother has a condition, but that condition has no untoward (negative) effect on the baby or fetus. Codes from these categories are to be used only when the maternal condition has affected the health of the newborn.

EXERCISE 15-31

CONGENITAL ANOMALIES AND CERTAIN CONDITIONS ORIGINATING IN THE PERINATAL PERIOD

Fill in the codes for the following:

1 Congenital absence of the earlobe

   Code(s): _____

2 Newborn male delivered in the hospital via vaginal delivery; undescended left testicle (will reevaluate in 6 weeks)

   Code(s): _____

3 Three-year-old diagnosed with fragile X syndrome

   Code(s): _____

4 Newborn transferred to a facility because of congenital dislocation of right hip

   Code(s): _____

Symptoms, Signs, and Ill-Defined Conditions

Chapter 16, Symptoms, Signs, and Ill-Defined Conditions, in the Tabular includes symptoms, signs, abnormal results of investigations and other ill-defined conditions.

You use the codes from Chapter 16 when

- no more specific diagnosis can be made after investigation
- signs and symptoms existing at the time of the initial encounter prove to be transient, or a cause cannot be determined
- a patient fails to return and all you have is a provisional diagnosis
- a case is referred elsewhere before a definitive diagnosis can be made
- a more precise diagnosis is not available for any other reason
- certain symptoms that represent important problems in medical care exist and it might be desirable to classify them in addition to the known cause

You do not code from Chapter 16 when a definitive diagnosis is available. Consider, for example, this diagnostic statement: "Right lower quadrant abdominal pain due to acute appendicitis." The code for right lower quadrant abdominal pain is 789.03, which is located in Chapter 16. But because the reason for the pain is the acute appendicitis, you would not include the code for the symptom of abdominal pain. The only code you would assign would be 540.9 for the acute appendicitis.

You do not code from Chapter 16 when the symptom is considered to be an integral part of the disease process. Consider, for example, this diagnostic statement: "Cough and fever with pneumonia." Both cough and fever are symptoms of the pneumonia; therefore, you would not assign codes for either symptom. The only code you would assign is 486 for the pneumonia.

STOP *A disease reference book comes in handy until you become more familiar with disease symptoms. If you do not know which symptoms are associated with a given disease, look them up in a reference or ask a colleague.*

Finding the codes for **abnormal investigations** in the Index is a little tricky. The codes are found under the main term "Findings, abnormal, without diagnosis (examination) (laboratory test)." Some entries may also be found under the main term "Elevation."

EXAMPLE

Diagnosis:	Abnormal liver scan
Index:	**Findings, abnormal, without diagnosis** (examination) (laboratory test) 796.4, scan NEC 794.9, liver 794.8
Tabular:	**794 Nonspecific abnormal results of function studies**
	794.8 Liver
Code:	794.8 Abnormal liver scan

EXERCISE
15-32

SYMPTOMS, SIGNS, AND ILL-DEFINED CONDITIONS

Fill in the codes for the following:

1 Presyncope

Code(s): _____

2 Pleuritic-type chest pain

Code(s): _____

3 Abnormal mammogram

Code(s): _____

4 Seizure disorder

Code(s): _____

5 Elevated blood pressure reading

Code(s): _____

Injury and Poisoning

Official Coding and Reporting Guidelines

11 GUIDELINES FOR CODING EXTERNAL CAUSES OF INJURIES, POISONINGS AND ADVERSE EFFECTS OF DRUGS (E CODES)

Introduction: These guidelines are provided for those who are currently collecting E codes in order that there will be standardization in the process. If your institution plans to begin collecting E codes, these guidelines are to be applied. The use of E codes is supplemental to the application of basic ICD-9-CM codes. E codes are never to be recorded as principal diagnosis (first listed in the outpatient setting) and are not required for reporting to the CMS.

Injuries are a major cause of mortality, morbidity, and disability. In the United States, the care of patients who suffer intentional and unintentional injuries and poisoning contributes significantly to the increase in medical care costs. External causes of injury and poisoning codes (E codes) are intended to provide data for injury research and evaluation of injury prevention strategies. E codes capture how the injury or poisoning happened (cause), the intent (unintentional or accidental; or intentional, such as suicide or assault), and the place where the event occurred. Some major categories of E codes include:

- transport accidents
- poisoning and adverse effects of drugs, medicinal substances and biologicals
- accidental falls
- accidents caused by fire and flames
- accidents due to natural and environmental factors
- late effects of accidents, assaults or self-injury
- assaults or purposely inflicted injury
- suicide or self-inflicted injury

These guidelines apply for the coding and collection of E codes from records in hospitals, outpatient clinics, emergency departments, other ambulatory care settings and physician offices except when other specific guidelines apply. (See Reporting Diagnostic Guidelines for Hospital-based Outpatient Services/ Reporting Requirements for Physician Billing.)

11.1 GENERAL E CODE CODING GUIDELINES

A. An E code may be used with any code in the range of 001–V82.9 which indicates an injury, poisoning, or adverse effect due to an external cause.
B. Assign the appropriate E code for all initial treatments of an injury, poisoning, or adverse effect of drugs.
C. Use a late effect E code for subsequent visits when a late effect of the initial injury or poisoning is being treated. There is no late effect E code for adverse effects of drugs.
D. Use the full range of E codes to completely describe the cause, the intent, and the place of the occurrence, if applicable, for all injuries, poisonings, and adverse effects of drugs.
E. Assign as many E codes as necessary to fully explain each cause. If only one E code can be recorded, assign the E code most related to the principal diagnosis.
F. The selection of the appropriate E code is guided by the Index to External Causes, which is located after the alphabetical index to diseases and by Inclusion and Exclusion notes in the Tabular List.
G. An E code can never be a principal (first listed) diagnosis.

11.2 PLACE OF OCCURRENCE GUIDELINE

Use an additional code from category E849 to indicate the Place of Occurrence for injuries and poisonings. The Place of Occurrence describes the place where the event occurred and not the patient's activity at the time of the event.

Do not use E849.9 if the place of occurrence is not stated.

11.3 POISONINGS AND ADVERSE EFFECTS OF DRUGS, MEDICINAL AND BIOLOGICAL SUBSTANCE GUIDELINES

A. Do not code directly from the Table of Drugs and Chemicals. Always refer back to the Tabular List.
B. Use as many codes as necessary to describe completely all drugs, medicinal or biological substances.
C. If the same E code would describe the causative agent for more than one adverse reaction, assign the code only once.
D. If two or more drugs, medicinal or biological substances are reported, code each individually unless the combination code is listed in the Table of Drugs and Chemicals. In that case, assign the E code for the combination.
E. When a reaction results from the interaction of a drug(s) and alcohol, use poisoning codes and E codes for both.
F. If the reporting format limits the number of E codes that can be used in reporting clinical data, code the one most related to the principal diagnosis. Include at least one from each category (cause, intent, place) if possible.

If there are different fourth-digit codes in the same three-digit category, use the code for "Other specified" of that category. If there is no "Other specified" code in that category, use the appropriate "Unspecified" code in that category.

If the codes are in different three-digit categories, assign the appropriate E code for other multiple drugs and medicinal substances.

11.4 MULTIPLE CAUSE E CODE CODING GUIDELINES

If two or more events cause separate injuries, an E code should be assigned for each cause. The first listed E code will be selected in the following order:

1. E codes for child and adult abuse take priority over all other E codes—see Child and Adult Abuse Guidelines
2. E codes for cataclysmic events take priority over all other E codes except child and adult abuse
3. E codes for transport accidents take priority over all other E codes except cataclysmic events and child and adult abuse

The first listed E code should correspond to the cause of the most serious diagnosis due to an assault, accident, or self-harm, following the order of hierarchy in the preceding list.

11.5 CHILD AND ADULT ABUSE GUIDELINES

A. When the cause of an injury or neglect is intentional child or adult abuse, the first listed E code should be assigned from categories E960–E968, Homicide and injury purposely inflicted by other persons (except category E967). An E code from category E967, Child and adult battering and other maltreatment, should be added as an additional code to identify the perpetrator, if known.
B. In cases of neglect when the intent is determined to be accidental, E code E904.0, Abandonment or neglect of infant and helpless person, should be the first listed E code.

11.6 UNKNOWN OR SUSPECTED INTENT GUIDELINES

A. If the intent (accident, self-harm, assault) of the cause of an injury or poisoning is unknown or unspecified, code the intent as undetermined E980–E989.

B. If the intent (accident, self-harm, assault) of the cause of an injury or poisoning is questionable, probable or suspected, code the intent as undetermined E980–E989.

11.7 UNDETERMINED CAUSE

When the intent of an injury or poisoning is known, but the cause is unknown, use codes E928.9, Unspecified accident, E958.9, Suicide and self-inflicted injury by unspecified means, and E968.9, Assault by unspecified means.

These E codes should rarely be used as the documentation in the medical record, in both the inpatient and outpatient settings, and should normally provide sufficient detail to determine the cause of the injury.

11.8 LATE EFFECTS OF EXTERNAL CAUSE GUIDELINES

A. Late effect E codes exist for injuries and poisonings but not for adverse effects of drugs, misadventures, and surgical complications.
B. A late effect E code (E929, E959, E969, E977, E989, or E999) should be used with any report of a late effect or sequela resulting from a previous injury or poisoning (905–909).
C. A late effect E code should never be used with a related current nature of injury code.

11.9 MISADVENTURES AND COMPLICATIONS OF CARE GUIDELINES

A. Assign a code in the range of E870–E876 if misadventures are stated by the physician.
B. Assign a code in the range of E878–E879 if the physician attributes an abnormal reaction or later complication to a surgical or medical procedure, but does not mention misadventure at the time of the procedure as the cause of the reaction.

Chapter 17, Injury and Poisoning, in the Tabular is a very long chapter that includes the codes that range from 800 to 999. At the beginning of this chapter there are notes that provide you with specific instructions for the entire chapter. A recent addition to this chapter is the statement that coders should "Use E code(s) to identify the cause and intent of the injury or poisoning (E800–E999)." You learned how to assign E codes in Chapter 14.

There are numerous guidelines that pertain to injuries and poisonings. See the following illustrations.

Official Coding and Reporting Guidelines

2.12 MULTIPLE INJURIES

When multiple injuries exist, the code for the most severe injury as determined by the attending physician is sequenced first.

2.11 MULTIPLE BURNS

Sequence first the code that reflects the highest degree of burn when more than one burn is present. (See also Burns Guideline 8.3)

8.3 CURRENT BURNS AND ENCOUNTERS FOR LATE EFFECTS OF BURNS

Current burns (940–948) are classified by depth, extent and, if desired, by agent (E code). By depth burns are classified as first degree (erythema), second degree (blistering), and third-degree (full-thickness involvement).

[Handwritten margin notes:]
normal burns 940
Not normal move the 30% on 3 degree code 948 site: often
Code most severe 1st
Seg the worst burn 1st. If in two places. But if in some area Seg most sever 1st
no healing burn are acute

A. All burns are coded with the highest degree of burn sequenced first.

B. Classify burns of the same local site (three-digit category level, 940–947) but of different degrees to the subcategory identifying the highest degree recorded in the diagnosis.

C. Non-healing burns are coded as acute burns. Necrosis of burned skin should be coded as a non-healed burn.

D. Assign code 958.3, Posttraumatic wound infection, not elsewhere classified, as an additional code for any documented infected burn site.

E. When coding multiple burns, assign separate codes for each burn site. Category 946, Burns of multiple specified sites, should only be used if the location of the burns is not documented. Category 949, Burn, unspecified, is extremely vague and should rarely be used.

F. Assign codes from category 948, Burns, classified according to extent of body surface involved, when the site of the burn is not specified or when there is a need for additional data. It is advisable to use category 948 as additional coding when needed to provide data for evaluating burn mortality, such as that needed by burn units. It is also advisable to use category 948 as an additional code for reporting purposes when there is mention of third-degree burn involving 20 percent or more of the body surface.

In assigning a code from category 948.

1. Fourth digit codes are used to identify the percentage of total body surface involved in a burn (all degrees).

2. Fifth digits are assigned to identify the percentage of body surface involved in a third-degree burn.

3. Fifth digit zero (0) is assigned when less than 10 percent or when no body surface is involved in a third-degree burn.

Category 948 is based on the classic rule of nines in estimating body surface involved: head and neck are assigned nine percent, each arm nine percent, each leg 18 percent, the anterior trunk 18 percent, posterior trunk 18 percent, and genitalia one percent. Physicians may change these percentage assignments when necessary to accommodate infants and children who have proportionately larger heads than adults and patients who have large buttocks, thighs, or abdomen that involve burns.

G. Encounters for the treatment of the late effects of burns (i.e., scars or joint contractures) should be coded to the residual condition (sequelae) followed by the appropriate late effect code (906.5–906.9). A late effect E code may also be used, if desired.

H. When appropriate, both a sequela with a late effect code, and a current burn code may be assigned on the same record.

8.4 DEBRIDEMENT OF WOUNDS, INFECTION, OR BURN

A. For coding purposes, excisional debridement, 86.22, is assigned only when the procedure is performed by a physician.

B. For coding purposes, nonexcisional debridement performed by the physician or nonphysician health care professional is assigned to 86.28. Any excisional type procedure performed by nonphysician is assigned to 86.28.

8.1 CODING FOR MULTIPLE INJURIES

When coding multiple injuries such as fracture of tibia and fibula, assign separate codes for each injury unless a combination code is provided, in which case the combination code is assigned. Multiple injury codes are provided in ICD-9-CM, but should not be assigned unless information for a more specific code is not available.

A. The code for the most serious injury, as determined by the physician, is sequenced first.

B. Superficial injuries such as abrasions or contusions are not coded when associated with more severe injuries of the same site.

C. When a primary injury results in minor damage to peripheral nerves or blood vessels, the primary injury is sequenced first with additional code(s) from categories 950–957, Injury to nerves and spinal cord, and/or 900–904, Injury to blood vessels. When the primary injury is to the blood vessels or nerves, that injury should be sequenced first.

8.2 MULTIPLE FRACTURES

The principle of multiple coding of injuries should be followed in coding multiple fractures. Multiple fractures of specified sites are coded individually by site in accordance with both the provisions within categories 800–829 and the level of detail furnished by medical record content. Combination categories for multiple fractures are provided for use when there is insufficient detail in the medical record (such as trauma cases transferred to another hospital); when the reporting form limits the number of codes that can be used in reporting pertinent clinical data; or when there is insufficient specificity at the fourth digit or fifth digit level. More specific guidelines are as follows:

A. Multiple fractures of same limb classifiable to the same three-digit or four-digit category are coded to that category.

B. Multiple unilateral or bilateral fractures of same bone(s) but classified to different fourth digit subdivisions (bone part) within the same three-digit category are coded individually by site.

C. Multiple fracture categories 819 and 828 classify bilateral fractures of both upper limbs (819) and both lower limbs (828), but without any detail at the fourth digit level other than open and closed type of fracture.

D. Multiple fractures are sequenced in accordance with the severity of the fracture and the physician should be asked to list the fracture diagnoses in the order of severity.

Fracture is the first section in the chapter and it contains the codes assigned for fractures caused by trauma. A fracture not indicated as closed or open should be classified as closed. If you have any doubt, check with the physician as to the nature of the fracture. A dislocation and fracture of the same bone would be coded to the fracture site. The cross-reference *"see"* is a mandatory instruction that tells you to go to Fracture and not to code the dislocation separately. When you locate the main term "dislocation" in the Index, you are directed to *"see* Fracture, by site." You locate Fracture in the Index on the basis of the anatomic location of the fracture.

EXAMPLES

Diagnosis:	Fracture, right patella with abrasions of the site
Index:	**Fracture,** patella (closed) 822.0
Tabular:	**822 Fracture of patella**
	822.0 Closed
Code(s):	822.0 Fracture, right patella with abrasions of the site

When a fracture is not specified as open or closed, assign a code that indicates a closed fracture. You would not assign a code for the abrasions when there is a more severe injury (the fracture) at the same site.

Diagnosis:	Fractured hip with dislocation
Index:	**Dislocation,** with fracture—*see* Fracture by site.

The "*see* Fracture by site" means the dislocation is included with the fracture code.

Index:	**Fracture,** hip (closed) 820.8
Tabular:	**820 Fracture of neck of femur**
	820.8 Unspecified part of neck of femur, closed
Code(s):	820.8 Fractured hip with dislocation

The guidelines for **burns** direct you to sequence the highest degree of burn first. If you are coding a third-degree burn of the hand and a second-degree burn of the chest wall, you would sequence the code for the third-degree burn of the hand first, followed by the second-degree burn of the chest.

If different degrees of burns are documented at the same site, assign a code to the highest degree only. If, for example, the patient has first- and second-degree burns to the hand, you would code only the second-degree burn or the second-degree burn to the hand.

Facilities may choose to capture data regarding the extent of body area burned. In this case, the rule of nines is applied (refer to Figs. 4–24 and 4–25). The Index entry is "Burn . . . 949.0" with a note indicating that the fifth digit is added to indicate the extent of body surface involved.

Burns are located in the Index by referring to the main term "Burn," to subterms according to the site (abdomen or thigh), and finally to the degree of burn (second or third).

Codes from the 948 category can be used alone or in combination with other specific burn codes. The inclusion of codes from 948 are important for statistical purposes and may affect reimbursement. The use of the three-digit code, 948, indicates a burn condition. The *fourth* digit indicates the total percentage of the body that has been burnt—including all first-, second-, and third-degree burns. The *fifth* digit (0–9) indicates the percentage of the body that has received third-degree burns. It is not the coder's job to calculate the percentages, but you should seek clarification from the physician if documentation is missing or unclear.

EXAMPLES

Diagnosis:	First- and second-degree burn to the back
Index:	**Burn,** back, second degree 942.24
Tabular:	**942 Burn of trunk**
	942.2 Blisters, epidermal [second degree]

A fifth digit is used to indicate the specific location of the burn to the trunk. In this case, the fifth digit 4 is used to indicate the location, back.

Code(s):	942.24 First- and second-degree burn to the back

Note that the diagnosis includes first- and second-degree burns and the code assigned indicates second-degree burns: You code only the highest degree when the burns are at the same site.

Diagnosis:	Second-degree burn, 1%, chin, and third-degree burn, 3%, scapular region, for a total of 4% of the body
Index:	**Burn,** chin, second 941.24
Tabular:	**941 Burn of face, head, and neck**
	941.2 Blisters, epidermal loss [second degree]

A fifth digit is used to indicate the specific location of the burn to the face, head, or neck. In this case, the fifth digit 4 is used to indicate the location, chin.

Index: **Burn,** scapular region, third degree 943.36

Tabular: **943 Burn of upper limb, except wrist and hand**

   943.3 Deep necrosis of underlying tissues [deep third degree] without mention of loss of body part

A fifth digit is used to indicate the specific location of the burn. In this case, the fifth digit 6 is used to indicate the location, scapular region.

Code(s):   943.36, 941.24, 948.00 Third-degree burn, scapular region, and second-degree burn, chin; and the 948.00 indicates that there is less than 10% third-degree burn on less than 10% of the body surface.

EXERCISE 15-33

BURNS

Code the burn, extent of the body surface involved, and percentage of body surface burned using the rule of nines.

1   A 3-year-old pulls a pan of hot grease off the stove and receives third-degree burns of the abdomen, 10%, and second-degree burns of the thigh, 5%

   Code(s): _____

2   Infected third-degree burn, left thigh, 4½%

   Code(s): _____

3   First- and second-degree burn, right foot, 2¼%, due to bonfire

   Code(s): _____

4   Non-healing burn, right hand, 2¼%; excisional debridement performed by physician

   Code(s): _____

5   Second-degree burn, right forearm, 2%; first-degree burn, right little finger, 4%; and third-degree burn, right chest wall, 5%

   Code(s): _____

Wounds (lacerations) are found under the main term "Wound." There are three subcategories in some of the wound codes. These injuries can be classified as

1. without mention of complication

2. complicated

3. with tendon involvement

A **complicated wound** is one that includes documentation of delayed healing, delayed treatment, foreign body, or major infection.

EXAMPLE

Diagnosis:	Infected wound of the right knee.
Index:	**Wound,** knee 891.0, complicated 891.1
Tabular:	**891 Open wound of knee, leg [except thigh], and ankle**
	891.1 Complicated
Codes:	891.1 Infected wound of the right knee

The coding of adverse effects and poisonings is probably the most difficult part of this chapter. It takes some practice to distinguish between an adverse effect and a poisoning. Because the physician is probably not going to use those specific terms in the diagnostic statement, you must question the physician if you are uncertain whether the diagnosis is an adverse effect or a poisoning.

Official Coding and Reporting Guidelines

9 ADVERSE EFFECTS AND POISONING

The properties of certain drugs, medicinal and biological substances, or combinations of such substances, may cause toxic reactions. The occurrence of drug toxicity is classified in ICD-9-CM as follows.

9.1 ADVERSE EFFECT

When the drug was correctly prescribed and properly administered, code the reaction plus the appropriate code from the E930–E949 series. Adverse effects of therapeutic substances correctly prescribed and properly administered (toxicity, synergistic reaction, side effect, and idiosyncratic reaction) may be due to (1) differences among patients, such as age, sex, disease, and genetic factors, and (2) drug-related factors, such as type of drug, route of administration, duration of therapy, dosage, and bioavailability. Codes from the E930–E949 series must be used to identify the causative substance for an adverse effect of drug, medicinal and biological substance, correctly prescribed and properly administered. The effect, such as tachycardia, delirium, gastrointestinal hemorrhaging, vomiting, hypokalemia, hepatitis, renal failure, or respiratory failure, is coded and followed by the appropriate code from the E930–E949 series.

An **adverse effect** occurs when a drug has been correctly prescribed and properly administered and the patient develops a reaction. Everything has been done correctly by the physician and the patient, but a reaction or adverse effect has occurred because of the drug.

When coding adverse effects, you code the effect first, followed by the E code from the therapeutic column on the Table of Drugs and Chemicals.

EXAMPLE

Diagnosis:	Urticaria due to penicillin (properly taken and prescribed)
Index:	**Urticaria** 708.9, due to, drugs 708.0
Tabular:	**708 Urticaria**
	708.0 Allergic urticaria
Drug Table:	Penicillin (any type) E930.0
Tabular:	**E930 Antibiotics**
	E930.0 Penicillins
Codes:	708.0, E930.0 Urticaria due to penicillin

The E codes from this section (E930–E949) are considered required E codes. Thus, therapeutic E codes for adverse effects must be assigned. E codes are never assigned as a principal diagnosis but are always considered an additional code.

There is a code available for an **unknown adverse effect.** If the physician has documented a reaction due to penicillin and you cannot determine from the record what the exact adverse effect has been, you would code unknown adverse effect. Adverse effects can be found in the Index under the main term "Effect, adverse," and the subterm "drugs and medicinals correct substance properly taken 995." The correct codes for adverse effect due to penicillin are 995.2 and E930.0.

A **poisoning** occurs when drugs or other chemical substances are taken not according to a physician's instruction. Poisonings occur in a variety of ways:

- The wrong dosage is given in error, either during medical treatment or by nonmedical personnel such as the mother or the patient herself or himself.

- The medication is given to the wrong person.

- The medication is taken by the wrong person.

- A medication overdose has occurred.

- Medications (prescription or over-the-counter) have been taken in combination with alcohol or other recreational drugs.

- Over-the-counter medications have been taken in combination with prescription medications without physician approval.

Official Coding and Reporting Guidelines

2.14 POISONING

When coding a poisoning or reaction to the improper use of a medication (e.g., wrong dose, wrong substance, wrong route of administration) the poisoning code is sequenced first, followed by a code for the manifestation. If there is also a diagnosis of drug abuse or dependence to the substance, the abuse or dependence is coded as an additional code.

9.2 POISONING (960–979)

For poisoning when an error was made in drug prescription or in the administration of the drug by a physician, nurse, patient, or other person, use the appropriate code from the 960–979 series. If an overdose of a drug was intentionally taken or administered and resulted in drug toxicity, it would be coded as a poisoning (960–979 series). If a nonprescription drug or medicinal agent was taken in combination with a correctly prescribed and properly administered drug, any drug toxicity or other reaction resulting from the interaction of the two drugs would be classified as a poisoning.

Poisoning codes are found in the Table of Drugs and Chemicals. You must always sequence the poisoning code first, then code any manifestation of the poisoning such as coma. You also assign the corresponding E code from the Table. If there is no documentation to indicate otherwise, you use the E code from the accidental column.

CAUTION *You CANNOT use an E code from the therapeutic column (E930–E940) with a poisoning code.*

EXAMPLE

Diagnosis: Coma due to accidental overdose of Valium

When you look up the main term "Overdose" in the Index, you are referred to the Table of Drugs and Chemicals.

Table of Drugs: Valium 969.4 (poisoning)

E853.2 (accidental)

Tabular: **969 Poisoning by psychotropic agents**

969.4 Benzodiazepine-based tranquilizers

Tabular: **E853 Accidental poisoning by tranquilizers**

E853.2 Benzodiazepine-based tranquilizers

Index: **Coma 780.01**

Tabular: **780 General symptoms**

780.01 Coma

Codes: 969.4, 780.01, E853.2 Coma due to accidental overdose of Valium

Note that the poisoning code is sequenced first, followed by the manifestation and then the E code.

If there has been no manifestation (coma, in the above case) of the poisoning, you would assign only the poisoning code with the appropriate E code. When a patient undergoes a poisoning that involves more than one drug or chemical, there could be a different poisoning code and E code for each drug or chemical. There are many codes to review when coding poisonings!

Official Coding and Reporting Guidelines

2.15 COMPLICATIONS OF SURGERY AND OTHER MEDICAL CARE

When the admission is for treatment of a complication resulting from surgery or other medical care, the complication code is sequenced as the principal diagnosis. If the complication is classified to the 996–999 series (complications), an additional code for the specific complication may be assigned.

When coding complications of surgical or medical care, you must be careful to be sure that actual complications are present. A surgical complication is one that takes place as a result of the procedure. Just because a complication occurs following a procedure does not mean the complication is a surgical complication. Do not assume a cause-and-effect relationship. Clarify any doubt or questions with the physician.

EXERCISE
15-34

INJURY/POISONING AND COMPLICATIONS

In the Index, you will find complications of medical and surgical procedures under the main term "Complications." Locate "Complications" in the Index.

What code does the Index direct you to for the following complications?

1   Breast implants, infection

Code(s): _____

2 Bone marrow graft, rejection

Code(s): _____

3 Surgical procedures, stitch abscess

Code(s): _____

4 Cardiac pacemaker, (device) mechanical complication

Code(s): _____

MORE GENERAL GUIDELINES

You have now reviewed all of the chapter-specific guidelines. However, there are a few more guidelines to consider.

Official Coding and Reporting Guidelines

Other diagnoses are defined as "all conditions that coexist at the time of admission, that develop subsequently, or that affect the treatment received and/or the length of stay. Diagnoses that relate to an earlier episode which have no bearing on the current hospital stay are to be excluded."

Reporting Other (Additional) Diagnoses

The general rule is that for reporting purposes, the term "other diagnoses" is interpreted to refer to additional conditions that affect patient care in terms of requiring

- clinical evaluation
- therapeutic treatment
- diagnostic procedures
- extended length of hospital stay, or
- increased nursing care and/or monitoring.

The listing of the diagnoses on the attestation statement is the responsibility of the attending physician.

Official Coding and Reporting Guidelines

3.1 PREVIOUS CONDITIONS

If the physician has included a diagnosis in the final diagnostic statement, such as the discharge summary or the face sheet, it should ordinarily be coded. Some physicians include in the diagnostic statement resolved conditions or diagnoses and status post procedures from previous admission that have no bearing on the current stay. Such conditions are not to be reported and are coded only if required by hospital policy.

However, history codes (V10–V19) may be used as secondary codes if the historical condition or family history has an impact on current care or influences treatment.

EXERCISE 15-35

PREVIOUS CONDITIONS

Circle the conditions in the following diagnostic lists that would not be coded:

1   Herpes zoster

    History of hysterectomy

    Diabetes

2   Influenza

    Hypertension (currently controlled by medication)

    History of peptic ulcer disease

Official Coding and Reporting Guidelines

3.2 DIAGNOSES NOT LISTED IN THE FINAL DIAGNOSTIC STATEMENT

When the physician has documented what appears to be a current diagnosis in the body of the record, but has not included the diagnosis in the final diagnostic statement, the physician should be asked whether the diagnosis should be added.

3.3 CONDITIONS THAT ARE AN INTEGRAL PART OF A DISEASE PROCESS

Conditions that are integral to the disease process should not be assigned as additional codes.

3.4 CONDITIONS THAT ARE NOT AN INTEGRAL PART OF A DISEASE PROCESS

Additional conditions that may not be associated routinely with a disease process should be coded when present.

3.5 ABNORMAL FINDINGS

Abnormal findings (laboratory, x-ray, pathologic, and other diagnostic results) are not coded and reported unless the physician indicates their clinical significance. If the findings are outside the normal range and the physician has ordered other tests to evaluate the condition or prescribed treatment, it is appropriate to ask the physician whether the diagnosis should be added.

EXERCISE 15-36

OTHER DIAGNOSES

Circle the diagnoses that should not be coded:

1   Acute myocardial infarction

    Chest pain

    Shortness of breath

    Congestive heart failure

2 Fractured hip

Hip pain

Contusion of hip

In the following cases, would anemia be coded?

3 A patient is admitted with a fractured femur and undergoes an open reduction. Laboratory values following surgery show a hemoglobin level of 8 mg/dL. No additional workup is done or treatment provided.

_____

4 A patient is admitted for reduction of a hip fracture but receives two units of blood following two reports of hemoglobin volumes of 7 and 8 mg/dL.

_____

In the following case, would the potassium level be coded?

5 A patient with gastroenteritis has a blood sample drawn that shows low levels of potassium. The physician initials the test result but does not order potassium supplements or additional laboratory studies.

_____

BASIC CODING GUIDELINES FOR OUTPATIENT SERVICES

The outpatient guidelines do not address specific sequencing or diseases as the inpatient guidelines do. Although it is not stated in the Guidelines, you will follow the inpatient coding guidelines in situations in which there are no clear outpatient coding guidelines. For example, in an outpatient setting, you would follow the hypertension guidelines and the sequencing of injuries according to severity as is done when following the inpatient guidelines.

Official Coding and Reporting Guidelines

DIAGNOSTIC CODING AND REPORTING GUIDELINES FOR OUTPATIENT SERVICES (HOSPITAL-BASED AND PHYSICIAN OFFICE)

Introduction
These revised coding guidelines for outpatient diagnoses have been approved for use by hospitals/physicians in coding and reporting hospital-based outpatient services and physician office visits.

Information about the use of certain abbreviations, punctuation, symbols, and other conventions used in the ICD-9-CM Tabular List (code numbers and titles) can be found in the section at the beginning of the ICD-9-CM on "Conventions Used in the Tabular List." Information about the correct sequence to use in finding a code is described in the Introduction to the Alphabetic Index of ICD-9-CM.

The terms encounter and visit are often used interchangeably in describing outpatient service contacts and, therefore, appear together in these guidelines without distinguishing one from the other.

Coding guidelines for outpatient and physician reporting of diagnoses will vary in a number of instances from those for inpatient diagnoses, recognizing that:

- The Uniform Hospital Discharge Data Set (UHDDS) definition of principal diagnosis applies only to inpatients in acute, short-term general hospitals.
- Coding guidelines for inconclusive diagnoses (probable, suspected, rule out, etc.) were developed for inpatient reporting and do not apply to outpatients.
- Diagnoses often are not established at the time of the initial encounter/ visit. It may take two or more visits before the diagnosis is confirmed.

The most critical rule involves beginning the search for the correct code assignment through the Alphabetic Index. Never begin searching initially in the Tabular List as this will lead to coding errors.

BASIC CODING GUIDELINES FOR OUTPATIENT SERVICES

A. The appropriate code or codes from 001.0 through V82.9 must be used to identify diagnoses, symptoms, conditions, problems, complaints, or other reason(s) for the encounter/visit.

B. For accurate reporting of ICD-9-CM diagnosis codes, the documentation should describe the patient's condition, using terminology which includes specific diagnoses as well as symptoms, problems, or reasons for the encounter. There are ICD-9-CM codes to describe all of these.

C. The selection of codes 001.0 through 999.9 will frequently be used to describe the reason for the encounter. These codes are from the section of ICD-9-CM for the classification of diseases and injuries (e.g., infectious and parasitic diseases; neoplasms; symptoms, signs, and ill-defined conditions, etc.)

D. Codes that describe symptoms and signs, as opposed to diagnoses, are acceptable for reporting purposes when an established diagnosis has not been diagnosed (confirmed) by the physician. Chapter 16 of ICD-9-CM, Symptoms, Signs, and Ill-Defined Conditions (codes 780.0–799.9), contains many but not all codes for symptoms.

E. ICD-9-CM provides codes to deal with encounters for circumstances other than a disease or injury. The Supplementary Classification of Factors Influencing Health Status and Contact with Health Services (V01.0–V82.9) is provided to deal with occasions when circumstances other than a disease or injury are recorded as diagnosis or problems.

F. ICD-9-CM is composed of codes with either 3, 4, or 5 digits. Codes with 3 digits are included in ICD-9-CM as the heading of a category of codes that may be further subdivided by the use of fourth and/or fifth digits which provide greater specificity.

A three-digit code is to be used only if it is not further subdivided. Where fourth-digit subcategories and/or fifth-digit subclassifications are provided, they must be assigned. A code is invalid if it has not been coded to the full number of digits for that code.

G. List first the ICD-9-CM code for the diagnosis, condition, problem, or other reason for encounter/visit shown in the medical record to be chiefly responsible for the services provided. List additional codes that describe any coexisting conditions.

H. Do not code diagnoses documented as "probable," "suspected," "questionable," "rule out," or "working diagnosis." Rather, code the condition(s) to the highest degree of certainty for that encounter/visit, such as symptoms, signs, abnormal test results, or other reason for the visit.

Please note: This is contrary to the coding practices used by hospitals and medical record departments for coding the diagnosis of hospital inpatients.

I. Chronic diseases treated on an ongoing basis may be coded and reported as many times as the patient receives treatment and care for the condition(s).

J. Code all documented conditions that coexist at the time of the encounter/visit, and require or affect patient care treatment or management. Do not code conditions that were previously treated and no longer exist. However, history codes (V10–V19) may be used as secondary codes if the historical condition or family history has an impact on current care or influences treatment.

K. For patients receiving diagnostic services only during an encounter/visit, sequence first the diagnosis, condition, problem, or other reason for encounter/visit shown in the medical record to be chiefly responsible for the outpatient services provided during the encounter/visit. Codes for other diagnoses (e.g., chronic conditions) may be sequenced as additional diagnoses.

L. For patients receiving therapeutic services only during an encounter/visit, sequence first the diagnosis, condition, problem, or other reason for encounter/visit shown in the medical record to be chiefly responsible for the outpatient services provided during the encounter/visit. Codes for other diagnoses (e.g., chronic conditions) may be sequenced as additional diagnoses.

M. The only exception to this rule is that for patients receiving chemotherapy, radiation therapy, or rehabilitation, the appropriate V code for the service is listed first, and the diagnosis or problem for which the service is being performed is listed second.

N. For patients receiving preoperative evaluations only, sequence a code from category V72.8, Other specified examinations, to describe the pre-op consultations. Assign a code for the condition to describe the reason for the surgery as an additional diagnosis. Code also any findings related to the pre-op evaluation.

O. For ambulatory surgery, code the diagnosis for which the surgery was performed. If the postoperative diagnosis is known to be different from the preoperative diagnosis at the time the diagnosis is confirmed, select the postoperative diagnosis for coding, since it is the most definitive.

OVERVIEW OF ICD-10-CM AND ICD-10-PCS

Development of the ICD-10

The tenth edition of the *International Classification of Diseases* (ICD-10) was issued in 1993 by the World Health Organization (WHO), and WHO is responsible for maintaining it. The ICD-10 does not include a procedure classification (Volume 3). Each world government is responsible for adapting the ICD-10 to suit its own country's needs. For example, Australia uses the ICD-10-AM, that is, the ICD-10-Australian Modification. Each government is responsible for ensuring that its modifications conform with the WHO's conventions in the ICD-10. In the United States, the Centers for Medicare and Medicaid Services is responsible for developing the procedure classification entitled the ICD-10-PCS (PCS stands for Procedure Coding System). The National Center for Health Statistics (NCHS) is responsible for the disease classification system (Volumes 1 and 2) entitled ICD-10-CM (CM stands for Clinical Modification). The ICD-10-CM and ICD-10-PCS are scheduled for introduction sometime after the year 2004.

The ICD-10 is already widely used in Europe, but conversion to the new edition in the United States has taken a great deal of time to implement. One reason for the additional time needed for conversion is that the ICD-9-CM is the basis for the hospital billing system in the United States. In addition, Diagnosis Related Groups (DRG) is the prospective payment system in place for reimbursement of Medicare hospital inpatient stays, and the DRG system is based on the ICD-9-CM.

At the time of publication of this textbook, the final versions of the ICD-10-CM and ICD-10-PCS had not been released. Therefore, all information presented here is based on the draft version of the ICD-10-CM.

Development of the ICD-10-CM to Replace the ICD-9-CM, Volumes 1 and 2

The ICD-10-CM will replace ICD-9-CM, Volumes 1 and 2. Prior to the implementation of the new edition, extensive consultation and review must take place with physician groups, clinical coders, and others. The NCHS has established a 20-member Technical Advisory Panel made up of representatives of the health care and coding communities to provide input during the development of the 10th edition.

Improvements in the ICD-10-CM

Notable improvements in the content and format of the ICD-10-CM include

- the addition of information relevant to ambulatory and managed care encounters

- the expansion of injury codes

    Extensive expansion of the injury codes allows for greater specificity. For example, S50.351 is the new code for Superficial foreign body of right elbow.

- the creation of combination diagnosis/symptom codes to reduce the number of codes needed to fully describe a condition

    For example, I25.12 is the new code for Atherosclerotic heart disease with unstable angina. Under the ICD-9-CM, two codes are required to classify both diagnoses.

- the addition of a sixth character

    For example, S06.336 is the new code for Contusion and laceration of brainstem with prolonged [> 24 hrs.] loss of consciousness. . . .

- the incorporation of common fourth and fifth digit subclassifications

    For example, F10.04 is the new code for Alcohol abuse with alcohol-induced mood disorder.

- the updating and greater specificity of diabetes mellitus codes

    For example, E11.21 is the new code for Type 2 diabetes mellitus with nephropathy.

- the facilitation of providing greater specificity when assigning

Structure of the System

ICD-10-CM contains 21 chapters and excludes the supplementary classifications found in ICD-9-CM. The E and V codes of ICD-9-CM have been incorporated throughout the ICD-10-CM. Chapter titles in the ICD-10-CM remain the same except for the presence of two new chapters: Chapter VII, Diseases of the Eye and Adnexa, and Chapter VIII, Diseases of the Ear and Mastoid Process.

Crosswalk

As a part of the conversion, a **crosswalk** has been developed. This crosswalk converts ICD-9-CM codes to ICD-10-CM codes. Figure 15–4 illustrates a section of the crosswalk. Sometimes, more than one ICD-10-CM code crosswalks from the ICD-9-CM code. In these instances, the possible matches are noted in a Best Match column. For example, in Figure 15–4

ICD-9-CM to ICD-10-CM Conversion Diseases of the Blood and Blood-forming Organs (pound sign (#) following ICD-10-CM code indicates the best match of one to many matches)				
ICD-9-CM Code	ICD-9-CM Abbreviated Title	ICD-10-CM Code	Best Match	ICD-10-CM Abbreviated Title
280	IRON DEFICIENCY ANEMIAS			
280.0	IRON DEF ANEM DT BL LOSS	D50.0		CHRONIC BLOOD LOSS ANEMIA
280.1	IRON DEF ANEM DT DIET	D50.8		FE DEFICIENCY ANEMIA NEC
280.8	IRON DEFICIT ANEMIAS NEC	D50.1		SIDEROPENIC DYSPHAGIA
280.8	IRON DEFICIT ANEMIAS NEC	D50.8	#b	FE DEFICIENCY ANEMIA NEC
280.9	IRON DEFICIT ANEMIA NOS	D50.9		FE DEFICIENCY ANEMIA NOS
281	OTHER DEFICIENCY ANEMIAS			
281.0	PERNICIOUS ANEMIA	D51.0		PERNICIOUS ANEMIA
281.1	VIT B12 DEFIC ANEMIA NEC	D51.1		HEREDIT MEGALOBLAST ANEM
281.1	VIT B12 DEFIC ANEMIA NEC	D51.2		TRANSCOBALAMIN DEF ANEM
281.1	VIT B12 DEFIC ANEMIA NEC	D51.3		DIETARY B12 DEF ANEM NEC
281.1	VIT B12 DEFIC ANEMIA NEC	D51.8		B12 DEFICIENC ANEM NEC
281.1	VIT B12 DEFIC ANEMIA NEC	D51.9	#a	B12 DEFICIENC ANEM NOS

ICD-10-CM Best Match for 281.1

Best Match Designation

Figure 15–4 ICD-9-CM to ICD-10-CM Conversion (crosswalk). (Courtesy of U.S. Department of Health and Human Services, Centers for Medicare and Medicaid Services.)

the ICD-9-CM code 281.1, Vitamin B_{12} deficiency anemia NEC, has five possible matches with ICD-10-CM codes. In the Best Match column, the symbol "#a" indicates that the best match for 281.1 is ICD-10-CM code D51.9. Every ICD-9-CM code is crosswalked to ICD-10-CM code(s) in this way.

Index

The Index for the ICD-10-CM is alphabetic, as illustrated in Figure 15–5. As in the ICD-9-CM, in the Index, the main terms are in bold type, and subterms are indented under the main term. After the index entry, a code is provided. Sometimes, only the first four digits of the code are given. To ensure that you have chosen the correct code and/or to obtain the remaining digits, you must refer to the Tabular.

Tabular

The 21 chapters of the Tabular are arranged in numeric order after the first letter assigned to the chapter. For example, the letter R is assigned to the chapter regarding symptoms. Figure 15–6 illustrates a portion of the chapter concerning symptoms. Note that in the index (Figure 15–5) the main entry is Abdomen, abdominal, and the first subterm is "acute," directing the coder to the Tabular location, R10.0. Now, note in the Tabular (Fig. 15–6) the location of R10.0 as Acute abdomen.

Development of the ICD-10-PCS to Replace the ICD-9-CM, Volume 3

The new structure will allow more expansion than was possible with the ICD-9-CM. Because the ICD-9-CM lacks specificity (exactness) and does not provide for sufficient expansion to support government payment systems and data needs, CMS contracted with 3M Health Information Systems to develop the ICD-10-PCS to replace the ICD-9-CM procedure codes for reporting inpatient procedures.

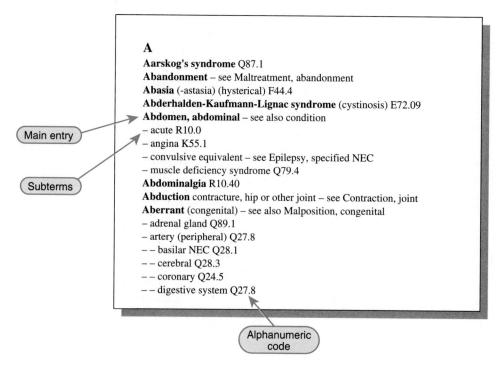

A

Aarskog's syndrome Q87.1
Abandonment – see Maltreatment, abandonment
Abasia (-astasia) (hysterical) F44.4
Abderhalden-Kaufmann-Lignac syndrome (cystinosis) E72.09
Abdomen, abdominal – see also condition
– acute R10.0
– angina K55.1
– convulsive equivalent – see Epilepsy, specified NEC
– muscle deficiency syndrome Q79.4
Abdominalgia R10.40
Abduction contracture, hip or other joint – see Contraction, joint
Aberrant (congenital) – see also Malposition, congenital
– adrenal gland Q89.1
– artery (peripheral) Q27.8
– – basilar NEC Q28.1
– – cerebral Q28.3
– – coronary Q24.5
– – digestive system Q27.8

Main entry

Subterms

Alphanumeric code

Figure 15–5 ICD-10-CM Index. (Courtesy of U.S. Department of Health and Human Services, Centers for Medicare and Medicaid Services.)

Four major objectives guided the development of ICD-10-PCS:

1. **Completeness.** There should be a unique code for all substantially different procedures. Currently, procedures performed on different body parts, using different approaches or of different types, are sometimes assigned the same code.

2. **Expandability.** As new procedures are developed, the structure of the ICD-10-PCS should allow for their incorporation as unique codes.

3. **Multiaxial.** ICD-10-PCS should have a structure such that each code character has, as much as possible, the same meaning, both within the specific procedure section and across procedure sections.

4. **Standardized terminology.** Although the meaning of a specific word can vary in common usage, ICD-10-PCS should not include multiple

Figure 15–6 ICD-10-CM Tabular. (Courtesy of U.S. Department of Health and Human Services, Centers for Medicare and Medicaid Services.)

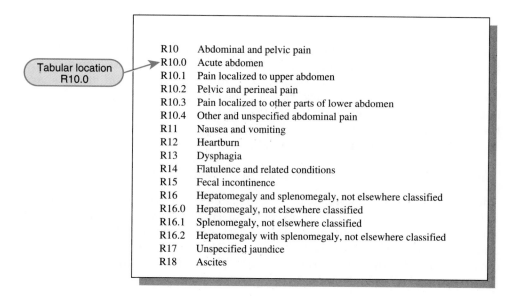

Tabular location R10.0

R10	Abdominal and pelvic pain
R10.0	Acute abdomen
R10.1	Pain localized to upper abdomen
R10.2	Pelvic and perineal pain
R10.3	Pain localized to other parts of lower abdomen
R10.4	Other and unspecified abdominal pain
R11	Nausea and vomiting
R12	Heartburn
R13	Dysphagia
R14	Flatulence and related conditions
R15	Fecal incontinence
R16	Hepatomegaly and splenomegaly, not elsewhere classified
R16.0	Hepatomegaly, not elsewhere classified
R16.1	Splenomegaly, not elsewhere classified
R16.2	Hepatomegaly with splenomegaly, not elsewhere classified
R17	Unspecified jaundice
R18	Ascites

meanings for the same term; each term should be assigned a specific meaning, and ICD-10-PCS should include definitions of the terminology.

A complete, expandable, multiaxial ICD-10-PCS with standardized terminology will allow coding specialists to determine accurate codes with minimal effort.

The Seven Characters of the ICD-10-PCS

The ICD-10-PCS has a seven-character alphanumeric code structure. Each character has as many as 34 different values: 10 digits (0–9) and 24 letters (A–H, J–N, and P–Z) may be assigned to each character. The letters O and I are not used in order to avoid confusion with the digits 0 and 1. In the ICD-10-PCS, the term "procedure" is used to refer to the complete designation of the seven characters. Procedures are divided into sections according to the type of procedure.

Character 1 Identifies the Section

The first character of the procedure code identifies the section. To assign an ICD-10-PCS code, the section where the procedure is coded must be identified. For example, a chest x-ray is in the Imaging section, a breast biopsy is in the Medical and Surgical section, and crisis intervention is in the Mental Health section. Each section is identified by a specific character—number or letter. Section titles and numbers/letters are shown in Figure 15–7.

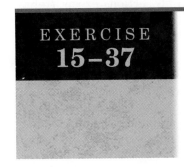

EXERCISE
15–37

ICD-10-PCS FIRST CHARACTER

Using Figure 15–7, identify the first character that would be assigned to the following procedures:

1 _____ Gait training (Rehabilitation)

2 _____ Cesarean section (Obstetrics)

3 _____ Computerized tomography, spine (Imaging)

Figure 15–7 Sections of ICD-10-PCS. (Courtesy of U.S. Department of Health and Human Services, Centers for Medicare and Medicaid Services.)

Sections

0	Medical and Surgical
1	Obstetrics
2	Placement
3	Administration
4	Measurement and Monitoring
5	Imaging
6	Nuclear Medicine
7	Radiation Oncology
8	Osteopathic
9	Rehabilitation and Diagnostic Audiology
B	Extracorporeal Assistance and Performance
C	Extracorporeal Therapies
D	Laboratory
F	Mental Health
G	Chiropractic
H	Miscellaneous

4 _____ Cholecystectomy (Medical/Surgical)

5 _____ Insertion of radium into cervix (brachytherapy) (Nuclear Medicine)

6 _____ Cranioplasty (Medical/Surgical)

Changing Characters

Characters 2 through 7 have a standard meaning within each section but may have different meanings across sections. The meanings for each character are described in each section. For example, Figure 15–8 shows the meanings of the seven characters for the Medical and Surgical sections, and Figure 15–9 shows the meanings for the Imaging section. Notice that several characters have different meanings across these sections. For instance, the third character in medical and surgical procedures (see Fig. 15–8) is used to define the root _operation_ (extraction, insertion, removal, etc.), whereas the third character in imaging procedures (see Fig. 15–9) is used to define the root _type_ (fluoroscopy, MRI, CT, ultrasonography, etc.).

STOP _Each code must include seven characters. If a character is not applicable to a specific procedure, the letter Z is used._

Character 2 Is the Body System

The second character identifies the body system in all sections except Rehabilitation and Mental Health. In these two sections, the second character identifies the type of procedure performed.

Character 3 Is the Root Operation

The third character identifies the root operation in all sections except Radiation Oncology, Rehabilitation, and Mental Health. In many sections, only a few root operations are performed, and these operations are defined for use in that section. The Medical and Surgical section uses an extensive list of root operations. The Obstetrics and Placement sections use some of these same root operations as well as section-specific root operations. See Table 15–1 for a list of the Medical and Surgical root operations definitions, explanations, and examples.

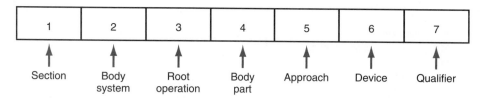

Figure 15–8 Medical and surgical procedures. (Courtesy of U.S. Department of Health and Human Services, Centers for Medicare and Medicaid Services.)

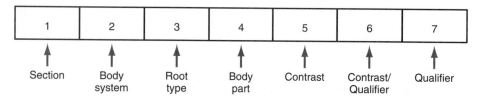

Figure 15–9 Imaging procedures. (Courtesy of U.S. Department of Health and Human Services, Centers for Medicare and Medicaid Services.)

TABLE 15–1   Medical and Surgical Root Operations

0	**Alteration**	**Definition:** Modifying the natural anatomic structure of a body part without affecting the function of the body part **Explanation:** Principal purpose is to improve appearance. **Examples:** Face lift Breast augmentation
1	**Bypass**	**Definition:** Altering the route of passage of the contents of a tubular body part **Explanation:** Rerouting contents around an area of a body part to another distal (downstream) area in the normal route; to another different but similar route and body part; or to an abnormal route and another dissimilar body part. **Encompasses:** Diversion, reroute, shunt **Examples:** Gastrojejunal bypass Coronary artery bypass
2	**Change**	**Definition:** Taking out or off a device from a body part and putting back an identical or similar device in or on the same body part without cutting or puncturing the skin or a mucous membrane **Explanation:** Requires no invasive intervention **Example:** Change of a drainage tube
3	**Control**	**Definition:** Stopping, or attempting to stop, postprocedural bleeding **Explanation:** Confined to postprocedural bleeding and limited to the Anatomic Regions, Upper Extremities, and Lower Extremities Body Systems **Examples:** Control of postprostatectomy bleeding Control of postpneumonectomy bleeding
4	**Creation**	**Definition:** Making a new structure that does not physically take the place of a body part **Explanation:** Confined to sex change operations in which genitalia are made **Encompasses:** Formation **Examples:** Creation of an artificial vagina in a male Creation of an artificial penis in a female
5	**Destruction**	**Definition:** Eradicating all or a portion of a body part **Explanation:** The actual physical destruction of all or a portion of a body part by the direct use of energy, force, or a destructive agent. No tissue is taken out. **Encompasses:** Ablation, cauterization, coagulation, crushing, electrocoagulation, fulguration, mashing, obliteration **Examples:** Fulguration of a rectal polyp Crushing of a fallopian tube
6	**Detachment**	**Definition:** Cutting off all or a portion of an extremity **Explanation:** Pertains only to extremities. The body part determines the level of the detachment. All of the body parts distal to the detachment level are detached. **Encompasses:** Amputation **Examples:** Shoulder disarticulation Below-knee amputation
7	**Dilation**	**Definition:** Expanding the orifice or the lumen of a tubular body part **Explanation:** Stretching by pressure using intraluminal instrumentation **Examples:** Dilation of the trachea Dilation of the anal sphincter

8	**Division**	**Definition:** Separating, without taking out, all or a portion of a body part
		Explanation: Separating into two or more portions by sharp or blunt dissection
		Encompasses: Bisection
		Examples: Bisection of an ovary
		      Spinal cordotomy
		      Division of a patent ductus

9	**Drainage**	**Definition:** Taking into or letting out of fluids and/or gases in a body part **Explanation:** The fluids or gases may be normal or abnormal. **Encompasses:** Aspiration, evacuation, marsupialization, needle puncture, rupture, stabbing, suction, taping, unbridling, undercutting, window formation **Examples:** I & D of an abscess Thoracentesis

B	**Excision**	**Definition:** Cutting out or off, without replacement, a portion of a body part
		Explanation: Involves the act of cutting using a sharp instrument or other method such as a hot knife or laser
		Encompasses: Biopsy, core needle biopsy, debridement, debulk, fine needle aspiration, punch, shuck, trim, wedge
		Examples: Partial nephrectomy
		      Wedge ostectomy
		      Pulmonary segmentectomy

Table continued on followng page

TABLE 15–1   Medical and Surgical Root Operations (Continued)

C	**Extirpation**	**Definition:** Taking or cutting out solid matter from a body part **Explanation:** Taking out solid matter (which may or may not have been broken up) by cutting with either a sharp instrument or other method such as a hot knife or laser, by blunt dissection, by pulling, by stripping, or by suctioning, with the intent not to take out any appreciable amount of the body part. The solid matter may be imbedded in the tissue of the body part or in the lumen of a tubular body part. **Examples:** Sequestrectomy Cholelithotomy
D	**Extraction**	**Definition:** Taking out or off all or a portion of a body part **Explanation:** The body part is not completely dissected free but is pulled or stripped by the use of force (manual, suction, etc.) from its location. **Encompasses:** Abrasion, avulsion, strip **Examples:** Tooth extraction Vein stripping Dermabrasion
F	**Fragmentation**	**Definition:** Breaking down solid matter in a body part **Explanation:** Physically breaking up solid matter not normally present in a body part, such as stones and foreign bodies. The breakup may be accomplished by direct physical force or by shock waves that are applied directly or indirectly through intervening layers. The resulting debris is not taken out but is passed from the body or absorbed by the body. The solid matter may be in the lumen of a tubular body part or in a body cavity. **Encompasses:** Pulverization **Examples:** Lithotripsy, urinary stones Lithotripsy, gallstones
G	**Fusion**	**Definition:** Joining together portions of an articular body part, rendering the articular body part immobile **Explanation:** Confined to joints **Examples:** Spinal fusion Ankle arthrodesis
H	**Insertion**	**Definition:** Putting into a body a nonbiologic appliance that monitors, assists, performs, or prevents a physiologic function, but does not physically take the place of a body part **Encompasses:** Cutdown, implantation, passage **Examples:** Implantation of a radioactive element Insertion of a diaphragmatic pacemaker
J	**Inspection**	**Definition:** Visually and/or manually exploring a body part **Explanation:** Looking at a body part directly or with an optical instrument or feeling the body part directly or through intervening body layers **Encompasses:** Checking, entering, examining, exploring, exposing, opening, probing **Examples:** Diagnostic arthroscopy Exploratory laparotomy
K	**Map**	**Definition:** Locating the route of passage of electrical impulses and/or locating functional areas in a body part **Explanation:** Confined to the cardiac conduction mechanism and the central nervous system **Encompasses:** Localization **Examples:** Mapping of cardiac conduction pathways Location of cortical areas
L	**Occlusion**	**Definition:** Completely closing the orifice or lumen of a tubular body part **Explanation:** Can be accomplished intraluminally or extraluminally **Encompasses:** Clamping, clipping, embolizing, interrupting, ligating, stopping, suturing **Examples:** Ligation of the vas deferens Fallopian tube ligation
M	**Reattachment**	**Definition:** Putting back into or onto a body all or a portion of a body part **Explanation:** Pertains only to body parts and appendages that have been severed; may or may not involve the reestablishment of vascular and nervous supplies **Encompasses:** Replantation **Examples:** Reattachment of penis Reattachment of a hand Replantation of parathyroids
N	**Release**	**Definition:** Freeing a body part **Explanation:** Eliminating abnormal compression or restraint by force or by sharp or blunt dissection. Some of the restraining tissue may be taken out, but none of the body part itself is taken out. **Encompasses:** Decompressing, freeing, lysing, mobilizing, relaxing, relieving, sectioning, taking down **Examples:** Lysing of peritoneal adhesions Freeing of median nerve
P	**Removal**	**Definition:** Taking out or off a device from a body part **Explanation:** May or may not involve invasive penetration **Examples:** Removal of a drainage tube Removal of a cardiac pacemaker

Q	**Repair**	**Definition:** Restoring, to the extent possible, a body part to its natural anatomic structure
		Explanation: An operation of exclusion. Most of the other operations are some type of repair, but if the objective of the procedure is one of the other operations, then that operation is coded. If none of the other operations is performed to accomplish the repair, then the operation "repair" is coded.
		Encompasses: Closure, correction, fixation, reconstruction, reduction, reformation, reinforcement, restoration, stitching, suturing
		Examples: Tracheoplasty
		Suture laceration
		Herniorrhaphy
R	**Replacement**	**Definition:** Putting into or onto a body biologic or synthetic material that physically takes the place of all or a portion of a body part
		Explanation: The biologic material may be living similar or dissimilar tissue from the same individual or nonliving similar or dissimilar tissue from the same individual, another individual, or an animal. The body part replaced may have been taken out previously or replaced previously or may be taken out concurrently with the replacement.
		Examples: Replacement of external ear with synthetic prosthesis
		Total hip replacement
		Replacement of part of the aorta
		Free skin graft
		Pedicle skin graft
S	**Reposition**	**Definition:** Moving to its normal location or other suitable location all or a portion of a body part
		Explanation: The body part repositioned is aberrant, compromised, or has been detached. If attached, it may or may not be detached to accomplish the repositioning.
		Examples: Repositioning of an undescended testicle
		Repositioning of an aberrant kidney
T	**Resection**	**Definition:** Cutting out or off, without replacement, all of a body part
		Explanation: Involves the act of cutting with a sharp instrument or other method such as a hot knife or laser
		Examples: Total gastrectomy
		Pneumonectomy
		Total nephrectomy
V	**Restriction**	**Definition:** Partially closing the orifice or lumen of a tubular body part
		Explanation: Can be accomplished intraluminally or extraluminally
		Encompasses: Banding, cerclage, collapse, compression, packing, tamponade
		Examples: Fundoplication
		Cervical cerclage
W	**Revision**	**Definition:** Correcting a portion of a previously performed procedure
		Explanation: Redoing a portion of a previously performed procedure that has failed to function as intended. Revisions exclude the complete redo of the procedure and procedures to correct complications that do not require the redoing of a portion of the original procedure, such as the control of bleeding.
		Examples: Revision of hip replacement
		Revision of gastroenterostomy
X	**Transfer**	**Definition:** Moving, without taking out, all or a portion of a body part to another location to take over the function of all or a portion of a body part
		Explanation: The body part transferred is not detached from the body. Its vascular and nerve supply remain intact. The body part whose function is taken over may or may not be similar.
		Encompasses: Transposition
		Examples: Never transfer
		Tendon transfer
Y	**Transplantation**	**Definition:** Putting in or on all or a portion of a living body part taken from another individual or animal to physically take the place and/or function of all or a portion of a similar body part
		Explanation: The native body part may or may not be taken out. The transplanted body part may physically take the place of the native body part or may simply take over all or a portion of its function.
		Examples: Lung transplant
		Kidney transplant

EXERCISE 15-38

ROOT OPERATION

Place the character for the root operation term before its definition:

1	____	Taking or letting out fluids and/or gases from a body part	1	Bypass
2	____	Freeing a body part	4	Destruction
3	____	Taking out or off a device from a body part	7	Drainage
4	____	Visually and/or manually exploring a body part	8	Excision
5	____	Restoring to the extent possible a body part to its natural anatomic structure	L	Release
6	____	Altering the route of passage of the contents of a tubular body part	M	Removal
7	____	Cutting out or off, without replacement, all of a body part	N	Repair
8	____	Eradicating all or a portion of a body part	R	Resection
9	____	Correcting a portion of a previously performed procedure	G	Inspection
10	____	Cutting out or off, without replacement, a portion of a body part	T	Revision

A Closer Look at Root Operations

The root operation is described by one of the main terms, as outlined in Table 15–1 (e.g., alteration, destruction, transfer). These root operations can be grouped into types of operations, such as operations that always involve devices: insertion, replacement, removal, change. Table 15–2 shows the root operations grouped by types.

EXERCISE 15-39

ROOT OPERATION TERMS

Using Table 15–2, identify the root operation term for each example:

1 _____ Tendon transfer

2 _____ Appendectomy

3 _____ Diagnostic bronchoscopy

4 _____ Kidney transplant

5 _____ Cardioverter-defibrillator implantation

6 _____ Removal of pulse generator for pacemaker

7 _____ Lithotripsy, bladder stone

8 _____ Fallopian tube ligation

9 _____ Elbow replacement revision

10 _____ Lysis peritoneal adhesions

TABLE 15-2   Root Operations by Type

Operation	Action	Object	Modification	Example
Operations that take out or eliminate all or a portion of a body part				
Excision	Cutting out or off	Portion of a body part	Without replacing the body part	Sigmoid polypectomy
Resection	Cutting out or off	All of a body part	Without replacing the body part	Total nephrectomy
Extraction	Taking out or off	All or a portion of a body part	Without replacing the body part	Tooth extraction
Destruction	Eradicating	All or a portion of a body part	Without taking out any of the body part Without replacing the body part	Fulguration of rectal polyp
Detachment	Cutting off	All or a portion of an extremity	Without replacing the extremity	Below-knee amputation
Operations that involve putting in or on, putting back, or moving living body parts				
Transplantation	Putting in or on	All or a portion of a living body part	Taking from other individual or animal; physically takes the place and/or function of all or a portion of a body part	Heart transplant
Reattachment	Putting back in or on	All or a portion of a body part	Attaching a body part that was detached	Reattachment of finger
Reposition	Moving	All or a portion of a body part	Putting into its normal or another suitable location; body part may or may not be detached	Repositioning of undescended testicle
Transfer	Moving	All or a portion of a body part	Without taking out the body part; takes over function of similar body part	Tendon transfer
Operations that take out or eliminate solid matter, fluids, or gases from a body part				
Drainage	Taking in or letting out	Fluid and/or gases of a body part	Without taking out any of the body part	I & D of an abscess
Extirpation	Taking in or cutting out	Solid matter in a body part	Without taking out any of the body part	Sequestrectomy
Fragmentation	Breaking down	Solid matter in a body part	Without taking out any of the body part or any of the solid matter	Lithotripsy, gallstones
Operations that only involve examination of body parts and regions				
Inspection	Visually and/or manually exploring	A body part		Diagnostic arthroscopy
Map	Locating	Route of passage of electrical impulses Functional areas in a body part		Cardiac conduction pathways Location of cortical areas
Operations that can be performed only on tubular body parts				
Bypass	Altering the route of passage	Contents of tubular body part	May include use of living tissue, nonliving biologic material or synthetic material that does not take the place of the body part	Gastrojejunal bypass
Dilation	Expanding	Orifice or lumen of a tubular body part	By applying pressure	Dilation of anal sphincter
Occlusion	Completely closing	Orifice or lumen of a tubular body part		Fallopian tube ligation
Restriction	Partially closing	Orifice or lumen of a tubular body part		Cervical cerclage
Operations that always involve devices				
Insertion	Putting in	Nonbiologic appliance	Does not physically take the place of body part	Pacemaker insertion
Replacement	Putting in or on	Biologic or synthetic material; living tissue taken from same individual	Physically takes the place of all or a portion of a body part	Total hip replacement
Removal	Taking out or off	Device		Removal of cardiac pacemaker

Table continued on following page

TABLE 15–2   Root Operations by Type (Continued)

Operation	Action	Object	Modification	Example
		Operations that always involve devices		
Change	Taking out or off and putting back	Identical or similar device	Without cutting or puncturing the skin or mucous membrane	Change of a drainage tube
		Miscellaneous operations		
Alteration	Modifying	Natural anatomic structures of a body part	Without affecting function of a body part	Face lift
Creation	Making	New structure	Does not physically take the place of a body part	Creation of an artificial vagina
Control	Stopping or attempting to stop	Postprocedural bleeding		Postprostatectomy bleeding
Division	Separating	A body part	Without taking out any of the body part	Bisection of ovary
Fusion	Joining together	An articular body part	Rendering a body part immobile	Spinal fusion
Release	Freeing	A body part	By eliminating compression or restriction; without taking out any of the body part	Lysing of peritoneal adhesions
Repair	Restoring	To the extent possible, a body part and its natural anatomic structure	May include use of living tissue, non-living biologic material, or synthetic material that does not take the place of or take over the function of the body part	Hernia repair
Revision	Correcting	Portion of a previously performed procedure	Procedure failing to function as intended	Revision hip replacement

The Index

ICD-10-PCS codes are described in both the Index and the Tabular List. The Index, which allows codes to be located by means of an alphabetic lookup, is divided into two parts. The first part of the Index includes the following sections:

- Medical and Surgical
- Obstetrics
- Placement
- Measurement and Monitoring
- Administration
- Extracorporeal Assistance and Performance
- Extracorporeal Therapies
- Miscellaneous Sections

The first part of the Index is arranged according to root operation terms and has subentries based on

- Body System
- Body Part
- Operation (for Revision)
- Device (for Change)

The Index may also be consulted for a specific operation term such as "Hysterectomy," where a cross-reference directs you to see "Resection, Female Reproductive System, OVT." Although you need to become very familiar with the root operations, you may be able to locate a code for a specific operation such as an appendectomy more rapidly by looking under the term "Appendectomy" than by consulting the root operation term "Resection," subterms "*by* Body Part," and "Appendix." See Figure 15–10 for an example of the Index of the ICD-10-PCS.

The second part of the Index covers the remaining sections. This part is also arranged by root operations. For example:

- Imaging—Fluoroscopy by Body System, by Body Part
- Nuclear Medicine—Nonimaging Assay by Body System, by Body Part
- Osteopathic—Treatment by Region

Codes may also be located in the second part of the Index by specific procedures such as Chest x-ray—see Plain Radiography, Anatomical Regions. The Index refers you to a specific entry in the Tabular List by providing the first three or four digits of the procedure code. It is always necessary to refer to the Tabular List to obtain the complete code because the Index contains only the first few numbers and letters.

The Tabular List Completes the Code

The Tabular List provides the remaining characters needed to complete the code given in the Index. The Tabular List is arranged by sections, and most sections are subdivided by body systems. For each body system, the Tabular List begins with a listing of the operations performed, that is, the root operations. When a procedure involves distinct parts, multiple codes are

```
Fasciectomy – see Resection, Bursa, Ligaments, Fascia 0MB....
Fasciectomy – see Excision, Bursa, Ligaments, Fascia 0MT....
Fascioplasty – see Repair, Bursa, Ligaments, Fascia 0MG....
Fine Needle Aspiration – see Excision
Fix – see Repair
Flushing – see Irrigation
Formation – see Creation
Fragmentation
    by Body System
        Anatomical Regions 0XF....
        Central Nervous System 00F...
        Eye 08F...
        Female Reproduction System 0VF....
        Gastrointestinal System 0DF...
        Heart & Great Vessels 02F....
        Hepatobiliary System & Pancreas 0FF....
        Mouth & Throat 0CF....
        Respiratory System 0BF....
        Urinary System 0TF....
    by Body Part
        Ampulla of Vater 0FFB....
        Anus 0DFQ....
        Appendix 0DFJ....
        Bladder 0TF8....
        Bladder Neck 0TF9....
        Bronchus
            Lingula 0BF9....
            Lower Lobe 0BF....
            Main 0BF....
            Middle Lobe, Right 0BF5....
            Segmental, Lingula 0BF9....
            Upper Lobe 0BF....
```

Figure 15–10 ICD-10-PCS Index. (Courtesy of U.S. Department of Health and Human Services, Centers for Medicare and Medicaid Services.)

provided. For example, a section of the listing of operations performed in respect to the central nervous system is as follows:

- Bypass
- Change
- Destruction
- Division
- Drainage
- Excision

The Tabular List for each body system also includes a listing of the body parts, approaches, devices, and qualifiers for that system. These listings are followed by separate tables for each root operation in the body system. At the top of each of the tables is the name of the section, body system, and root operation as well as the definition of the root operation. The list is formatted as a grid, with rows and columns. The four columns in the grid represent the last four characters of the code (which are labeled Body Part, Approach, Device, and Qualifier in the Obstetrics and Medical and Surgical sections). Each row in the grid specifies the allowable combinations of the last four characters. For example, looking at the grid in Figure 15–11, you can see that the code for delivery of retained products of conception is 10Y1BZZ:

1	Obstetrics
0	Pregnancy
Y	Delivery
1	Products of Conception, Retained
B	Transorifice Intraluminal
Z	None
Z	None

Code 10Y1BZZ would be the only allowable code for Products of Conception, Retained, because you may not complete a code by choosing entries from different rows (a row may consist of multiple entries in a box). Thus the code 10Y1BZ6 is not permitted because the qualifier 6 can be used only with the body part 0; it cannot be used with body part 1. If you begin the

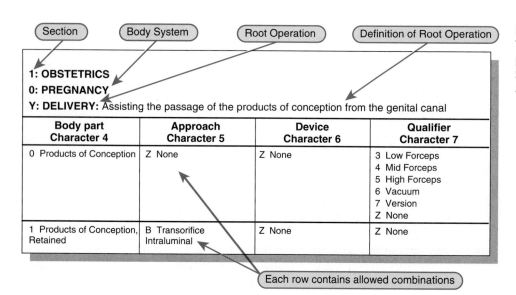

Figure   15–11 ICD-10-PCS Tabular. (Courtesy of U.S. Department of Health and Human Services, Centers for Medicare and Medicaid Services.)

code with 0, Products of Conception, you must continue to choose from the available numbers or letters in that same line. So, with the qualifier 6, the code would have to be 10Y0ZZ6.

EXERCISE 15–40

ICD-10-PCS FORMAT

Complete the following:

Achievement of the four major objectives guiding the development of the ICD-10-PCS will result in a classification system that is

1 _____

2 _____

3 _____

4 _____

Provide the requested information about the ICD-10-PCS code structure:

5 The ICD-10-PCS has a _____ character code structure.

6 The characters in ICD-10-PCS are _____ .

7 Each character has up to _____ different values.

8 The letters _____ are not used as character values.

9 The complete specification of seven characters describes a(n) _____ _____ in the ICD-10-PCS.

CHAPTER GLOSSARY

AHA: American Hospital Association

AHIMA: American Health Information Management Association

anomaly: abnormality

asymptomatic: not showing any of the typical symptoms of a disease or condition

benign: not progressive or recurrent

benign hypertension: hypertensive condition with a continuous, mild blood pressure elevation

combination code: single five-digit code used to identify etiology and manifestation of a disease

comparative conditions: patient conditions that are documented as "either/or" in the patient record

congenital: existing from birth

Crohn's disease: regional enteritis

debridement: cleansing of or removal of dead tissue from a wound

HCFA: Health Care Financing Administration, now known as Centers for Medicare and Medicaid Services (CMS)

Hodgkin's disease: malignant lymphoma

hypertension, uncontrolled: untreated hypertension or hypertension that is not responding to the therapeutic regimen

hypertensive heart disease: secondary effects on the heart of prolonged, sustained systemic hypertension; the heart has to work against greatly increased resistance, causing increased blood pressure

in situ: malignancy that is within the original site of development

italicized code: an ICD-9-CM code that can never be sequenced as the principal diagnosis

late effect: residual effect (condition produced) after the acute phase of an illness or injury has terminated

lesion: abnormal or altered tissue, e.g., wound, cyst, abscess, or boil

malignancy: used in reference to a cancerous tumor

malignant: used to describe a cancerous tumor that grows worse over time

malignant hypertension: accelerated, severe

form of hypertension, manifested by headaches, blurred vision, dyspnea, and uremia; usually causes permanent organ damage

morphology: study of neoplasms

myocardial infarction (MI): necrosis of the myocardium resulting from interrupted blood supply

NEC: not elsewhere classified

neoplasm: new tumor growth that can be benign or malignant

NOS: not otherwise specified

Official Coding and Reporting Guidelines: rules of coding diagnosis codes (ICD-9-CM) published by the Editorial Advisory Board of Coding Clinic

pericarditis: swelling of the sac surrounding the great vessels and the heart

principal diagnosis: defined in the Uniform Hospital Discharge Data Set (UHDDS) as "that condition established after study to be chiefly responsible for occasioning the admission of the patient to the hospital for care": the principal diagnosis is sequenced first

prophylactic: substance or agent that offers some protection from disease

residual: that which is left behind or remains

rule of nines: rule used to estimate burned body surface in burn patients

RUQ: right upper quadrant

secondary site: place to which a malignant tumor has spread; metastatic site

sequela: a condition that follows an illness

slanted brackets: indicate that the ICD-9-CM code can never be sequenced as the principal diagnosis

thyroiditis: a thyroid gland inflammation

UHDDS: Uniform Hospital Discharge Data Set

uncertain behavior: refers to the behavior of a neoplasm as being neither malignant nor benign but having characteristics of both kinds of activity

uncertain diagnosis: diagnosis documented at the time of discharge as "probable," "suspected," "likely," "questionable," "possible," or "rule out"

unspecified hypertension: hypertensive condition that has not been specified as either benign or malignant hypertension

unspecified nature: when the behavior or histology of a neoplasm is not known or is not specified

CHAPTER REVIEW

CHAPTER 15, PART I, THEORY

List, define, or describe the following, as directed:

1   The UHDDS definition of a Principal Diagnosis

is _____

_____

_____

_____

2   List two of the four cooperating parties that

agree on coding principles: _____

_____

CHAPTER 15, PART II, PRACTICAL

Using the ICD-9-CM and coding guidelines, fill in the codes for the following:

1   Combined spinal cord degeneration with pernicious anemia

Code(s): _____

2   Carcinoma, in situ, of skin of lip, vermilion border

Code(s): _____

3   Bilateral occlusion of carotid arteries

Code(s): _____

4   Subacute bacterial endocarditis

Code(s): _____

5   Nephrogenic diabetes insipidus

Code(s): _____

6   Ovarian cyst

Code(s): _____

7   Uterine fibroids complicating pregnancy, 23 weeks' gestation

Code(s): _____

8   Acute and chronic bronchitis

Code(s): _____

9   Group B streptococcal pneumonia

Code(s): _____

10 Obstructed labor caused by cephalopelvic disproportion, delivered liveborn male

Code(s): _____

11 Term birth, delivered by cesarean section, with intrauterine growth retardation

Code(s): _____

12 Alzheimer's disease

Code(s): _____

13 Hypertension with end-stage renal disease

Code(s): _____

14 Anal fistula

Code(s): _____

Fill in the ICD-9-CM codes for the following cases:

15 Mr. Jones presents to the emergency department with acute abdominal pain. After a thorough examination and diagnostic x-ray film, Mr. Jones is diagnosed with acute small bowel obstruction and taken immediately to surgery.

Code(s): _____

16 Mrs. Smith is at 32 weeks' gestation and is admitted with severe bleeding with abdominal cramping. An emergency ultrasound is done and fetal monitors are applied. She is diagnosed with total placenta previa with indications of fetal distress. An emergency cesarean section is done, with delivery of a viable male infant.

Code(s): _____

17 Mr. Jensen is status post colon resection 3 months ago for sigmoid colon cancer and is now admitted for adjunct chemotherapy.

Code(s): _____

18 Miss Halliday is an 80-year-old woman who presents to the emergency department with a history of abdominal pain, fever, and burning with urination. Urine culture is obtained, and Miss Halliday is admitted for workup to rule out urosepsis.

Code(s): _____

19 Mr. Johnson is admitted to the hospital with chest and epigastric pain. He is evaluated by the emergency department physician with a diagnosis of Rule out myocardial infarction. Mr. Johnson is then transferred to a larger facility for further workup.

Code(s): _____

In the following cases, identify the principal diagnosis and all other diagnoses. Assign the appropriate ICD-9-CM codes.

CASE STUDY 1

History of Present Illness

The patient is a 68-year-old female, status post motor vehicle accident 3 months ago. The patient had an open fracture that was treated initially with traction for 6 to 8 weeks. After initial treatment with traction, the patient was placed in a cast brace. She presents with a complaint of pain in the left femur and inability to bear weight on her leg. The patient was referred from an orthopedic surgeon. The past medical history was significant for no history of myocardial infarction or renal disease and no asthma. The patient had undergone no previous procedures with the exception of debridement of the open fracture. Otherwise the patient's history was unremarkable. The patient was taking no medications and had no known allergies. She underwent a preoperative workup that included a gallium scan.

Physical Examination

The heart, lungs, and abdomen were benign. The left knee had a 30-degree extension lag. There was motion with the knee approximately 30 degrees from horizontal axis to 90 degrees of flexion. The patella was difficult to palpate, and it was very difficult to tell at the time of examination whether motion was occurring at the fracture or whether it was occurring at the knee joint. The vascular examination was unremarkable.

Laboratory Data and Course in Hospital

The x-ray film showed nonunion of the left femur. The gallium scan obtained preoperatively was unremarkable, and there was no evidence of infection.

Treatment

On May 14, the patient underwent open reduction and internal fixation of the left femur fracture with a 90-degree dynamic condylar screw and side plate. The patient tolerated the procedure well. She received two units of her own autologous blood at the time of surgery. Postoperatively she was quite anemic, with hemoglobin of 6 to 7 mg/dL. The patient was asymptomatic clinically, and her vascular examination was intact. On postoperative day 2, she had motion in the left knee from 0 to 30 degrees of flexion. She was placed in continuous passive motion and was up with physical therapy but non–weight-bearing on the left leg. Physical therapy was tolerated well. The hospital course was benign. The wound was clean and dry, and the neurovascular examination was unchanged. The x-ray films obtained before discharge showed maintenance of alignment of the left femur. The patient's staples were removed on postoperative day 7. She was placed in a cast brace and was discharged home after being independent in physical therapy.

Final Diagnosis

Nonunion of the left femur

Procedure

Open reduction and internal fixation of the left femur with 90-degree screw and site plate.

20 Code(s): _____

CASE STUDY 2

History of Present Illness

This 50-year-old disabled male is a resident of a nursing home who has been admitted because of marked congestion and respiratory distress. He is known to have mental retardation and frequent urinary tract and pulmonary infections. He has a recurrent epileptic disorder that is well controlled on Dilantin.

Physical Examination

On admission, vital signs include a temperature of 101°F, respiratory rate of 32 breaths per minute, heart rate of 82 beats per minute, and blood pressure of 120/70 mm Hg. Examination of the chest reveals bilateral crepitations. There is moderate redness and edema of the scrotal skin.

Laboratory Data and Course in Hospital

His white blood cell count is 8.5; hemoglobin, 12.9 g/dL; polymorphonuclear leukocytes, 64; bands, 19; lymphocytes, 10; monocytes, 6; and eosinophils, 1. Urinalysis shows moderate bacterial and 1 + white blood cell count. Urine culture shows mixed flora. The repeat urine culture shows *Providencia stuartii* sensitive to Fortaz. Sputum culture reveals the presence of methicillin-resistant *Staphylococcus aureus,* sensitive to vancomycin. Chest x-ray film shows bilateral pulmonary infiltrates. Arterial blood gases on room air show a PO_2 of 48, PCO_2 of 30, and pH of 7.50. When repeated with the patient on oxygen, PO_2 is 66, PCO_2 is 36, and pH is 7.45. The patient is treated with intravenous vancomycin and intravenous Fortaz. His pulmonary infiltrate decreases. His oral intake has been somewhat poor, and he has been given intravenous fluids off and on. The nursing staff at the nursing home note that his intake, in terms of eating and taking fluids, is much better. His medications at the nursing home include Dilantin, 200 mg twice a day; Tegretol, 400 mg at 8 AM and 4 PM, and 200 mg at 8 PM; and Cipro, 500 mg twice a day; and his maintenance medications are continued. This patient is being discharged today.

Final Diagnosis

Acute respiratory insufficiency

Bilateral pneumonia

Mental retardation

Epilepsy

21 Code(s): _____

CASE STUDY 3

History of Present Illness

The patient is an 80-year-old female with a known history of advanced metastatic carcinoma of the breast. The patient has been admitted because of increased shortness of breath and severe pain. The pain is worse in her left chest, and this is associated with increased shortness of breath. At the time of admission, the patient is in so much pain that she is unable to remember her history. The patient initially presented for congestive heart failure more than a year earlier. This was subsequently found to be secondary to metastatic breast cancer, after left mastectomy, 3 years ago. The patient had previously been on chemotherapy.

Course in Hospital

The patient is treated initially with intravenous pain medication to control her pain, and subsequently her condition becomes stable on oral medication. By the time of discharge, the patient is stable on oral Vicodin. She is able to eat. Admission blood urea nitrogen (BUN) was 38 mg/dL with creatinine of 1.3 mg/dL secondary to dehydration. By the time of discharge, these levels have improved. Admission glucose of 225 mg/dL is down to 110 mg/dL at discharge.

Discharge Diagnoses

Uncontrolled pain, secondary to widely metastatic breast carcinoma

Dehydration

Type II diabetes mellitus, uncontrolled

22 What is the principal diagnosis and the code for the principal diagnosis for this patient?

Diagnosis and code(s): _____

23 What are the other diagnoses for this patient and what are the codes for these other diagnoses?

Diagnosis and code(s): _____

_____

_____

unit III

An Overview of
Reimbursement

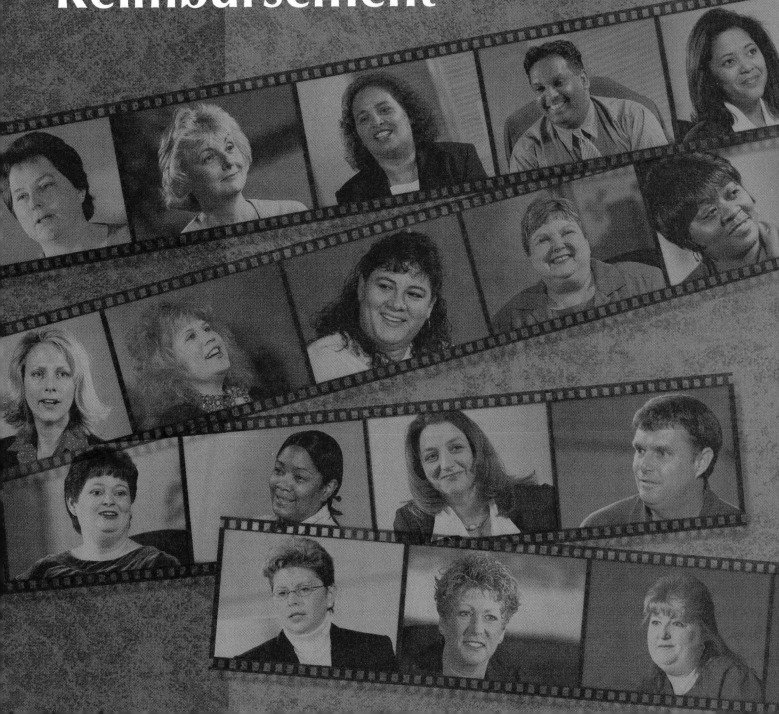

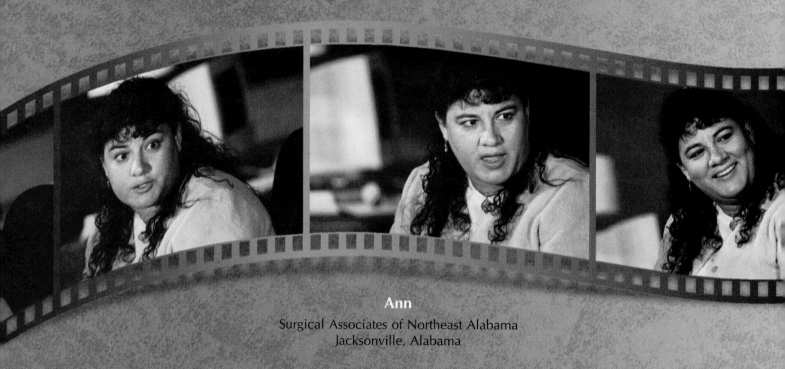

Ann
Surgical Associates of Northeast Alabama
Jacksonville, Alabama

chapter 16

Third-Party Reimbursement Issues

CHAPTER TOPICS

LEARNING OBJECTIVES

After completing this chapter you should be able to

1 Distinguish between Medicare Part A and Part B.

2 Define a "participating provider."

3 Locate information in the *Federal Register.*

4 Identify major elements of the DRG system.

5 Choose the correct DRG.

6 Explain the purpose of PROs.

7 Explain the RBRVS system.

8 State the structure of the APC system.

9 Understand the framework of Medicare Fraud and Abuse.

10 Identify the major components of Managed Health Care.

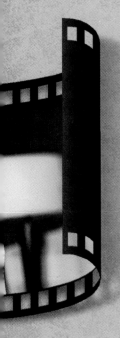

INTRODUCTION

You now have an understanding of the coding systems used in the outpatient and inpatient health care settings. Each of the coding systems plays a key role in the reimbursement of providers of patient health care services. In your role as a medical coder, it is your responsibility to ensure that you code accurately and completely to optimize reimbursement for services provided.

Today, the elderly compose the fastest growing segment of our population. Medical advances allow people to live longer and healthier lives than ever before. Consider that in 1949 there were four persons age 19 and younger for every one person age 65 and older; in 2030 there will be one person age 19 and younger for every one person older than age 65.[1]

Persons enrolled in Medicare coverage increased from 19.5 million in 1967 to 38.1 million in 1996, a 95% increase.[2] Medicare is big business, with Medicare spending at $159.9 billion in 1997[3] and projected to be $364.5 billion in 2008.

RATIO OF CHILDREN 18 AND YOUNGER TO PERSONS 65 AND OLDER[1,2]

- 4:1   1949
- 2:1   1988
- 1:1   2030

Increasing numbers of elderly people, technologic advances, and improved access to health care have increased consumer use of health care services. As more people use health care services, coding becomes even more important to appropriate reimbursement and cost control.

You must understand that your responsibility is to ensure that the data are as accurate as possible, not only for classification and study purposes but also to obtain appropriate reimbursement. Ethical issues surface and must be dealt with by coding personnel. Guidelines must always be followed in the assignment of codes. Instruction from internal and external sources (e.g., administration, peer review organizations, third-party payers) that may increase reimbursement but that conflict with coding guidelines must be discussed and resolved. The principal diagnosis must match the documentation. The sequencing in diagnosis-related group (DRG) payment must always be substantiated by the medical records. Upcoding (maximizing), assigning comorbidity/complications based only on laboratory values, and using nonphysician impressions/assessments without physician agreement are all clearly fraudulent, prompting ethical concerns when coding for reimbursement.

Reimbursement usually comes from third-party payers. By far, the largest third-party payer is the government through the Medicare program. Because the Medicare program plays such an important role in reimbursement, the rules and regulations that govern Medicare reimbursement will be your first topic of study.

THE BASIC STRUCTURE OF THE MEDICARE PROGRAM

The Medicare program was established in 1965 with the passage of the Social Security Act. The Medicare Program dramatically increased the involvement of the government in health care. The program consists of Part A (Hospital Insurance) and Part B (Supplemental Medical Insurance). Part A pays for the cost of hospital/facility care, and Part B pays for physician services and durable medical equipment that are not paid for under Part A.[4,5]

Medicare was originally designed for people 65 and over, but later, people who were eligible for disability benefits from Social Security were also covered under the Medicare program, along with those experiencing permanent kidney failure. Individuals covered under Medicare are called **beneficiaries.**

The Secretary of the Department of Health and Human Services (DHHS) is responsible for the administration of the federal Medicare program. Within the Department, the operation of Medicare is delegated to the Centers for Medicare and Medicaid Services (CMS), formerly the Health Care Financing Administration (HCFA). The funds to run Medicare are generated from payroll taxes paid by employers and employees. The Social Security Administration is responsible for collecting and handling the funds. CMS's function is to promote the general welfare of the public. Its stated goals are to

1. Protect and improve beneficiary health and satisfaction

2. Promote the fiscal integrity of CMS programs

3. Purchase the best-value health care for beneficiaries

4. Promote beneficiary and public understanding of CMS and its programs

5. Foster excellence in the design and administration of CMS's programs

6. Provide leadership in the broader public interest in improving health

CMS handles the daily operation of the Medicare program through the use of fiscal intermediaries. The **fiscal intermediary** does the paperwork for Medicare. A fiscal intermediary is usually an insurance company that bids for a contract with CMS to handle the Medicare program in a specific area. The monies for Medicare flow from the Social Security Administration through the CMS to the fiscal intermediary and, finally, are paid to beneficiaries and providers.

Physicians, hospitals, and other suppliers that furnish care or supplies to Medicare patients are called **providers.** Providers must be licensed by local and state health agencies to be eligible to provide Medicare patients services or supplies. Providers must also meet various additional Medicare requirements before payment can be made for their services.

Medicare pays for 80% of covered charges, and the beneficiary pays the remaining 20%. The beneficiary pays deductibles, premiums, and coinsurance payments. (The 2002 deductible for Part A was $812[6] and for Part B, $54.[7]) The **coinsurance** is the 20% that Medicare does not pay. Often, beneficiaries have additional insurance to cover out-of-pocket expenses. The maximum out-of-pocket amounts are set each year according to formulas established by Congress and published in the *Federal Register*. New amounts usually take effect each January 1.

What Is a Participating Provider?

Claims sent in by the providers of services are processed by fiscal intermediaries according to Medicare guidelines. Providers can sign a **participating provider (PAR) agreement** with a fiscal intermediary to accept assignment on all claims submitted to Medicare.[5] *Accepting assignment* means that the provider will accept what Medicare pays and not bill the patient for the difference between what the service costs and what Medicare pays. For example, a PAR renders a service that costs $100 and bills Medicare for the service; Medicare pays $58; and the provider accepts the Medicare payment as payment in full. Now, you are probably asking yourself why anyone would agree to this. The patient does not pay the $42 difference, nor does Medicare. The amount is written off by the provider as if the service really cost only $58 to provide. This is a good deal for Medicare and the patient, but what about the provider? Why would he or she agree to decreased payments?

Incentives have been established to encourage providers to become PARs. Congress has mandated the following incentives.

For participating providers:

- Direct payment is made on all claims.

- A 5% higher fee schedule than that for nonparticipating providers is in effect.

- Faster processing of assigned claims is offered.

- The provider's name is listed in the PAR directory, which is made available to each Medicare patient, along with identification as a PAR provider who accepts assignment on all claims.

- Hospital referrals for outpatient care must provide the patient with the name and address of at least one participating provider.

For nonparticipating providers:

- Payment goes to the patient on all claims.

- A 5% lower fee schedule than that for participating providers is in effect.

- Slower processing of nonassigned claims is the norm.

- A statement on the Explanation of Benefits (EOB) sent to the patient reminds the patient that the use of a participating physician will lower his or her out-of-pocket expenses.

For fiscal intermediaries:

- A bonus is offered for each recruited and enrolled participating provider.

There are incentives for providers to participate in the Medicare program! Incentives backed by Congress. Currently, half of all physicians in the nation are participating providers.

Part A: Hospital Insurance

Hospitals submit bills for Part A services by using ICD-9-CM codes and the DRG assignment. DRGs are discussed later in this chapter. Beneficiaries are automatically eligible for Part A, hospital insurance, when they are eligible for Medicare benefits.

During a hospital inpatient stay, Part A pays for a semiprivate room (two to four beds), meals and special diet, plus all other medically necessary services except personal-convenience items and private-duty nurses.[5] Part A can also help pay for inpatient care in a Medicare-certified skilled nursing facility if the patient's condition requires daily skilled nursing or rehabilitation services that can be provided only in a skilled nursing facility. Skilled nursing care means care that can be performed only by or under the supervision of licensed nursing personnel. Skilled rehabilitation services may include such services as physical therapy performed by or under the supervision of a professional therapist. The skilled nursing care and skilled rehabilitation services received must be based on a physician's orders. Part A pays for a semiprivate room in the skilled nursing facility, plus meals, nursing services, and drugs. Personal-convenience items, private-duty nurses, and custodial nursing home services are provided to covered beneficiaries who have chronic long-term illnesses or disabilities.[5]

Part A can pay for covered home health care visits from a participating home health agency. The visits can include part-time skilled nursing care and physical therapy or speech therapy when the services are approved by a physician.

Hospice provides relief (palliative) care and support care to terminally ill patients. Part A also pays for hospice care for terminally ill patients when a physician has certified that the patient is terminally ill, the patient has elected to receive care from a hospice rather than the standard Medicare benefits, and the hospice is Medicare-certified. Items covered include nursing services, physician services, and certain other medically necessary services.[5]

Part B: Supplementary Insurance

Part B is not automatically provided to beneficiaries when they become eligible for Medicare. Instead, beneficiaries must purchase the benefits with a monthly premium ($54.00 in 2002).[7] Part B helps to pay for medically necessary physicians' services, outpatient hospital services, home health care, and a number of other medical services and supplies that are not covered by Part A. These Part B services are billed using the ICD-9-CM codes for the diagnosis, the CPT codes for the procedure (service), and HCPCS codes (national codes) for the additional supplies and services.

EXERCISE 16-1

MEDICARE

Using the information presented in this chapter, complete the following:

1 The major third-party reimburser in the United States is

_____ .

2 The Medicare program was established in what year? _____ .

3 Hospital Insurance is Medicare, Part _____ .

4 Supplemental Medical Insurance is Medicare, Part _____ .

Check This Out! ☞ The CMS Website is located at http://www.hcfa.gov. It contains information about the Medicare program, and through it, you can link to the Public Use Files (PUFs), which house useful information concerning providers in the Medicare program.

THE IMPORTANCE OF THE *FEDERAL REGISTER*

The *Federal Register* is the official publication for all "Presidential Documents," "Rules and Regulations," "Proposed Rules," and "Notices." When the government institutes national changes, those changes are published in the *Federal Register*. You must be aware of the changes listed in the *Federal Register* that relate to reimbursement of Medicare so as to submit Medicare

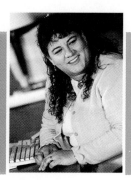

charges correctly. Most of the information in this chapter is about rules that the government has developed and introduced through the *Federal Register*. You might wonder why so much time is to be spent on learning how to follow the guidelines set by the government for reimbursement when it is only one third-party payer. The answer is simple: Because the government is the largest third-party payer in the nation, even a slight change in the rules governing reimbursement to providers can have a major consequence. For example, there was a 45% decrease in the number of inpatient hospital beds between 1975 and 1996.[2] Many of the reasons for this decrease are directly related to the government-implemented inpatient reimbursement system that you will learn about in this chapter—DRGs. Often, more than 33% of the patients in a hospital are Medicare patients. Because the government is such an important payer in the health care system, you must know how to interpret the government's directives published in the *Federal Register*. In addition, many commercial insurers are adopting Medicare payment philosophies for their own reimbursement policies. The government has changed health care reimbursement through the Medicare program, and even more changes are promised.

If you have the *Federal Register* available to you through a library, locating and reviewing some of the issues would be an excellent educational activity for you.

Check This Out! ☞ You can access the *Federal Register* on the Web-site for the National Archives and Records Administration at http://www.access.gpo.gov/nara. This site houses issues of the *Federal Register* from 1994 to the present.

The October editions of the *Federal Register* are of special interest to **hospital** facilities because the hospital updates are released in that edition. **Outpatient** facilities are especially interested in the November or December edition of the *Federal Register* because Medicare reimbursements for outpatient services are published in that edition. Each year, when changes to the various payment systems are proposed, those proposed changes are published early in the year, and a period of several months is offered to interested parties so they can comment and make suggestions on the proposed changes. The final rules are published in the fall editions. The changes presented in fall editions of the *Federal Register* are implemented in the following calendar year.

Figure 16–1 shows a copy of a portion of a *Federal Register;* it is marked to indicate the location of the following details:[8]

1. The regulation's issuing office

2. The subject of the notice

8. Further information

9. Supplementary information

60366 Federal Register/Vol. 65, No. 197/Wednesday, October 11, 2000/Rules and Regulations

1. Issuing office

DEPARTMENT OF HEALTH AND HUMAN SERVICES

Health Care Financing Administration

42 CFR Part 424

[HCFA–6004–FC]

RIN 0938–AH19

2. Subject

Medicare Program; Additional Supplier Standards.

3. Agency

AGENCY: Health Care Financing Administration (HCFA), HHS.

4. Action

ACTION: Final rule with comment period.

5. Summary

SUMMARY: This final rule establishes additional standards for an entity to qualify as a Medicare supplier for purposes of submitting claims and receiving payment for durable medical equipment, prosthetics, orthotics, and supplies (DMEPOS). These regulations will ensure that suppliers of DMEPOS are qualified to provide the appropriate health care services and will help safeguard the Medicare program and its beneficiaries from any instances of fraudulent or obusive billing practices.

6. Dates

DATES: *Effective Date:* These regulations are effective on December 11, 2000.

Comment Date: We will accept comments on the policies discussed in section IV of the **SUPPLEMENTARY INFORMATION** section of this document. Comments will be considered if we receive them at the appropriate address, as provided below, no later than 5 p.m. on December 11, 2000.

7. Address

ADDRESSES: Mail an original and 3 copies of written comments to the following address only:

Health Care Financing Administration, Department of Health and Human Services, Attention: 6004–FC, P.O. Box 8013, Baltimore, MD 21244–8013 Room 443–G, Hubert H. Humphrey Building, 200 Independence Avenue, SW., Washington, D.C. 20201, or Room C5–16–03, 7500 Security Boulevard, Baltimore, MD 21244–1850.

To ensure that mailed comments are received in time for us to consider them, please allow for possible delays in delivering them.

Comments mailed to the above addresses may be delayed and received too late for us to consider them.

Because of staff and resource limitations, we cannot accept comments by facsimile (FAX) transmission. In commenting, please refer to file code HCFA–6004–FC. Comments received timely will be available for public

inspection as they are received, generally beginning approximately 3 weeks after publication of a document, in Room 443–G of the Department's office at 200 Independence Avenue, SW., Washington, D.C., on Monday through Friday of each week from 8:30 a.m. to 5 p.m. (phone: (202) 690–7890).

FOR FURTHER INFORMATION CONTACT: Charles Waldhauser (410) 786–6140.

SUPPLEMENTARY INFORMATION: *Copies:* To order copies of the **Federal Register** containing this document, send your request to: New Orders, Superintendent of Documents, P.O. Box 371954, Pittsburgh, PA 15250–7954. Specify the date of the issue requested and enclose a check or money order payable to the Superintendent of Documents, or enclose your Visa or Master Card number and expiration date. Credit card orders can also be placed by calling the order desk at (202) 512–1800 or by faxing to (202) 512–2250. The cost for each copy is $8. As an alternative, you can view and photocopy the **Federal Register** document at most libraries designated as Federal Depository Libraries and at many other public and academic libraries throughout the country that receive the **Federal Register**.

This **Federal Register** document is also available from the **Federal Register** online database through GPO Access, a service of the U.S. Government Printing Office. The Website address is: http://www.access.gpo.gov/nara/index.html

I. Background

A. General

Medicare services are furnished by two types of entities, providers and suppliers. The term "provider," as defined in our regulations at 42 CFR 400.202, means a hospital, a critical access hospital, a skilled nursing facility, a comprehensive outpatient rehabilitation facility, a home health agency, or a hospice, that has in effect an agreement to participate in Medicare. A clinic, a rehabilitation agency, or a public health agency that has in effect a similar agreement but only to furnish outpatient physical therapy or speech pathology services, or a community mental health center with a similar agreement to furnish partial hospitalization services, is also considered a provider (see sections 1861(u) and 1866(e) of the Social Security Act (the Act) concerning definitions and provider agreements, respectively).

Generally, a Medicare "supplier" is an individual or entity that furnishes certain types of medical and other health items and services under Medicare Part B.

There are different types of suppliers and thus, different definitions of the term "supplier," as well as specific regulations governing the different types of suppliers. A supplier that furnishes durable medical equipment, prosthetics, orthotics, and supplies (DMEPOS) is one category of supplier known as a DMEPOS supplier.

In current regulations at § 424.57(a) concerning payment rules for items furnished by DMEPOS suppliers, we define the term "supplier" as an entity or individual, including a physician or Part A provider, that sells or rents Part B covered items to Medicare beneficiaries, and that meets certain standards. The Part B covered items to which the definition refers are DMEPOS.

B. Legislative History

Section 131 of the Social Security Act Amendments of 1994 (Public Law 103–432, enacted on October 31, 1994) made changes to section 1834 of the Act, "Special Payment Rules for Particular Items and Services." Specifically, it added a new subsection (j) to section 1834 of the Act that established additional requirements that a DMEPOS supplier must meet in order to obtain a supplier number. (A "supplier number" is the equivalent of a "billing number" that a supplier must have in order to submit claims and receive payment for items and services furnished under Medicare.) In section 1834(j)(1)(B)(ii)(IV) of the Act, the Congress also expressly delegated authority to the Secretary to specify any other requirements that a supplier must meet.

II. Provisions of the Proposed Regulations

On January 20, 1998, we published in the **Federal Register** (63 FR 2926) a proposed rule that would require DMEPOS suppliers to meet additional standards in order to submit claims and receive payment. We issued the proposal on the basis of section 1834(j)(1)(B)(ii)(IV) of the Act that authorizes the Secretary to specify additional requirements a DMEPOS supplier must meet. We note that we consulted with representatives of medical equipment and supply companies, carriers, and consumers before issuing the proposal.

As we stated in the proposed rule, we believe it was the Congress' intent in enacting section 131 of the Social Security Act Amendments of 1994 to

Figure 16–1 Example of a page from the *Federal Register*. (From Fed Regist Oct 11;65(197):60366, 2000.)

3. The agency

4. The action

5. A summary

6. The dates

7. The addresses

8. Contacts for further information

9. Supplementary information

Items 1 through 9 are always placed before the Final Rule, which is the official statement of the entire rule.

EXERCISE
16-2

FEDERAL REGISTER

Answer the following questions:

1 Which edition of the *Federal Register* is of special interest to hospital facilities? _____

2 Which edition of the *Federal Register* is of special interest to outpatient facilities? _____

Using Figure 16–1, answer the following questions:

3 What is the issuing office? _____

4 What is the last date for comment to be received on this proposal?

_____

5 According to the Summary section in Figure 16–1, what does DMEPOS mean? _____

_____

6 According to the For Further Information Contact section in Figure 16–1, who could give you further information related to the issue addressed in this *Federal Register*? _____

UNDERSTANDING INPATIENT DIAGNOSIS-RELATED GROUPS (DRGs)

The system of classifying patients into DRGs[9] provides a means of relating the types of patients, the types of illnesses, and the volume treated by a hospital to the costs incurred by the hospital. The complexity of a hospital's case load is referred to as a hospital's **case mix.**

The design and development of the DRGs began in the late 1960s at Yale University. The initial motivation for developing the DRGs was to create a framework for monitoring the quality of care and the utilization of services in a hospital setting. The first large-scale application of the DRGs was in the late 1970s in New Jersey. The New Jersey State Department of Health used DRGs as the basis of a prospective payment system in which hospitals were reimbursed a fixed DRG-specific amount for each patient treated. In 1982, the Tax Equity and Fiscal Responsibility Act (TEFRA) modified the Medicare hospital reimbursement limits to include a system based on DRGs. In 1983, Congress amended the Social Security Act to include a national DRG-based hospital prospective payment system for all Medicare patients.

Prospective payment rates based on DRGs have been established as the basis of the Medicare's hospital reimbursement system. The evolution of the DRGs and their use as the basic unit of payment in Medicare's hospital reimbursement system represents a recognition of the basic role that a hospital's case mix plays in determining its costs. Currently, hospitals are paid according to the DRG and a hospital payment rate. The hospital payment rate for Medicare patients is based on the type of hospital, the geographic area, the designation of urban or rural, and other factors that affect the cost of providing care. In the past, hospital characteristics such as teaching status and number of beds were used to explain the cost differences among hospitals. However, such characteristics failed to account for the cost impact of a hospital's case mix. Individual hospitals have often attempted to justify higher cost by stating that they treated a more complex mix of patients or that the patients they treated were simply "sicker." Everyone agreed that more complicated cases cost a hospital more to treat, but exactly how to define and measure a hospital's case mix was a very difficult matter. The concept of case mix complexity has been used to refer to a set of patient attributes that includes

- Severity of illness
- Prognosis
- Treatment difficulty
- Need for intervention
- Resource intensity

Each of these attributes has an exact meaning that describes a particular aspect of a hospital case mix.

- *Severity of illness* refers to the levels of loss of function and likelihood of mortality that may be experienced by patients with particular diseases.

- *Prognosis* refers to the probable outcome of illnesses, including the likelihood of improvement or deterioration in the severity of an illness, the likelihood of recurrence, and the probable life span.

- *Treatment difficulty* refers to the patient management problems that a particular illness presents to the health care provider. Such management problems are associated with illnesses without clear patterns of symptoms, illnesses requiring sophisticated and technically difficult procedures, and illnesses requiring close monitoring and supervision.

- *Need for intervention* relates to the consequences to the patient that lack of immediate or continuing care would produce.

- *Resource intensity* refers to the volume and type of diagnostic, therapeutic, and bed services used in the management of particular illnesses.

There are two ways to use the term "case mix complexity." Clinicians use it to mean that the patient has a greater severity of illness, presents greater treatment difficulty, has a poorer prognosis, or has a greater need for intervention. *Administrators and regulators,* however, usually use the term "case mix complexity" to indicate a patient's need for more resources and thus the higher cost of providing care. Often the two interpretations of case mix complexity are closely related, but they can be very different for certain kinds of patients. For example, terminal cancer patients are severely ill and have poor prognoses, but in the end stages, they commonly require few hospital resources beyond basic nursing care.

Because the purpose of the DRGs is to relate a hospital's case mix to the resource demands and associated costs experienced by the hospital, when a hospital is said to have a more complex case mix, from a DRG perspective that means that the hospital treats patients who require more hospital resources—not necessarily that the hospital treats patients who have greater severity of illness, have illnesses that present greater treatment difficulty, have poorer prognoses, or have greater needs for intervention.

Major Diagnostic Categories

The process of forming the DRGs was begun by dividing all possible principal diagnoses into 23 principal diagnosis areas referred to as major diagnostic categories (MDCs). Two new MDCs were created in the eighth version of the DRGs, for a total of 25 MDCs. The MDCs are displayed in Figure 16–2. Physician panels developed the diagnoses in each MDC to correspond to a single organ system (respiratory system, circulatory system, digestive sys-

Major Diagnostic Categories

1 - Diseases and Disorders of the Nervous System
2 - Diseases and Disorders of the Eye
3 - Diseases and Disorders of the Ear, Nose, Mouth and Throat
4 - Diseases and Disorders of the Respiratory System
5 - Diseases and Disorders of the Circulatory System
6 - Diseases and Disorders of the Digestive System
7 - Diseases and Disorders of the Hepatobiliary System and Pancreas
8 - Diseases and Disorders of the Musculoskeletal System and Connective Tissue
9 - Diseases and Disorders of the Skin, Subcutaneous Tissue and Breast
10 - Endocrine, Nutritional and Metabolic Diseases and Disorders
11 - Diseases and Disorders of the Kidney and Urinary Tract
12 - Diseases and Disorders of the Male Reproductive System
13 - Diseases and Disorders of the Female Reproductive System
14 - Pregnancy, Childbirth and the Puerperium
15 - Newborns and Other Neonates with Conditions Originating in the Perinatal Period
16 - Diseases and Disorders of the Blood and Blood Forming Organs and Immunological Disorders
17 - Myeloproliferative Diseases and Disorders, and Poorly Differentiated Neoplasms
18 - Infectious and Parasitic Diseases (Systemic or Unspecified Sites)
19 - Mental Diseases and Disorders
20 - Alcohol/Drug Use and Alcohol/Drug Induced Organic Mental Disorders
21 - Injuries, Poisonings and Toxic Effects of Drugs
22 - Burns
23 - Factors Influencing Health Status and Other Contacts with Health Services
24 - Multiple Significant Trauma
25 - Human Immunodeficiency Virus Infections

Figure 16–2 Major Diagnostic Categories of the Diagnosis-Related Groups. (From Diagnosis Related Groups, Version 14.0, Definitions Manual, 3M Health Information Systems.)

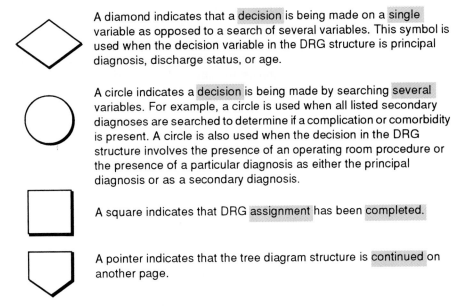

A diamond indicates that a decision is being made on a single variable as opposed to a search of several variables. This symbol is used when the decision variable in the DRG structure is principal diagnosis, discharge status, or age.

A circle indicates a decision is being made by searching several variables. For example, a circle is used when all listed secondary diagnoses are searched to determine if a complication or comorbidity is present. A circle is also used when the decision in the DRG structure involves the presence of an operating room procedure or the presence of a particular diagnosis as either the principal diagnosis or as a secondary diagnosis.

A square indicates that DRG assignment has been completed.

A pointer indicates that the tree diagram structure is continued on another page.

Figure 16–3 DRG symbols used in tree diagrams for each Major Diagnostic Category. (From Diagnosis Related Groups, Version 14.0, Definitions Manual, 3M Health Information Systems.)

tem, etc.) and generally to be associated with a particular medical specialty. This was done because most clinical care is organized around medical specialties. Not all diseases and disorders can be assigned to an organ system (e.g., systemic infections), so a number of non–organ system categories exist: Systemic Infectious Diseases, Myeloproliferative Diseases, and Poorly Differentiated Neoplasms. Each of the DRGs is defined by a particular set of patient attributes:

- Principal diagnosis
- Secondary diagnosis
- Procedures
- Age
- Sex
- Discharge status

A tree diagram (flow chart) depicts the DRG structure for each MDC. Tree diagrams use several symbols to describe the various types of decisions made when determining DRG assignment. Figure 16–3 indicates the symbols and the definitions of each.

Every classification of a patient begins with the diagnosis and the pre-MDC flow chart, or tree diagram, as shown in Figure 16–4. For example, if a patient is admitted to the hospital for a tracheostomy, DRG 483 is assigned; if for a liver transplant, DRG 480 is assigned. If the patient was not admitted for a tracheostomy or a liver transplant, the next question in the tree diagram asks if the patient was admitted for a bone marrow transplant (481), and so on down the tree diagram. If the patient was not admitted for one of the principal diagnoses noted on the flow chart of pre-MDCs, the classification of the patient moves on to one of the remaining 23 MDCs. When surgical procedures are classified, the additional hospital resources used are indicated by employing the surgical-procedure MDCs (e.g., operating room, recovery room, anesthesia). For this reason most MDCs were initially divided into medical and surgical groups. Figure 16–5 shows the typical division, depending on whether a surgical procedure was performed.

A patient is placed in the surgical-procedure category if he or she undergoes a procedure that requires the use of an operating room. If a patient has multiple surgical procedures, the DRG assignment is based on a ranking of most to least resource-intensive surgeries (surgical hierarchy). For example, if a patient undergoes both a dilation and curettage and a hysterectomy, the hysterectomy would use more resources and so would be the basis for the DRG selection. A principal diagnosis is one that is performed

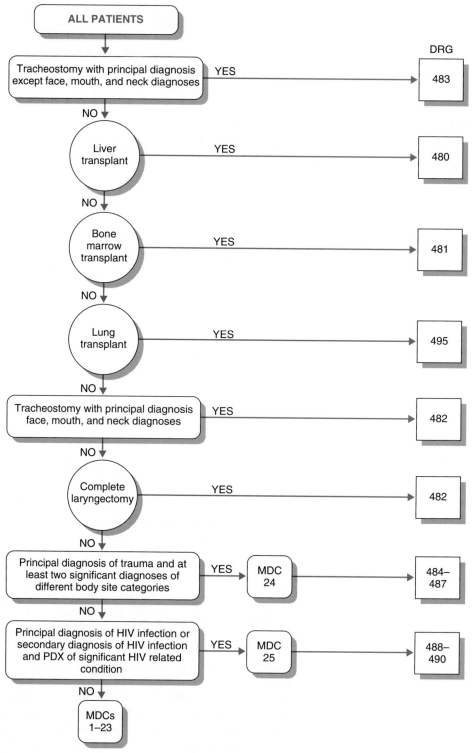

Figure 16–4 Pre-MDC flow chart, CMS Grouper. (From Diagnosis Related Groups, Version 14.0, Definitions Manual, 3M Health Information Systems.)

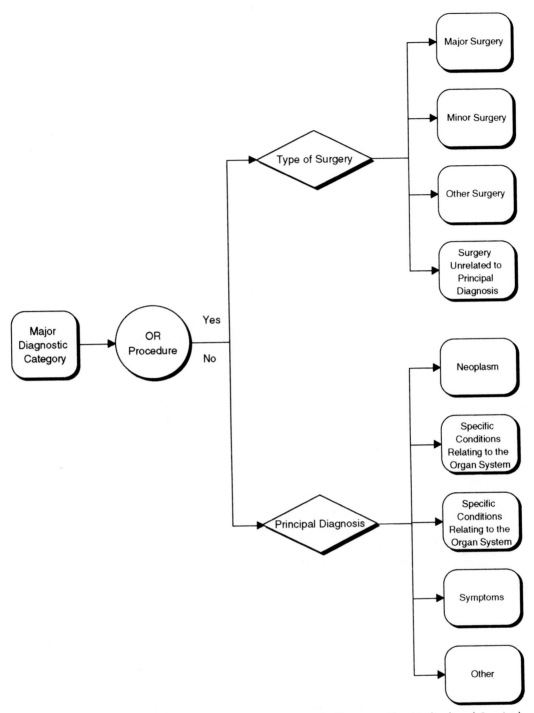

Figure 16–5 Typical DRG structure for a Major Diagnostic Category. The Medical and Surgical Classes are further divided based on the age of the patient or the presence of complications or comorbidities. (From Diagnosis Related Groups, Version 14.0, Definitions Manual, 3M Health Information Systems.)

for definitive treatment rather than one that is performed for diagnostic or exploratory purposes or one that was necessary in order to take care of a complication.

DRG selection is based on selection of the principal diagnosis if no surgery is performed. DRG selection is also based on complications, comorbidities, and the patient's age. Panels of physicians have classified each diagnosis code on the basis of whether the diagnosis, when presented with a secondary condition, would be considered a substantial complication or comorbidity. A substantial complication or comorbidity is considered a condition that increases the length of stay in the hospital by at least 1 day in at least 75% of patients. For example, pneumonia is considered a substantial complication or comorbidity, whereas benign hypertension is not. The same basic list of complications and comorbidities is used in most DRGs.

The patient's age is sometimes used in the definition of the DRGs. Pediatric patients are often assigned to separate DRGs. Age is used because extremely young and extremely old patients often require more resources. Also, patient discharge status is a consideration in assignment of a DRG. For example, separate DRGs were formed for burn patients and newborns if the patients were transferred to another acute care facility. Separate DRGs were also formed for patients with alcoholism or drug abuse who left the facility against medical advice, for patients with acute myocardial infarction, and for newborns who died.

There are also five DRGs that are used for patients whose records contain inconsistent or invalid information. DRGs 468, 476, and 477 are used for records that indicate that the patient underwent a surgical procedure unrelated to the diagnosis. Typically, such patient has been admitted with a diagnosis requiring no surgery but then develops a complication unrelated to the principal diagnosis and requires the performance of an operating-room procedure; or the patient may undergo a diagnostic procedure for a concurrent principal diagnosis. For example, a patient who has a principal diagnosis of congestive heart failure and develops acute cholecystitis and whose only procedure is a cholecystectomy is assigned to DRG 468 because the cholecystectomy is considered an extensive procedure and is unrelated to the reason for admission.

A patient is assigned to DRG 469 when a selected principal diagnosis, although a valid ICD-9-CM code, is not precise enough to allow the patient to be assigned to a DRG. For example, ICD-9-CM code 646.90 is an unspecified complication of pregnancy, with the episode of care unspecified. The diagnosis code indicates neither the type of complication nor whether the episode of care was antepartum, postpartum, or for delivery. Because DRG definitions assign patients to different DRGs depending on whether the episode of care was antepartum, postpartum, or for delivery, a patient with a principal diagnosis that does not indicate the specificity would be assigned to DRG 469 as the principal diagnosis. DRG 470 is for certain types of record errors that may affect the DRG assignment. For example, a patient who is 154 years of age would be assigned to 470 if the correct choice of DRG depends on the age of the patient because the age is an obvious error.

With the principal diagnosis of the patient, you can locate the correct DRG. A computer program, called a grouper, is used to input the principal diagnosis and other critical information about a patient (secondary diagnosis, procedures, age, sex, discharge status). The grouper then provides the correct DRG assignment for the case on the basis of the information the coder provides. For now, you are going to use the best computer of all to calculate a DRG—your brain. Did you know that it would take a computer that was as tall as a 33-story building to hold all of the capability your brain has? You have tremendous potential! The computer is only as smart as the operator. You will be the operator of the grouper, and the quality of the information you input will determine the quality of the information that is output. Understanding how the grouper works will help you to identify the correct information to input into the computer.

Tree Diagrams Guide You

Each MDC has a flow chart called a tree. In each flow chart, the codes available for selection are located within symbols that have particular meanings. The tree diagram uses decision symbols to guide you through the diagram. The symbols are like road signs that make sure you stay on the right path.

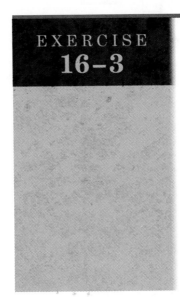

EXERCISE
16-3

TERMINAL DRG

Using Figure 16–6, the flow chart for Diseases and Disorders of the Respiratory System, let's locate a DRG together.

A 72-year-old patient is admitted to the hospital because of pneumonia.

You begin on the left side of Figure 16–6, at the circle labeled OR Procedure. This patient has not had surgery, so move on down the No path until you arrive at the question that asks whether ventilator support has been used. There is no indication of ventilator support, so you continue down the No path to the off-page connector 1 symbol, which tells you that there is another page. Figure 16–7 shows that next page. From the pointer 1, you arrive at the decision symbol labeled Principal Diagnosis. You have five principal diagnosis categories from which to choose on this medical page: Pulmonary Embolism, Infections and Inflammations, Neoplasm, Major Chest Trauma, and Pleural Effusion. This patient has an infection of the lungs, so you follow the line down from the principal diagnosis category of Infections and Inflammations. The decision operation Age > 17 asks

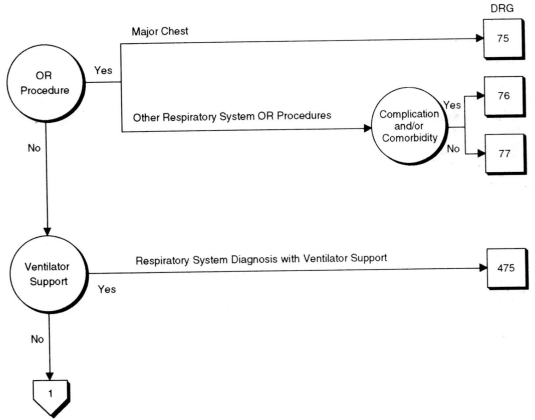

Figure 16–6 Major Diagnostic Category 4, Diseases and Disorders of the Respiratory System, Surgical Partitioning. (From Diagnosis Related Groups, Version 14.0, Definitions Manual, 3M Health Information Systems.)

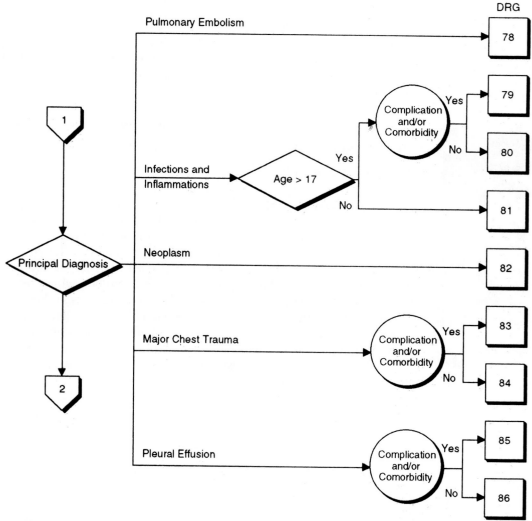

Figure 16-7 Major Diagnostic Category 4, Diseases and Disorders of the Respiratory System, Medical Partitioning. (From Diagnosis Related Groups, Version 14.0, Definitions Manual, 3M Health Information Systems.)

whether the age of the patient is greater than 17, yes or no. This patient is 72, so you follow the line down the Yes path. Next, you are presented with the question of whether the patient has any Complication and/or Comorbidity. There is no indication of any comorbidity or complication. You proceed along the No path and arrive at the correct DRG for this case—80.

Now you do one. Using Figure 16–7, locate the correct DRG for the following:

1 The patient is an 82-year-old who has been admitted with the principal diagnosis of iatrogenic pulmonary embolism and infarction (iatrogenic means physician-induced) (ICD-9-CM 415.11).

   DRG: _____

2 A 42-year-old patient is admitted with the principal diagnosis of major chest trauma (without complications)—three fractured ribs, larynx, and trachea (ICD-9-CM code 807.03).

   DRG: _____

Connecting the ICD-9-CM and the DRG

In the DRG manual, each of the DRG numbers has assigned to it a group of ICD-9-CM codes along with the principal diagnosis statement. For example, question 1 in Exercise 16–3 indicates a principal diagnosis of iatrogenic pulmonary embolism and infarction, which is identified by ICD-9-CM code 415.11. Figure 16–8 shows this diagnosis code as it appears in the ICD-9-CM. The DRG manual also lists 415.11 under DRG 78, Pulmonary Embolism (Figure 16–9). (Note that in the DRG manual, the decimal point used in the ICD-9-CM code is deleted because the computer does not need the decimal point.) Therefore, in question 1, the patient's diagnosis of iatrogenic pulmonary embolism and infarction, 415.11, is automatically classified to DRG 78 by the grouper. All of the principal diagnoses listed under DRG 78 (Fig. 16–9) are automatically assigned to DRG 78 on the basis of the ICD-9-CM code you input into the computer.

Question 2 in Exercise 16–3 has an ICD-9-CM code of 807.03 (three fractured ribs, larynx, and trachea). Figure 16–10 shows the diagnosis code as it appears in the ICD-9-CM. The ICD-9-CM code 807.03 is listed in the group of codes for DRG 84 in the description of DRGs (Fig. 16–11).

As you can see from this exercise, your coding ability and the completeness of the medical record are critical to correct DRG assignment. The computer follows the flow charts just as you did when you assigned the DRGs in questions 1 and 2. The advantage is that the computer can quickly accomplish the task of DRG assignment for you. However, the assignment

---

DISEASES OF PULMONARY CIRCULATION (415-417)

415 Acute pulmonary heart disease

  415.0 Acute cor pulmonale

  |Excludes:| *cor pulmonale NOS (416.9)*

  415.1 Pulmonary embolism and infarction
  Pulmonary (artery) (vein):
    apoplexy
    embolism
    infarction (hemorrhagic)
    thrombosis
  |Excludes:| *that complicating:*
        abortion (634-638 with .6, 639.6)
        ectopic or molar pregnancy (639.6)
        pregnancy, childbirth, or the puerperium
                (673.0-673.8)

  (ICD-9-CM code) → **415.11 Iatrogenic pulmonary embolism and infarction**

  415.19 Other

Figure 16–8 ICD-9-CM diagnosis code for iatrogenic pulmonary embolism and infarction. (From International Classification of Diseases, 9th Revision. U.S. Department of Health and Human Services, Public Health Service, Centers for Medicare and Medicaid Services.)

DRG 78 PULMONARY EMBOLISM

PRINCIPAL DIAGNOSIS

ICD-9-CM code ──→ 41511   Iatrogen pulm emb/infarc   9581   Fat embolism
                  41519   Pulm embolism/infarct NEC   9991   Air embol comp med care
                  9580   Air embolism

Figure 16–9 Section on MDC 4 Definition of DRGs showing ICD-9-CM code for iatrogenic pulmonary embolism and infarction. (From Diagnosis Related Groups, Version 14.0, Definitions Manual, 3M Health Information Systems.)

will only be as accurate as the information you input. What a difference the correct DRG assignment can make in the reimbursement received by the hospital for patients' care!

As an example of how the sequencing of complications and comorbidity can affect the reimbursement amount, consider the following actual case:

---

807   Fracture of rib(s), sternum, larynx, and trachea

The following fifth-digit subclassification is for use with codes 807.0-807.1:

0   rib(s), unspecified
1   one rib
2   two ribs
3   three ribs
4   four ribs
5   five ribs
6   six ribs
7   seven ribs
8   eight or more ribs
9   multiple ribs, unspecified

ICD-9-CM code ──→ **807.0 Rib(s), closed**

807.1 Rib(s), open

807.2 Sternum, closed

807.3 Sternum, open

807.4 Flail chest

807.5 Larynx and trachea, closed
       Hyoid bone   Trachea
       Thyroid cartilage

807.6 Larynx and trachea, open

Figure 16–10 ICD-9-CM diagnosis code for three fractured ribs—closed. (From International Classification of Diseases, 9th Revision. U.S. Department of Health and Human Services, Public Health Service, Centers for Medicare and Medicaid Services.)

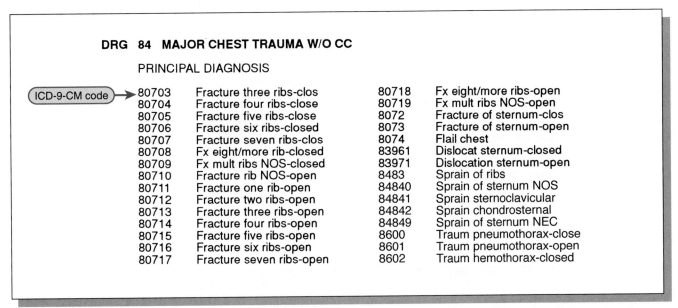

Figure 16–11 Section on MDC 4 Definition of DRGs showing ICD-9-CM code for three fractured ribs—closed. (From Diagnosis Related Groups, Version 14.0, Definitions Manual, 3M Health Information Systems.)

CASE STUDY ONE

The principal diagnosis is congestive heart failure (428.0). Additional diagnoses are morbid obesity (278.01), diabetes (250.00), coronary atherosclerosis (414.0), psoriasis (696.1), depressive disorder (311), unspecified personality disorder (301.9), hypercholesterolemia (272.0), cardiomegaly (429.3), and initial episode, subendocardial infarction (410.71). The result of code 410.71's being listed as the tenth diagnosis was a reimbursement of $4,702. If 410.71 is within the top nine diagnoses, the reimbursement is $7,055. This is a $2,353 loss to the hospital because of the incorrect sequencing of a complication.

Correct DRG assignment makes good "cents."

All ICD-9-CM codes considered to be complications or comorbidities (C/C) of a DRG are a part of the DRG system and are listed in Appendix C of the DRG manual. Figure 16–12 shows a page of Appendix C, Diagnoses Defined as Complications or Comorbidities, in the Diagnosis-Related Groups, Definition Manual. The complication/comorbidity ICD-9-CM code is displayed in bold type, and an abbreviated diagnosis statement follows the code. For example, in Figure 16–13, ICD-9-CM code 83914, dislocation of the fourth cervical vertebra—open (top of the second column, "83914 Disloc 4th cerv vert-opn") is listed as a complication/comorbidity. The codes listed under 83914 are the principal diagnoses for which a dislocation of the fourth cervical vertebra (open) is not considered a complication.

For example, the first range of principal diagnosis codes listed under 83914 is 80500 to 80518. Code 805 identifies Fractures of the vertebral column; the fourth digit identifies cervical, thoracic, lumbar, or other location; and the fifth digit specifies which cervical vertebra was fractured—first, second, third, and so on. Code 805.14 represents the diagnosis of "fracture of the fourth cervical vertebral (open)." A "fracture of the fourth cervical vertebra" (80514) cannot be a complication/comorbidity for "dislocation of the fourth cervical vertebra" (83914).

As another example, codes 80600 to 80619 are listed as principal diagnoses that also cannot use 83914 as a complication/comorbidity. Codes in the

APPENDIX C - DIAGNOSES DEFINED AS COMPLICATIONS OR COMORBIDITIES

83901   Disloc 1st cerv vert-cl
80500-80518,80600-80619,
8068-8069,83900-83918,8470,
8488-8489,8798-8799,9290-9299,
95200-95209,9588,9598-9599

83902   Disloc 2nd cerv vert-cl
80500-80518,80600-80619,
8068-8069,83900-83918,8470,
8488-8489,8798-8799,9290-9299,
95200-95209,9588,9598-9599

83903   Disloc 3rd cerv vert-cl
80500-80518,80600-80619,
8068-8069,83900-83918,8470,
8488-8489,8798-8799,9290-9299,
95200-95209,9588,9598-9599

83904   Disloc 4th cerv vert-cl
80500-80518,80600-80619,
8068-8069,83900-83918,8470,
8488-8489,8798-8799,9290-9299,
95200-95209,9588,9598-9599

83905   Disloc 5th cerv vert-cl
80500-80518,80600-80619,
8068-8069,83900-83918,8470,
8488-8489,8798-8799,9290-9299,
95200-95209,9588,9598-9599

83906   Disloc 6th cerv vert-cl
80500-80518,80600-80619,
8068-8069,83900-83918,8470,
8488-8489,8798-8799,9290-9299,
95200-95209,9588,9598-9599

83907   Disloc 7th cerv vert-cl
80500-80518,80600-80619,
8068-8069,83900-83918,8470,
8488-8489,8798-8799,9290-9299,
95200-95209,9588,9598-9599

83908   Disloc mult cerv vert-cl
80500-80518,80600-80619,
8068-8069,83900-83918,8470,
8488-8489,8798-8799,9290-9299,
95200-95209,9588,9598-9599

83910   Disloc cerv vert NOS-opn
80500-80518,80600-80619,
8068-8069,83900-83918,8470,
8488-8489,8798-8799,9290-9299,
95200-95209,9588,9598-9599

83911   Disloc lst cerv vert-opn
80500-80518,80600-80619,
8068-8069,83900-83918,8470,
8488-8489,8798-8799,9290-9299,
95200-95209,9588,9598-9599

83912   Disloc 2nd cerv vert-opn
80500-80518,80600-80619,
8068-8069,83900-83918,8470,
8488-8489,8798-8799,9290-9299,
95200-95209,9588,9598-9599

83913   Disloc 3rd cerv vert-opn
80500-80518,80600-80619,
8068-8069,83900-83918,8470,
8488-8489,8798-8799,9290-9299,
95200-95209,9588,9598-9599

83914   Disloc 4th cerv vert-opn
80500-80518,80600-80619,
8068-8069,83900-83918,8470,
8488-8489,8798-8799,9290-9299,
95200-95209,9588,9598-9599

83915   Disloc 5th cerv vert-opn
80500-80518,80600-80619,
8068-8069,83900-83918,8470,
8488-8489,8798-8799,9290-9299,
95200-95209,9588,9598-9599

83916   Disloc 6th cerv vert-opn
80500-80518,80600-80619,
8068-8069,83900-83918,8470,
8488-8489,8798-8799,9290-9299,
95200-95209,9588,9598-9599

83917   Disloc 7th cerv vert-opn
80500-80518,80600-80619,
8068-8069,83900-83918,8470,
8488-8489,8798-8799,9290-9299,
95200-95209,9588,9598-9599

83918   Disloc mlt cerv vert-opn
80500-80518,80600-80619,
8068-8069,83900-83918,8470,
8488-8489,8798-8799,9290-9299,
95200-95209,9588,9598-9599

8500   Concussion w/o coma
80000-80199,80300-80499,
8500-85219,85221-85419,
8738-8739,8798-8799,9050,
9251-9252,9290-9299,9588-9590,
9598-9599

8501   Concussion-brief coma
80000-80199,80300-80499,
8500-85219,85221-85419,
8738-8739,8798-8799,9050,
9251-9252,9290-9299,9588-9590,
9598-9599

8502   Concussion-moderate coma
80000-80199,80300-80499,
8500-85219,85221-85419,
8738-8739,8798-8799,9050,
9251-9252,9290-9299,9588-9590,
9598-9599

8503   Concussion-prolong coma
80000-80199,80300-80499,
8500-85219,85221-85419,
8738-8739,8798-8799,9050,
9251-9252,9290-9299,9588-9590,
9598-9599

8504   Concussion-deep coma
80000-80199,80300-80499,
8500-85219,85221-85419,
8738-8739,8798-8799,9050,
9251-9252,9290-9299,9588-9590,
9598-9599

8505   Concussion w coma NOS
80000-80199,80300-80499,
8500-85219,85221-85419,
8738-8739,8798-8799,9050,
9251-9252,9290-9299,9588-9590,
9598-9599

C
C

Figure 16–12   Appendix C, Diagnoses Defined as Complications or Comorbidities. (From Diagnosis Related Groups, Version 14.0, Definitions Manual, 3M Health Information Systems.)

CMS's guidelines for PRO quality criteria

Admissions for acute medical conditions

1. Initial assessment—adequacy of initial assessment of:
   a. respiratory function
   b. cardiac function
   c. neurologic function
   d. biochemical/metabolic status
   e. gastrointestinal status
2. Stabilization—restoration of:
   a. respiratory function
   b. cardiac function
   c. fluid volume and chemical balance
3. Definitive diagnosis—identification of:
   a. the immediate cause of hospitalization:
      i. failure of organ system
      ii. infectious process
   b. significant comorbidities
   c. other major reversible problems
   d. adequate diagnostic workup
   e. documentation
   f. comments
   g. complications
4. Definitive therapy—
   a. physiologic support
   b. pharmacologic intervention:
      i. selection of agents
      ii. determination of proper doses
      iii. consideration of toxicity drug interactions
      iv. consideration of interactions with comorbidities
   c. surgical evaluation—specialty consultation
   d. provision of device:
      i. selection and fitting
      ii. training
   e. referral/transfer
5. Recovery—
   a. titration of therapeutic agents and supports
   b. mgmt. of intercurrent infections
   c. mgmt. of complications related to comorbidities
6. Discharge—
   a. physiologic stability sufficient for ambulatory care
   b. plan for followup and aftercare/sociologic setting
   c. rehabilitation

Chronic medical conditions

1. Adequacy of assessment of deterioration of function—
   a. measures of deficit and residual function/reserve
      i. vital organs
      ii. biochem/metabolic status
      iii. motor capability
      iv. sensory limitation pain
      v. psychologic
      vi. social situation
   b. comorbidities
2. Management—
   a. pharmacologic
      i. agent selection
      ii. dosage titration
      iii. drug interactions
      iv. interactions with comorbidities
   b. device
      i. selection and fitting
      ii. training
   c. surgical evaluation/referral
3. Discharge—
   a. assessment of restoration of function/physiologic stability
   b. plan for followup and aftercare/sociologic setting

Elective surgical admissions

1. Adequacy of assessment of physiologic/functional impairment—
   a. underlying disorder and stage of progression
   b. comorbidities
   c. evaluation of medical/interventional radiologic mgmt. alternatives
   d. need for procedures
   e. documentation
2. Preoperative evaluation—
   a. cardiac
   b. pulmonary
   c. neurologic
   d. renal
   e. endocrine metabolic
   f. hydration and electrolytes (anesthetic staging)
   g. radiologic assessment
3. Operative protocol—
   a. preparation
      i. gastrointestinal
      ii. antibiotic prophylaxis
      iii. sedation
   b. anesthesia
      i. agent route
      ii. ventilation
      iii. hemodynamic monitor
      iv. intravenous fluids (volume electrolytes)
   c. surgical procedure
      i. appropriateness and adequacy
      ii. support staff
      iii. operative complications
4. Post-operative mgmt.—
   a. vital signs
   b. stabilization
      i. ventilation
      ii. hemodynamics
   c. neurologic status/sensorium
5. Recovery—
   a. physiologic support
   b. wound management

Figure 16–13 CMS guidelines for peer review organization quality criteria. (From Fed Regist Jan 18;54:1965–1966, 1989.)

Illustration continued on following page

80600 to 80619 range are for vertebra fractures with spinal cord injury; the fourth digit identifies a cervical, thoracic, lumbar, or sacrum/coccyx location, and the fifth digit specifies the extent and level of the spinal injury. Again, complication involving a dislocation of the fourth cervical vertebra would not be considered a complication of the fracture of the same vertebra because the complication/comorbidity is closely related to the principal diagnosis. So, even though complications increase the reimbursement for a diagnosis, the DRG system specifies which complications cannot be considered in combination with a given principal diagnosis, and all complications must be adequately documented in the medical record.

c. mgmt. of current infections
d. mgmt. of comorbidities
e. other postop complications
6. Discharge—
a. physiologic stability
b. wound stability
c. management of temporary functional deficit
d. plan for followup and aftercare/sociological setting

Acute surgical admissions

1. Initial assessment—adequacy of initial assessment of:
a. cardiac output/blood volume
b. ventilation
c. biochemical/metabolic balance
d. neurologic status/sensorium
2. Stabilization—
a. respiration
b. cardiac output/blood volume
c. biochemical/metabolic balance
3. Identification of affected organ/lesion—
a. history/physical
b. radiology (imaging)
c. laboratory
d. other diagnostic procedures
e. documentation
4. Preoperative evaluation management—
a. cardiac

b. pulmonary
c. neurologic
d. electrolytes/hematology
e. renal function
f. assessment of medical or interventional radiologic alternatives

5. Operative protocol—
a. preparation
i. gastrointestinal
ii. antibiotic prophylaxis
iii. sedation
b. anesthesia
i. agent route
ii. ventilation
iii. hemodynamic cardiovascular
iv. intravenous fluids (volume, electrolytes)
c. surgical procedure
i. appropriateness, adequacy
ii. support staff
iii. operative complications
6. Post-operative mgmt.—
a. vital signs
b. stabilization
i. ventilation
ii. hemodynamics
c. neurologic status/sensorium
7. Recovery—
a. physiologic support
b. wound management
c. mgmt. of intercurrent infections
d. mgmt. of comorbidities
e. other postoperative complications

8. Discharge—
a. physiologic ability
b. wound stability
c. mgmt. of temporary functional deficit
d. plan for followup and aftercare sociologic setting

Admissions for trauma

1. Initial assessment—adequacy of initial assessment of:
a. anatomic damage
b. respiratory function
c. cardiac function, blood volume
d. neurologic status
e. biochemical/metabolic
2. Stabilization—
a. correction of stabilization of anatomic injury
b. respiratory function
c. cardiac function/blood volume
3. Evaluation/diagnosis—
a. collateral injuries
i. radiology
ii. invasive procedures
b. comorbidities
4. Corrective treatment—
a. surgical (see acute surgical admissions)
b. physiologic support
c. physical therapy/rehab.
5. Discharge—
a. stability of injury
b. physiologic stability
c. functional capacity
d. followup and aftercare
e. rehabilitation

f. sociologic evaluation support

Acute psychiatric admissions

1. Assessment—adequacy of initial assessment of:
a. degree of functional impairment
b. underlying physiologic disorder
c. comorbidities
d. history
e. medical status
f. documentation
g. mental status
h. assessment for potential harm to self or others
2. Management—
a. underlying physiologic disorder
b. pharmacologic
i. agent
ii. titration of dosage
iii. drug interactions
iv. interactions with comorbidities
c. surgical
d. other therapy: electric shock therapy, analysis, psychotherapy, rehab, etc.
3. Disposition—
a. functional capacity
b. followup monitoring
c. aftercare/sociologic support

Federal Register, Jan. 18, 1989. pp. 1965–1966

Figure 16–13   *Continued*

EXERCISE
16-4

DRG INFORMATION

After locating the principal diagnosis in your ICD-9-CM, use Figure 16–12 to answer the following:

1 Can a complication/comorbidity of a concussion with a brief coma be used with a principal diagnosis of a cerebral laceration with open intracranial wound?

_____

2 Can a complication/comorbidity of a dislocation of the third cervical vertebra (closed) be used as a complication/comorbidity with the principal diagnosis of whiplash?

_____

3 Can the complication/comorbidity of dislocation of the sixth cervical vertebra (open) be used as a complication/comorbidity with the principal diagnosis of injury to the external carotid artery?

_____

Fill in the blanks with the correct word(s):

4 The design and development of the DRGs began in the late 1960s at which university?

_____

5 The first large-scale application of the DRGs was in the late 1970s in which state?

_____

6 The types of illnesses and volume of patients treated by a hospital represent the complexity of the hospital's

_____

7 The concept of case mix complexity refers to a set of patient attributes that include these five elements:

_____

_____

_____

_____

_____

THE PURPOSE OF PEER REVIEW ORGANIZATIONS (PROs)

An attempt to monitor payment and ensure quality care for hospital services came about when Congress amended the Social Security Act of 1972 and established the Professional Standards Review Organization (PSRO). The PSRO was a voluntary group of physicians who monitored the necessity of hospital admissions and reviewed the treatment costs and medical records of hospitals. But the cost of operating the PSRO was more than the amount the program saved each year. Congress wanted a program that had stricter controls over Medicare reimbursement for inpatient costs. Congress was concerned that within the Prospective Payment System of DRGs there was an incentive for hospitals to increase admissions, increase readmissions, and code hospital stays into higher-priced diagnostic categories so as to receive higher payments. So Congress created control peer review organi-

from the trenches

What is the one personality trait that all coders should have?
"A can-do attitude!"

ANN

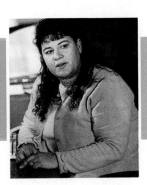

zations (PROs).[5] The creation of the PROs (also known as quality improvement organizations) was made possible under the provision of TEFRA, which gave the CMS the right to contract with private organizations for peer review purposes.

The review services of the PROs are intended to determine

1. Whether the services provided or proposed are reasonable and medically necessary for (A) the diagnosis and treatment of an illness or injury; (B) improving the function of the patient; (C) the prevention of illness; or (D) the management of a terminal illness.

2. Whether the services proposed to be provided on an inpatient basis could actually be provided on an outpatient basis.

3. The medical necessity, reasonableness, and appropriateness of the care.

4. Whether a hospital has misrepresented admission or discharge information or has taken action that has resulted in (A) unnecessary admission; (B) unnecessary multiple admissions; (C) any other inappropriate medical practices with respect to the beneficiary; or (D) the potential of premature discharge.

5. The validity of all information supplied by the provider.

6. The completeness and adequacy of the hospital care provided.

7. The quality of services meets professionally recognized standards of health care.

The review obligations of the PROs are outlined in the CMS's Scope of Work document, which defines the type and number of health records that must be reviewed. The focus of the Scope of Work includes

• Increased educational and focused review

• Patterns of care and outcome

• Differences that occur regularly versus isolated cases

• Identification of patterns and variations

• Cooperation with the community (education and reports)

Six types of reviews are performed by the PROs:

1. Admission

2. Discharge

3. Quality

4. DRG validation

5. Coverage

6. Procedure

The review begins with a nonphysician reviewer, usually a nurse, who screens the records according to guidelines established by CMS. For example, an elective surgical admission is reviewed on the basis of six criteria: (1) adequacy of assessment of physiologic functional impairment, (2) preoperative evaluation, (3) operative protocol, (4) postoperative management, (5) recovery, and (6) discharge. Each includes items that are to be reviewed (e.g., operative protocol requires a review of the patient's preparation for surgery, anesthesia, and surgical procedure). See Figure 16–13 for an excerpt from the CMS guidelines for the PRO quality criteria. The PRO quality criteria were originally published in the *Federal Register* on January 18, 1989.

The nonphysician reviewer forwards cases that do not meet the criteria to a physician. The physician then reviews the records to identify whether any unnecessary services were provided and whether the services were provided on an inpatient basis when they could have been provided in an outpatient setting. If the physician reviewer believes that the care was inappropriate, a letter outlining the problem with the record is sent to the attending physician and to the hospital. Both the attending physician and the hospital must respond to the problems identified in the letter within 20 days. The PRO can either dismiss the case and approve the admission or deny reimbursement for the admission and declare medical mismanagement.

Medical mismanagement problems are classified into three levels of severity:

1. Without the potential for significant adverse effects on the patient
2. With the potential for significant adverse effects on the patient
3. With significant adverse effects on the patient

Adverse effects are defined by the CMS as (1) unnecessarily prolonged treatment, complications, or readmissions; and (2) patient management that results in anatomic or physiologic impairment or disability.

Each of the levels of severity is assigned a score, and a record of the providers, physicians, and hospitals indicates the number and the severity of occurrences. At preset levels, the PRO intervenes. Interventions can include education, intensified review, denial of payments, other corrective interventions, notification of licensing and accreditation bodies, and sanctions. Ultimately, sanctions may be levied in two situations: (1) when substantial violations have occurred in a substantial number of cases; or (2) when a gross or flagrant violation has taken place, causing danger to the health, safety, or well-being of a patient.

EXERCISE 16-5

PEER REVIEW ORGANIZATIONS

Fill in the blanks with the correct word(s):

1 The creation of Peer Review Organizations was made possible under the provision of what act?

_____

2 What is the name of the document produced by the CMS that defines the type and number of health records that must be reviewed?

_____

3 What are the six types of review that are performed by the PROs?

_____

_____

_____

_____

_____

_____

4 What are the three levels of medical mismanagement?

_____

_____

_____

WHAT IS THE OUTPATIENT RESOURCE-BASED RELATIVE VALUE SCALE (RBRVS)?

Physician payment reform was implemented to

1. Decrease Medicare expenditures
2. Redistribute physicians' payments more equitably
3. Ensure quality health care at a reasonable rate

Before January 1, 1992, payment under Medicare Part B for physicians' services was based on a reasonable charge that, under the Social Security Act, could not exceed the lowest of (1) the physician's actual charge for the service, (2) the physician's customary charge for the service, or (3) the prevailing charges of physicians for similar services in the locality.

The act also required that the local prevailing charge for a physician's service not exceed the level in effect for that service in the locality for the fiscal year ending on June 30, 1973. Some provision was made for changes in the level on the basis of economic changes. When there were economic changes in the country, the Medicare Economic Index (MEI) reflected these changes. Until 1992, the MEI tied increases in the Medicare prevailing charges to increases in the costs of physicians' practice and general wage rates throughout the economy as compared with the index base year. The MEI was first published in the *Federal Register* on June 16, 1975, and has been recalculated annually since then.

Congress mandated the MEI as part of the 1972 Amendments to the Social Security Act. The 1972 Amendment to the Act did not specify the particular type of index to be used; however, the present form of the MEI follows the recommendations outlined by the Senate Finance Committee in its report accompanying the legislation. The MEI attempts to present an equitable measure for changes in the costs of physicians' time and operating expenses.

A major change took place in Medicare in 1989 with the enactment of the Omnibus Budget Reconciliation Act of 1989 (OBRA), Public Law 101-239. Section 6102 of PL 101-239 amended Title XVIII of the Social Security Act by adding Section 1848, Payment for Physician Services. The new section contained three major elements:

1. Establishment of standard rates of increase of expenditures for physicians' services
2. Replacement of the reasonable charge payment mechanism by a fee schedule for physicians' services
3. Replacement of the maximum actual allowable charge (MAAC), which limits the total amount nonparticipating physicians can charge

Revisions were made and a new Omnibus Budget Reconciliation Act of 1990 was passed. OBRA 1990 contained several modifications and clarifications of the PL 101-239 provisions establishing the physician fee schedule. This final rule required that before January 1 of each year, beginning with 1992, the Secretary shall establish, by regulation, fee schedules that determine payment amounts for all physicians' services furnished in all fee schedule areas for the year.

The physician fee schedule is updated each April 15 and is composed of three basic elements:

1. The relative value units for each service
2. A geographic adjustment factor to adjust for regional variations in the cost of operating a health care facility
3. A national conversion factor

Medicare volume performance standards have been developed to be used as a tool to monitor annual increases in Part B expenditures for physicians' services and, when appropriate, to adjust payment levels to reflect the success or failure in meeting the performance standards. Various financial protections have been designed and instituted on behalf of the Medicare beneficiary. Uniformity of administration and standardization of procedures, policies, and coding have been implemented so that all Medicare carriers communicate on the same level and use the same language.

National Fee Schedule

Beginning January 1, 1992, the Medicare Fee Schedule (MFS) replaced the reasonable-charge payment system.[5] All physicians' services are paid on the basis of the amounts indicated in the new MFS. Reimbursement is made at 80% of the fee schedule amount, subject to the annual Part B Medicare deductible. The fee schedule applies to Medicare payment for physicians' services and supplies furnished "incidental to" physicians' services, outpatient physical and occupational therapy services, diagnostic tests, and radiology services. The fee schedule applies when payment is made to either physicians or suppliers.

Relative Value Unit

Nationally, unit values have been assigned for each service (CPT code), and they are determined on the basis of the resources necessary to the physician's performance of the service. By analyzing a service, a Harvard team was able to identify its separate parts and assign each part a relative value unit (RVU). These parts or components are as follows:

1. Work. The work component is identified as the amount of time, the intensity of effort, and the technical expertise required for the physician to provide the service.

2. Overhead. The overhead component is identified as the allocation of costs associated with the physician's practice (e.g., rent, staffing, supplies) that must be expended in order to provide a service.

3. Malpractice. The malpractice component is identified as the cost of the medical malpractice insurance coverage associated with providing service.

The sum of the units established for each component of the service equals the total RVUs of a service.

A relative value of 1 has been established for a midlevel, established-patient office visit (99213). All other services are valued at, above, or below this service relative to the work, overhead, and malpractice expenses associated with the service.

Geographic Practice Cost Index

The Urban Institute developed scales that measure cost differences in various areas. The Geographic Practice Cost Indices (GPCIs) have been established for each of the prevailing charge localities.[5] An entire state may be considered a locality for purposes of physician payment reform. The GPCIs reflect the relative costs of practice in a given locality compared with the national average. The national average is 1. A separate GPCI has been established and is applied to each component of a service. For example, the GPCIs for Minnesota are .999 for work, .971 for overhead, and .748 for malpractice insurance.

Conversion Factor

The conversion factor (CF) is a national dollar amount that is applied to all services paid on the basis of the Medicare Fee Schedule.[5] Congress provided a CF to be used to convert RVUs to dollars. The CF is updated annually on the basis of the data sources, which indicate

- Percent changes to the Medicare Economic Index (MEI)
- Percent changes in physician expenditures
- The relationship of expenditures to volume performance standards
- Change in access and quality

The CF varies according to the type of service provided (e.g., medical, surgical, nonsurgical).

The Transition

To prevent extreme fluctuation in Medicare reimbursement amounts, some of the fee schedule amounts are subject to a 5-year transitional phase-in.[5] A historical payment base charge (HPBC) was established for all services so it could be used in a comparison with the fee schedule allowance. Simply put, this means that Medicare allowed 5 years to bring the prices for services to the fee schedule amounts. Those prices that were higher than the fee schedule slowly dropped during this period, and those that were lower were slowly raised. By 1996, all prices for services reflected the fee schedule amount.

Medicare Volume Performance Standards

The Medicare Volume Performance Standards (MVPS) are best thought of as an object. "It" represents the government's estimate of how much growth is appropriate for nationwide physician expenditures paid by the Part B Medicare program. The purpose of MVPS is to guide Congress in its consideration of the appropriate annual payment update.[5]

The Secretary of Health and Human Services must make MVPS recommendations to Congress by April 15 for the upcoming fiscal year, and by May 15, the Physician Payment Review Commission (PPRC) must make its recommendations for the fiscal year. Congress has until October 15 to establish the MVPS by either accepting or modifying the two proposed MVPS recommendations.

If Congress does not react by October 15, the MVPS rate is established by using a default mechanism. If the default mechanism is used, the Secretary is then required to publish a notice in the *Federal Register* that provides the formula for deriving the MVPS.

Variations in health care usage by Medicare patients occur every year. Because Medicare strives for balanced billing, if CMS agrees to pay for additional services not previously paid for or increases the weights of CPT codes, thus increasing reimbursement, then discounts are taken across the board so that more money than authorized is not spent and the budget is balanced.

Beneficiary Protection

Several provisions in the Physician Payment Reform were designed to protect Medicare beneficiaries:[5]

1. As of September 1, 1990, all providers must file claims for their Medicare patients (free of charge). In addition, claims must be submitted within 1 year of the date of service or they will be subject to a 10% reduction in payment.

2. The Omnibus Budget Reconciliation Act of 1989 requires the physician to accept the amount paid for eligible Medicaid services (mandatory assignment).

3. Effective January 1, 1991, the Maximum Actual Allowable Charge (MAAC) limitations that applied to unassigned physician charges were replaced by new billing limits called limiting charges. The provisions of the new limitations state that nonparticipating physicians and suppliers cannot charge more than the stated limiting charge on unassigned claims.

Limiting Charge

In 1991 and 1992, the limiting charge was specific to each physician. Beginning in 1993, the limiting charge for a service has been the same for all physicians within a locality, regardless of specialty. The limiting charge for each service also appears on the beneficiary's Explanation of Medicare Benefits.[5]

The limiting charge applies to every service listed in the Medicare Physicians' Fee Schedule that is performed by a nonparticipating physician. This includes global, professional, and technical services performed by a physician. When a nonphysician provider (e.g., portable x-ray supplier, laboratory technician) provides the technical component of a service that is on the fee schedule, the limiting charge does not apply. CPT codes are assigned many different prices. The amount determined by multiplying the RVU weight by the geographic index and the conversion factor is called the fee schedule amount. If a physician is participating, he or she receives the fee schedule amount. If the physician is not participating, the fee schedule amount or the allowable payment is slightly less than the participating physician's payment. The limiting amount is a percentage over the allowable (e.g., 115% times the allowable amount). The limiting charge is important because that is the maximum amount a Medicare patient can be billed for a service. For covered services, Medicare usually pays 80% of the allowable amount. The beneficiary is then balance-billed, which means that the patient is billed the difference between what Medicare pays and the limiting charge.

EXAMPLE

Limiting charge is	$115	(Maximum charge)
Allowable is	$100	
Medicare pays	$80	(Medicare pays 80%)
Patient is billed	$35	($20, 20% of $100, and $15, the remainder of the limiting charge maximum)

Physicians may round the limiting charge to the nearest dollar if they do this consistently for all services.

Uniformity Provision

Equitable use of the Medicare fee schedule requires a payment system with a uniform policy and uniform procedures.[5] Because the relative value of the work component of a service is the same nationwide (except for a geographic practice cost adjustment), it is important that when physicians across the country are paid for a service they be paid for the same amount, or "package," of work. For example, the preoperative and postoperative periods included in the payment must be the same. To prevent variation in interpretation, standard definitions of services are required.

A comprehensive survey of carrier policies resulted in CMS's issuing a standardization policy for the following items:

- Evaluation and management services
- Visits and procedures on the same day
- Global surgical packages
- Starred procedures
- Endoscopies
- Multiple/bilateral/incidental surgeries
- Assistant/team surgeon
- Outpatient limits
- Inpatient visits—concurrent care
- Site of service differentials
- Travel/mileage charges
- Specimen handling
- Injections and other "incident-to" services
- Modifiers used for payment differential purposes
- Place and type of service

Adjustments

Whenever an adjustment of the full fee schedule amount is made to a service, the limiting charge for that service must be adjusted.[5] Medicare has provided adjusted limiting charges to providers for services to which the site-of-service limitation applies, the assistant-at-surgery limitation applies, and multiple surgery limitations apply, and when only a portion of the global surgical package is being provided. These adjustments are identified on the physician disclosure, which is provided to all physicians during the participating enrollment period each year.

Adjustments to the limiting charge must be manually calculated before submitting unassigned claims for all services in which a fee schedule limitation applies.

Payments to nonparticipating physicians will not exceed 95% of the physician fee schedule for a service.

Site-of-Service Limitations

Services that are performed primarily in office settings are subject to a payment discount if they are performed in outpatient hospital departments. There is a national list of procedures that are performed 50% of the time in the office setting.[5] These procedures are subject to site-of-service limitations, which means that a discount is taken on any service that is performed in a setting other than a clinic setting. For instance, an arthrocentesis is normally performed in the office. If a physician provides this service in a hospital outpatient setting, the limiting charge will be less than that for the office setting. This is because the hospital will also be billing Medicare for the use of the room and the supplies. Medicare has a built-in practice expense, or overhead, for the clinic setting (the RVU weight for practice expense), and Medicare doesn't want to pay twice for the overhead. So part of the overhead is reduced from the physician's payment to make up for the hospital payment. For these procedures, the practice expense RVU is reduced by 50%. Payment is the lower of the actual charge or the reduced fee schedule amount. Physicians who bill an emergency department visit are not subject to the outpatient limit on these services.

Surgical Modifier Circumstances

Multiple Surgery

General

If a surgeon performs more than one procedure on the same patient on the same day, discounts are made on all subsequent procedures. Medicare will pay 100% of the fee for the highest value procedure, 50% for the second most expensive procedure, and 25% for the third, fourth, and fifth procedures. Discounting is why the service (CPT code) that you place the modifier on is so important! Each procedure after the fifth procedure requires documentation and special carrier review to determine the payment amount. These discount amounts are subject to review every year by the CMS.

Commercial insurers often follow discount limits different from those of Medicare, as established by their own individual reimbursement policies.

Endoscopic Procedures

In the case of multiple endoscopic procedures, Medicare allows the full value of the highest valued endoscopy, plus the difference between the next highest endoscopy and the base endoscopy.[5] As in all other reimbursement issues, some non-Medicare carriers follow this pricing method, whereas others follow their own multiple-procedure discounting policies.

Dermatologic Surgery

For certain dermatology services, there are CPT codes that indicate that multiple surgical procedures have been performed. When the CPT code description states "additional," the general multiple-procedure rules do not apply.

Providers Furnishing Part of the Global Fee Package

Under the fee schedule, Medicare pays the same amount for surgical services furnished by several physicians as it pays if only one physician furnished all of the services in the global package.

Medicare pays each physician directly for his or her part of the global surgical services. The policy is written with the assumption that the surgeon always furnishes the usual and necessary preoperative and intraoperative services and also, with a few exceptions, in-hospital postoperative services. In most cases, the surgeon also furnishes the postoperative office services necessary to ensure normal recovery from the surgery. Recognizing that there are cases in which the surgeon turns over the out-of-hospital recovery care to another physician, Medicare has determined percentages for families of procedures for paying usual out-of-hospital postoperative care if furnished by someone other than the surgeon. These are weighted percentages based on the percentage of total global surgical work.

Again, become familiar with individual third-party payer policies, because some may not split their global payments in this manner.

Physicians Who Assist at Surgery

Physicians assisting the primary physician in a procedure receive a set percentage of the total fee for the service. Medicare sets the payment level for assistants-at-surgery at 16% of the fee schedule amount for the global surgical service. Non-Medicare payers may set this percentage at 20% or more.

Two Surgeons and Surgical Team

When two surgeons of different specialties perform a procedure, each is paid an equal percentage of the global fee. For co-surgeons, Medicare pays 125%

of the global fee, dividing the payment equally between the two surgeons (or each will receive 62.5% of the global fee). No payment is made for an assistant-at-surgery in these cases.

For team surgery, a medical director determines the payment amounts on an individual basis.

Purchased Diagnostic Services

For physicians who bill for a diagnostic test performed by an outside supplier, the fee schedule amount is limited to the lower of the billing physician's fee schedule amount or the price he or she paid for the service.

Reoperations

The amount paid by Medicare for a return trip to the operating room for treatment of a complication is limited to the intraoperative portion of the code that best describes the treatment of the complications.

When an unlisted procedure is billed because no other code exists to describe the treatment, payment is based on a maximum of 50% of the value of the intraoperative services originally performed.

Commercial insurance companies again have their own guidelines. Many do not take discounts for these subsequent surgical procedures.

EXERCISE 16–6

RBRVS

Fill in the blanks with the correct words:

1 What does RBRVS stand for? _____

_____

2 The Medicare Economic Index is published in what publication? _____

_____

3 In 1989, a major change took place in Medicare with the enactment of

_____

_____ .

Check This Out! ☞ CMS publishes the RVUs on their Website (www.hcfa.gov) under the Public Use files (PUFs). Click on "Students" and then on "Public Use Files." In the medical office, you may be responsible for downloading the new RVUs when they are posted, usually in October of each year.

THE PROSPECTIVE PAYMENT SYSTEM FOR THE SKILLED NURSING FACILITY

Effective July 1, 1998, a per diem prospective payment system (PPS) for skilled nursing facilities (SNFs) was implemented to cover all costs (routine, ancillary, and capital) related to services provided to Medicare Part A beneficiaries. Federal rates were established using fiscal year (FY) 1995 cost reports, and per diem payments are case-mix–adjusted according to a classification system entitled Resource Utilization Groups III (RUGS III).

Information collected by completing the Minimum Data Set 2.0 (MDS 2.0) resident assessment instrument (RAI) determines the amount of per diem payments for each SNF admission. Payments are case-mix–adjusted on the basis of data from the MDS 2.0 and relative weights determined by SNF staff time. The per diem rate is adjusted for geographic variation in wages, using the hospital wage index, and rates are expected to increase each federal fiscal year using a "SNF market-basket index (minus 1 percentage point in FY 2000 through FY 2002)." A blending of the facility-specific payment rate and the federal case-mix–adjusted rate applies during the three-year phase-in period.

OUTPATIENT MEDICARE REIMBURSEMENT SYSTEM—APC

Medicare payments for hospital services, both inpatient and outpatient, were historically based on the customary and reasonable cost of a service. In 1983, the law that governs Medicare was revised to move from this cost-based payment to a prospective payment system (PPS) for hospital inpatients. Outpatient hospital services continued to operate on the cost-based system. Advances in medical technology and changes in practices (such as more outpatient surgery) brought a shift in the site of medical care from the inpatient to the outpatient setting. In the years that followed, Congress enacted many laws to try to curb this shift to outpatient-based services, but to no avail. OBRA 1986 (the Omnibus Budget Reconciliation Act of 1986) contained a requirement to replace the existing outpatient hospital cost-based system with a PPS. Also with OBRA 1986 came the ability to require hospitals to report claims for services under the CMS Common Procedure Coding System (HCPCS). This coding requirement provided data to CMS about the specific services being provided on an outpatient basis. These data were used to develop the outpatient PPS.

CMS conducted research into ways to classify outpatient services for the purposes of developing the outpatient PPS. The resulting report cited the Ambulatory Patient Groups (APGs), developed by 3M Health Information Systems under a cooperative grant with CMS, as the most promising classification system for grouping outpatient services, and recommended that APG-like groups be used in the hospital PPS. The APG-like groups were named Ambulatory Patient Classifications (APCs) and were scheduled for implementation on January 1, 1999. However, that date was delayed owing to concerns with year 2000 (Y2K) computer issues. Implementation was final on August 1, 2000.

Introduction to Ambulatory Patient Classifications

APCs are a system for reimbursing facilities for Medicare outpatient health care. They are mandatory for all hospital outpatient services. They include inpatient services covered under Part B for beneficiaries who are entitled to Part A benefits but who have exhausted their Part A benefits or otherwise are not involved in a hospital stay covered by Part A. Patients who receive partial hospitalization services furnished by community mental health centers also qualify to have their services paid for under the PPS of APCs. In general, the definition of a hospital outpatient is an individual who is not an inpatient of the hospital but who is registered as an outpatient.

A coinsurance amount is calculated for each APC based on 20% of the national median charge for services in the APC. The coinsurance amount for an APC will not change until such time as the amount becomes 20% of the total APC payment.

ADDENDUM F. — STATUS INDICATORS:
HOW VARIOUS SERVICES ARE TREATED UNDER OUTPATIENT PPS

Indicator	Service	Status
A............	Pulmonary Rehabilitation Clinical Trial..........................	Not paid under PPS
C............	Inpatient Procedures...	Admit patient; bill as inpatient
A............	Durable Medical Equipment, Prosthetics and Orthotics.....	DMEPOS Fee Schedule
E............	Non-covered Items and Services..................................	Non-paid
A............	Physical, Occupational and Speech Therapy	Rehabilitation Fee Schedule
A............	Ambulance...	Ambulance Fee Schedule
A............	EPO for ESRD patients..	National Rate
A............	Clinical Diagnostic Laboratory Services........................	Laboratory Fee Schedule
A............	Physician Services for ESRD patients..........................	Not paid under PPS
A............	Screening Mammography..	National Rate
N............	Incidental Services, packaged into APC rate..............	Packaged
P............	Partial Hospitalization...	Paid per diem APC
S............	Significant Procedure, not discounted when..................	Paid
T............	Procedure, multiple when discount applies..................	Paid
V............	Visit to Clinic or Emergency Department	Paid
X............	Ancillary Service..	Paid

Figure 16–14 A listing of groups of services and the payment status for each group. (From Fed Regist Apr 7;65(68):18787, 2000.)

18552   **Federal Register**/Vol. 65, No. 68/Friday, April 7, 2000/Rules and Regulations

ADDENDUM A. – LIST OF HOSPITAL OUTPATIENT AMBULATORY PAYMENT CLASSES WITH STATUS INDICATORS, RELATIVE WEIGHTS, PAYMENT RATES, AND COINSURANCE AMOUNTS – Continued

APC	Group Title	Status Indicator	Relative Weight	Payment Rate	National Unadjusted Coinsurance	Minimum Unadjusted Coinsurance
0057	Bunion Procedures...	T	21.00	$1,018.23	$496.65	$203.65
0058	Level I Strapping and Cast Application	S	1.09	$52.85	$19.27	$10.57
0059	Level II Strapping and Cast Application	S	1.74	$84.37	$29.59	$16.87
0060	Manipulation Therapy...	S	0.77	$37.34	$7.80	$7.47
0070	Thoracentesis/Lavage Procedures	T	3.64	$176.49	$79.60	$35.30
0071	Level I Endoscopy Upper Airway..	T	0.55	$26.67	$14.22	$5.33
0072	Level II Endoscopy Upper Airway.......................................	T	1.26	$61.09	$41.52	$12.22
0073	Level III Endoscopy Upper Airway......................................	T	4.11	$199.28	$91.07	$39.86
0074	Level IV Endoscopy Upper Airway......................................	T	13.61	$659.91	$347.54	$131.98
0075	Level V Endoscopy Upper Airway.......................................	T	18.55	$899.44	$467.29	$179.89
0076	Endoscopy Lower Airway..	T	8.06	$390.81	$197.05	$78.16
0077	Level I Pulmonary Treatment...	S	0.43	$20.85	$12.62	$4.17
0078	Level II Pulmonary Treatment..	S	1.34	$64.97	$29.13	$12.99
0079	Ventilation Initiation and Management.................................	S	3.18	$154.19	$107.70	$30.84
0080	Diagnostic Cardiac Catheterization....................................	T	25.77	$1,249.51	$713.89	$249.90
0081	Non-coronary Angioplasty or Atherectomy..........................	T	19.36	$938.71	$434.25	$187.74
0082	Coronary Atherectomy...	T	40.34	$1,955.97	$859.56	$391.19
0083	Coronary Angioplasty..	T	45.79	$2,220.22	$1,322.95	$444.04
0084	Level I Electrophysiologic Evaluation..................................	S	10.70	$518.81	$177.79	$103.76
0085	Level II Electrophysiologic Evaluation.................................	S	27.06	$1,312.06	$654.48	$262.41
0086	Ablate Heart Dysrhythm Focus..	S	47.62	$2,308.95	$1,265.37	$461.79
0087	Cardiac Electrophysiologic Recording/Mapping....................	S	9.53	$462.08	$214.72	$92.42
0088	Thrombectomy...	T	26.49	$1,284.42	$678.68	$256.88
0089	Level I Implantation/Removal/Revision of Pacemaker, AICD or Vascular Device	T	6.49	$314.68	$130.07	$62.94
0090	Level II Implantation/Removal/Revision of Pacemaker, AICD or Vascular Device	T	20.96	$1,016.29	$573.04	$203.26
0091	Level I Vascular Ligation..	T	14.79	$717.12	$348.23	$143.42
0092	Level II Vascular Ligation...	T	20.21	$979.92	$505.37	$195.98

APC number   Service Description   Payment Rate   Payment Coinsurance Rate

Figure 16–15 APCs with group titles and payment rates. (From Fed Regist Apr 7;65(68):18552, 2000.)

ADDENDUM B. – PROPOSED HOSPITAL OUTPATIENT DEPARTMENT (HOPD) PAYMENT STATUS BY HCPCS CODE AND RELATED INFORMATION – Continued

CPT/ HCPCS	HOPD Status Indicator	Description	APC	Relative Weight	Proposed Payment Rate	National Unadjusted Coinsurance	Minimum Unadjusted Coinsurance
D0473	S	Micro exam, prep & report	0330	1.51	$73.22	$14.64	$14.64
D0474	S	Micro w exam of surg margins	0330	1.51	$73.22	$14.64	$14.64
D0480	S	Cytopath smear prep & report	0330	1.51	$73.22	$14.64	$14.64
D4268	S	Surgical revision procedure	0330	1.51	$73.22	$14.64	$14.64
G0104	S	CA screen; flexible sigmoidscope	0159	2.83	$137.22	....	$34.31
G0105	S	Colorectal screen; high risk ind	0158	7.98	$386.93	....	$96.73
G0122	S	Colon ca scrn; barium enema	0157	1.79	$86.79	....	$17.36
G0125	S	Lung image (PET)	0981	46.40	$2,249.80	....	$449.96
G0126	S	Lung image (PET) staging	0981	46.40	$2,249.80	....	$449.96
G0163	S	PET for rec of colorectal cancer	0981	46.40	$2,249.80	....	$449.96
G0164	S	PET for lymphoma staging	0981	46.40	$2,249.80	....	$449.96
G0165	S	PET, rec of melanoma/met cancer	0981	46.40	$2,249.80	....	$449.96
G0168	T	Wound closure by adhesive	0970	0.52	$25.21	....	$5.04
G0169	T	Removal tissue; no anesthesia	0013	0.91	$44.12	$17.66	$8.82
G0170	T	Skin biograft	0025	3.74	$181.34	$70.66	$36.27
G0171	T	Skin biograft add-on	0025	3.74	$181.34	$70.66	$36.27

HCPCS or CPT Code for Service   Description   Payment Rate   Patient Coinsurance Rate

Figure 16–16 Individual HCPCS or CPT codes assigned to payment rate. (From Fed Regist Apr 7; 65(68):18551, 2000.)

Figure 16–14 shows the broad range of categories of services provided under the Medicare program and which categories are paid according to the APC rate. The APC system consists of 346 groups of services that are covered under this hospital outpatient prospective payment system (OPPS). Each procedure is then assigned into a group of APCs, and the payment rate and beneficiary coinsurance portion are identified (Fig. 16–15). The services are identified by HCPCS codes and descriptions, as illustrated in Figure 16–16. The APCs identify the packaged services that are included in each APC. Packaged services are those that are recognized as contributing to the cost of the services in the APC, but that Medicare does not pay for separately. Under the APC system, packaged services include the operating room, recovery room, anesthesia, medical/surgical supplies, pharmaceuticals, observation, blood, intraocular lenses, casts and splints, donor tissue, and various incidental services such as venipuncture. Also bundled into the APC is any medical visit that takes place on the same date of service as a scheduled outpatient surgery. Registration of the patient, taking of vital signs, insertion of an IV, preparation for surgery, and so forth, are packaged into and paid for as a part of the APC group to which the surgical procedure or service is classified.

EXERCISE 16-7

APCs

Fill in the blanks:

1 APC stands for _____

_____ .

2 APCs were implemented on August 1 of what year? _____

3 The coinsurance amount for the beneficiaries under the APC system is _____ percent.

4 The APC system has how many groups that are covered under the outpatient hospital prospective payment system? _____

MEDICARE FRAUD AND ABUSE

What Are Fraud and Abuse?

The Medicare program is subject to fraud and abuse, as is any third-party payer program. But because Medicare is the largest third-party payer, it has the most comprehensive anti–fraud and abuse program. You must understand the specifics of this program because you will be filing Medicare claims. CMS is responsible for establishing the regulations that monitor the Medicare program for fraud and abuse.

Medicare defines fraud as "the intentional deception or misrepresentation that an individual knows to be false or does not believe to be true and makes it knowing that the deception could result in some unauthorized benefit to himself/herself or some other person."[10] So fraud involves both deliberate intention to deceive and an expectation of an unauthorized benefit. By this definition, it is fraud if a claim is filed for a service rendered to a Medicare patient when that service was not actually provided. How could this type of fraud happen? The fact is that most Medicare patients sign a standing approval, which is kept in the patient's file in the medical office. Having a standing approval is convenient for the patient and for the coding staff: After the patient has received a service, the Medicare claim is filed automatically, without the patient's having to sign the form again. But a standing approval also makes it easy for unscrupulous persons to submit charges for services never provided. This circumstance also makes it possible for extra services to be submitted in addition to services that were provided (upcoding). Suppose, for example, a patient came in for an office visit and a claim was submitted for an in-office surgical procedure. That's also fraud.

STOP *The most common kind of fraud arises from a false statement or misrepresentation made, or caused to be made, that results in additional payment by the Medicare program.*

Who Are the Violators?

The violator may be a physician or other practitioner, a hospital or other institutional provider, a clinical laboratory or other supplier, an employee of any provider, a billing service, a beneficiary, a Medicare carrier employee, or any person in a position to file a claim for Medicare benefits. You will be the person filing Medicare claims so you have to be careful about the claims you submit—it's important to validate that the service was provided by consulting the medical record or the physician.

Fraud schemes range from those committed by individuals acting alone to broad-based activities perpetrated by institutions or groups of individuals, sometimes employing sophisticated telemarketing and other promotional techniques to lure consumers into serving as unwitting tools in the schemes. Seldom do such perpetrators target just one insurer; nor do they focus exclusively on either the public or the private sector. Rather, most are found to be defrauding several private- and public-sector victims such as Medicare simultaneously.

What Forms Does Fraud Take?

The most common forms of Medicare fraud are

- Billing for services not furnished
- Misrepresenting a diagnosis to justify a payment
- Soliciting, offering, or receiving a kickback
- Unbundling, or "exploding," charges
- Falsifying certificates of medical necessity, plans of treatment, and medical records to justify payment
- Billing for additional services not furnished as billed—that is, upcoding
- Routine waiver of copayment

Who Says What Is Fraudulent?

CMS administers the Medicare program. CMS's responsibilities include managing contractor claims payment, overseeing fiscal audit and/or overpayment prevention and recovery, and developing and monitoring the payment safeguards necessary to detect and respond to payment errors or abusive patterns of service delivery. Within CMS's Bureau of Program Operations is the Office of Benefits Integrity (OBI), which oversees Medicare's payment safeguard program, including carrier and intermediary operations related to fraud, audit, medical review, the collection of overpayments, and the imposition of civil monetary penalties (CMPs) for certain violations of Medicare law.

The Office of the Inspector General (OIG), Department of Health and Human Services, is responsible for developing an annual work plan that outlines the ways in which the Medicare program is monitored to identify fraud and abuse. The plan is a published public document that provides the evaluation methods and approaches that will be taken the following year to monitor the Medicare program. For example, in the 2001 Work Plan, the following is listed as the review for critical care services:

Critical Care Codes

We will examine the use of two critical care codes that may be billed to Medicare only if the patient is critically ill and requires constant attention by the physician. Payment for critical care is based on the time spent with the patient. We will examine claim data to determine whether some physicians may be billing inappropriately for critical care as well as identify any other potential vulnerabilities.[11]

This excerpt from OIG Work Plan identifies critical care service as a specific area to be monitored in that year. The OIG charges the fiscal intermediaries (carriers) with doing the actual monitoring. (Recall that insurance companies bid for the opportunity to be the fiscal intermediary for Medicare and handle the payments to providers for Medicare services.) The OIG Work Plan sets the broad boundaries for monitoring the Medicare program for fraud and abuse.

The Specific Regulations Are in the MCM

CMS establishes the specific regulations in the *Medicare Carriers Manual* (MCM) for the carriers to follow. You will deal with MCM regulations as you code Medicare claims in order to know what is allowable. The MCM regulations that deal with Medicare fraud and abuse are numbered 14000 to 14032. The following are selected excerpts from these regulations addressed to the carriers:

14000. Fraud and Abuse—Background

The effort to prevent and detect fraud, abuse, and waste is a cooperative one that involves beneficiaries, Medicare contractors, providers, Peer Review Organizations (PROs), State Medicaid Fraud Control Units (MFCUs), and Federal agencies such as HCFA, Office of Inspector General (OIG), DHHS, the Federal Bureau of Investigation (FBI), and the Department of Justice (DOJ).

You are responsible for assisting Medicare in protecting the program's Trust Fund from those persons and entities that would seek payment for items and services under false or fraudulent circumstances. This includes effectively developing cases of suspected fraud to the fullest potential possible before you refer them to the OIG, Office of Investigations (OI) Field Office. OI is responsible for determining if federal and/or civil statutes have been violated. Ensure that you make only appropriate payments and that you take appropriate steps to recover any mistaken payments. This can be accomplished through actions such as suspension of payments, denial of payments, and recovery of overpayments. These options are discussed in more detail in 14004, 14008, 14017, and 14018.

This chapter explains the actions you are to take to protect the Medicare Trust Funds and applies to all Medicare carriers, including Durable Medical Equipment Regional Carriers (DMERCs). It provides general guidelines and suggestions for preventing and detecting fraud and abuse, and for developing incidents of suspected fraud and abuse.

Each investigation is unique and should be tailored to the specific circumstances involved. The guidelines provided here should not be interpreted as requiring a specific course of action or establishing any specific requirements on the part of the government or its agents with respect to any investigation. Similarly, these guidelines should not be interpreted as creating any rights in favor of any person, including the subject of an investigation.[10]

MCMs Referring to Part B Fraud

14001. Part B Medicare Fraud

Fraud is the intentional deception or misrepresentation that an individual knows to be false or does not believe to be true and makes it, knowing that the deception could result in some unauthorized benefit to himself/herself or some other person. The most frequent kind of fraud arises from a false statement or misrepresentation made, or caused to be made, that is material to entitlement or payment under the Medicare program. The violator may be a physician or other practitioner, a supplier of durable medical equipment, an employee of a physician or supplier, a carrier employee, a billing service, a beneficiary, or any other person or business entity in a position to bill the Medicare program or to otherwise benefit from such billing.

Attempts to defraud the Medicare program may take a variety of forms. The following are some examples of how fraud may be perpetrated in the Medicare medical insurance program:

- Billing for services or supplies that were not provided. This includes billings for "no shows," ie billing Medicare for services that were not actually furnished because patients failed to keep their appointments;

- Misrepresenting the diagnosis for the patient to justify the services or equipment furnished;

- Altering claim forms to obtain a higher payment amount;

- Deliberately applying for duplicate payment, eg billing both Medicare and the beneficiary for the same service or billing both Medicare and another insurer in an attempt to get paid twice;

- Soliciting, offering, or receiving a kickback, bribe, or rebate, eg paying for a referral of patients in exchange for the ordering of diagnostic tests and other services or medical equipment;

- Unbundling or "exploding" charges, eg the billing of a multichannel set of lab tests to appear as if the individual tests had been performed.
- Completing Certificates of Medical Necessity (CMNs) for patients not personally and professionally known by the provider;
- Misrepresenting the services rendered (upcoding or the use of procedure codes not appropriate for the item or service actually furnished), amounts charged for services rendered, identity of the person receiving the services, dates of services, etc;
- Billing for noncovered services, eg routine foot care billed as a more involved form of foot care to obtain payment;
- Participating in schemes that involve collusion between a provider and a beneficiary, or between a supplier and a provider, and result in higher costs or charges to the Medicare program;
- Using another person's Medicare card to obtain medical care;
- Utilizing split billing schemes (eg billing procedures over a period of days when all treatment occurred during one visit);
- Participating in schemes that involve collusion between a provider and a carrier employee where the claim is assigned, eg, the provider deliberately overbills for services, and the carrier employee then generates adjustments with little or no awareness on the part of the beneficiary;
- Manipulating claims data on unassigned claims for one's own benefit, eg through manipulation of beneficiary address or the claims history record, a carrier employee could generate adjustment payments against many beneficiary records and cause payments to be mailed to an address known only to him/her; and
- Billing based on "gang visits," eg a physician visits a nursing home and bills for 20 nursing home visits without furnishing any specific service to, or on behalf of, individual patients.

Although some of the preceding practices initially may be considered abusive rather than fraudulent activities, they may evolve into fraud. Note that the term "provider" means physicians, practitioners, and other suppliers of health care services/supplies.[10]

Some of the Ways Reviews Are Conducted

The reviews of Medicare claims take a wide variety of methods; the following excerpt is from the MCM and concerns ideas for reviews.

> **E. Conduct Reviews.**—Conduct a variety of reviews to determine the appropriateness of payments even when there is no evidence of fraud. Some or all of the following reviews are to be done, depending on your funding level. They include:
>
> - Sampling of claims for a variety of items and services to determine propriety of payments;
> - Telephone contacts with beneficiaries to verify the delivery of items and services;
> - Random validation checks of physician licensure;
> - Reviews of original certificates of medical necessity. . . .[10]

How Does Medicare Find Out About Suspected Fraud?

The MCMs identify a number of ways in which leads on fraud can come to Medicare carriers.

14005. Fraud Detection Leads

A variety of sources may be used to identify potential fraud and abuse situations. They include but are not limited to:

- Referrals from MR or carrier quality assurance (QA) staff;

- Suggestions/referrals from HCFA components, other Federal agencies, State agencies, contractors, PROs, or other sources, concerning areas where they have experienced problems or identified program matters that do not seem to be properly addressed in current policy. These suggestions may be provided directly or may be implicit in various reports and other materials produced in the course of evaluation and audit activities, eg, contractor evaluations, State assessment, HCFA-directed surveys, contractor or State audits of providers;

- Leads developed through data analysis, pattern detection, or link analysis methods, or produced by State and contractor systems or other sources that indicate aberrancies such as excessive costs, upcoding, or questionable charging practices;

- Complaints or questions from providers, beneficiaries, Medicaid recipients, or private citizens;

- Referrals from the RO, SSA, HCFA and/or from any component of OIG;

- Aberrancies detected through internal controls, postpayment and other reviews, audits, or inspections;

- OI and HCFA fraud alerts;

- Investigative leads from ongoing fraud and abuse case review activity; and

- Ideas stemming from ongoing or completed inspections.[10]

Two Types of Medicare Alerts

Medicare distributes alerts on fraud and abuse to carriers, providers, and beneficiaries throughout the year. As part of the MCM, the following are the current alerts:

14019. Fraud and Abuse Alerts.

14019.1 Types of Fraud Alerts.—There are two types of fraud alerts, National Medicare Fraud Alerts (NMFAs) and Restricted Medicare Fraud Alerts (RFAs).

A. National Medicare Fraud Alerts.—The most commonly issued alert is the NMFA. These alerts do not identify specific providers or other entities suspected of committing fraud. They focus on a particular scheme or scam and are intended to serve as a fraud detection lead.[10]

The following is a sample of Unrestricted Fraud Alert.

Unrestricted National Medicare Fraud Alert (UMFA 9605: Billing Protective Pads As Hip Abduction Orthotics)

Supplier submitted claims for hip abduction orthotic devices when it was actually supplying a protective pad unit. In addition, claims were submitted for a large number of the supplies which were refused and returned.

A survey of several nursing/residential facilities indicated the following:

1. The item provided is not a "hip orthotic," but is a set of cushioned plastic pads, designed to protect the hip from fracture, in the event of a fall, and was so marketed by the representative of the supplier;

2. Many of the units known as "Hip guards," were returned to the supplier upon receipt and examination by the beneficiaries and/or facility staff;

3. The certificates of medical necessity provided by the supplier failed to support the need for a genuine hip orthotic.[12]

The following is a sample of Restricted Fraud Alert.

Restricted National Medicare Fraud Alert (RMFA 9612: Fraudulent Billing for 24-Hour Cardiac Monitoring)

Provider was billing Medicare for 24-hour attended monitoring, receipt of transmissions, and 24-hour attended monitoring, recording, for beneficiaries residing in New Jersey, New York, Puerto Rico and Florida. The Florida and Puerto Rico beneficiaries reported to the Florida carrier that they are visited by a nurse in their home, the equipment (event recorder) is hooked up for approximately 20 minutes to 30 minutes, then the equipment is removed and the nurse takes it with her when she leaves. This continues on a monthly basis.

Provider billed for patient demand single or multiple event recording with presymptom memory loop and 24-hour attended monitoring, (G0006), 24-hour attended monitoring, recording (G0005), and postsymptom telephone transmission of EKG rhythm strip; 24-hour attended monitoring (G0015). Eighty-six percent of the beneficiaries being billed in New York resided in Florida while only 6% lived in New York. The majority of beneficiaries contacted stated they did not know this provider nor the address of the provider.

Medical Policy for 24-hour monitoring requires that the event recorder be attached to the patient in the doctor's office and the patient wears the monitor home. This permits the patient to record an EKG at the onset of symptoms (ie, dizziness, palpitations, or syncope) or in response to a doctor's order (ie, immediately following strong exertion). Most devices also permit the patient to simultaneously voice-record in order to describe symptoms and/or activity. A supplier of the service must be capable of receiving and recording transmissions. This includes receipt of the EKG signal as well as voice transmission relating any associated services. The person receiving the transmission must be a technician, nurse or physician trained in interpreting EKGs and abnormal rhythms. A physician must be available for immediate consultation to review the transmission in case of significant symptoms or EKG abnormalities. The provider of the service must maintain hard copy documentation of test results and interpretation along with copies of the ordering/referring physician's order for the study.[13]

Who Makes Complaints of Fraud and Abuse?

The definition of a complaint of fraud or abuse is as follows:

14020.1 Definition of a Complaint of Fraud or Abuse.—A complaint is a statement, oral or written, alleging that a provider, supplier, or beneficiary received a Medicare benefit of monetary value, directly or indirectly, overtly or covertly, in cash or in kind, to which he or she is not entitled under current Medicare law, regulations, or policy. Included are allegations of misrepresentation and violations of Medicare requirements applicable to persons or entities that bill for covered items and services. Use this definition for workload reporting purposes on Schedule G. Examples of complaints include:

- Allegations that items or services were not received;
- Allegations that services received are inconsistent with the services billed (as indicated on the Explanation of Medicare Benefits (EOMB));
- Allegations that a provider or supplier has billed both the beneficiary and Medicare for the same item or service;
- Allegations regarding waiver of copayments or deductibles;
- Allegations that a supplier or provider has misrepresented itself as having an affiliation with an agency or department of the State, local, or Federal government, whether expressed or implied; and
- Beneficiary inquiries concerning payment for an item or service, that in his/her opinion, far exceeds reasonable payment for the item or service that the beneficiary received (eg, the supplier or physician has "upcoded" to receive higher payment).[10]

Not all complaints made to Medicare are considered fraud or abuse; the following are not fraud or abuse complaints:

- Complaints (or inquiries) regarding Medicare coverage policy;
- Complaints (or inquiries) regarding the status of claims;
- Requests for claims appeal;
- Complaints regarding the appeals process; or
- Complaints concerning providers or suppliers (other than those complaints meeting the criteria established above) that are general in nature and are policy or program oriented.[10]

What Is the Difference between Abuse and Fraud?

Abuse is different from fraud, although the two words have been used together throughout the MCM. The following defines abuse:

14022. Development of Abuse Cases

14022.1 General.—Correcting and preventing program abuse are functions of the MR Unit. The difference between abuse reviews and fraud reviews is essentially that the abuse situation involves a review of the propriety or medical necessity of services that are billed. **Fraud reviews** are geared towards determining, for example, whether or not billed services were, in fact, furnished. **Abuse reviews** generally occur after your claims processing activity, although they may arise as a result of information obtained during the claims processing cycle.[10]

What Is a Kickback?

Kickbacks are not allowable under the Medicare and Medicaid programs. The following is the law that defines what a kickback is and indicates the penalties for kickbacks that involve the Medicare program:

B. Anti-Kickback Statute Implications.—The Medicare and Medicaid anti-kickback statute provides the following:

Whoever knowingly and willfully solicits or receives any remuneration (including any kickback, bribe, or rebate) directly or indirectly, overtly or covertly, in cash or in kind, in return for referring a patient to a person for the furnishing or arranging for the furnishing of any item or service for which payment may be made in whole or in part under Medicare, Medicaid or a State health care program, or in return for purchasing, leasing, or ordering or arranging for or recommending purchasing, leasing, or ordering any good facility, service, or item for which payment may be made in whole or in part under Medicare, Medicaid or a State health program, shall be guilty of a felony and upon conviction thereof, shall be fined not more than $25,000 or imprisoned for not more than five years, or both. 42 U.S.C. 1320a-7b(b), Section 1128B(b) of the Act.[10]

There is a "safe harbor" clause in the statute that protects certain types of discounting of medical services. For example, an HMO might contract with a laboratory for all laboratory services and receive a discounted price for those services. Not all discounts are protected.

The following types of discounts are *not* protected:

- Rebates offered to beneficiaries;
- Cash payments;
- Furnishing an item or service free of charge or at a reduced charge in exchange for any agreement to buy a different item or service;
- Reduction in price applicable to one payer but not to Medicare or a State health care program; and
- Routine reduction or waiver of any coinsurance or deductible amount owed by a program beneficiary.[10]

Out of Compliance Is Not a Good Place to Be!

If an organization or individual is found to be not in compliance with any of the fraud and abuse regulations, the carrier can impose a number of remedies. The following remedies are addressed to the fiscal intermediaries:

14029.2 Administrative Remedies Considered Initially

A. Educational Contact and/or Warning.—Inform the provider of questionable or improper practices, the correct procedure to be followed, and that continuation of the improper practice may result in administrative sanctions.

B. Revocation of Assignment Privileges.—Revocation of a provider's assignment privileges is a possible administrative action that may be taken in appropriate situations. Use revocation of assignment privileges as an administrative sanction to deny payment while criminal prosecution is being considered or is in process.

C. Withholding of Payments/Recovery of Overpayments.—In cases involving abuse, OIG may, in conjunction with HCFA, ask you to notify the provider or other supplier of your intention to suspend payment, in whole or in part, and the reasons for making the suspension (42 CFR 405.371(a)). The provider or other supplier has 15 days following the date of notification to submit additional evidence, unless an extension is granted.

D. Referral of Situations to State Licensing Boards or Medical/Professional Societies.—Refer instances of apparent unethical or improper practices or unprofessional conduct to State licensing authorities, medical boards, the PRO, or professional societies for review and possible disciplinary action. It may be appropriate to refer a provider to the PRO for action by a State licensing agency or medical society. If a case requires immediate attention, refer it directly to the State licensing agency or medical society and send a copy of the referral to the PRO. (See 14013.C.)[10]

Review the following list of violations for which the Secretary of Health may impose financial penalties on individuals or organizations that are found guilty of fraud or abuse.

The Secretary may also impose a civil monetary penalty against a person who presents or causes to be presented a request for payment in violation of:

- A Medicare assignment agreement;
- An agreement with the State Medicaid agency not to charge a person in excess of permitted limits;
- A Medicare participating physician or supplier agreement; or
- An agreement not to charge patients for services denied as a result of a determination of an abuse of PPS. A person that gives false or misleading information regarding PPS that could reasonably be expected to influence a discharge decision is also subject to the imposition of a civil monetary penalty.

Other situations where civil monetary penalties may be applied include:

- Violation of assignment requirements for certain diagnostic clinical lab tests (1833(h));
- Violation of assignment requirements for nurse-anesthetist services (1833(1));
- Any supplier who refuses to supply rented DME supplies without charge after rental payments may no longer be made (effective January 1, 1989) (1834(a));
- Nonparticipating physician or supplier violation of charge limitation provisions for radiology services (effective January 1, 1989) (1834(b));
- Violation of assignment requirement for physician assistant services (1842(b));

- Medicare nonparticipating physician's violation of limiting charge limits;
- Nonparticipating physician's violation of charge limitations (1842(j));
- Nonparticipating physician's violation of charge limitation provision for services to inherent reasonableness provisions, specified overpriced procedures, specified cataract procedures, A-mode ophthalmic ultrasound procedures, medical direction of nurse-anesthetists, and for certain purchased diagnostic procedures where mark-up is prohibited (effective July 1, 1988 for cataract procedures) (1842(j));
- Physician billing for assistants at cataract surgery without prior approval of PRO (1842(k));
- Nonparticipating physician's violation of refund requirements for medically unnecessary services (1842(l));
- Nonparticipating physician's violation of refund provision for unassigned claims for elective surgery (1842(m));
- Physician charges in violation of assignment provision for certain purchased diagnostic procedures where mark-up is prohibited or where a payment is prohibited for these procedures due to failure to disclose required information (1842(n));
- Hospital unbundling of outpatient surgery costs (1866(g)); and
- Hospital and responsible physician "dumping" of patients (1867).[10]

How to Protect Yourself

As you can see from the preceding information about Medicare fraud and abuse, CMS is very serious about identifying those who try to take advantage of the program. As the person submitting the Medicare claims, you are one of those whom the CMS holds responsible for submitting truthful and accurate claims. If you are unsure about a charge or a request, check with the physician or other supervisory personnel to ensure that you are submitting the correct charges for each patient. In this way, you protect the Medicare program, your facility, and yourself.

THE MANAGED HEALTH CARE CONCEPT

Health care in the United States is the best in the world, and people come from all over the world to access the health care that U.S. residents take for granted. Physicians and health care have traditionally been held in high esteem by U.S. citizens. Whatever it took to provide access to high-quality health care is what these citizens demanded. Historically, the government responded to these demands by funding the research, facilities, and services necessary to keep the U.S. health system on the cutting edge of medical advances. But the research, facilities, and services are extremely expensive, and many U.S. citizens are also demanding a balanced federal budget.

Health care services in the United States are undergoing rapid change. The U.S. health care system has been financed through traditional health insurance systems, which paid providers on a fee-for-service basis and allowed beneficiaries relative freedom in their selection of health care providers. Health insurance has become an important benefit of employment. Employers became the primary purchasers of health insurance, and the rising cost of health care is reflected in the premiums employers pay and the subsequent decrease in employer-sponsored coverage. Private purchasers of health insurance have also seen a steady increase in their health insurance premiums, until many are forced to go "bare," forgoing health insurance due to the high costs. Fewer people now have health insurance coverage as a benefit of their employment. The number of uninsured people increased from 36 million in 1990 to nearly 40 million in 1994,[14] and the number of uninsured continues to rise as employers and individuals find health care insurance out of their reach. "People who are uninsured, under-insured, chronically ill, or disabled are likely to have increasing difficulties gaining access to health care as the ability of institutions to subsidize care continues to erode."[15] Today there are 42.6 million Americans without health insurance, including 10 million children. One way of containing health care costs that is gaining widespread popularity is managed health care.

The term "managed health care" refers to the concept of establishing networks of health care providers that offer an array of health care services under the umbrella of a single organization. A managed health care organization may be a group of physicians, hospitals, and health plans responsible for the health services for an enrolled individual or group. The organization coordinates the total health care services required by its enrollees. The purpose of managed health care is to provide cost-effectiveness of services and theoretically to improve the health care services provided to the enrollee by ensuring access to all required health services.

Many models are used to deliver managed health care: Health Maintenance Organizations (HMOs), Individual Practice Associations (IPAs), Group Practice, Multiple Option Plan, Medicare Risk HMOs, Preferred Provider Organizations (PPOs), and the Staff model. Each of these models delivers managed health care using a different structure.

In 1994, about 18% of the U.S. population (47 million persons) were enrolled in HMOs and about 23% of the population (60 million) received coverage through PPOs.[15] HMO and PPO enrollees make up 41% of the U.S. population. The use of the managed health care approach varies widely with geography. Many regions have little managed care and others have enrollment that represents more than 50% of the population. In 1994, 65% of employees of large and medium-sized companies were in managed care. In 1996, 70% of workers in firms with more than 200 employees were in managed care.[16] In 1997, more than 85% of the enrolled workforce was in some type of a managed care plan.[2] In 2001, there continued to be a rising percentage of employers opting for a managed care health plan for their employees; this indicates the employers' search for cost containment while offering the benefit of health coverage to employees.

The managed care industry has evolved from small, regional nonprofit plans to large, national, for-profit companies. Eleven national managed care companies now account for half of all HMO enrollment.

The pressure on the government to cut expenses and balance the budget guarantees the continued increases in market share for managed care. The government mandated the use of managed care within the Medicaid program, and the number of Medicaid beneficiaries enrolled in managed care continues to increase.

In the early stages of development, the managed care market included networks that allowed the enrollees a broad choice of providers. As the market segments for managed care expand, choice for the enrollees decreased.

Types of HMOs

A **Managed Care Organization (MCO)** is a group that is responsible for the health care services offered to an enrolled group or person. The organization coordinates or manages the care of the enrollee. The MCO contains costs by negotiating with various health care entities—hospitals, clinics, laboratories, and so forth—for a discounted rate for services provided to its enrollees. Providers of the health care services must receive prior approval from the MCO before services are rendered. For example, a physician may want to conduct a certain high-cost diagnostic test in a patient, but before the test can be conducted, the MCO must give the physician approval. The MCO uses a gatekeeper, usually the primary care physician of the patient, who can authorize the patient's need to seek health care services outside of the established organization. For example, a certain specialist may not be available within the MCO, and the primary care physician can recommend that the enrollee be referred to such a specialist. If the enrollee were to see the specialist without the recommendation of the primary care physician and the approval of the MCO, the enrollee would be responsible for all charges incurred. MCOs develop practice guidelines that evaluate the appropriateness and medical necessity of medical care provided to the enrollee by the physicians, which gives the MCO control over what care is provided to the enrollee.

A **Preferred Provider Organization (PPO)** is a group of providers who form a network and who have agreed to provide services to enrollees at a discounted rate. Enrollees are usually responsible for paying a portion of the costs (cost sharing) when using a PPO provider. Enrollees who seek health care outside of the PPO providers pay an additional out-of-pocket cost. The out-of-pocket costs are established by the PPO to discourage the use of outside providers. The PPOs do not use a gatekeeper, but they do have strict guidelines that denote approved expenses and how much the enrollee will pay.

A **Health Maintenance Organization (HMO)** is a delivery system that allows the enrollee access to all health care services. The HMO is the "total package" approach to health care organizations, and the out-of-pocket expenses are minimal. However, the enrollee is assigned a primary care physician who manages all the health care needs of the enrollee and acts as the gatekeeper for the enrollee. Services are prepaid by the HMO. For example, the HMO pays a laboratory to provide services at a negotiated price and the services are prepaid by the HMO. The gatekeeper has authority to allow the enrollee access to the services available or authorize services outside of those the HMO has available. The gatekeeper has strong incentives to contain costs for the HMO by controlling and managing the health care services provided to the enrollee. The HMO can directly employ the physician in the **Staff Model** HMO or contract the physician through the **Individual Practice Associations (IPA)** model in which the physician provides services for a set fee. Either way, the physician has an incentive to service the cost containment needs of the HMO.

An **Exclusive Provider Organization (EPO)** has many of the same features as an HMO except that the providers of the services are not prepaid. Instead, the providers are paid on a fee-for-service basis. The **Group Practice Model (GPM)** is a form of HMO in which an organization of physicians contracts with the HMO to provide services to the enrollees of the HMO. A payment is negotiated, the HMO pays the group, and then the group pays the individual physicians.

Medicare + Choice (M+C) is a Medicare-funded alternative to the standard Medicare supplemental coverage. M+C is a standard HMO; however, it is provided to Medicare beneficiaries rather than the traditional fee-for-service model historically used by Medicare. The enrollees pay out of pocket if they choose to go outside the network of providers. **Point-of-Service (POS)** benefits allow enrollees to receive services outside of the HMO's health care network, but at increased cost in copayments, in coinsurance, or in a deductible. The POS benefit is one that the HMO may choose to offer, but it is not required, and the CMS does not provide any additional funding for this benefit. However, the HMO that offers this option is more attractive to a potential enrollee, because the lack of access to providers outside of a predefined network is the one reason people do not join a managed health care organization. The POS benefit option is also referred to as an *open-ended HMO* or a *self-referral option*. The POS benefit is attractive not only to Medicare enrollees who wish to be treated by providers not available in their plan's network but also to those who travel and would like access to routine medical care while temporarily (for fewer than 90 days) out of their plan's service area. The supplemental benefit of coverage of prescription drugs is a major reason Medicare beneficiaries are attracted to M+C; approximately 70% of all providers under M+C offer this benefit. Total Medicare managed care enrollment more than doubled between 1995 and 1999.

Managed health care is now part of the fabric of the U.S. health care system. The "richer" plans of traditional insurance companies are often no longer an option to a great segment of the population.

Drawbacks of the HMO

There are some significant drawbacks to the HMO concept in terms of access to health care. Consider that providers (physicians in particular) have an incentive to keep treatment costs to a minimum. Traditionally, a physician's primary concern was what was in the best interest of the patient, not what was in the best interest of containment of cost. This fundamental change transformed physicians into gatekeepers for third-party payers and transformed third-party payers into developers of guidelines that ultimately control the services patients can and do receive. The patient-physician relationship has shifted to a physician/third-party-payer relationship, which leaves the patient at the mercy of the third-party payer. Many lawsuits have been brought by patients who allege that lack of treatment caused harm and sometimes death. Cost-containment issues, and hence HMOs, raise many ethical and legal issues that will continue to involve patients, providers, and third-party payers.

CHAPTER GLOSSARY

APCs (Ambulatory Patient Categories): patient classification that provides a payment system for outpatients

assignment: Medicare's payment for the service, which participating physicians agree to accept as payment in full

CF (conversion factor): national dollar amount that is applied to all services paid on the Medicare Fee Schedule basis

CMS: Centers for Medicare and Medicaid Services, formerly HCFA, Health Care Financing Administration

DHHS: Department of Health and Human Services

DRGs (Diagnosis-Related Groups): a disease classification system that relates the type of inpatients a hospital treats (case mix) to the costs incurred by the hospital

Exclusive Provider Organization (EPO): similar to a Health Maintenance Organization except that the providers of the services are not prepaid, but rather are paid on a fee-for-service basis

Federal Register: official publication of all "Presidential Documents," "Rules and Regulations," "Proposed Rules," and "Notices"; government-instituted national changes are published in the *Federal Register*

Group Practice Model: an organization of physicians who contract with a Health Maintenance Organization to provide services to the enrollees of the HMO

grouper: computer used to input the principal diagnosis and other critical information about a patient and then provide the correct DRG code

HCFA: Health Care Financing Administration, now known as Centers for Medicare and Medicaid Services (CMS)

Health Maintenance Organization (HMO): a health care delivery system in which an enrollee is assigned a primary care physician who manages all the health care needs of the enrollee

Individual Practice Association (IPA): an organization of physicians who provide services for a set fee; Health Maintenance Organizations often contract with the IPA for services to their enrollees

MAAC (Maximum Actual Allowable Charge): limitation on the total amount that can be charged by physicians who are not participants in Medicare

Managed Care Organization (MCO): a group that is responsible for the health care services offered to an enrolled group of persons

MDC (Major Diagnostic Categories): the division of all principal diagnoses into 25 mutually exclusive principal diagnosis areas within the DRG system

Medicare Risk HMO: a Medicare-funded alternative to the standard Medicare supplemental coverage

MEI (Medicare Economic Index): government-mandated index that ties increases in the Medicare prevailing charges to economic indicators

MFS (Medicare Fee Schedule): schedule that listed the allowable charges for Medicare services; was replaced by the Medicare reasonable charge payment system

MVPS (Medical Volume Performance Standards): government's estimate of how much growth is appropriate for nationwide physician expenditures paid by the Part B Medicare program

OBRA (Omnibus Budget Reconciliation Act of 1989): act that established new rules for Medicare reimbursement

Part A: Medicare's Hospital Insurance; covers hospital/facility care

Part B: Medicare's Supplemental Medical Insurance; covers physician services and durable medical equipment that are not paid for under Part A

participating provider program: Medicare providers who have agreed in advance to accept assignment on all Medicare claims

Preferred Provider Organization (PPO): a group of providers who form a network and who have agreed to provide services to enrollees at a discounted rate

prognosis: probable outcome of an illness

PROs (Peer Review Organizations): groups established to review hospital admission and care

PSRO (Professional Standards Review Organization): voluntary physicians' organization designed to monitor the necessity of hospital admissions, treatment costs, and medical records of hospitals

RBRVS (Resource-Based Relative Value Scale): scale designed to decrease Medicare expenditures, redistribute physician payment, and ensure quality health care at reasonable rates

resource intensity: refers to the relative volume and type of diagnostic, therapeutic, and bed services used in the management of a particular illness

RVU (Relative Value Unit): unit value that has been assigned for each service

severity of illness: refers to the levels of loss of function and mortality that may be experienced by patients with a particular disease

Staff Model: a Health Maintenance Organization that directly employs the physicians who provide services to enrollees

TEFRA (Tax Equity and Fiscal Responsibility Act): act that contains language to reward cost-conscious health care providers

CHAPTER REVIEW

CHAPTER 16, PART I, THEORY

Complete the following:

1 What two insurance programs were established in 1965 by amendments to the Social Security Act?

2 The Secretary of DHHS has delegated responsibility for Medicare to which department?

3 Who administers funds for Medicare?

4 Who is eligible for Medicare? _____

5 What are the six types of reviews defined in the Scope of Work that are performed by the PROs?

6 List three goals of Physician Payment Reform:

_____

_____

_____

7 List the three components of the relative value unit:

_____

_____

_____

8 What does UHDDS stand for?

_____

9 What is the fastest growing segment of our population today?

_____

10 What is the name given to the groups that handle the daily operations of the Medicare program?

_____

REFERENCES

1. Resident Population of the United States: Middle Series Projections, p. 2015–2030, by Age and Sex; U.S. Bureau of the Census; March 1996.
2. 1996 HCFA Statistics. Bureau of Data Management, HCFA Pub. No. 03394, Sept. 1996.
3. Highlights, National Health Expenditures, 1997, Health Care Financing Administration, p. 1.
4. *Federal Register* 59(121), Friday, June 24, 1994, p. 32753.
5. Blue Cross and Blue Shield of Minnesota. *Medicare Coding Manual.* St. Paul, Minn.
6. *Federal Register* 63 (203), October 21, 1998, p. 56199.
7. Program Memorandum, Department of HCFA, transmittal AB-00-98, October 20, 2000.
8. *Federal Register* 63 (211), November 2, 1998, p. 58814.
9. Diagnosis-Related Groups, Version 14.0, Definitions Manual.
10. 2000 Medicare Carriers Manual, Fraud and Abuse, Health Care Financing Administration, p. 14000–14032.
11. Department of Health and Human Services, Office of the Inspector General, Fiscal Year 2001 Work Plan, Health Care Financing Administration, p. 14.
12. Unrestricted Medicare Fraud Alert 9605, July 12, 1996, Health Care Financing Administration.
13. Restricted Medicare Fraud Alert 9612, October 1996, Health Care Financing Administration.
14. Mechanic R, Dobson A, Yu S: *The Impact of Managed Care on Clinical Research: A Preliminary Investigation:* The Commonwealth Fund, January 1996, p 570.
15. Health Care Coverage and Access Program. Picker/Commonwealth Program on Health Care Quality and Managed Care, March 1996.
16. Davis K: Health Services Research and the Changing Health Care system. Briefing, Notes: The Commonwealth Fund, March 1996.

Official ICD-9-CM Guidelines for Coding and Reporting

The Public Health Service and the Center for Medicare and Medicaid Services of the U.S. Department of Health and Human Services present the following guidelines for coding and reporting using the International Classification of Diseases, 9th Revision, Clinical Modification (ICD-9-CM). These guidelines should be used as a companion document to the official versions of the ICD-9-CM.

These guidelines for coding and reporting have been developed and approved by the cooperating parties for ICD-9-CM: American Hospital Association, American Health Information Management Association, Centers for Medicare and Medicaid Services, and the National Center for Health Statistics. These guidelines previously appeared in the Coding Clinic for ICD-9-CM, published by the American Hospital Association.

These guidelines have been developed to assist the user in coding and reporting in situations where the ICD-9-CM manual does not provide direction. Coding and sequencing instructions in the three ICD-9-CM manuals take precedence over any guidelines.

These guidelines are not exhaustive. The cooperating parties are continuing to conduct review of these guidelines and develop new guidelines as needed. Users of the ICD-9-CM should be aware that only guidelines approved by the cooperating parties are official. Revision of these guidelines and new guidelines will be published by the U.S. Department of Health and Human Services when they are approved by the cooperating parties.

Table of Contents

1. GENERAL INPATIENT CODING GUIDELINES

1.1 Use of Both Alphabetic Index and Tabular List

    A. Use both the Alphabetic Index and the Tabular List when locating and assigning a code. Reliance on only the Alphabetic Index or the Tabular List leads to errors in code assignments and less specificity in code selection.

    B. Locate each term in the Alphabetic Index and verify the code selected in the Tabular List. Read and be guided by instructional notations that appear in both the Alphabetic Index and the Tabular List.

1.2 Level of Specificity in Coding

Diagnostic and procedure codes are to be used at their highest level of specificity:

    Assign three-digit codes only if there are no four-digit codes within that code category.

    Assign four-digit codes only if there is no fifth digit subclassification for that category.

    Assign the fifth digit subclassification code for those categories where it exists.

1.3 Other (NEC) and Unspecified (NOS) Code Titles

Codes labeled "other specified" (NEC not elsewhere classified) or "unspecified" (NOS not otherwise specified) are used only when neither the diagnostic statement nor a thorough review of the medical record provides adequate information to permit assignment of a more specific code.

Use the code assignment for "other" or NEC when the information at hand specifies a condition but no separate code for that condition is provided.

Use "unspecified" (NOS) when the information at hand does not permit either a more specific or "other" code assignment.

When the Alphabetic Index assigns a code to a category labeled "other (NEC)" or to a category labeled "unspecified (NOS)," refer to the Tabular List and review the titles and inclusion terms in the subdivisions under that particular three-digit category (or subdivision under the four-digit code) to determine if the information at hand can be appropriately assigned to a more specific code.

1.4 Acute and Chronic Conditions

If the same condition is described as both acute (subacute) and chronic and separate subentries exist in the Alphabetic Index at the same indentation level, code both and sequence the acute (sub-acute) code first.

1.5 Combination Code

A single code used to classify two diagnoses or a diagnosis with an associated secondary process (manifestation) or an associated complication is called a combination code. Combination codes are identified by referring to subterm entries in the Alphabetic Index and by reading the inclusion and exclusion notes in the Tabular List.

A. Assign only the combination code when that code fully identifies the diagnostic conditions involved or when the Alphabetic Index so directs. Multiple coding should not be used when the classification provides a combination code that clearly identifies all of the elements documented in the diagnosis. When the combination code lacks necessary specificity in describing the manifestation or complication, an additional code may be used as a secondary code.

1.6 Multiple Coding of Diagnoses

Multiple coding is required for certain conditions not subject to the rules for combination codes.

Instructions for conditions that require multiple coding appear in the Alphabetic Index and the Tabular List.

A. Alphabetic Index: Codes for both etiology and manifestation of a disease appear following the subentry term, with the second code in brackets. Assign both codes in the same sequence in which they appear in the Alphabetic Index.

B. Tabular List: Instructional terms, such as "Code first . . . ," "Use additional code for any . . . ," and "Note . . . ," indicate when to use more than one code.

"Code first underlying disease"—Assign the codes for both the manifestation and underlying cause. The codes for manifestations cannot be used (designated) as principal diagnosis.

"Use additional code to identify manifestation, as . . ."—Assign also the code that identifies the manifestation, such as, but not limited to, the examples listed. The codes for manifestations cannot be used (designated) as principal diagnosis.

C. Apply multiple coding instructions throughout the classification where appropriate, whether or not multiple coding directions appear in the Alphabetic Index or the Tabular List. Avoid indiscriminate multiple coding or irrelevant information, such as symptoms or signs characteristic of the diagnosis.

1.7 Late Effect

A late effect is the residual effect (condition produced) after the acute phase of an illness or injury has terminated. There is no time limit on when a late effect code can be used. The residual may be apparent early, such as in cerebrovascular accident cases, or it may occur months or years later, such as that due to a previous injury.

Coding of late effects requires two codes:

The residual condition or nature of the late effect
The cause of the late effect

The residual condition or nature of the late effect is sequenced first, followed by the cause of the late effect, except in those few instances where the code for late effect is followed by a manifestation code identified in the Tabular List and title or the late effect code has been expanded (at the fourth and fifth digit levels) to include the manifestation(s).

The code for the acute phase of an illness or injury that led to the late effect is never used with a code for the cause of the late effect.

A. Late Effects of Cerebrovascular Disease

Category 438 is used to indicate conditions classifiable to categories 430-437 as the causes of late effects (neurologic deficits), themselves classified elsewhere. These "late effects" include neurologic deficits that persist after initial onset of conditions classifiable to 430-437. The neurologic deficits caused by cerebrovascular disease may be present from the onset or may arise at any time after the onset of the condition classifiable to 430-437.

Codes from category 438 may be assigned on a health care record with codes from 430-437, if the patient has a current CVA and deficits from an old CVA.

Assign code V12.59 (and not a code from category 438) as an additional code for history of cerebrovascular disease when no neurologic deficits are present.

1.8 Uncertain Diagnosis

If the diagnosis documented at the time of discharge is qualified as "probable," "suspected," "likely," "questionable," "possible," or "still to be ruled out," code the condition as if it existed or was established. The bases for these guidelines are the diagnostic workup, arrangements for further workup or observation, and initial therapeutic approach that correspond most closely with the established diagnosis.

1.9 Impending or Threatened Condition

Code any condition described at the time of discharge as "impending" or "threatened" as follows:

If it did occur, code as confirmed diagnosis.

If it did not occur, reference the Alphabetic Index to determine if the condition has a subentry term for "impending" or "threatened" and also reference main term entries for Impending and for Threatened.

If the subterms are listed, assign the given code.

If the subterms are not listed, code the existing forerunner condition(s) and not the condition described as impending or threatened.

2. SELECTION OF PRINCIPAL DIAGNOSIS

The circumstances of inpatient admission always govern the selection of principal diagnosis. The principal diagnosis is defined in the Uniform Hospital Discharge Data Set (UHDDS) as "that condition established after study to be chiefly responsible for occasioning the admission of the patient to the hospital for care."

In determining principal diagnosis the coding directives in the ICD-9-CM manuals, Volumes I, II, and III, take precedence over all other guidelines.

The importance of consistent, complete documentation in the medical record cannot be overemphasized. Without such documentation the application of all coding guidelines is a difficult, if not impossible, task.

2.1 Codes for symptoms, signs, and ill-defined conditions.

Codes for symptoms, signs, and ill-defined conditions from Chapter 16 are not to be used as principal diagnosis when a related definitive diagnosis has been established.

2.2 Codes in brackets.

Codes in brackets in the Alphabetic Index can never be sequenced as principal diagnosis. Coding directives require that the codes in brackets be sequenced in the order as they appear in the Alphabetic Index.

2.3 Acute and chronic conditions.

If the same condition is described as both acute (subacute) and chronic and separate subentries exist in the Alphabetic Index at the same indentation level, code both and sequence the acute (subacute) code first.

2.4 Two or more interrelated conditions, each potentially meeting the definition for principal diagnosis.

When there are two or more interrelated conditions (such as diseases in the same ICD-9-CM chapter or manifestations characteristically associated with a certain disease) potentially meeting the definition of principal diagnosis, either condition may be sequenced first, unless the circumstances of the admission, the therapy provided, the Tabular List, or the Alphabetic Index indicates otherwise.

2.5 Two or more diagnoses that equally meet the definition for principal diagnosis.

In the unusual instance when two or more diagnoses equally meet the criteria for principal diagnosis as determined by the circumstances of admission, diagnostic workup and/or therapy provided, and the Alphabetic Index, Tabular List, or another coding guideline does not provide sequencing direction, any one of the diagnoses may be sequenced first.

2.6 Two or more comparative or contrasting conditions.

In those rare instances when two or more contrasting or comparative diagnoses are documented as "either/or" (or similar terminology), they are coded as if the diagnoses were confirmed and the diagnoses are sequenced according to the circumstances of the admission. If no further determination can be made as to which diagnosis should be principal, either diagnosis may be sequenced first.

2.7 A symptom(s) followed by contrasting/comparative diagnoses.

When a symptom(s) is followed by contrasting/comparative diagnoses, the symptom code is sequenced first. All the contrasting/comparative diagnoses should be coded as suspected conditions.

2.8 Codes from the V71.0-V71.9 series, Observation and evaluation for suspected conditions.

Codes from the V71.0-V71.9 series are assigned as principal diagnoses for encounters or admissions to evaluate the patient's condition when there is some evidence to suggest the existence of an abnormal condition or following an accident or other incident that ordinarily results in a health problem, and where no supporting evidence for the suspected condition is found and no treatment is currently required. The fact that the patient may be scheduled for continuing observation in the office/clinic setting following discharge does not limit the use of this category.

2.9 Original treatment plan not carried out.

Sequence as the principal diagnosis the condition which after study occasioned the admission to the hospital, even though treatment may not have been carried out due to unforeseen circumstances.

2.10 Residual condition or nature of late effect.

The residual condition or nature of the late effect is sequenced first, followed by the late effect code for the cause of the residual condition, except in a few instances where the Alphabetic Index or Tabular List directs otherwise.

2.11 Multiple burns.

Sequence first the code that reflects the highest degree of burn when more than one burn is present. (See also Burns guideline 8.3.)

2.12 Multiple injuries.

When multiple injuries exist, the code for the most severe injury as determined by the attending physician is sequenced first.

2.13 Neoplasms.

A. If the treatment is directed at the malignancy, designate the malignancy as the principal diagnosis, except when the purpose of the encounter or hospital admission is for radiotherapy session(s), V58.0, or for chemotherapy session(s), V58.1, in which instance the malignancy is coded and sequenced second.

B. When a patient is admitted for the purpose of radiotherapy or chemotherapy and develops complications such as uncontrolled nausea and vomiting or dehydration, the principal diagnosis is Encounter for radiotherapy, V58.0, or Encounter for chemotherapy, V58.1.

C. When an episode of inpatient care involves surgical removal of a primary site or secondary site malignancy followed by adjunct chemotherapy or radiotherapy, code the malignancy as the principal diagnosis, using codes in the 140-198 series or where appropriate in the 200-203 series.

D. When the reason for admission is to determine the extent of the malignancy, or for a procedure such as paracentesis or thoracentesis, the primary malignancy or appropriate metastatic site is designed as the principal diagnosis, even though chemotherapy or radiotherapy is administered.

E. When the primary malignancy has been previously excised or eradicated from its site and there is no adjunct treatment directed to that site and no evidence of any remaining malignancy at the primary site, use the appropriate code from the V10 series to indicate the former site of primary malignancy. Any mention of extension, invasion, or metastasis to a nearby structure or organ or to a distant site is coded as a secondary malignant neoplasm to that site and may be the principal diagnosis in the absence of the primary site.

F. When a patient is admitted because of a primary neoplasm with metastasis and treatment is directed toward the secondary site only, the secondary neoplasm is designated as the principal diagnosis even though the primary malignancy is still present.

G. Symptoms, signs, and ill-defined conditions listed in Chapter 16 characteristic of, or associated with, an existing primary or secondary site malignancy cannot be used to replace the malignancy as principal diagnosis, regardless of the number of admissions or encounters for treatment and care of the neoplasm.

H. Coding and sequencing of complications associated with the malignant neoplasm or with the therapy thereof are subject to the following guidelines:

When admission is for management of an anemia associated with the malignancy, and the treatment is only for anemia, the anemia is designated as the principal diagnosis and is followed by the appropriate code(s) for the malignancy.

When the admission is for management of an anemia associated with chemotherapy or radiotherapy and the only treatment is for the anemia, the anemia is designated as the principal diagnosis followed by the appropriate code(s) for the malignancy.

When the admission is for management of dehydration due to the malignancy or the therapy, or a combination of both, and only the dehydration is being treated (intravenous rehydration), the dehydration is designed as the principal diagnosis, followed by the code(s) for the malignancy.

When the admission is for treatment of a complication resulting from a surgical procedure performed for the treatment of an intestinal malignancy, designate the complication as the principal diagnosis if treatment is directed at resolving the complication.

2.14 Poisoning.

When coding a poisoning or reaction to the improper use of a medication (e.g., wrong dose, wrong substance, wrong route of administration) the poisoning code is sequenced first, followed by a code for the manifestation. If there is also a diagnosis of drug abuse or dependence to the substance, the abuse or dependence is coded as an additional code.

2.15 Complications of surgery and other medical care.

When the admission is for treatment of a complication resulting from surgery or other medical care, the complication code is sequenced as the principal diagnosis. If the complication is classified to the 996-999 series, an additional code for the specific complication may be assigned.

2.16 Complication of pregnancy.

When a patient is admitted because of a condition that is either a complication of pregnancy or that is complicating the pregnancy, the code for the obstetric complication is the principal diagnosis. An additional code may be assigned as needed to provide specificity.

3. REPORTING OTHER (ADDITIONAL) DIAGNOSES

A joint effort between the attending physician and coder is essential to achieve complete and accurate documentation, code assignment, and reporting of diagnoses and procedures.

These guidelines have been developed and approved by the Cooperating Parties to assure both the physician and the coder in identifying those diagnoses that are to be reported in addition to the principal diagnosis. Hospitals may record other diagnoses as needed for internal data use.

The UHDDS definitions are used by acute care short-term hospitals to report inpatient data elements in a standardized manner. These data elements and their definitions can be found in the July 31, 1985 *Federal Register* (Vol. 50, No. 147), pp. 31038-40.

The UHDDS item #11-b defines Other Diagnoses as "all conditions that coexist at the time of admission, that develop subsequently, or that affect the treatment received and/or the length of stay. Diagnoses that relate to an earlier episode which have no bearing on the current hospital stay are to be excluded."

General Rule

For reporting purposes the definition for "other diagnoses" is interpreted as additional conditions that affect patient care in terms of requiring:

clinical evaluation; or

therapeutic treatment; or

diagnostic procedures; or

extended length of hospital stay; or

increased nursing care and/or monitoring.

The following guidelines are to be applied in designating "other diagnoses" when neither the Alphabetic Index nor the Tabular List in ICD-9-CM provides direction.

The listing of the diagnoses on the attestation statement is the responsibility of the attending physician.

3.1 Previous conditions.

If the physician has included a diagnosis in the final diagnostic statement, such as the discharge summary or the face sheet, it should ordinarily be coded. Some physicians include in the diagnostic statement resolved conditions or diagnoses and status-post procedures from previous admission that have no bearing on the current stay. Such conditions are not to be reported and are coded only if required by hospital policy.

However, history codes (V10-V19) may be used as secondary codes if the historical condition or family history has an impact on current care or influences treatment.

3.2 Diagnoses not listed in the final diagnostic statement.

When the physician has documented what appears to be a current diagnosis in the body of the record, but has not included the diagnosis in the final diagnostic statement, the physician should be asked whether the diagnosis should be added.

3.3 Conditions that are an integral part of a disease process.

Conditions that are integral to the disease process should not be assigned as additional codes.

3.4 Conditions that are not an integral part of a disease process.

Additional conditions that may not be associated routinely with a disease process should be coded when present.

3.5 Abnormal findings.

Abnormal findings (laboratory, x-ray, pathologic, and other diagnostic results) are not coded and reported unless the physician indicates their clinical significance. If the findings are outside the normal range and the physician has ordered other tests to evaluate the condition or prescribed treatment, it is appropriate to ask the physician whether the diagnosis should be added.

4. HYPERTENSION

4.1 Hypertension, Essential, or NOS

Assign hypertension (arterial) (essential) (primary) (systemic) (NOS) to category code 401 with the appropriate fourth digit to indicate malignant (.0), benign (.1), or unspecified (.9). Do not use either .0 malignant or .1 benign unless medical record documentation supports such a designation.

4.2 Hypertension with Heart Disease

Certain heart conditions (425.8, 428, 429.0-429.3, 429.8, 429.9) are assigned to a code from category 402 when a causal relationship is stated (due to hypertension) or implied (hypertensive). Use only the code from category 402.

The same heart conditions (425.8, 428, 429.0-429.3, 429.8, 429.9) with hypertension, but without a stated casual relationship, are coded separately. Sequence according to the circumstances of the admission.

4.3 Hypertensive Renal Disease with Chronic Renal Failure

Assign codes from category 403, Hypertensive renal disease, when conditions classified to categories 585-587 are present. Unlike hypertension with heart disease, ICD-9-CM presumes a cause-and-effect relationship and classifies renal failure with hypertension as hypertensive renal disease.

4.4 Hypertensive Heart and Renal Disease

Assign codes from combination category 404, Hypertensive heart and renal disease, when both hypertensive renal disease and hypertensive heart disease are stated in the diagnosis. Assume a relationship between the hypertension and the renal disease, whether or not the condition is so designated.

4.5 Hypertensive Cerebrovascular Disease.

First assign codes from 430-438, Cerebrovascular disease, then the appropriate hypertension code from categories 401-405.

4.6 Hypertensive Retinopathy

Two codes are necessary to identify the condition. First assign the code from subcategory 362.11, Hypertensive retinopathy, then the appropriate code from categories 401-405 to indicate the type of hypertension.

4.7 Hypertension, Secondary

Two codes are required: one to identify the underlying condition and one from category 405 to identify the hypertension. Sequencing of codes is determined by the reason for admission to the hospital.

4.8 Hypertension, Transient

Assign code 796.2, Elevated blood pressure reading without diagnosis of hypertension, unless patient has an established diagnosis of hypertension. Assign code 642.3x for transient hypertension of pregnancy.

4.9 Hypertension, Controlled

Assign appropriate code from categories 401-405. This diagnostic statement usually refers to an existing state of hypertension under control by therapy.

4.10 Hypertension, Uncontrolled

Uncontrolled hypertension may refer to untreated hypertension or hypertension not responding to current therapeutic regimen. In either case, assign the appropriate code from categories 401-405 to designate the stage and type of hypertension. Code to the type of hypertension.

4.11 Elevated Blood Pressure

For a statement of elevated blood pressure without further specificity, assign code 796.2, Elevated blood pressure reading without diagnosis of hypertension, rather than a code from category 401.

5. OBSTETRICS

Introduction

These guidelines have been developed and approved by the Cooperating Parties in conjunction with the Editorial Advisory Board of Coding Clinic and the American College of Obstetricians and Gynecologists, to assist the coder in coding and reporting obstetric cases. Where feasible, previously published advice has been incorporated. Some advice in these new guidelines may supersede previous advice. The guidelines are provided for reporting purposes. Health care facilities may record additional diagnoses as needed for internal data needs.

5.1 General Rules

   A. Obstetric cases require codes from chapter 11, codes in the range 630-677, Complications of Pregnancy, Childbirth, and the Puerperium. Should the physician document that the pregnancy is incidental to the encounter, then code V22.2 should be used in place of any chapter 11 codes. It is the physician's responsibility to state that the condition being treated is not affecting the pregnancy.

   B. Chapter 11 codes have sequencing priority over codes from other chapters. Additional codes from other chapters may be used in conjunction with chapter 11 codes to further specify conditions.

   C. Chapter 11 codes are to be used only on the maternal record, never on the record of the newborn.

   D. An outcome of delivery code, V27.0-V27.9, should be included on every maternal record when a delivery has occurred. These codes are not to be used on subsequent records or on the newborn record.

5.2 Selection of Principal Diagnosis

   A. The circumstances of the encounter govern the selection of the principal diagnosis.

   B. In episodes when no delivery occurs the principal diagnosis should correspond to the principal complication of the pregnancy which necessitated the encounter. Should more than one complication exist, all of which are treated or monitored, any of the complications codes may be sequenced first.

   C. When a delivery occurs the principal diagnosis should correspond to the main circumstances or complication of the delivery. In cases of cesarean deliveries, the principal diagnosis should correspond to the reason the cesarean was performed, unless the reason for admission was unrelated to the condition resulting in the cesarean delivery.

   D. For routine prenatal visits when no complications are present codes V22.0, Supervision of normal first pregnancy, and V22.1, Supervision of other normal pregnancy, should be used as principal diagnoses. These codes should not be used in conjunction with chapter 11 codes.

   E. For prenatal outpatient visits for patients with high-risk pregnancies, a code from category V23, Supervision of high-risk pregnancy, should be used as the principal diagnosis. Secondary chapter 11 codes may be used in conjunction with these codes if appropriate. A thorough review of any pertinent excludes note is necessary to be certain that these V codes are being used properly.

5.3 Chapter 11 Fifth digits
   A. Categories 640-648, 651-676 have required fifth digits which indicate whether the encounter is antepartum, postpartum and whether a delivery has also occurred.
   B. The fifth digits which are appropriate for each code number are listed in brackets under each code. The fifth digits on each code should all be consistent with each other. That is, should a delivery occur all of the fifth digits should indicate the delivery.

5.4 Fetal Conditions Affecting the Management of the Mother.
   Codes from category 655, Known or suspected fetal abnormality affecting management of the mother, and category 656, Other fetal and placental problems affecting the management of the mother, are assigned only when the fetal condition is actually responsible for modifying the management of the mother, i.e., by requiring diagnostic studies, additional observation, special care, or termination of pregnancy. The fact that the fetal condition exists does not justify assigning a code from this series to the mother's record.

5.5 Normal Delivery, 650
   A. Code 650 is for use in cases when a woman is admitted for a full-term normal delivery and delivers a single, healthy infant without any complications antepartum, during the delivery, or postpartum during the delivery episode.
   B. 650 may be used if the patient had a complication at some point during her pregnancy but the complication is not present at the time of the admission for delivery.
   C. Code 650 is always a principal diagnosis. It is not to be used if any other code from chapter 11 is needed to describe a current complication of the antenatal, delivery, or perinatal period. Additional codes from other chapters may be used with code 650 if they are not related to or are in any way complicating the pregnancy.
   D. V27.0, Single liveborn, is the only outcome of delivery code appropriate for use with 650.

5.6 Procedure Codes
   A. In cases of cesarean delivery, the selection of the principal diagnosis should correspond to the reason the cesarean delivery was performed unless the reason for admission was unrelated to the condition resulting in the cesarean delivery.
   B. A delivery procedure code should not be used for a woman who has delivered prior to admission to the hospital. Any postpartum repairs should be coded.

5.7 The Postpartum Period
   A. The postpartum period begins immediately after delivery and continues for 6 weeks following delivery.
   B. A postpartum complication is any complication occurring within the 6 week period.
   C. Chapter 11 codes may also be used to describe pregnancy-related complications after the 6 week period should the physician document that a condition is pregnancy related.
   D. Postpartum complications that occur during the same admission as the delivery are identified with a fifth digit of "2." Subsequent admissions for postpartum complications should be identified with a fifth digit of "4."
   E. When the mother delivers outside the hospital prior to admission and is admitted for routine postpartum care and no complications are noted, code V24.0, Postpartum care and examina-

tion immediately after delivery, should be assigned as the principal diagnosis.

5.8 Abortions

A. Fifth digits are required for abortion categories 634-637. Fifth digit 1, incomplete, indicates that all of the products of conception have not been expelled from the uterus. Fifth digit 2, complete, indicates that all products of conception have been expelled from the uterus prior to the episode of care.

B. A code from categories 640-648 and 651-657 may be used as additional codes with an abortion code to indicate the complication leading to the abortion.

Fifth digit 3 is assigned with codes from these categories when used with an abortion code because the other fifth digits will not apply. Codes from the 660-669 series are not to be used for complications of abortion.

C. Code 639 is to be used for all complications following abortion. Code 639 cannot be assigned with codes from categories 634-638.

D. Abortion with Liveborn Fetus. When an attempted termination of pregnancy results in a liveborn fetus assign code 644.21, Early onset of delivery, with an appropriate code from category V27, Outcome of Delivery. The procedure code for the attempted termination of pregnancy should also be assigned.

E. Retained Products of Conception following an abortion. Subsequent admissions for retained products of conception following a spontaneous or legally induced abortion are assigned the appropriate code from category 634, Spontaneous abortion, or legally induced abortion, with a fifth digit of "1" (incomplete). This advice is appropriate even when the patient was discharged previously with a discharge diagnosis of complete abortion.

5.9 Code 677, Late effect of complication of pregnancy, childbirth, and the puerperium

A. Code 677, Late effect of complication of pregnancy, childbirth, and the puerperium, is for use in those cases when an initial complication of a pregnancy develops a sequela requiring care or treatment at a future date.

B. This code may be used at any time after the initial postpartum period.

C. This code, like all late effect codes, is to be sequenced following the code describing the sequela of the complication.

6. NEWBORN GUIDELINES

Definition

The newborn period is defined as beginning at birth and lasting through the 28th day following birth.

The following guidelines are provided for reporting purposes. Hospitals may record other diagnoses as needed for internal data use.

General Rule

All clinically significant conditions noted on routine newborn examination should be coded. A condition is clinically significant if it requires:

• clinical evaluation; or

• therapeutic treatment; or

- diagnostic procedures; or
- extended length of hospital stay; or
- increased nursing care and/or monitoring; or
- has implications for future health care needs.

Note: The preceding list of newborn guidelines are the same as the general coding guidelines for "other diagnoses," except for the final bullet regarding implications for future health care needs. Whether or not a condition is clinically significant can only be determined by the physician.

6.1 Use of Codes V30-V39

When coding the birth of an infant, assign a code from categories V30-V39, according to the type of birth. A code from this series is assigned as a principal diagnosis, and assigned only once to a newborn at the time of birth.

6.2 Newborn Transfers

If the newborn is transferred to another institution, the V30 series is not used.

6.3 Use of Category V29

A. Assign a code from category V29, Observation and evaluation of newborns and infants for suspected conditions not found, to identify those instances when a healthy newborn is evaluated for a suspected condition that is determined after study not to be present. Do not use a code from category V29 when the patient has identified signs or symptoms of a suspected problem; in such cases, code the sign or symptom.

B. A V29 code is to be used as a secondary code after the V30, Outcome of delivery, code. It may also be assigned as a principal code for readmissions or encounters when the V30 code no longer applies. It is for use only for healthy newborns and infants for which no condition after study is found to be present.

6.4 Maternal Causes of Perinatal Morbidity

Codes from categories 760-763, Maternal causes of perinatal morbidity and mortality, are assigned only when the maternal condition has actually affected the fetus or newborn. The fact that the mother has an associated medical condition or experiences some complication of pregnancy, labor or delivery does not justify the routine assignment of codes from these categories to the newborn record.

6.5 Congenital Anomalies

Assign an appropriate code from categories 740-759, Congenital Anomalies, when a specific abnormality is diagnosed for an infant. Such abnormalities may occur as a set of symptoms or multiple malformations. A code should be assigned for each presenting manifestation of the syndrome if the syndrome is not specifically indexed in ICD-9-CM.

6.6 Coding of Other (Additional) Diagnoses

A. Assign codes for conditions that require treatment or further investigation, prolong the length of stay, or require resource utilization.

B. Assign codes for conditions that have been specified by the physician as having implications for future health care needs.

Note: This guideline should not be used for adult patients.

C. Assign a code for Newborn conditions originating in the perinatal period (categories 760-779), as well as complications arising during the current episode of care classified in other chapters, only if the diagnoses have been documented by the responsible physician at the time of transfer or discharge as having affected the fetus or newborn.

D. Insignificant conditions or signs or symptoms that resolve without treatment are not coded.

6.7 Prematurity and Fetal Growth Retardation

Codes from categories 764 and 765 should not be assigned based solely on recorded birthweight or estimated gestational age, but upon the attending physician's clinical assessment of maturity of the infant.

Note: Since physicians may utilize different criteria in determining prematurity, do not code the diagnosis of prematurity unless the physician documents this condition.

7. SEPTICEMIA AND SEPTIC SHOCK

When the diagnosis of septicemia with shock or the diagnosis of general sepsis with septic shock is documented, code and list the septicemia first and report the septic shock code as a secondary condition. The septicemia code assignment should identify the type of bacteria if it is known.

Sepsis and septic shock associated with abortion, ectopic pregnancy, and molar pregnancy are classified to category codes in chapter 11 (630-639).

Negative or inconclusive blood cultures do not preclude a diagnosis of septicemia in patients with clinical evidence of the condition.

8. TRAUMA

8.1 Coding for Multiple Injuries

When coding multiple injuries such as fracture of tibia and fibula, assign separate codes for each injury unless a combination code is provided, in which case the combination code is assigned. Multiple injury codes are provided in ICD-9-CM, but should not be assigned unless information for a more specific code is not available.

A. The code for the most serious injury, as determined by the physician, is sequenced first.

B. Superficial injuries such as abrasions or contusions are not coded when associated with more severe injuries of the same site.

C. When a primary injury results in minor damage to peripheral nerves or blood vessels, the primary injury is sequenced first with additional code(s) from categories 950-957, Injury to nerves and spinal cord, and/or 900-904, Injury to blood vessels. When the primary injury is to the blood vessels or nerves, that injury should be sequenced first.

8.2 Coding for Multiple Fractures

The principle of multiple coding of injuries should be followed in coding multiple fractures. Multiple fractures of specified sites are coded individually by site in accordance with both the provisions within categories 800-829 and the level of detail furnished by medical record content. Combination categories for multiple fractures are provided for use when there is insufficient detail in the medical record (such as trauma cases transferred to another hospital), when the reporting form limits the number of codes that can be used in reporting pertinent clinical data, or when there is insufficient specificity at the fourth digit or fifth digit level. More specific guidelines are as follows:

A. Multiple fractures of same limb classifiable to the same three-digit or four-digit category are coded to that category.

B. Multiple unilateral or bilateral fractures of same bone(s) but classified to different fourth digit subdivisions (bone part) within the same three-digit category are coded individually by site.

C. Multiple fracture categories 819 and 828 classify bilateral fractures of both upper limbs (819) and both lower limbs (828), but without any detail at the fourth digit level other than open and closed type of fractures.

D. Multiple fractures are sequenced in accordance with the severity of the fracture and the physician should be asked to list the fracture diagnoses in the order of severity.

8.3 Current Burns and Encounters for Late Effects of Burns

Current burns (940-948) are classified by depth, extent and, if desired, by agent (E code). By depth burns are classified as first degree (erythema), second degree (blistering), and third degree (full-thickness involvement).

A. All burns are coded with the highest degree of burn sequenced first.

B. Classify burns of the same local site (three-digit category level, (940-947) but of different degrees to the subcategory identifying the highest degree recorded in the diagnosis.

C. Non-healing burns are coded as acute burns. Necrosis of burned skin should be coded as a non-healed burn.

D. Assign code 958.3, Posttraumatic wound infection, not elsewhere classified, as an additional code for any documented infected burn site.

E. When coding multiple burns, assign separate codes for each burn site.

Category 946, Burns of multiple specified sites, should only be used if the location[s] of the burns are not documented.

Category 949, Burn, unspecified, is extremely vague and should rarely be used.

F. Assign codes from category 948, Burns classified according to extent of body surface involved, when the site of the burn is not specified or when there is a need for additional data. It is advisable to use category 948 as additional coding when needed to provide data for evaluating burn mortality, such as that needed by burn units. It is also advisable to use category 948 as an additional code for reporting purposes when there is mention of a third-degree burn involving 20 percent or more of the body surface. In assigning a code from category 948:

Fourth digit codes are used to identify the percentage of total body surface involved in a burn (all degree).

Fifth digits are assigned to identify the percentage of body surface involved in third-degree burn.

Fifth digit zero (0) is assigned when less than 10 percent or when no body surface is involved in a third-degree burn.

Category 948 is based on the classic "rule of nines" in estimating body surface involved: head and neck are assigned nine percent, each arm nine percent, each leg 18 percent, the anterior trunk 18 percent, posterior trunk 18 percent, and genitalia one percent. Physicians may change these percentage assignments where necessary to accommodate infants and children, who have proportionately larger heads than adults and patients who have large buttocks, thighs, or abdomen that involve burns.

G. Encounters for the treatment of the late effects of burns (i.e., scars or joint contractures) should be coded to the residual condition (sequelae) followed by the appropriate late effect code (906.5-906.9). A late effect E code may also be used, if desired.

H. When appropriate, both a sequela with a late effect code, and a current burn code may be assigned on the same record.

8.4 Debridement of Wound, Infection, or Burn

A. For coding purposes, excisional debridement, 86.22, is assigned only when the procedure is performed by a physician.

B. For coding purposes, nonexcisional debridement performed by the physician or nonphysician health care professional is assigned to 86.28. Any "excisional" type procedure performed by a nonphysician is assigned to 86.28.

9. ADVERSE EFFECTS AND POISONING

The properties of certain drugs, medicinal and biological substances or combinations of such substances, may cause toxic reactions. The occurrence of drug toxicity is classified in ICD-9-CM as follows:

9.1 Adverse Effect

When the drug was correctly prescribed and properly administered, code the reaction plus the appropriate code from the E930-E949 series.

Adverse effects of therapeutic substances correctly prescribed and properly administered (toxicity, synergistic reaction, side effect, and idiosyncratic reaction) may be due to (1) differences among patients, such as age, sex, disease, and genetic factors, and (2) drug-related factors, such as type of drug, route of administration, duration of therapy, dosage, and bioavailability.

Codes from the E930-E949 series must be used to identify the causative substance for an adverse effect of drug, medicinal and biological substances, correctly prescribed and properly administered. The effect, such as tachycardia, delirium, gastrointestinal hemorrhaging, vomiting, hypokalemia, hepatitis, renal failure, or respiratory failure, is coded and followed by the appropriate code from the E930-E949 series.

9.2 Poisoning

Poisoning when an error was made in drug prescription or in the administration of the drug by physician, nurse, patient, or other person, use the appropriate code from the 960-979 series. If an overdose of a drug was intentionally taken or administered and resulted in drug toxicity, it would be coded as a poisoning (960-979 series). If a nonprescribed drug or medicinal agent was taken in combination with a correctly prescribed and properly administered drug, any drug toxicity or other reaction resulting from the interaction of the two drugs would be classified as a poisoning.

10. HUMAN IMMUNODEFICIENCY VIRUS (HIV) INFECTIONS

10.1 Code only confirmed cases of HIV infection/illness.

This is an exception to guideline 1.8 which states "If the diagnosis documented at the time of discharge is qualified as 'probable,' 'suspected,' 'likely,' 'questionable,' 'possible,' or 'still to be ruled out,' code the condition as if it existed or was established. . . . "

In this context, "confirmation" does not require documentation of positive serology or culture for HIV; the physician's diagnostic statement that the patient is HIV positive, or has an HIV-related illness is sufficient.

10.2 Selection of HIV code

042   Human Immunodeficiency Virus [HIV] Disease
Patients with an HIV-related illness should be coded to 042, Human Immunodeficiency Virus [HIV] Disease.

V08   Asymptomatic Human Immunodeficiency Virus [HIV] Infection
Patients with physician-documented asymptomatic HIV infections who have never had an HIV-related illness should be coded to V08, Asymptomatic Human Immunodeficiency Virus [HIV] Infection.

795.71 Nonspecific Serologic Evidence of Human Immunodeficiency Virus [HIV]
Code 795.71, Nonspecific serologic evidence of human immunodeficiency virus [HIV], should be used for patients (including infants) with inconclusive HIV test results.

10.3 Previously diagnosed HIV-related illness
Patients with any known prior diagnosis of an HIV-related illness should be coded to 042. Once a patient has developed an HIV-related illness, the patient should always be assigned code 042 on every subsequent admission. Patients previously diagnosed with any HIV illness (042) should never be assigned to 795.71 or V08.

10.4 Sequencing
The sequencing of diagnoses for patients with HIV-related illnesses follows guideline 2 for selection of principal diagnosis. That is, the circumstances of admission govern the selection of principal diagnosis, "that condition established after study to be chiefly responsible for occasioning the admission of the patient to the hospital for care."

Patients who are admitted for an HIV-related illness should be assigned a minimum of two codes: first assign code 042 to identify the HIV disease and then sequence additional codes to identify the other diagnoses. If a patient is admitted for an HIV-related condition, the principal diagnosis should be 042, followed by additional diagnosis codes for all reported HIV-related conditions.

If a patient with HIV disease is admitted for an unrelated condition (such as a traumatic injury), the code for the unrelated condition (e.g., the nature of injury code) should be the principal diagnosis. Other diagnoses would be 042 followed by additional diagnosis codes for all reported HIV-related conditions.

Whether the patient is newly diagnosed or has had previous admissions for HIV conditions (or has expired) is irrelevant to the sequencing decision.

10.5 HIV Infection in Pregnancy, Childbirth, and the Puerperium
During pregnancy, childbirth or the puerperium, a patient admitted because of an HIV-related illness should receive a principal diagnosis of 647.6X, Other specified infectious and parasitic diseases in the mother classifiable elsewhere, but complicating the

pregnancy, childbirth or the puerperium, followed by 042 and the code(s) for the HIV-related illness(es). This is an exception to the sequencing rule found in 10.4 above.

Patients with asymptomatic HIV infection status admitted during pregnancy, childbirth, or the puerperium should receive codes of 647.6X and V08.

10.6 Asymptomatic HIV Infection

V08 Asymptomatic human immunodeficiency virus [HIV] infection, is to be applied when the patient without any documentation of symptoms is listed as being "HIV positive," "known HIV," "HIV test positive," or similar terminology. Do not use this code if the term "AIDS" is used or if the patient is treated for any HIV-related illness or is described as having any condition(s) resulting from his/her HIV positive status; use 042 in these cases.

10.7 Inconclusive Laboratory Test for HIV

Patients with inconclusive HIV serology, but no definitive diagnosis or manifestations of the illness may be assigned code 795.71, Inconclusive serologic test for Human Immunodeficiency Virus [HIV]

10.8 Testing for HIV

If the patient is asymptomatic but wishes to know his/her HIV status, use code V73.89, Screening for other specified viral disease. Use code V69.8, Other problems related to lifestyle, as a secondary code if an asymptomatic patient is in a known high-risk group for HIV. Should a patient with signs or symptoms or illness, or a confirmed HIV-related diagnosis be tested for HIV, code the signs and symptoms or the diagnosis. An additional counseling code V65.44 may be used if counseling is provided during the encounter for the test.

When the patient returns to be informed of his/her HIV test results use code V65.44, HIV counseling, if the results of the test are negative. If the results are positive but the patient is asymptomatic use code V08, Asymptomatic HIV infection. If the results are positive and the patient is asymptomatic use code 042, HIV infection, with codes for the HIV-related symptoms or diagnosis. The HIV counseling code may also be used if counseling is provided for patients with positive test results.

11. GUIDELINES FOR CODING EXTERNAL CAUSES OF INJURIES, POISONINGS, AND ADVERSE EFFECTS OF DRUGS (E Codes)

Introduction

These guidelines are provided for those who are currently collecting E codes in order that there will be standardization in the process. If your institution plans to begin collecting E codes, these guidelines are to be applied. The use of E codes is supplemental to the application of basic ICD-9-CM codes. E codes are never to be recorded as principal diagnosis (first listed in the outpatient setting) and are not required for reporting to the Centers for Medicare and Medicaid Services.

Injuries are a major cause of mortality, morbidity, and disability. In the United States, the care of patients who suffer intentional and unintentional injuries and poisonings contributes significantly to the increase in medical care costs. External causes of injury and poisoning codes (E codes) are intended to provide data for injury research and evaluation of injury prevention strategies. E codes capture how the injury or poisoning happened (cause), the intent (unintentional or accidental; or intentional, such as suicide or assault), and the place where the event occurred. Some major categories of E codes include:

transport accidents

poisoning and adverse effects of drugs, medicinal substances and biologicals

accidental falls

accidents caused by fire and flames

accidents due to natural and environmental factors

late effects of accidents, assaults, or self-injury

assaults or purposely inflicted injury

suicide or self-inflicted injury

These guidelines apply for the coding and collection of E code from records in hospitals, outpatient clinics, emergency departments, other ambulatory care settings and physician offices except when other specific guidelines apply. (See Reporting Diagnostic Guidelines for Hospital-based Outpatient Services/Reporting Requirements for Physician Billing.)

11.1 General E Code Coding Guidelines

A. An E code may be used with any code in the range of 001-V82.9 which indicates an injury, poisoning, or adverse effect due to an external cause.

B. Assign the appropriate E-code for all initial treatments of an injury, poisoning, or adverse effect of drugs.

C. Use a late effect E code for subsequent visits when a late effect of the initial injury or poisoning is being treated. There is no late effect E code for adverse effects of drugs.

D. Use the full range of E codes to completely describe the cause, the intent and the place of occurrence, if applicable, for all injuries, poisonings, and adverse effects of drugs.

E. Assign as many E codes as necessary to fully explain each cause. If only one E code can be recorded, assign the E code most related to the principal diagnosis.

F. The selection of the appropriate E code is guided by the Index to External Causes which is located after the Alphabetic Index to diseases and by Inclusion and Exclusion notes in the Tabular List.

G. An E code can never be a principal (first listed) diagnosis.

11.2 Place of Occurrence Guideline

Use an additional code from category E849 to indicate the Place of Occurrence for injuries and poisonings. The Place of Occurrence describes the place where the event occurred and not the patient's activity at the time of the event.

Do not use E849.9 if the place of occurrence is not stated.

11.3 Poisonings and Adverse Effects of Drugs, Medicinal and Biological Substances Guidelines

A. Do not code directly from the Table of Drugs and Chemicals. Always refer back to the Tabular List.

B. Use as many codes as necessary to describe completely all drugs, medicinal or biological substances.

C. If the same E code would describe the causative agent for more than one adverse reaction, assign the code only once.

D. If two or more drugs, medicinal or biological substances are reported, code each individually unless the combination code is listed in the Table of Drugs and Chemicals. In that case, assign the E code for the combination.

E. When a reaction results from the interaction of a drug(s) and alcohol, use poisoning codes and E codes for both.

F. If the reporting format limits the number of E codes that can be used in reporting clinical data, code the one most related to the principal diagnosis. Include at least one from each category (cause, intent, place) if possible.

If there are different fourth digit codes in the same three digit category, use the code for "Other specified" of that category. If there is no "Other specified" code in that category, use the appropriate "Unspecified" code in that category.

If the codes are in different three digit categories, assign the appropriate E code for other multiple drugs and medicinal substances.

11.4 Multiple Cause E Code Coding Guidelines

If two or more events cause separate injuries, an E code should be assigned for each cause. The first listed E code will be selected in the following order:

E codes for child and adult abuse take priority over all other E codes—see Child and Adult abuse guidelines

E codes for cataclysmic events take priority over all other E codes except child and adult abuse

E codes for transport accidents take priority over all other E codes except cataclysmic events and child and adult abuse

The first list E code should correspond to the cause of the most serious diagnosis due to an assault, accident, or self-harm, following the order of hierarchy in the preceding list.

11.5 Child and Adult Abuse Guideline

A. When the cause of an injury or neglect is intentional child or adult abuse, the first listed E code should be assigned from categories E960-E968, Homicide and injury purposely inflicted by other persons (except category E967). An E code from category E967, Child and adult battering and other maltreatment, should be added as an additional code to identify the perpetrator, if known.

B. In cases of neglect when the intent is determined to be accidental E code E904.0, Abandonment or neglect of infant and helpless person, should be the first listed E code.

11.6 Unknown or Suspected Intent Guideline

A. If the intent (accident, self-harm, assault) of the cause of an injury or poisoning is unknown or unspecified, code the intent as undetermined E980-E989.

B. If the intent (accident, self-harm, assault) of the cause of an injury or poisoning is questionable, probable or suspected, code the intent as undetermined E980-E989.

11.7 Undetermined Cause

When the intent of an injury or poisoning is known, but the cause is unknown, use codes: E928.9, Unspecified accident, E958.9, Suicide and self-inflicted injury by unspecified means, and E968.9, Assault by unspecified means.

These E codes should rarely be used as the documentation in the medical record, in both the inpatient and outpatient settings, should normally provide sufficient detail to determine the cause of the injury.

11.8 Late Effects of External Cause Guidelines

A. Late effect E codes exist for injuries and poisonings but not for adverse effects of drugs, misadventures, and surgical complications.

B. A late effect E code (E929, E959, E969, E977, E989, or E999) should be used with any report of a late effect or sequela resulting from a previous injury or poisoning (905-909).

C. A late effect E code should never be used with a related current nature of injury code.

11.9 Misadventures and Complications of Care Guidelines

A. Assign a code in the range of E870-E876 if misadventures are stated by the physician.

B. Assign a code in the range of E878-E879 if the physician attributes an abnormal reaction or later complication to a surgical or medical procedure, but does not mention misadventure at the time of the procedure as the cause of the reaction.

12. DIAGNOSTIC CODING AND REPORTING GUIDELINES FOR OUTPATIENT SERVICES (HOSPITAL-BASED AND PHYSICIAN OFFICE) Revised October 1, 1995

Introduction

These revised coding guidelines for outpatient diagnoses have been approved for use by hospitals/physicians in coding and reporting hospital-based outpatient services and physician office visits. These guidelines replace the official guidelines on the October 1, 1994 CD-ROM.

Information about the use of certain abbreviations, punctuation, symbols, and other conventions used in the ICD-9-CM Tabular List (code numbers and titles), can be found in the section at the beginning of the ICD-9-CM on "Conventions Used in the Tabular List." Information about the correct sequence to use in finding a code is described in the "Introduction" to the Alphabetic Index of ICD-9-CM.

The terms encounter and visit are often used interchangeably in describing outpatient service contacts and, therefore, appear together in these guidelines without distinguishing one from the other.

Coding guidelines for outpatient and physician reporting of diagnoses will vary in a number of instances from those for inpatient diagnoses, recognizing that

The Uniform Hospital Discharge Data Set (UHDDS) definition of principal diagnosis applies only to inpatients in acute, short-term, general hospitals.

Coding guidelines for inconclusive diagnoses (probable, suspected, rule out, etc.) were developed for inpatient reporting and do not apply to outpatients.

Diagnoses often are not established at the time of the initial encounter/ visit. It may take two or more visits before the diagnosis is confirmed.

The most critical rule involves beginning the search for the correct code assignment through the Alphabetic Index. Never begin searching initially in the Tabular List as this will lead to coding errors.

Basic Coding Guidelines for Outpatient Services

A. The appropriate code or codes from 001.0 through V82.9 must be used to identify diagnoses, symptoms, conditions, problems, complaints, or other reason(s) for the encounter/visit.

B. For accurate reporting of ICD-9-CM diagnosis codes, the documentation should describe the patient's condition, using terminology which includes specific diagnoses as well as symptoms, problems, or reasons for the encounter. There are ICD-9-CM codes to describe all of these.

C. The selection of codes 001.0 through 999.9 will frequently be used to describe the reason for the encounter. These codes are from the section of ICD-9-CM for the classification of diseases and injuries (e.g., infectious and parasitic diseases; neoplasms; symptoms, signs, and ill-defined conditions, etc.).

D. Codes that describe symptoms and signs, as opposed to diagnoses, are acceptable for reporting purposes when an established diagnosis has not been diagnosed (confirmed) by the physician. Chapter 16 of ICD-9-CM, Symptoms, Signs, and Ill-Defined Conditions (codes 780.0-799.9) contain many, but not all codes for symptoms.

E. ICD-9-CM provides codes to deal with encounters for circumstances other than a disease or injury. The Supplementary Classification of Factors Influencing Health Status and Contact with Health Services (V01.0-V82.9) is provided to deal with occasions when circumstances other than a disease or injury are recorded as diagnosis or problems.

F. ICD-9-CM is composed of codes with either 3, 4, or 5 digits. Codes with 3 digits are included in ICD-9-CM as the heading of a category of codes that may be further subdivided by the use of fourth and/or fifth digits which provide greater specificity.

A three-digit code is to be used only if it is not further subdivided. Where fourth-digit subcategories and/or fifth-digit subclassifications are provided, they must be assigned. A code is invalid if it has not been coded to the full number of digits required for that code.

G. List first the ICD-9-CM code for the diagnosis, condition, problem, or other reason for encounter/visit shown in the medical record to be chiefly responsible for the services provided. List additional codes that describe any coexisting conditions.

H. Do not code diagnoses documented as "probable," "suspected," "questionable," "rule out," or "working diagnosis." Rather, code the condition(s) to the highest degree of certainty for that encounter/visit, such as symptoms, signs, abnormal test results, or other reason for the visit.

Please note: This is contrary to the coding practices used by hospitals and medical record departments for coding the diagnosis of hospital inpatients.

I. Chronic diseases treated on an ongoing basis may be coded and reported as many times as the patient receives treatment and care for the condition(s).

J. Code all documented conditions that coexist at the time of the encounter/visit, and require or affect patient care treatment or management. Do not code conditions that were previously treated and no longer exist. However, history codes (V10-V19) may be used as secondary codes if the historical condition or family history has an impact on current care or influences treatment.

K. For patients receiving diagnostic services only during an encounter/visit, sequence first the diagnosis, condition, problem, or other reason for encounter/visit shown in the medical record to be chiefly responsible for the outpatient services provided during the encounter/visit. Codes for other diagnoses (e.g., chronic conditions) may be sequenced as additional diagnoses.

L. For patients receiving therapeutic services only during an encounter/visit, sequence first the diagnosis, condition, problem, or other reason for encounter/visit shown in the medical record to be chiefly responsible for the outpatient services provided during the encounter/visit. Codes for other diagnoses (e.g., chronic conditions) may be sequenced as additional diagnoses.

M. The only exception to this rule is that for patients receiving chemotherapy, radiation therapy, or rehabilitation, the appropriate V code for the service is listed first, and the diagnosis or problem for which the service is being performed listed second.

N. For patients receiving preoperative evaluations only, sequence a code from category V72.8, Other specified examinations, to describe the pre-op consultations. Assign a code for the condition to describe the reason for the surgery as an additional diagnosis. Code also any findings related to the pre-op evaluation.

O. For ambulatory surgery, code the diagnosis for which the surgery was performed. If the postoperative diagnosis is known to be different from the preoperative diagnosis at the time the diagnosis is confirmed, select the postoperative diagnosis for coding, since it is the most definitive.

Exercise Answers

Chapter 1

Exercise 1–1

1. American Medical Association
2. Current Procedural Terminology
3. services
4. 1966
5. 1983

Exercise 1–2

1. c
2. a
3. e
4. b
5. d
6. Appendix B
7. Appendix F
8. Appendix E

Exercise 1–3

1. Surgery
2. Respiratory System
3. Nose
4. Excision

Exercise 1–4

1. A concise statement describing the symptom, problem, condition, diagnosis, or other factor that is the reason for the encounter, usually stated in the patient's words
2. yes
3. interpreting physician
4. a physician
5. 99070

Exercise 1–5

1. those codes that have full description (or similar wording)
2. those codes that include their own description as well as that portion of the stand-alone code description found before the semicolon in a preceding code (or similar wording)

3. alternative anatomic site, alternative procedure, or description of the extent of service (in any order and similar wording)

Exercise 1–6

1. 09962

2. 43820-62 or 43820 and 09962

3. -50, 09950

4. -78, 09978

5. -57, 09957

6. -51, 09951

7. -66, 09966

8. -80, 09980

Exercise 1–7

1. 69799, 29909 (note that this code ends in 09, not the standard 99), 43499

2. 88299, 81099, 84999

3. 99199

4. 77799, 78999

Exercise 1–8

no answer necessary

Exercise 1–9

1.

   a. Emergency

   b. 99288 (Emergency Department Services, Physician Direction of Advanced Life Support)

2.

   a. fracture

   b. 27238 (Fracture, Femur, Intertrochanteric, Closed Treatment)

3.

   a. removal

   b. 47480 (Removal, Calculi, Gallbladder)

4.

   a. lung

   b. 32141 (Lung, Bullae, Excision)

Exercise 1–10

1. *See* Dialysis

2. *See* Antinuclear Antibodies (ANA)

3. *See* Radius; Ulna; Wrist

Chapter 2

Exercise 2–1

1. office

2. office visit or other outpatient service

3. new

4. 99201

5. five

6. five

Exercise 2–2

1. problem focused

2. expanded problem focused

3. detailed

4. comprehensive

5. comprehensive

Exercise 2–3

1. problem focused

2. expanded problem focused

3. detailed

4. comprehensive

5. comprehensive

Exercise 2–4

1. OS

2. BA

3. OS

4. OS

5. OS

6. OS

7. OS

8. BA

9. BA

10. BA

11. OS

12. OS

13. BA

14. OS

15. BA

16. BA

17. OS

18. OS

19. OS

20. OS

Note: Some terms—thorax, lungs, heart, vagina, blood vessels, neurologic—are specifically presented in the text as being a body area or an organ system. For other terms, you have to make the connection; for example, the thorax is examined as a body area but the lungs are examined as an organ system.

21.

    a. problem focused (or expanded problem focused if you believe the aching and ringing are pertinent components of a system review)

    b. problem focused

22.

CC:	Cold
HPI:	Dry, hacking cough and nasal congestion for the past 6 days and a fever the past 3 days. (Note that duration is 9 days, quality is dry, hacking.)
PFSH:	Personal and family history negative for respiratory problems
ROS:	Respiratory system (lungs clear to percussion and auscultation) and ENT (ears, normal; nose, mucous membranes inflamed with postnasal [throat] phlegm) (two organ systems); chest and head (two body areas)

    a. expanded problem focused (Note: There were the CC, expanded HPI, extended ROS, and pertinent family history.)

General survey:	In minor distress
Vital signs:	Temperature, 100°F; blood pressure, 150/90; pulse 93 and regular.
Body Areas/Organ Systems:	Head and neck (two body areas) and respiratory and ears (two organ systems)

    b. problem focused or expanded problem focused

Exercise 2–5

1. limited

2. limited (The data could be moderate if the patient has brought records that the physician would have to review.)

3. moderate

4. low

5. 99203

6. straightforward or low

7. low, as it could be bronchitis, influenza, an upper respiratory infection, etc. Risks are increased for the elderly.

Exercise 2–6

1. b

2. e

3. d

4. c

5. a

Exercise 2–7

1. detailed, detailed, low

2. comprehensive, comprehensive, moderate

3. comprehensive, comprehensive, high

4. 99203 (Office and/or Other Outpatient Services, Office Visit, New Patient)

5. 99201 (Office and/or Other Outpatient Services, Office Visit, New Patient)

6. 99205 (Office and/or Other Outpatient Services, Office Visit, New Patient) (Note that some coders may use 90801, Psychiatric Diagnostic or Evaluation Interview Procedures.)

7. 99203 or 99204 (Office and/or Other Outpatient Services, Office Visit, New Patient)

8. 99202 (Office and/or Other Outpatient Services, Office Visit, New Patient)

Exercise 2–8

1. yes

2. 99212 (Office and/or Other Outpatient Services, Office Visit, Established Patient)

3. 99211 (Office and/or Other Outpatient Services, Office Visit, Established Patient)

4. 99215 (Office and/or Other Outpatient Services, Office Visit, Established Patient)

5. 99213 (Office and/or Other Outpatient Services, Office Visit, Established Patient) (Note: Although the MDM complexity is at the level of code 99214, the history and examination were at the level of code 99213; because two of the three key components must be documented in order to use 99214, you must assign the lower level, 99213.)

6. 99212 (Office and/or Other Outpatient Services, Office Visit, Established Patient)

7. 99213 (Office and/or Other Outpatient Services, Office Visit, Established Patient)

Exercise 2–9

1. 99219 (E/M, Hospital Services, Observation Care)

Exercise 2–10

1. 99221 (Hospital Service, Initial Hospital Care)

2. 99223 (Hospital Service, Initial Hospital Care)

3. comprehensive, moderate

4. 99221 (Hospital Service, Inpatient Services, Initial Hospital Care)

Exercise 2–11

1. 30 minutes or less, more than 30 minutes

2. no

Exercise 2–12

1. 99244 (Consultation, Office and/or Other Outpatient)

2. 99241 (Consultation, Office and/or Other Outpatient)

3. 99242 (Consultation, Office and/or Other Outpatient)

4. 99241 (Consultation, Office and/or Other Outpatient)

5. 99244 (Consultation, Office and/or Other Outpatient)

6. 99252 (Consultation, Inpatient, Initial)

7. 99255 (Consultation, Inpatient, Initial) (Modifier -57 would also be used to indicate the decision to perform surgery.)

8. 99252 (Consultation, Inpatient, Initial)

9. 99255 (Consultation, Inpatient, Initial)

10. 99263 (Consultation, Follow-up, Inpatient; Established Patient)

11. 99263 (Consultation, Follow-up, Inpatient; Established Patient)

12. 99274 (Consultation, Confirmatory) (Modifier -32 would also be used to indicate a mandatory confirmatory consultation.)
13. 99272 (Consultation, Confirmatory)
14. 99274 (Consultation, Confirmatory) (Modifier -32 would also be used to indicate a mandatory confirmatory consultation.)

Exercise 2–13

1. self-limited or minor
2. high
3. low to moderate
4. moderate
5. 99285 (Emergency Department Services)
6. 99285 (Emergency Department Services)
7. 99283 (Emergency Department Services)
8. 99288 (Emergency Department, Physician Direction of Advanced Life Support)

Exercise 2–14

1. 99291 (Critical Care Services)
2. no
3. 99291 × 1 and 99292 × 4 (80 minutes of care) (Critical Care Services)

Exercise 2–15

1. very low birth weight
2. Subsequent Hospital Care
3. 99295 (Critical Care Services, Neonatal, Initial)
4. yes
5. 99295 (Critical Care Services, Neonatal, Initial)

Exercise 2–16

1. 50 minutes
2. 99303 (Nursing Facility Services, Comprehensive Assessment, New or Established Patient)
3. b
4. c
5. a
6. 99312 (Nursing Facility Services, Subsequent Care, New or Established Patient)

Exercise 2–17

1. 99347 (Home Services, Established Patient)

Exercise 2–18

1. no
2. no
3. no
4. whether the patient is an inpatient or an outpatient
5. no
6. no

Exercise 2–19

1. approximately 30 minutes and approximately 60 minutes
2. (a) simple or brief; (b) intermediate; (c) complex or lengthy

Exercise 2–20

1. Age
2. -25

Exercise 2–21

1. Basic Life and/or Disability Evaluation Services
2. Work-Related or Medical Disability Evaluation Services
3. whether the treating physician or a physician other than the treating physician conducted the evaluation
4. 99455 (E/M, Insurance Exam)

Exercise 2–22

1. 99201 (Office and/or Other Outpatient Services, Office Visits, New Patient)
2. 99212 (Office and Other Outpatient Visits, Office Visits, Established Patient)
3. 99211 (Office and/or Other Outpatient Services, Office Visits, Established Patient)
4. 99303 (Nursing Facility Services, Comprehensive Assessment, New or Established Patient)
5. 99202 (Office and/or Other Outpatient Services, Office Visits, New Patient)
6. 99211 (Office and/or Other Outpatient Services, Office Visits, Established Patient)
7. 99285 (Emergency Department Services)
8. 99291 (Critical Care Services)
9. 99291 × 1 (Critical Care Services) and 99292 × 1 (Critical Care Services)
10. 99214 (Office and/or Other Outpatient Services)
11. 99255 (Consultation, Initial Inpatient)

Chapter 3

Exercise 3–1

1. Head; Neck; Thorax; Intrathoracic; Spine and Spinal Cord; Upper Abdomen; Lower Abdomen; Perineum; Pelvis; Upper Leg; Knee and Popliteal Area; Lower Leg; Shoulder and Axilla; Upper Arm and Elbow; Forearm, Wrist, and Hand; Radiological Procedures; Burn Excision or Debridement; Obstetrics; Other Procedures.
2. Radiologic Procedures, Burn Excisions or Debridement, Obstetrics, and Other Procedures
3. absence of pain
4. induction or administration of a drug to obtain partial or complete loss of sensation (or similar wording)
5. general, regional, and local
6. conscious
7. Medicine

Exercise 3–2

1. -22
2. -23
3. -22
4. -23
5. -47

Exercise 3–3

1. P2
2. P3
3. 99116

Exercise 3–4

1. 01999 (Anesthesia, Unlisted Services and Procedures)
2. Anesthesia, Thyroid, 00322
3. Anesthesia, Cesarean Delivery, 01961
4. Anesthesia, Prostate, 00914
5. Anesthesia, Cleft Palate Repair, 00172
6. Anesthesia, Ankle, 01472
7. $78.85 (B = 3, T = 1, M = 1; total = 5; 5 × $15.77)
8.
    a. $184.32 (B = 5, T = 4, M = 0; total = 9; 9 × $20.48)
    b. $144.09 (B = 5, T = 4, M = 0; total = 9; 9 × $16.01)
9.
    a. $151.56 (B = 7, T = 2, M = 0; total = 9; 9 × $16.84)
    b. $168.40 (B = 7, T = 3, M = 0; total = 10; 10 × $16.84)

Exercise 3–5

1. 17274 (Destruction, Skin, Lesion, Malignant) (Note that 17274 is more resource-intensive and therefore is listed first and without the modifier.) 17264-51 (Destruction, Skin, Lesion, Malignant)
2. 58150 (Hysterectomy, Abdominal, Total); 57250-51 (Vagina, Repair, Rectocele, Posterior)
3. 28450 × 2 units or 28450 and 28450-51 (Tarsal Joint, Fracture, without Manipulation)
4. 99215-21 (Office and/or Other Outpatient Services, Office Visit, Established Patient)
5. 99215 (Office and/or Other Outpatient Services, Office Visit, Established Patient)
6. -26
7. -50
8. 27447 (Arthroplasty, Knee)
9. 27447 × 2 or 27447 and 27447-50
10. 19200 × 2 or 19200 and 19200-50

Exercise 3–6

1. 43124-54 (Esophagectomy, Total)
2. 19220-55 (Mastectomy, Radical)

3. 19220-56 (Mastectomy, Radical)
4. -52

Exercise 3–7
1. -91
2. -62
3. -66
4. -80
5. -81

Exercise 3–8
1. -78
2. -47
3. -23
4. -78

Exercise 3–9
1. -79
2. -58
3. -99
4. -90
5. -24
6. -25
7. -77
8. -32

Chapter 4
Exercise 4–1
1. General
2. Integumentary System
3. Musculoskeletal System
4. Respiratory System
5. Cardiovascular System
6. Hemic and Lymphatic Systems
7. Mediastinum and Diaphragm
8. Digestive System
9. Urinary System
10. Male Genital System
11. Intersex Surgery
12. Female Genital System
13. Maternity Care and Delivery
14. Endocrine System
15. Nervous System
16. Eye and Ocular Adnexa
17. Auditory System
18. Operating Microscope

Exercise 4–2

1. 20999
2. 69949
3. 17999
4. 27899
5. 64999
6. 67999

Exercise 4–3

1. pre-, intra-, and postoperative services, or similar wording
2. no
3. no

Exercise 4–4

1. 11056 (Lesion, Skin, Paring/Curettement)
2. 11200 (Lesion, Skin Tags, Removal)
3. 11311 (Lesion, Skin, Shaving)

Exercise 4–5

1. 13121 (Repair, Wound, Complex)
2. 13101 for complex repair of abdomen (Repair, Wound, Complex); 12004-51 for 12-cm simple repair of back, forearm, and neck added together (Repair, Wound, Simple). (Note that the same types of repair are combined—back (trunk), forearm (extremities), and neck are all included in the code description for 12004.)
3. 12034 for the 10.7-cm intermediate forearm repair (Wound, Repair, Intermediate); 12002-51 for the 3.1-cm scalp repair (Repair, Wound, Simple).
4. 15120 for the cheek graft (Skin Graft and Flap, Split Graft); 15100-51 and 15101 for the upper chest graft (Skin Graft and Flaps, Split Graft) (Also, note that 15101 is an add-on code and does not have a modifier -51.) 15000 for site preparation of first 100 cm² and 15001 × 2 for the second 200 cm² of site preparation.
5. 14041 (Skin, Adjacent Tissue Transfer)
6. 14040 (Skin, Adjacent Tissue Transfer) (Note that a Z-plasty is a form of adjacent tissue transfer. The excision is included in the adjacent tissue transfer code.)
7. 15732 (Skin, Myocutaneous Flaps) (Note that modifier -58 could also be used to indicate staged procedure.)
8. 16015 × 5 debridement with anesthesia for each day of the first week, and 16030 × 6 for debridement without anesthesia for every other day of the next 2 weeks (Burn, Dressings)

Exercise 4–6

1. 17000 (Destruction, Skin, Benign)
2. 17000 (Destruction, Skin, Benign), 17003 × 13 (Destruction, Skin, Benign)
3. 17310 (Mohs' Micrographic Surgery)

Exercise 4–7

1. 19000 (Breast, Cyst, Puncture Aspiration)
2. 19180 and 19180-50 (Breast; Removal; Simple, Complete)
3. 19240 (Breast, Removal, Modified Radical)
4. 19290 (Breast, Needle Wire Placement)
5. 19350 (Breast, Reconstruction, Nipple, Areola)

Chapter 5

Exercise 5–1

1. 21310 (Nasal Bone, Closed Treatment)
2. 21800 (Rib, Closed Treatment)
3. 28675 (Dislocation, Interphalangeal, Open Treatment)
4. 27792 (Fracture, Fibula, Open Treatment)
5. 27500 (Fracture, Femur, Closed Treatment)
6. 27235 (Fracture, Femur, Percutaneous Fixation)
7. 23670 (Fracture, Humerus, with Dislocation, Open Treatment)
8. 21453 (Fracture, Mandible, Closed Treatment, Interdental Fixation)
9. 25611 (Colles Fracture)
10. 27840 (Ankle, Dislocation, Closed Treatment)

Exercise 5–2

1. 20103 (Wound, Exploration, Extremity)
2. 20838 (Replantation, Foot)
3. 21015 (Tumor, Resection, Face)
4. 20974 (Electrical Stimulation, Bone Healing, Noninvasive)
5. 20206 (Biopsy, Muscle)
6. 20600 (Aspiration, Joint)

Exercise 5–3

1. 20965 (Cast, Long Arm); 90070 (Supply, Materials), or A4590 (Special Casting Materials)
2. 29425 (Cast, Walking)
3. 29705 (Cast, Removal)
4. 29530 (Strapping, Knee)
5. 29345 (Cast, Long Leg)

Exercise 5–4

1. 29898 (Arthroscopy, Surgical, Ankle)
2. 29870 (Arthroscopy, Diagnostic, Knee)
3. 29805 (Arthroscopy, Shoulder)
4. 29850 (Fracture, Knee, Arthroscopic Treatment)
5. 29891 (Arthroscopy, Surgical, Ankle)

Chapter 6

Exercise 6–1

1. 31256 (Antrostomy, Sinus, Maxillary)
2. 31530 (Laryngoscopy, Direct)

3. 31628 (Bronchoscopy, Biopsy)

4. 32605 (Thoracoscopy, Diagnostic, without Biopsy)

5. 32663 (Thoracoscopy, Surgical, with Lobectomy)

Exercise 6–2

1. 30100 (Biopsy, Nose, Intranasal)

2. 30420 (Rhinoplasty, Primary)

3. 30901 (Epistaxis)

4. 30520 (Septoplasty)

5. 30300 (Removal, Foreign Bodies, Nose)

Exercise 6–3

1. 31000 × 2 or 31000 and 31000-50 (Sinuses, Maxillary, Irrigation)

2. 31070 (Sinusotomy, Frontal Sinus, Exploratory)

3. 31090 (Sinusotomy, Combined)

4. 31030 (Sinusotomy, Maxillary, Incision)

5. 31201 (Ethmoidectomy)

Exercise 6–4

1. 31320 (Laryngotomy, Diagnostic)

2. 31580 (Laryngoplasty, Laryngeal Web)

3. 31500 (Endotracheal Tube, Intubation)

4. 31368 (Laryngectomy, Partial)

5. 31390 (Pharyngolaryngectomy)

Exercise 6–5

1. 31605 (Tracheostomy, Emergency)

2. 31785 (Trachea; Tumor; Excision, Cervical)

3. 31715 (Bronchography; Injection, Transtracheal)

4. 31600 (Tracheostomy, Planned)

5. 31717 (Bronchial Brush Biopsy, with Catheterization)

Exercise 6–6

1. 32095 (Biopsy, Lung, Thoracotomy)

2. 32405 (Biopsy, Lung, Needle)

3. 32480 (Lobectomy, Lung) and 32501 (Bronchoplasty). (Note that code 32501 is an add-on code and does not need modifier -51.)

4. 32520 (Reconstruction, Lung)

5. 32200 (Pneumonostomy)

Chapter 7

Exercise 7–1

1. Pericardium, Veins

2. internal

3. Medicine, Surgery, Radiology

4. invasive or interventional

5. electrophysiology

6. nuclear

Exercise 7–2

1. 33207 (Pacemaker, Insertion)
2. This is not coded because the notes above the pacemaker codes state that procedure includes repositioning or replacement within the first 14 days.
3. 33214 (Pacemaker, Conversion)
4. 33010 (Pericardiocentesis)
5. 33120 (Tumor, Heart, Excision)

Exercise 7–3

1. 33430 (Mitral Valve, Replacement)
2. 33405 (Aorta, Valve, Replacement) (Note that a prosthetic valve, and not a homograft valve, is used.)
3. 33251 (Heart, Arrhythmogenic Focus, Destruction)
4. 33282 (Implantation, Cardiac Event Recorder)

Exercise 7–4

1. 33511 (Bypass Graft, Coronary Artery, Venous Graft)
2. 33534 (Coronary Artery Bypass Graft, Arterial)
3. 33519 (Coronary Artery Bypass Graft, Arterial Venous)

Exercise 7–5

1. 34201 (Thrombectomy, Popliteal Artery)
2. 34001 (Embolectomy, Carotid Artery)
3. 35875 (Thrombectomy, Bypass Graft, Other Than Hemodialysis Graft or Fistula)

Exercise 7–6

1. 35506 (Bypass Graft, Carotid Artery)
2. 35556 (Bypass Graft, Femoral Artery)
3. 35650 (Bypass Graft, Axillary Artery)
4. 35141 (Aneurysm Repair, Femoral Artery)
5. 36246 and 36248 (Catheterization, Abdominal Artery) (Note that modifier -51 is not used with add-on code 36248.)

Exercise 7–7

1. 92950 (CPR)
2. 93015 (Stress Tests, Cardiovascular)
3. 92982 and 92984 × 2 (Angioplasty, Percutaneous Transluminal Angioplasty)
4. 93278-26 (Electrocardiography, Signal-Averaged)

Exercise 7–8

1. Catheterization procedure 93501 (Catheterization, Cardiac, Right Heart); Injection procedure 93542 (Catheterization, Cardiac, Injection); Supervision, interpretation, and report for injection procedure 93555 (Catheterization, Cardiac, Imaging)
2. 93511 (Catheterization, Cardiac, Left Heart); 93543 (Catheterization, Cardiac, Injection); 93555 (Catheterization, Cardiac, Imaging)
3. False; they are already bundled into the codes.
4. True
5. False; most codes are modifier -5–exempt.

Exercise 7–9

1. 93600 (Electrophysiology Procedures)
2. 93622 (Electrophysiology Procedures)
3. 93720 (Plethysmography, Total Body)

Exercise 7–10

1. Injection procedure for angiography 36215 (Catheterization, Brachiocephalic Artery); angiography 75658 (Angiography, Brachial Artery); contrast material 99070 (Supply, Material)
2. 36215 (Artery, Thoracic, Catheterization); 75658 (Angiography, Brachial, Artery)
3. 36246, injection (Artery, Abdomen, Catheterization); 75625, abdominal angiography (Aortography, Serial); 99070, supply of contrast material (Supply, Materials)
4. 75553 (MRI, Heart)

Chapter 8

Exercise 8–1

1. 57061 (Destroy, Vaginal Lesions, Simple)
2. 56605, 56606 × 2 or 56606 and 56606 (Vulva, Perineum, Biopsy) (Note that the code 56605 is for the first lesion, and 56606 is for *each* additional lesion.)
3. 57305 (Vagina, Repair, Fistula, Rectovaginal)
4. 57520 (Cervix, Conization) (Note that dilation and curettage is not coded separately because it is included in the description of the conization.)
5. 58940 (Oophorectomy) (Note that the salpingectomy is not coded because the words "separate procedure" appear after code 58700 in the CPT manual, and since the salpingectomy was done as a part of a more major procedure [oophorectomy], the salpingectomy is bundled into the more major procedure.)
6. c
7. b
8. d
9. a

Exercise 8–2

1. 59151 (Laparoscopy, Ectopic Pregnancy with Salpingectomy and/or Oophorectomy)
2. 59409 (Vaginal Delivery, Delivery only); 59412 (External Cephalic Version) (Note that the version is stated "list in addition", therefore, modifier -51 is not necessary.)
3. 59320 (Cerclage, Cervix, Vaginal)

Chapter 9

Exercise 9–1

1. 54520 (Orchiectomy, Simple) (Note that the terms "simple" and "radical" are based on the interpretation of the physician.)
2. 54820 (Epididymis, Exploration, Biopsy)
3. 55000 (Tunica Vaginalis, Hydrocele, Aspiration)

4. 54065 (Penis, Lesion, Destruction, Extensive)

5. 55400 (Vas Deferens, Repair, Suture)

Exercise 9–2

1. 51000 (Aspiration, Bladder)

2. 52332 (Cystourethroscopy, Insertion, Indwelling Urethral Stent)

3. 50065 (Nephrolithotomy) (Note that the term "secondary" means that the procedure is being repeated. Some may code this 50060-76.)

4. 53520 (Urethra, Repair, Fistula)

5. 53405 (Urethra, Repair, Fistula)

Exercise 9–3

1. 43255 (Hemorrhage; Gastrointestinal, Upper; Endoscopic Control); 43239-51 (Endoscopy, Gastrointestinal, Upper, Biopsy) (Note that you must remember to code to the farthest extent of the procedure.)

2. 45331 (Sigmoidoscopy, Biopsy); the description states biopsy, single or multiple, so only one code is used for multiple (three) biopsies.

3. 45385 (Colonoscopy, Removal, Polyp)

Exercise 9–4

1. surgical communication from the colon to the rectum

2. surgical communication from the ileum to the body surface

3. surgical communication from the large intestine to the body surface

4. surgical communication between segments of intestine

5. 44141 (Colon, Excision, Partial)

6. 44120 (Enterectomy)

Exercise 9–5

1. 47600 (Cholecystectomy) (Note that the exploratory laparotomy is not coded, as it turns into the surgical approach once the cholecystectomy is performed.)

2. 47480 (Cholecystotomy)

3. 49565 (Hernia, Repair, Abdominal Incisional); 49568 (Implantation, Mesh, Hernia Repair) (Note that the mesh code can be used only with incisional hernias and it is stated to "list in addition," so a -51 modifier is not necessary.)

4. 49507 (Hernia, Repair, Inguinal, Incarcerated)

5. 40490 (Biopsy, Lip)

Exercise 9–6

1. 39502 (Diaphragm, Repair, Hernia)

2. 39000 (Mediastinum, Exploration)

3. 39220 (Mediastinum, Tumor, Excision)

4. 39520 (Diaphragm, Repair, Hernia)

Chapter 10

Exercise 10–1

1. 38550 (Lymph Nodes, Hygroma Cystic Axillary/Cervical, Excision)

2. 38100 (Splenectomy, Total)

3. 38200 (Splenoportography, Injection Procedure)

Exercise 10–2

1. 60200 (Thyroid Gland, Cyst, Excision)
2. 60280 (Thyroglossal Duct, Cyst, Excision)
3. 60522 (Thymectomy, Sternal Split/Transthoracic Approach)
4. 60600 (Carotid Body, Lesion, Excision)
5. 60212 (Thyroid Gland, Excision, Partial)

Exercise 10–3

1. 61154 (Burr Hole, Skull, Drainage, Hematoma)
2. 61312 (Craniectomy, Surgical)
3. 61607 (Skull Base Surgery, Middle Cranial Fossa, Extradural); and 61590-51 (Skull Base Surgery, Middle Cranial Fossa, Infratemporal Approach)
4. 62258 (Shunt, Brain, Replacement)

Exercise 10–4

1. 65930 (Eye, Removal, Blood Clot)
2. 67318 (Strabismus, Repair, Superior Oblique Muscle)
3. 67415 (Retina, Repair, Prophylaxis, Detachment)
4. 65772 (Cornea, Repair, Astigmatism)
5. 65105 (Eye, with Muscle or Myocutaneous Flap, Muscles Attached)

Exercise 10–5

1. 69801 (Labyrinthotomy, with/without Cryosurgery)
2. 69436 × 2 or 69436 and 69436-50 (Eustachian Tube, Catheterization)
3. 69950 (Vestibular Nerve, Section, Transcranial Approach)
4. 69310 (Meatoplasty)
5. 69820 (Ear, Inner, Incision)

Chapter 11

Exercise 11–1

1. aorta
2. joint
3. biliary system or pancreas
4. bile ducts
5. urinary bladder
6. lacrimal sac or tear duct sac
7. duodenum or first part of the small intestine
8. heart or heart walls or neighboring tissues
9. subarachnoid space and ventricles of the brain
10. epididymis with contrast material
11. liver
12. uterine cavity and fallopian tubes
13. larynx
14. lymphatic vessels and node
15. spinal cord
16. ureter and renal pelvis

17. salivary duct and branches
18. sinus or sinus tract
19. spleen
20. any part of the urinary system
21. vein and tributaries
22. seminal vesicles

Exercise 11–2

1. position
2. projection
3. anteroposterior
4. posteroanterior
5. right anterior oblique
6. left posterior oblique
7. dorsal
8. ventral
9. right lateral recumbent
10. dorsal decubitus, right lateral

Exercise 11–3

1. separate
2. multiple
3. Diagnostic Radiology, Diagnostic Ultrasound, Radiation Oncology, and Nuclear Medicine (in any order)

Exercise 11–4

1. 76091 (Mammography)
2. 76499 (Radiology, Diagnostic; Unlisted); also see Unlisted Service or Procedure in the index listing.
3. 75605 (Aortography)

Exercise 11–5

1. Head and Neck
2. Chest
3. Abdomen and Retroperitoneum
4. Spinal Canal
5. Pelvis
6. Genitalia
7. Extremities
8. Vascular Studies, no codes
9. Ultrasonic Guidance Procedures

Exercise 11–6

1. 76800 (Ultrasound, Spine)
2. 76604 (Ultrasound, Chest)
3. 76700 (Ultrasound, Abdomen)
4. 76816 (Ultrasound, Pregnant Uterus)
5. 76818 (Ultrasound, Fetus)

Exercise 11–7

1. 77290 (Radiology, Therapeutic, Field Set-Up)
2. 77261 (Radiology, Therapeutic, Planning)

Exercise 11–8

1. 77333 (Radiation Therapy, Treatment Device)
2. 77326 (Radiation Therapy, Dose Plan, Brachytherapy)
3. 77305 (Radiation Therapy, Dose Plan, Teletherapy)

Exercise 11–9

1. 77402 (Radiation Therapy, Treatment Delivery, Single)
2. 77401 (Radiation Therapy, Treatment Delivery, Superficial)
3. 77412 (Radiation Therapy, Treatment Delivery, Three or More Areas)
4. 77407 (Radiation Therapy, Treatment Delivery, Two Areas)
5. 77412 (Radiation Therapy, Treatment Delivery, Three or More Areas)

Exercise 11–10

1. 77427 (Radiation Therapy, Treatment Delivery, Weekly)
2. 77499 (Radiation Therapy, Management, Unlisted Services and Procedures)

Exercise 11–11

1. 77761 (Brachytherapy)
2. 77776 (Brachytherapy)
3. 77789 (Brachytherapy)

Exercise 11–12

1. Gastrointestinal System
2. Endocrine System
3. Hematopoietic, Reticuloendothelial, and Lymphatic System
4. Musculoskeletal System
5. Nervous System

Chapter 12

Exercise 12–1

1. 80076 (Organ or Disease Oriented Panel, Hepatic Function Panel)
2. seven (Blood Tests, Panel, Hepatic Function)
3. yes (Blood Tests, Panel, Obstetric Panel)
4. yes

Exercise 12–2

1. 80102 (Drug, Confirmation)
2. 80162 (Drug Assay, Digoxin)
3. 80150 (Drug Assay, Amikacin)
4. 80178 (Drug Assay, Lithium)

Exercise 12–3

1. 81003 (Urinalysis, Automated)
2. 81015 (Urinalysis, Microscopic)
3. 82040 (Albumin, Serum)

4. 82247 total (Bilirubin, Blood)

5. 82800 (Blood Gases, pH)

6. 84300 (Sodium, Urine)

7. 84550 (Uric Acid, Blood)

Exercise 12–4

1. 85021 (Hemogram, Automated)

2. 85025 (Hemogram, Automated)

3. 85031 (Hemogram, Manual)

4. 85097 (Bone Marrow, Smear)

Exercise 12–5

1. 86039 (Antibody, Antinuclear)

2. 86063 (Antibody, Antistreptolysin O)

3. 86156 (Cold, Agglutinin)

Exercise 12–6

1. 86900 (Blood Typing, ABO only); 86901 (Blood Typing, Rh(O))

2. 86945 × 3 (Blood Products, Irradiation)

Exercise 12–7

1. 87536 (Microbiology)

2. 87651 (Microbiology)

3. 87512 (Microbiology); 87530 (Microbiology); 87482 (Microbiology)

4. 87555 (Microbiology); 87528 (Microbiology); 87490 (Microbiology)

5. 87086 (Microbiology)

6. to identify each organism present in a microbacterial culture

Exercise 12–8

1. 88309 (Pathology, Surgical, Level VI)

2. 88309 (Pathology, Surgical, Level VI)

3. 88305 (Pathology, Surgical, Level IV)

4. 88302 (Pathology, Surgical, Level II)

Chapter 13

Exercise 13–1

1. 90712 (Poliovirus, Vaccine); 90473 (Immunization Administration). (Note that no E/M code is used because the injection is the only service provided to the patient.)

2.

a. 90701 (Vaccines, Diphtheria); 90712 (Poliovirus, Vaccine); 90471 for first injection; and 90473 for the administration service (Immunization Administration) (Note that no E/M code is used because no significant service other than the immunizations were provided.)

b. 99392 (Preventive Medicine, New Patient); 90712 (Poliovirus, Vaccine); 90702 (Vaccines, Diphtheria); 90471 for the first injection; and 90472 for the second injection (Immunization Administration) (Note that E/M code 99392 is used here because the well-baby checkup service provided is significant and separate from the injection service. Modifier -25 would also be added to 99392.)

    c. 90658 (Vaccines, Influenza); 90471 (Immunization Administration, One Vaccine/Toxoid) (Note that no E/M code is used because no other significant service was provided beyond the injection.)

    d. 99202 (Office and/or Other Outpatient Services, New Patient); 90720, combination code for DTP and Hib (Vaccines, Diphtheria); and 90471 (Immunization Administration) (Note: E/M code 99202 is used here because the E/M service provided was significant and separate from the injection service. Modifier -25 would also be added to 99392.)

3. 99392 (Preventive Medicine, Established Patient); 90702 (Vaccines, Diphtheria, Tetanus); 90471 (Immunization Administration, One Vaccine/Toxoid) (Note that an E/M code, 99392, is used here because the E/M service provided was significant and was separate from the injection service. Modifier -25 would also be added to 99392.)

Exercise 13–2

1. 90782 (Injection, IM, Therapeutic) (Note that the injection code does not include the drug provided, so 99070 would also be used to identify the drug supplied (Note that an E/M code is not used here because the service provided is not a significant and separate service from the injection service.)

2. 90780 (Infusion Therapy, Intravenous) (Note that 99070 [Supplies/Materials] would also be coded for the provision of the drug, which in this case is not stated. An E/M code would be reported only if the physician also provides a significant and separately identifiable service in addition to the infusion service.)

Exercise 13–3

1. 90804 (Psychiatric Treatment, Individual Insight-Oriented, Office or Outpatient)

2. 96100 × 2 (Psychiatric Diagnosis, Psychological Testing)

3. 90885 (Psychiatric Diagnosis, Evaluation of Records or Reports)

4. 90801 (Psychiatric Diagnosis, Interview and Evaluation)

Exercise 13–4

1. 90875 (Biofeedback, Psychiatric Treatment)

2. 90901 (Training, Biofeedback)

Exercise 13–5

1. 90919 (Dialysis, End-Stage Renal Disease)

2. 90935 (Dialysis, Hemodialysis)

3. 90947 (Dialysis, Peritoneal)

4. within the lining of the abdominal cavity

5. filtration of blood and waste products through a filter outside the body

6. end-stage renal disease

Exercise 13–6

1. 91032 (Esophagus, Acid Reflux Tests)

2. 91100 (Bleeding Tube, Passage and Placement)

3. 91055 (Intubation, Specimen Collection, Stomach)

4. spontaneous movement study

5. pressure measurements

Exercise 13–7

1. 92014 (Ophthalmology, Diagnostic; Eye Exam; Established Patient)
2. 92070 (Contact Lens Services, Fitting and Prescription)
3. 92120 (Ophthalmology, Diagnostic; Tonography)
4. 92004 (Ophthalmology, Diagnostic; Eye Exam, New Patient)

Exercise 13–8

1. 92592 (Hearing Aid, Check)
2. 92551 (Audiologic Function Tests, Screening)
3. 92511 (Nasopharyngoscopy)
4. 92512 (Nasal Function Study)

Exercise 13–9

1. 93922 (Plethysmography, Extremities) (Note that modifier -52, reduced service, would also be used because the code specifies bilateral service.)
2. 93980 (Vascular Studies, Penile Vessels)

Exercise 13–10

1. 94620 (Pulmonology, Diagnostic; Stress Test, Pulmonary)
2. 94150 (Vital Capacity Measurement)
3. 94060 (Pulmonology, Diagnostic; Spirometry)

Exercise 13–11

1. 95065 (Allergy Tests, Nose Allergy)
2. 95004 × 10 (Allergy Tests, Skin Tests, Allergen Extract) (Note that one unit is used for each test.)
3. 95115 (Allergen Immunotherapy, Allergen, Injection)

Exercise 13–12

1. nasal continuous position airway pressure
2. electroencephalogram
3. electromyogram
4. electro-oculogram
5. 95816 (Electroencephalography)
6. 95863 (Electromyography, Needle; Extremities)
7. 95851 × 2 (both legs) (Range of Motion Test, Extremities)

Exercise 13–13

1. 96110 (Developmental Testing)
2. 96100 (MMPI)
3. 96115 (Cognitive Function Tests)

Exercise 13–14

1. 96440 (Chemotherapy, Pleural Cavity); 96545 (Chemotherapy, Supply of Agent)
2. 96520 (Chemotherapy, Pump Services, Portable); 96545 (Chemotherapy, Supply of Agent)
3. 96400 (Chemotherapy, Subcutaneous); 96545 (Chemotherapy, Supply of Agent)

4. 96410 (Chemotherapy, Intravenous); 96545 (Chemotherapy, Supply of Agent)

5. 96450 (Chemotherapy, CNS); 96545 (Chemotherapy, Supply of Agent)

Exercise 13–15

1. 99241-25 (Consultation, Office and/or Other Outpatient); 96900 (Ultraviolet Light Therapy, for Dermatology)

2. 99244-25 (Consultation, Office and/or Other Outpatient); 96913 (Photochemotherapy)

Exercise 13–16

1. 97010 (Physical Medicine/Therapy/Occupational Therapy, Modality, Hot or Cold Packs)

2. 97520 × 2 (Physical Medicine/Therapy/Occupational Therapy, Prosthetic Training)

3. 97116 × 2 (Physical Medicine/Therapy/Occupational Therapy, Procedures, Gait Training) (Note that the stand-alone code 97110 specifies "each 15 minutes.")

Exercise 13–17

1. 98940 (Chiropractic Treatment, Spinal, Extraspinal)

2. 98925 (Osteopathic Manipulation)

Exercise 13–18

1. 99054 (Special Services, After Hours Medical Services)

2. 99000 (Special Services, Specimen Handling)

3. 99070 (Special Services, Supply of Materials)

Exercise 13–19

1. into the subarachnoid space

2. into a vein

3. into a muscle

4. under the skin

5. through the respiratory system

Exercise 13–20

1.
   a. Current Procedural Terminology, Level I
   b. National Codes, Level II
   c. Local Codes, Level III

2. G, K, Q

3. No

4. J codes

5. oral

6. E codes

7. J7010-J7020

8.
   a. NU
   b. E2
   c. AM

9. IM

10. up to 5 mg

11. J1730

12. E0965

Chapter 14

Exercise 14–1

1. morbidity or sickness; mortality or death rate.

2. ICD-9

3. Clinical Modification

4. Any four of the following six:

    a. facilitate payment of health services

    b. evaluate patients' use of health care facilities (utilization patterns)

    c. study health care costs

    d. research the quality of health care

    e. predict health care trends

    f. plan for future health care needs

5. diagnosis, procedure

Exercise 14–2

1. f

2. g

3. a

4. i

5. h

6. l

7. j

8. e

9. d

10. k

11. b

12. c

13. false

14. true

Exercise 14–3

1. g

2. b

3. i

4. e

5. c

6. d

7. a

8. f

9. h

10. Not Elsewhere Classified (NEC)

11. *See also*

Exercise 14–4

1. 198.81
2. 217

Exercise 14–5

1. 980.0, E980.9
2. 989.89, E980.9
3. 976.0, E858.7
4. due to drug and medicines

Exercise 14–6

1. Endocrine, Nutritional and Metabolic Disease, and Immunity Disorders
2. Disorders of Thyroid Gland
3. Simple and unspecified goiter
4. Goiter, specified as simple

Exercise 14–7

1. 711.06
2. no
3. by adding fourth and fifth digits to the codes

Exercise 14–8

1. Contact, smallpox; V01.3
2. Vaccination, prophylactic, smallpox; V04.1
3. History, malignant neoplasm, tongue; V10.01

Exercise 14–9

1. Derailment, railway; E802.0
2. Accident, machine, not involving collision; E816.0
3. Collision, pedal cycle, nonmotor road vehicle; E821.6
4. Collision, animal being ridden, nonmotor vehicle; E828.2
5. Collision, watercraft, causing, injury; E831.1

Exercise 14–10

1.
   a. Appendix B
   b. Appendix D
   c. Appendix A
   d. Appendix E
   e. Appendix C
2. Appendix D: Industrial Accidents

Exercise 14–11

1. Obstetrical Procedures
2. Miscellaneous Diagnostic and Therapeutic Procedures

Exercise 14–12

1. referring to a vein
2. pertaining to the lungs or pulmonary artery

3. the joining together of two openings

4. pertaining to the heart and lungs

5. circulation that occurs outside of the body

6. a surgical procedure that joins the superior vena cava and pulmonary artery

7. takes over the heart and lung functions of the patient during the surgical procedure

Exercise 14–13

1. 45.24 (Sigmoidoscopy, flexible)

2. 63.73 (Vasectomy)

3. 76.73 (Reduction, fracture, maxilla)

4. 99.04 (Transfusion, packed cells)

5. 21.03 (Cauterization, nose)

Chapter 15

Exercise 15–1

1. category code, subcategory code, subclassification code

2. category code, subcategory code, subclassification code

Exercise 15–2

1. 482.2 (Pneumonia, due to, *Haemophilus influenzae*)

2. 112.0 (Thrush)

3. 008.45 (Enteritis, *Clostridium, difficile*)

4. 437.2 (Hypertension, cerebrovascular disease NEC)

5. 823.82 (Fracture, tibia (closed), with fibula)

Exercise 15–3

1. 601.1 (Prostatitis, chronic); 041.00 (Infection, streptococcal) [in this order]

2. 466.0 (Bronchitis, with acute or subacute); 041.7 (Infection, *Pseudomonas* NEC) [in this order]

3. 250.71 (Diabetes, with gangrene); 785.4 (Gangrene) [in this order]

4. 599.0 (Infection, urinary [tract] NEC); 041.4 (Infection, *Escherichia coli* NEC) [in this order]

5. 277.3 (Cardiomyopathy, amyloid); 425.7 (Cardiomyopathy, metabolic NEC, amyloid)

Exercise 15–4

1. 435.9 (Stroke, in evolution)

2. 291.0 (Impending, delirium tremens) [Check record for documentation of alcoholism.]

3. 640.03 (Threatened, miscarriage)

4. 644.1 (Labor, threatened)

5. 411.1 (Impending, coronary, syndrome)

Exercise 15–5

1. No answer required

2.
   a. Pyelonephritis, acute
   b. Acute, 590.10

  c. 590, Infections of kidney

  d. no

  e. 590.10

  f. because flank pain and hematuria are symptoms of pyelonephritis

Exercise 15–6

1. No answer required
2.

  a. see condition

  b. 710.0 [517.8] This is more specific than the entry under the main term "Erythema."

  c. Diffuse Disease of Connective Tissue

  d. all collagen diseases whose effects are not confined mainly to a single system

  e. lung involvement (517.8) and myopathy (359.6)

  f. 710.**0**

  g. 710.0, 517.8

Exercise 15–7

1. No answer required
2.

  a. open fracture of the right humerus and distal femur

  b. Fracture

  c. humerus

  d. (closed); 812.30 (Note that "open 812.54" is a subterm under "humerus (closed), condyle(s), open 812.54," which is not humerus open but instead is the lower end of the humerus. The diagnosis does not indicate "lower end," so this is not likely to be the correct code. You need to continue down the index list to "open," the subterm of humerus.)

  e. Yes, because the patient record did not specify the exact location of the fracture of the humerus, so the "unspecified part of the humerus, NOS" is as specific as you can get with the information that you have available.

  f. femur

  g. (closed)

  h. distal or distal end

  i. see Fracture, femur, lower end

  j. open

  k. 821.30

  l. yes

Exercise 15–8

1. No answer necessary
2.

  a. menometrorrhagia

  b. 626.2

  c. anemia

  d. 285.1

Exercise 15–9

1. No answer necessary
2.
   a. Fracture
   b. *see also* Fracture, by site; yes
   c. 198.5

Exercise 15–10

1.
   a. 719.46
   b. 717.0
   c. 717.6

Exercise 15–11

1.
   a. V71.4
   b. 913.0
2.
   a. V71.5 (Rape)

Exercise 15–12

1.
   a. 574.10 (Cholecystitis, chronic, with, calculus, gallbladder)
   b. 486 (Pneumonia)
   c. Contraindicated
   d. V64.1 (Surgery, not done because of, contraindicated)
2.
   a. 2; sterilization and surgery not done
   b. V25.2 (Sterilization, admission for)
   c. V64.2 (Surgery, not done because of, patient's decision)

Exercise 15–13

1. V53.31 (Cardiac, device, pacemaker, cardiac, fitting or adjustment)
2. V25.5 (Insertion, subdermal implantable contraceptive)
3. V10.46 (History, malignant neoplasm, prostate)
4. V06.4 (Vaccination, mumps, with measles and rubella [MMR])
5. V76.12 (Screening, mammogram)
6. V70.5 (Examination, medical, pre-employment)

Exercise 15–14

1. scars, face; third-degree burns
2. constrictive pericarditis; tuberculosis infection
3. foreign body, femur; gunshot injury, femur
4. mental retardation; poliomyelitis
5. leg pain; fracture, femur

Exercise 15–15

1. arthritis, ankle, traumatic, 716.17 (Arthritis, traumatic); fracture, ankle, 905.4 (Late, effect(s) (of), fracture, extremity, lower)

2. aphasia (Note that there is no code for residual because there is one code for residual and cause.); cerebrovascular accident, 438.11 (Late effect(s) (of), cerebrovascular disease with aphasia)

3. deafness, sensorineural, 389.10 (Deafness, sensorineural); meningitis, 326 (Late effect(s) (of), Meningitis, unspecified cause)

Exercise 15–16

1. 008.8 (Gastroenteritis, viral NEC)

2. 038.43 (Septicemia, *Pseudomonas*); 785.59 (Septic, shock)

3. 045.90 (Poliomyelitis, unspecified type)

4. 112.1 (Candidiasis, vagina)

Exercise 15–17

1. i

2. c

3. h

4. g

5. a

6. b

7. e

8. f

9. d

Exercise 15–18

1. V58.1 (Chemotherapy, encounter for); 183.0 (Neoplasm, ovary, primary) (Although you were not directed to code the procedure, the code for the injection of the chemotherapy agent would be 99.25.)

2. V58.0 (Admission, radiation management); 198.5 (Neoplasm, bone, secondary); V10.3 (History (of), malignant neoplasm (of), breast) (Although you were not directed to code the procedure, the code for the radiation would be 99.29.)

3.

   a. metastatic carcinoma of bronchus

   b. primary, unknown

   c. secondary

   d. 197.0 (Neoplasm, lung, main bronchus, secondary); 199.1 (Neoplasm, unknown site or unspecified, primary); 33.27 (Biopsy, lung, endoscopic)

4.

   a. Two, plus an E code

   b. Uncontrolled nausea and vomiting

   c. Lung cancer

   d. 787.01 (Nausea, with vomiting)

   e. 162.9 (Neoplasm, lung, primary); E933.1 (Table of Drugs and Chemicals, Antineoplastic agents, Therapeutic Use)

Exercise 15–19

1. 203.00 (Myeloma, multiple); M9730/3 (Myeloma)

2. 233.1 (Neoplasm, cervix); M8010/2 (Carcinoma, in situ)

3. 153.3 (Neoplasm, intestinal, colon, sigmoid, primary); M8000/3 (Cancer); 197.6 (Neoplasm, peritoneum, secondary); M8000/6 (Metastasis, cancer, to specified site)

4. 185 (Neoplasm, prostate, primary); M8140/3 (Adenocarcinoma, primary); 198.5 (Neoplasm, bone, secondary); M8140/6 (Adenocarcinoma)

5. 199.1 (Neoplasm, unknown, primary); M8000/3 (Cancer, primary); 198.3 (Neoplasm, brain, secondary); M8000/6 (Metastasis, cancer, to specified site) (Note that the active primary neoplasm should be sequenced first unless treatment is directed to the secondary neoplasm.)

6. 197.0 (Neoplasm, lung, secondary); V10.3 (History (of), malignant neoplasm (of), breast); M8010/6 (Carcinoma, secondary)

Exercise 15–20

1. 255.4 (Disease, Addison's)

2. 276.5 (Dehydration)

3. 250.30 (Diabetes, coma, hypoglycemic)

4. 242.01 (Goiter, toxic, with mention of thyrotoxic crisis or storm)

Exercise 15–21

1. 281.0 (Anemia, pernicious)

2. 286.6 (Coagulation, intravascular)

3. 286.0 (Hemophilia)

4. 285.1 (Anemia, blood loss, acute)

5. 289.6 (Polycythemia, familial)

Exercise 15–22

1. 331.0 (Alzheimer's, disease or sclerosis); 294.11 (Alzheimer's, dementia, with behavior disturbance) [in this order]

2. 300.4 (Depression, anxiety)

3. 318.2 (Retardation, mental, profound, IQ under 20)

4. 307.1 (Anorexia, nervosa)

5. 291.0 (Delirium, withdrawal, alcoholic, chronic); 303.91 (Dependence, alcohol, alcoholic)

Exercise 15–23

1. 320.82 (Meningitis, *E. Coli*)

2. 340 (Sclerosis, multiple)

3. 382.9 (Otitis, media, acute)

4. 365.11 (Glaucoma, chronic, open angle, primary)

5. 351.0 (Palsy, Bell's)

Exercise 15–24

1. 428.0 (Failure, heart, congestive)

2. 410.71 (Infarction, subendocardial)

3. 446.0 (Periarteritis); 405.99 (Hypertension, due to, periarteritis nodosa)

4. 434.01 (Infarction, brain, thrombotic)

5. 430 (Hemorrhage, subarachnoid)

Exercise 15–25

1. 464.4 (Croup)
2. 428.0 (Disease, heart, congestive); 518.81 (Respiratory, failure) [in this order]
3. 491.20 (Disease, lung, obstructive with, bronchitis)
4. 487.1 (Influenza, with, bronchitis)
5. 482.2 (Pneumonia, due to, *Hemophilus influenzae*)

Exercise 15–26

1. 540.0 (Appendicitis, with perforation, peritonitis or rupture)
2. 532.00 (Ulcer, duodenum, acute, with hemorrhage)
3. 574.00 (Cholecystitis, with, cholelithiasis, acute); 574.10 (Cholecystitis, with, cholelithiasis, chronic)
4. 558.9 (Gastroenteritis)
5. 530.81 (Reflux, gastroesophageal)

Exercise 15–27

1. 614.9 (Disease, pelvis, inflammatory)
2. 599.7 (Hematuria)
3. 590.10 (Pyelonephritis, acute); 590.00 (Pyelonephritis, chronic)
4. 600 (Hypertrophy, prostatic, benign)
5. 610.1 (Disease, breast, fibrocystic)

Exercise 15–28

1. 631 (Blighted ovum)
2. 634.91 (Abortion, spontaneous); 69.02 (Dilation and curettage, uterus, after, abortion)
3. 644.13 (Labor, false)
4. 664.31 (Laceration, perineum, complicating delivery, fourth degree); V27.0 (Outcome of delivery, single, liveborn); 75.69 (Repair, perineum, laceration, obstetric, current)
5. 660.11 (Delivery, complicated by, deformity, fetus, causing obstructed labor); 653.41 (Delivery, complicated, cephalopelvic disproportion); V27.0 (Outcome of delivery, single, liveborn); 74.1 (Cesarean section, lower uterine segment)

Exercise 15–29

1. 698.9 (Pruritus NOS)
2. 705.1 (Rash, heat)
3. 696.1 (Psoriasis)
4. 707.0 (Ulcer, skin, decubitus)
5. 692.6 (Dermatitis, due to, poison, ivy)

Exercise 15–30

1. 714.0 (Arthritis, rheumatoid)
2. 723.1 (Pain, neck)
3. 718.31 (Dislocation, shoulder, recurrent)
4. 710.0 (Lupus); 517.8 (Lupus, erythematosus, systemic, with lung involvement) [in this order]

5. 733.11 (Fracture, pathologic, humerus); 198.5 (Neoplasm, bone, secondary); V10.3 (History (of), malignant neoplasm, breast)

Exercise 15–31

1. 744.21 (Absence, ear, lobe)

2. V30.00 (Newborn, single, born in hospital, without mention of cesarean delivery or section); 752.51 (Undescended, testis)

3. 759.83 (Syndrome, fragile X)

4. 754.30 (Dislocation, hip, congenital)

Exercise 15–32

1. 780.2 (Presyncope)

2. 786.52 (Pain, chest, wall)

3. 793.80 (Abnormal, mammogram)

4. 780.39 (Disorder, seizure)

5. 796.2 (Blood, pressure, high, incidental reading, without diagnosis of hypertension)

Exercise 15–33

1. 942.33 (Burn, abdomen, third degree); 945.26 (Burn, thigh, second degree); E924.0 (Burn, hot, liquid); 948.11—15%

2. 945.36 (Burn, thigh, third degree); 958.3 (Burn, infected); 948.00—4½%

3. 945.22 (Burn, foot, second degree) (Note that only the highest level burn is coded when burns are in the same area); E897 (Fire, controlled, bonfire); 948.00—2¼%

4. 944.00 (Burn, hand); 86.22 (Debridement, burn, excisional); 948.00 for 2¼%

5. 942.32 (Burn, chest wall, third degree); 943.21 (Burn, forearm, second degree); 944.11 (Burn, finger, first degree); 948.10—11% [in this order]

Exercise 15–34

1. 996.69 (Complications, breast implants, infection or inflammation)

2. 996.85 (Rejection, transplant, bone marrow)

3. 998.59 (Abscess, stitch)

4. 996.01 (Complications, mechanical, implant, pacemaker, cardiac)

Exercise 15–35

1. history of hysterectomy

2. history of peptic ulcer disease

Exercise 15–36

1. chest pain, shortness of breath

2. hip pain, contusion of hip

3. No; the patient did not require any of the five items that would substantiate use of additional resources (unless hospital policy dictates otherwise).

4. Yes; additional laboratory studies were done, and treatment (transfusion) was provided.

5. No; diagnoses are not made from laboratory values

Exercise 15–37

1. 9

2. 1

3. 5
4. 0
5. 7
6. 0

Exercise 15–38

1. 7
2. L
3. M
4. G
5. N
6. 1
7. R
8. 4
9. T
10. 8

Exercise 15–39

1. transfer
2. resection
3. inspection
4. transplantation
5. insertion
6. removal
7. fragmentation
8. occlusion
9. revision
10. release

Exercise 15–40

1. complete
2. expandable
3. multiaxial
4. standardized in terminology
5. 7
6. alphanumeric
7. 34
8. O and I
9. procedure

Chapter 16

Exercise 16–1

1. the government
2. 1965
3. A
4. B

Exercise 16–2

1. October
2. November or December
3. Department of Health and Human Services
4. December 11, 2000
5. durable medical equipment, prosthetics, orthotics, and supplies
6. Charles Waldhouser

Exercise 16–3

1. 78
2. 84

Exercise 16–4

1. No
2. No
3. Yes
4. Yale
5. New Jersey
6. case mix
7. severity of illness, prognosis, treatment difficulty, need for intervention, and resource intensity

Exercise 16–5

1. TEFRA
2. Scope of Work
3. admission, discharge, quality, DRG validation, coverage, and procedure
4. without the potential for significant adverse effects on the patient, with the potential for significant adverse effects on the patient, and with significant adverse effects on the patient

Exercise 16–6

1. Resource-Based Relative Value Scale
2. the *Federal Register*
3. OBRA

Exercise 16–7

1. Ambulatory Patient Classification
2. 2000
3. 20%
4. 346

Glossary

A-mode: one-dimensional ultrasonic display reflecting the time it takes a sound wave to reach a structure and reflect back; maps the structure's outline

ablation: removal by cutting

abortion: termination of pregnancy

abscess: localized collection of pus that will result in the disintegration of tissue over time

abuse: misuse of substance

acquired: not genetic

actinotherapy: treatment of acne using ultraviolet rays

acute: of sudden onset and short duration

addiction: dependence on a drug

admission: attention to an acute illness or injury resulting in admission to a hospital

adrenal: glands, located at the top of the kidneys, that produce steroid hormones

AHA: American Hospital Association

AHIMA: American Health Information Management Association

allogenic: of the same species, but genetically different

allograft: tissue graft between individuals who are not of the same genotype

allotransplantation: transplantation between individuals who are not of the same genotype

amniocentesis: percutaneous aspiration of amniotic fluid

anastomosis: surgical connection of two tubular structures, such as two pieces of the intestine

aneurysm: sac of clotted blood or fluid formed in the circulatory system, i.e., vein or artery

angiography: taking of x-ray films of vessels after injection of contrast material

angioplasty: surgical or percutaneous procedure in a vessel to dilate the vessel opening; used in the treatment of atherosclerotic disease

anomaly: abnormality

anomaloscope: instrument used to test color vision

anoscopy: procedure that uses a scope to examine the anus

antepartum: before childbirth

anterior (ventral): in front of

anterior segment: those parts of the eye in the front of and including the lens, orbit, extraocular muscles, and eyelid

anteroposterior: from front to back

antrotomy: cutting through the antrum wall to make an opening in the sinus

antrum: maxillary sinus

aortography: radiographic recording of the aorta

apexcardiography: recording of the movement of the chest wall

APCs (Ambulatory Patient Categories): a patient classification that provides a payment system for outpatients

aphakia: absence of the lens of the eye

apicectomy: excision of a portion of the temporal bone

Appendix A: located near the back of the CPT manual; lists all modifiers with complete explanations for use

Appendix B: located near the back of the CPT manual; contains a complete list of additions to, deletions from, and revisions of the previous edition

Appendix C: located near the back of the CPT manual; contains the list of updates to the electronic version of the CPT

Appendix D: located near the back of the CPT manual; presents clinical examples of Evaluation and Management (E/M) Procedures

Appendix E: located near the back of the CPT manual; contains a list of the CPT add-on codes

Appendix F: located near the back of the CPT manual; contains a list of modifier -51 exempt codes

arteriovenous fistula: direct communication (passage) between an artery and vein

artery: vessel that carries oxygenated blood from the heart to body tissues

arthrodesis: surgical immobilization of a joint

arthrography: radiographic recording of a joint

arthroplasty: reshaping or reconstruction of a joint

aspiration: use of a needle and a syringe to withdraw fluid

assignment: Medicare's payment for the service, which participating physicians agree to accept as payment in full

astigmatism: condition in which the refractive surfaces of the eye are unequal

asymptomatic: not showing any of the typical symptoms of a disease or condition

atrium: chamber in the upper part of the heart

attending physician: the physician with the primary responsibility for care of the patient

audi-: prefix meaning hearing

audiometry: hearing testing

aur-: prefix meaning ear

aural atresia: congenital absence of the external auditory canal

autogenous, autologous: from oneself

axillary nodes: lymph nodes located in the armpit

B-scan: two-dimensional display of tissues and organs

barium enema: radiographic contrast medium—enhanced examination of the colon

benign: not progressive or recurrent

benign hypertension: hypertensive condition with a continuous, mild blood pressure elevation

bifocal: two focuses in eyeglasses, one usually for close work and the other for improvement of distance vision

bilateral: occurring on two sides

bilobectomy: surgical removal of two lobes of a lung

biofeedback: process of giving a person self-information

biometry: application of a statistical measure to a biologic fact

biopsy: removal of a small piece of living tissue for diagnostic purposes

blephar(o)-: prefix meaning eyelid

block: frozen piece of a sample

brachytherapy: therapy using radioactive sources that are placed inside the body

bronchography: radiographic recording of the lungs

bronchoplasty: surgical repair of the bronchi

bronchoscopy: inspection of the bronchial tree using a bronchoscope

bulbocavernosus: muscle that constricts the vagina in a female and the urethra in a male

bulbourethral gland: rounded mass of the urethra

bypass: to go around

calculus: concretion of mineral salts, also called a stone

calycoplasty: surgical reconstruction of a recess of the renal pelvis

calyx: recess of the renal pelvis

cannulation: insertion of a tube into a duct or cavity

cardiopulmonary: refers to the heart and lungs

cardiopulmonary bypass: blood bypasses the heart through a heart-lung machine during open-heart surgery

cardioversion: electric shock to the heart to restore normal rhythm

cardioverter-defibrillator: surgically placed device that directs an electric current shock to the heart to restore rhythm

cataract: opaque covering on or in the lens

catheter: tube placed into the body to put fluid in or take fluid out

caudal: same as inferior; away from the head, or the lower part of the body

cauterization: destruction of tissue by the use of cautery

cavernosa–corpus spongiosum shunt: creation of a connection between a cavity of the penis and the urethra

cavernosa–glans penis fistulization: creation of a connection between a cavity of the penis and the glans penis, which overlaps the penis cavity

cavernosa–saphenous vein shunt: creation of a connection between the cavity of the penis and a vein

cavernosography: radiographic recording of a cavity, e.g., the pulmonary cavity or the main part of the penis

cavernosometry: measurement of the pressure in a cavity, e.g., the penis

-centesis: suffix meaning puncture of a cavity

central nervous system: brain and spinal cord

cervical: pertaining to the neck or to the cervix of the uterus

cervix uteri: rounded, cone-shaped neck of the uterus

cesarean: surgical opening through abdominal wall for delivery

CF (conversion factor): national dollar amount that is applied to all services paid on the Medicare Fee Schedule basis

cholangiography: radiographic recording of the bile ducts

cholangiopancreatography (ERCP): radiographic recording of the biliary system or pancreas

chole-: prefix meaning bile

cholecystectomy: surgical removal of the gallbladder

cholecystoenterostomy: creation of a connection between the gallbladder and intestine

cholecystography: radiographic recording of the gallbladder

chordee: condition resulting in the penis' being bent downward

chorionic villus sampling (CVS): biopsy of the outermost part of the placenta

chronic: of long duration

Cloquet's node: also called a gland; it is the highest of the deep groin lymph nodes

closed treatment: fracture site that is not surgically opened and visualized

CMS: Centers for Medicare and Medicaid Services, formerly HCFA, Health Care Financing Administration

colonoscopy: fiberscopic examination of the entire colon that may include part of the terminal ileum

colostomy: artificial opening between the colon and the abdominal wall

combination code: single five-digit code used to identify etiology and manifestation of a disease

communicable disease: disease that can be transmitted from one person to another or one species to another

comparative conditions: patient conditions that are documented as "either/or" in the patient record

component: part

computed axial tomography (CAT or CT): procedure by which selected planes of tissue are pinpointed through computer enhancement, and images may be reconstructed by analysis of variance in absorption of the tissue

concurrent care: the provision of similar services (e.g., hospital visits) to the same patient by more than one physician on the same day. Each physician provides services for a separate condition, not reasonably expected to be managed by the attending physician. When concurrent care is provided, the diagnosis must reflect the medical necessity of different specialties

congenital: existing from birth

conjunctiva: the lining of the eyelids and the covering of the sclerae

conscious sedation: a decreased level of consciousness in which the patient is not completely asleep

consultation: includes those services rendered by a physician whose opinion or advice is requested by another physician or agency concerning the evaluation and/or treatment of a patient; a consultant is not an attending physician

contralateral: affecting the opposite side

contributing factors: counseling, coordination of care, nature of the presenting problem, and time of an E/M service

cordectomy: surgical removal of the vocal cord(s)

cor/o-: prefix meaning pupil

cordocentesis: procedure to obtain a fetal blood sample; also called a percutaneous umbilical blood sampling

corneosclera: cornea and sclera of the eye

corpora cavernosa: the two cavities of the penis

corpus uteri: uterus

counseling: a discussion with a patient and/or family concerning one or more of the following areas: diagnostic results, impressions, and/or recommended diagnostic studies; prognosis; risks and benefits of treatment; instructions for treatment; importance of compliance with treatment; risk factor reduction; and patient and family education

CPT (Current Procedural Terminology): a coding system developed by the American Medical Association (AMA) to convert widely accepted, uniform descriptions of medical, surgical, and diagnostic services rendered by health care providers into five-digit numeric codes

cranium: that part of the skeleton that encloses the brain

critical care: the care of critically ill patients in medical emergencies that requires the constant attendance of the physician (e.g., cardiac arrest, shock, bleeding, respiratory failure); critical care is usually, but not always, given in a critical care area, such as the coronary care unit (CCU) or the intensive care unit (ICU)

CRNA: certified registered nurse anesthetist

Crohn's disease: regional enteritis

cryosurgery: destruction of lesions using extreme cold

curettage: scraping of a cavity using a spoon-shaped instrument

cycl/o-: prefix meaning ciliary body or eye muscle

cyst: closed sac containing matter or fluid

cystic hygroma: congenital deformity or benign tumor of the lymphatic system

cystocele: herniation of the bladder into the vagina

cystography: radiographic recording of the urinary bladder

cystolithectomy: removal of a calculus (stone) from the urinary bladder

cystolithotomy: cystolithectomy

cystometrogram (CMG): measurement of the pressures and capacity of the urinary bladder

cystoplasty: surgical reconstruction of the bladder

cystorrhaphy: suture of the bladder

cystoscopy: use of a scope to view the bladder

cystostomy: surgical creation of an opening into the bladder

cystotomy: incision into the bladder

cystourethroplasty: surgical reconstruction of the bladder and urethra

cystourethroscopy: use of a scope to view the bladder and urethra

cytopathology: study of the diseases of cells

dacry/o-: prefix meaning tear or tear duct

dacryocyst/o-: prefix meaning pertaining to the lacrimal sac

dacryocystography: radiographic recording of the lacrimal sac or tear duct sac

debridement: cleansing of or removal of dead tissue from a wound

delivery: childbirth

Demerol: a narcotic analgesic

dermatoplasty: surgical repair of the skin

dermis: second layer of skin, holding blood vessels, nerve endings, sweat glands, and hair follicles

destruction: killing of tissue by means of electrocautery, laser, chemicals, or other means

DHHS: Department of Health and Human Services

diaphragm: muscular wall that separates the thoracic and abdominal cavities

diaphragmatic hernia: hernia of the diaphragm

dilation: expansion (of the cervix)

diskography: radiographic recording of an intervertebral joint

dislocation: placement in a location other than the original location

distal: farther from the point of attachment or origin

distinct procedure: one service or procedure that has no relationship to another service or procedure

Doppler: ultrasonic measure of blood movement

dosimetry: scientific calculation of radiation emitted from various radioactive sources

drainage: free flow or withdrawal of fluids from a wound or cavity

DRGs (Diagnosis-Related Groups): a disease classification system that relates the type of inpatients a hospital treats (case mix) to the costs incurred by the hospital

dual chamber pacemaker: electrodes of the pacemaker are placed in both the atria and the ventricles of the heart

duodenography: radiographic recording of the duodenum or first part of the small intestine

ear, parts of the external: auricle, pinna, external acoustic, and meatus

ear, parts of the inner: vestibule, semicircular canals, and cochlea

ear, parts of the middle: malleus, incus, and stapes

ECG: *see* electrocardiogram

echocardiography: radiographic recording of the heart or heart walls or surrounding tissues

echoencephalography: ultrasound of the brain

echography: ultrasound procedure in which sound waves are bounced off an internal organ and the resulting image is recorded

-ectomy: suffix meaning removal of part or all of an organ of the body

ectopic: pregnancy outside the uterus (i.e., in the fallopian tube)

EEG: *see* electroencephalogram

electrocardiogram (ECG): written record of the electrical activity of the heart

electrocochleography: test to measure the eighth cranial nerve (hearing test)

electrode: lead attached to a generator that carries the electric current from the generator to the atria or ventricles

electrodesiccation: destruction of a lesion by the use of electric current radiated through a needle

electroencephalogram (EEG): written record of the electrical activity of the brain

electromyogram (EMG): written record of the electrical activity of the skeletal muscles

electromyography (EMG): recording of the electrical impulses of muscles

electro-oculogram (EOG): written record of the electrical activity of the eye

electrophysiology: the study of the electrical system of the heart, including the study of arrhythmias

embolectomy: removal of blockage (embolism) from vessels

embolism: blockage of a blood vessel by a blood clot or other matter that has moved from another area of the body through the circulatory system

emergency care services: services that are provided by the physician in the emergency department for unplanned patient encounters; no distinction is made between new and established patients who are seen in the emergency department

encephalography: radiographic recording of the subarachnoid space and ventricles of the brain

endarterectomy: incision into an artery to remove the inner lining so as to eliminate disease or blockage

endomyocardial: pertaining to the inner and middle layers of the heart

endopyelotomy: procedure involving the bladder and ureters, including the insertion of a stent

endoscopy: inspection of body organs or cavities using a lighted scope that may be inserted through an existing opening or through a small incision

enterocystoplasty: surgical reconstruction of the

small intestine after the removal of a cyst and usually including a bowel anastomosis

enucleation: removal of an organ or organs from a body cavity

epicardial: over the heart

epidermis: outer layer of skin

epididymectomy: surgical removal of the epididymis

epididymis: tube located at the top of the testes that stores sperm

epididymovasostomy: creation of a new connection between the vas deferens and epididymis

epididymography: radiographic recording of the epididymis

epiglottidectomy: excision of the covering of the larynx

ESRD: end-stage renal disease

established patient: a patient who has received professional services from the physician or another physician of the same specialty in the same group within the past 3 years

etiology: study of causes of diseases

eventration: protrusion of the bowel through the viscera of the abdomen

evisceration: pulling the viscera outside of the body through an incision

excision: cutting or taking away (in reference to lesion removal, it is full-thickness removal of a lesion that may include simple closure)

excisional: removal of an entire lesion for biopsy

Exclusive Provider Organization (EPO): similar to a Health Maintenance Organization except that the providers of the services are not prepaid, but rather are paid on a fee-for-service basis

exenteration: removal of an organ all in one piece

exostosis: bony growth

exstrophy: condition in which an organ is turned inside out

false aneurysm: sac of clotted blood that has completely destroyed the vessel and is being contained by the tissue that surrounds the vessel

Federal Register: official publication of all "Presidential Documents," "Rules and Regulations," "Proposed Rules," and "Notices"; government-instituted national changes are published in the *Federal Register*

fenestration: creation of a new opening in the inner wall of the middle ear

fimbrioplasty: surgical repair of the fringe of the uterine tube

fistula: abnormal opening from one area to another area or to the outside of the body

fluoroscopy: procedure for viewing the interior of the body using x-rays and projecting the image onto a television screen

fracture: break in a bone

fulguration: use of electric current to destroy tissue

fundoplasty: repair of the bottom of an organ or muscle

gastro-: prefix meaning stomach

gastrointestinal: pertaining to the stomach and intestine

gastroplasty: operation on the stomach for repair or reconfiguration

gastrostomy: artificial opening between the stomach and the abdominal wall

gloss(o)-: prefix meaning tongue

gonioscopy: use of a scope to examine the angles of the eye

Group Practice Model: an organization of physicians who contract with a Health Maintenance Organization to provide services to the enrollees of the HMO

grouper: computer used to input the principal diagnosis and other critical information about a patient and then provide the correct DRG code

Guidelines: provide specific instructions about coding for each section; the Guidelines contain definitions of terms, applicable modifiers, explanation of notes, subsection information, unlisted services, special reports information, and clinical examples

HCFA: Health Care Financing Administration, now known as Centers for Medicare and Medicaid Services (CMS)

Health Maintenance Organization (HMO): a health care delivery system in which an enrollee is assigned a primary care physician who manages all the health care needs of the enrollee

hemodialysis: cleansing of the blood outside of the body

hepat(o)-: prefix meaning liver

hepatography: radiographic recording of the liver

hernia: organ or tissue protruding through the wall or cavity that usually contains it

histology: study of the minute structures, composition, and function of tissues

Hodgkin's disease: malignant lymphoma

hydrocele: sac of fluid

hypertension, uncontrolled: untreated hypertension or hypertension that is not responding to the therapeutic regimen

hypertensive heart disease: secondary effects on the heart of prolonged, sustained systemic hypertension; the heart has to work against greatly increased resistance, causing increased blood pressure

hypogastric: lowest middle abdominal area

hyposensitization: decreased sensitivity

hypospadias: congenital deformity of the urethra in which the urethral opening is on the underside of the penis rather than at the end

hypotension: abnormally low blood pressure

hypothermia: low body temperature; sometimes induced during surgical procedures

hysterectomy: surgical removal of the uterus

hysterorrhaphy: suturing of the uterus

hysterosalpingography: radiographic recording of the uterine cavity and fallopian tubes

hysteroscopy: visualization of the canal of the uterine cervix and cavity of the uterus using a scope placed through the vagina

hysterotomy: incision into the uterus

ileostomy: artificial opening between the ileum and the abdominal wall

imbrication: overlapping

immunotherapy: therapy to increase immunity

incarcerated: regarding hernias, a constricted, irreducible hernia that may cause obstruction of an intestine

incision: surgically cutting into

incision and drainage: to cut and withdraw fluid

incisional: *see* incision

Individual Practice Association (IPA): an organization of physicians who provide services for a set fee; Health Maintenance Organizations often contract with the IPA for services to their enrollees

infectious disease carrier: person who has a communicable disease

infectious disease contact: encounter with a person who has a disease that can be communicated or transmitted

inferior: away from the head or the lower part of the body; also known as caudal

inguinofemoral: referring to the groin and thigh

injection: forcing of a fluid into a vessel or cavity

inpatient: one who has been formally admitted to a health care facility

in situ: malignancy that is within the original site of development

internal/external fixation: application of pins, wires, screws, and so on to immobilize a body part; they can be placed externally or internally

intracardiac: inside the heart

intramural: within the organ wall

intramuscular: into a muscle

intraoperative: period of time during which a surgical procedure is being performed

intravenous: into a vein

intravenous pyelography (IVP): radiographic recording of the urinary system

introitus: opening or entrance to the vagina from the uterus

intubation: insertion of a tube

invasive: entering the body, breaking the skin

iontophoresis: introduction of ions into the body

ischemia: deficient blood supply due to obstruction of the circulatory system

isthmus: connection of two regions or structures

isthmus, thyroid: tissue connection between right and left thyroid lobes

isthmusectomy: surgical removal of the isthmus

italicized code: an ICD-9-CM code that can never be sequenced as the principal diagnosis

jejunostomy: artificial opening between the jejunum and the abdominal wall

jugular nodes: lymph nodes located next to the large vein in the neck

kerat/o-: prefix meaning cornea

keratoplasty: surgical repair of the cornea

key components: the history, examination, and medical decision-making complexity of an E/M service

Kock pouch: surgical creation of a urinary bladder from a segment of the ileum

labyrinth: inner connecting cavities, such as the internal ear

laminectomy: surgical excision of the lamina

laparoscopy: exploration of the abdomen and pelvic cavities using a scope placed through a small incision in the abdominal wall

laryngeal web: congenital abnormality of connective tissue between the vocal cords

laryngectomy: surgical removal of the larynx

laryngo-: prefix meaning larynx

laryngography: radiographic recording of the larynx

laryngoplasty: surgical repair of the larynx

laryngoscope: fiberoptic scope used to view the inside of the larynx

laryngoscopy: viewing of the larynx using a fiberoptic scope

laryngotomy: incision into the larynx

late effect: residual effect (condition produced) after the acute phase of an illness or injury has terminated

lateral: away from the midline of the body (to the side)

lavage: washing out of an organ

lesion: abnormal or altered tissue, e.g., wound, cyst, abscess, or boil

ligation: binding or tying off, as in constricting the bloodflow of a vessel or binding fallopian tubes for sterilization

litholapaxy: lithotripsy

lithotomy: incision into an organ or a duct for the purpose of removing a stone

lithotripsy: crushing of a gallbladder or urinary bladder stone followed by irrigation to wash the fragment out

lobectomy: surgical excision of a lobe of the lung

lymph node: station along the lymphatic system

lymphadenectomy: excision of a lymph node or nodes

lymphadenitis: inflammation of a lymph node

lymphangiography: radiographic recording of the lymphatic vessels and nodes

lymphangiotomy: incision into a lymphatic vessel

lysis: releasing

M-mode: one-dimensional display of movement of structures

MAAC (Maximum Actual Allowable Charge): limitation on the total amount that can be charged by physicians who are not participants in Medicare

magnetic resonance imaging (MRI): procedure that uses nonionizing radiation to view the body in a cross-sectional view

malignancy: used in reference to a cancerous tumor

malignant: used to describe a cancerous tumor that grows worse over time

malignant hypertension: accelerated, severe form of hypertension, manifested by headaches, blurred vision, dyspnea, and uremia; usually causes permanent organ damage

mammography: radiographic recording of the breasts

Managed Care Organization (MCO): a group that is responsible for the health care services offered to an enrolled group of persons

mandated service: a service required by an agency or organization to be performed for a patient; usually the agency or organization pays all or a portion of the patient's medical bills

manifestation: sign of a disease

manipulation or reduction: words used interchangeably to mean the attempted restoration of a fracture or joint dislocation to its normal anatomic position

marsupialization: surgical procedure that creates an exterior pouch from an internal abscess

mast-: prefix meaning breast

mastoid-: prefix meaning posterior temporal bone

MDC (Major Diagnostic Categories): the division of all principal diagnoses into 25 mutually exclusive principal diagnosis areas within the DRG system

meatotomy: surgical enlargement of the opening of the urinary meatus

medial: toward the midline of the body

mediastinoscopy: use of an endoscope inserted through a small incision to view the mediastinum

mediastinotomy: cutting into the mediastinum

mediastinum: area between the lungs that contains the heart, aorta, trachea, lymph nodes, thymus gland, esophagus, and bronchial tubes

Medicare risk HMO: a Medicare-funded alternative to the standard Medicare supplemental coverage

MEI (Medicare Economic Index): government-mandated index that ties increases in the Medicare prevailing charges to economic indicators

MeV: megaelectron volt

MFS (Medicare Fee Schedule): schedule that listed the allowable charges for Medicare services; was replaced by the Medicare reasonable charge payment system

modality: treatment method

modifiers: two- or five-digit numbers added to CPT codes to supply more specific information about the services provided to the patient

monofocal: eyeglasses with one vision correction

morbidity: condition of being diseased or morbid

morphine: a narcotic analgesic

morphology: study of neoplasms

mortality: death

MSLT: multiple sleep latency testing

multiple coding: use of more than one code to identify both etiology and manifestation of a disease, as contrasted with combination coding

MVPS (Medical Volume Performance Standards): government's estimate of how much growth is appropriate for nationwide physician expenditures paid by the Part B Medicare program

myasthenia gravis: syndrome characterized by muscle weakness

myelography: radiographic recording of the subarachnoid space of the spine

myocardial infarction (MI): necrosis of the myocardium resulting from interrupted blood supply

myring-: prefix meaning eardrum

nasal button: a synthetic circular disk used to cover a hole in the nasal septum

nasopharyngoscopy: use of a scope to visualize the nose and pharynx

NCPAP: nasal continuous positive airway pressure

NEC: not elsewhere classified

neoplasm: new tumor growth that can be benign or malignant

nephrectomy, paraperitoneal: kidney transplant

nephro-: prefix meaning kidney

nephrocutaneous fistula: a channel from the kidney to the skin

nephrolithotomy: removal of a kidney stone through an incision made into the kidney

nephrorrhaphy: suturing of the kidney

nephrostolithotomy: creation of an artificial channel to the kidney

nephrostolithotomy, percutaneous: procedure to establish an artificial channel between the skin and the kidney

nephrostomy: creation of a channel into the renal pelvis of the kidney

nephrostomy, percutaneous: creation of a channel from the skin to the renal pelvis

nephrotomy: incision into the kidney

new patient: a patient who has not received any professional services from the physician or another physician of the same specialty in the same group within the past 3 years

newborn care: the evaluation and determination of care management of a newly born infant

noninvasive: not entering the body, not breaking the skin

NOS: not otherwise specified

nuclear cardiology: diagnostic specialty that uses radiologic procedures to aid in the diagnosis of cardiologic conditions

nystagmus: rapid involuntary eye movements

OBRA (Omnibus Budget Reconciliation Act of 1989): act that established new rules for Medicare reimbursement

ocul/o-: prefix meaning eye

ocular adnexa: orbit, extraocular muscles, and eyelid

office visit: a face-to-face encounter between a physician and a patient to allow for primary management of a patient's health care status

Official Coding and Reporting Guidelines: rules of coding diagnosis codes (ICD-9-CM) published by the Editorial Advisory Board of Coding Clinic

omentum: peritoneal connection between the stomach and other internal organs

oophor-: prefix meaning ovary

oophorectomy: surgical removal of the ovary(ies)

opacification: area that has become opaque (milky)

open treatment: fracture site that is surgically opened and visualized

ophthalmodynamometry: test of the blood pressure of the eye

ophthalmology: body of knowledge regarding the eyes

optokinetic: movement of the eyes to objects moving in the visual field

orchiectomy: castration

orchiopexy: surgical procedure to release undescended testis

orthoptic: corrective; in the correct place

ostomy: artificial opening

oto-: prefix meaning ear

-otomy: suffix meaning incision into

outpatient: a patient who receives services in an ambulatory health care facility and is currently not an inpatient

overdose: excessive dose

oviduct: fallopian tube

pacemaker: electrical device that controls the beating of the heart by electrical impulses

paraesophageal hiatus hernia: hernia that is near the esophagus

parathyroid: produces a hormone to mobilize calcium from the bones to the blood

paring: removal of thin layers of skin by peeling or scraping

Part A: Medicare's Hospital Insurance; covers hospital/facility care

Part B: Medicare's Supplemental Medical Insurance; covers physician services and durable medical equipment that are not paid for under Part A

participating provider program: Medicare providers who have agreed in advance to accept assignment on all Medicare claims

pelviolithotomy: pyeloplasty

penoscrotal: referring to the penis and scrotum

percutaneous: through the skin

percutaneous skeletal fixation: considered neither open nor closed; the fracture is not visualized, but fixation is placed across the fracture site under x-ray imaging

pericardiocentesis: procedure in which a surgeon withdraws fluid from the pericardial space by means of a needle inserted percutaneously into the space

pericarditis: swelling of the sac surrounding the great vessels and the heart

pericardium: membranous sac enclosing the heart and the ends of the great vessels

perineal approach: surgical approach in the area between the thighs

perinephric cyst: cyst in the tissue around the kidney

perineum: area between the vulva and anus; also known as the pelvic floor

peripheral nerves: 12 pairs of cranial nerves, 31 pairs of spinal nerves, and autonomic nervous system; connects peripheral receptors to the brain and spinal cord

perirenal: around the kidney

peritoneal: within the lining of the abdominal cavity

peritoneoscopy: visualization of the abdominal cavity using one scope placed through a small incision in the abdominal wall and another scope placed in the vagina

perivesical: around the bladder

periviceral: around an organ

pharyngolaryngectomy: surgical removal of the pharynx and larynx

phlebotomy: cutting into a vein

phonocardiogram: recording of heart sounds

photochemotherapy: treatment by means of drugs that react to ultraviolet radiation or sunlight

physical status modifiers: modifying units in the Anesthesia section of the CPT that describe a patient's condition at the time anesthesia is administered

physics: scientific study of energy

-plasty: suffix meaning technique involving molding or surgically forming

plethysmography: determining the changes in volume of an organ part or body

pleura: covering of the lungs and thoracic cavity that is moistened with serous fluid to reduce friction during respiratory movements of the lungs

pleurectomy: surgical excision of the pleura

pneumo-: prefix meaning lung or air

pneumoncentesis: surgical puncturing of a lung to withdraw fluid

pneumonolysis: surgical separation of the lung from the chest wall to allow the lung to collapse

pneumonostomy: surgical procedure in which the chest cavity is exposed and the lung is incised

pneumonotomy: incision of the lung

pneumoplethysmography: determining the changes in the volume of the lung

polyp: tumor on a pedicle that bleeds easily and may become malignant

posterior (dorsal): in back of

posterior segment: those parts of the eye behind the lens

posteroanterior: from back to front

postoperative: period of time after a surgical procedure

postpartum: after childbirth

Preferred Provider Organization (PPO): a group of providers who form a network and who have agreed to provide services to enrollees at a discounted rate

preoperative: period of time prior to a surgical procedure

priapism: painful condition in which the penis is constantly erect

primary site: site of origin or where the tumor originated

principal diagnosis: defined in the Uniform Hospital Discharge Data Set (UHDDS) as "that condition established after study to be chiefly responsible for occasioning the admission of the patient to the hospital for care"; the principal diagnosis is sequenced first

proctosigmoidoscopy: fiberscopic examination of the sigmoid colon and rectum

professional component: term used in describing radiology services provided by a radiologist

prognosis: probable outcome of an illness

prophylactic: substance or agent that offers some protection from disease

PROs (Peer Review Organizations): groups established to review hospital admission and care

prostatotomy: incision into the prostate

PSRO (Professional Standards Review Organization): voluntary physicians' organization designed to monitor the necessity of hospital admissions, treatment costs, and medical records of hospitals

punch: use of a small hollow instrument to puncture a lesion

pyelo-: prefix meaning renal pelvis

pyelocutaneous: from the renal pelvis to the skin

pyelography: radiographic recording of the kidneys, renal pelvis, ureters, and bladder

pyelolithotomy: surgical removal of a kidney stone from the renal pelvis

pyeloplasty: surgical reconstruction of the renal pelvis

pyeloscopy: viewing of the renal pelvis using a fluoroscope after injection of contrast material

pyelostolithotomy: removal of a kidney stone and establishment of a stoma

pyelostomy: surgical creation of a temporary diversion around the ureter

pyelotomy: incision into the renal pelvis

pyloroplasty: incision and repair of the pyloric channel

qualifying circumstances: five-digit CPT codes that describe situations or conditions that make the administration of anesthesia more difficult than is normal

qualitative: measuring the presence or absence of

quantitative: measuring the presence or absence of and the amount of

rad: radiation absorption dose, the energy deposited in patients' tissues

radiation oncology: branch of medicine concerned with the application of radiation to a tumor site for treatment (destruction) of cancerous tumors

radiograph: film on which an image is produced through exposure to x-radiation

radiologist: physician who specializes in the use of radioactive materials in the diagnosis and treatment of diseases and illnesses

radiology: branch of medicine concerned with the use of radioactive substances for diagnosis and therapy

RBRVS (Resource-Based Relative Value Scale): scale designed to decrease Medicare expenditures, redistribute physician payment, and ensure quality health care at reasonable rates

real time: two-dimensional display of both the structures and the motion of tissues and organs, with the length of time also recorded as part of the study

reanastomosis: reconnection of a previous connection between two places, organs, or spaces

rectocele: herniation of the rectal wall through the posterior wall of the vagina

reducible: able to be corrected or put back into a normal position

referral: the transfer of the total or a specific portion of care of a patient from one physician to another that does not constitute a consultation

Relative Value Guide: comparison of anesthesia services; published by the American Society of Anesthesiologists (ASA)

renal pelvis: funnel-shaped sac in the kidney where urine is received

repair: to remedy, replace, or heal (in the Integumentary subsection pertains to suturing a wound)

residual: that which is left behind or remains

resource intensity: refers to the relative volume and type of diagnostic, therapeutic, and bed services used in the management of a particular illness

retrograde: moving backward or against the usual direction of flow

retroperitoneal: behind the sac holding the abdominal organs and viscera (peritoneum)

rhino-: prefix meaning nose

rhinoplasty: surgical repair of the nose

-rrhaphy: suffix meaning suturing

rubric: heading used as a direction or explanation as to what follows and the way in which the information is to be used. In ICD-9-CM coding, the rubric is the three-digit code that precedes the four- and five-digit codes

rule of nines: rule used to estimate burned body surface in burn patients

RUQ: right upper quadrant

RVU (Relative Value Unit): unit value that has been assigned for each service

salpingectomy: surgical removal of the uterine tube

salping(o)-: prefix meaning tube

salpingostomy: creation of a fistula into the uterine tube

scan: mapping of emissions of radioactive substances after they have been introduced into the body; the density can determine normal or abnormal conditions

sclera: outer covering of the eye

secondary site: place to which a malignant tumor has spread; metastatic site

section: slice of a frozen block

sections: the seven major areas into which all CPT codes and descriptions are categorized

See: a cross-reference system within the index of the CPT manual used to direct the coder to another term or other terms. The *See* indicates that the correct code will be found elsewhere

segmentectomy: surgical removal of a portion of a lung

seminal vesicle: gland that secretes fluid into the vas deferens

separate procedures: minor procedures that when done by themselves are coded as a procedure, but when performed at the same time as a major procedure are considered incidental and not coded separately

septoplasty: surgical repair of the nasal septum

sequela: a condition that follows an illness

severity of illness: refers to the levels of loss of function and mortality that may be experienced by patients with a particular disease

shaving: horizontal or transverse removal of dermal or epidermal lesions, without full-thickness excision

shunt: divert or make an artificial passage

sialography: radiographic recording of the salivary duct and branches

sigmoidoscopy: fiberscopic examination of the entire rectum and sigmoid colon that may include a portion of the descending colon

single chamber pacemaker: the electrode of the pacemaker is placed only in the atrium or only in the ventricle, but not in both places

sinography: radiographic recording of the sinus or sinus tract

sinuses: cavities within the nasal bones

sinusotomy: surgical incision into a sinus

skin graft: transplantation of tissue to repair a defect

skull: entire skeletal framework of the head

slanted brackets: indicate that the ICD-9-CM code can never be sequenced as the principal diagnosis

soft tissue: tissues (fascia, connective tissue, muscle, and so forth) surrounding a bone

somatic nerve: sensory or motor nerve

special reports: detailed reports that include adequate definitions or descriptions of the nature, extent, and need for the procedure and the time, effort, and equipment necessary to provide the services

specimen: sample of tissue or fluid

spermatocele: cyst filled with spermatozoa

spirometry: measurement of breathing capacity

splenectomy: excision of the spleen

splenography: radiographic recording of the spleen

splenoportography: radiographic procedure to allow visualization of the splenic and portal veins of the spleen

Staff Model: a Health Maintenance Organization that directly employs the physicians who provide services to enrollees

starred procedures: procedures and services that do not include various preoperative or post-operative services

stem cell: immature blood cell

stent: mold that holds a surgically placed graft in place

stereotaxis: method of identifying a specific area or point in the brain

strabismus: extraocular muscle deviation resulting in unequal visual axes

subcutaneous: tissue below the dermis, primarily fat cells that insulate the body

subsections: the further division of sections into smaller units, usually by body systems

superior: toward the head or the upper part of the body; also known as cephalic

supine: lying on the back

surgical package: bundling together of time, effort, and services for a specific procedure into one code instead of billing separately for each component

suture: to unite parts by stitching them together

Swan-Ganz catheter: central venous catheter

symbols: special guides that help the coder compare codes and descriptors with the previous edition. A bullet (●) is used to indicate a new procedure or service code added since the previous edition of the CPT manual. A solid triangle (▲) placed in front of a code number indicates that the code has been changed or modified since the last edition. A star (✳) placed after a code number indicates a minor procedure. A plus (+) is used to indicate an add-on code. A circle with a line through it (⊘) is used to identify a modifier -51 exempt code. A right and left triangle (► ◄) indicate the beginning and end of the text changes

sympathetic nerve: part of the peripheral nervous system that controls automatic body function and sympathetic nerves activated under stress

symphysiotomy: cutting of the pubis cartilage to help in birthing

systemic: affecting the entire body

tarsorrhaphy: suturing together of the eyelids

technical component: term used in describing radiology services provided by a technician

TEFRA (Tax Equity and Fiscal Responsibility Act): act that contains language to reward cost-conscious health care providers

term location methods: service/procedure, anatomic site/body organ, condition/disease, synonym, eponym, and abbreviation

thermogram: written record of temperature variation

thoracentesis: surgical puncture of the thoracic cavity, usually using a needle, to remove fluids

thoracic duct: collection and distribution point for lymph, and the largest lymph vessel located in the chest

thoracoplasty: surgical procedure that removes rib(s) and thereby allows the collapse of a lung

thoracoscopy: use of a lighted endoscope to view the pleural spaces and thoracic cavity or perform surgical procedures

thoracostomy: surgical incision into the chest wall and insertion of a chest tube

thoracotomy: surgical incision into the chest wall

thrombosis: blood clot

thymectomy: surgical removal of the thymus

thymus: gland that produces hormones important to the immune response

thyroglossal duct: connection between the thyroid and the pharynx

thyroid: part of the endocrine system that produces hormones that regulate metabolism

thyroidectomy: surgical removal of the thyroid

thyroiditis: a thyroid gland inflammation

tissue transfer: piece of skin for grafting that is still partially attached to the original blood supply and is used to cover an adjacent wound area

tocolysis: repression of uterine contractions

tomography: procedure that allows viewing of a single plane of the body by blurring out all but that particular level

tonography: recording of changes in intraocular pressure in response to sustained pressure on the eyeball

tonometry: measurement of pressure or tension

total pneumonectomy: surgical removal of an entire lobe of a lung

tracheostomy: creation of an opening into the trachea

tracheotomy: incision into the trachea

traction: application of force to a limb

transabdominal: across the abdomen

transcutaneous: entering by way of the skin

transesophageal echocardiogram (TEE): echocardiogram performed by placing a probe down the esophagus and sending out sound waves to obtain images of the heart and its movement

transfer order: official document that transfers the care of a patient from one physician to another; often required by third-party payers to transfer the care of a patient legally

transglottictracheoplasty: surgical repair of the vocal apparatus and trachea

transhepatic: across the liver

transmastoid antrostomy: called a simple mastoidectomy, it creates an opening in the mastoid for drainage

transplantation: grafting of tissue from one source to another

transseptal: through the septum

transthoracic: across the thorax

transtracheal: across the trachea

transvenous: across a vein

transverse: horizontal

transureteroureterostomy: surgical connection of one ureter to the other ureter

transurethral resection, prostate: procedure performed through the urethra by means of a cystoscopy to remove part or all of the prostate

transvenous: across a vein

transvesical ureterolithotomy: removal of a ureter stone (calculus) through the bladder

trocar needle: needle with a tube on the end; used to puncture and withdraw fluid from a cavity

tumescence: state of being swollen

tumor: swelling or enlargement; a spontaneous growth of tissue that forms an abnormal mass

tunica vaginalis: covering of the testes

tympanic neurectomy: excision of the tympanic nerve

tympanometry: test of the inner ear using air pressure

UHDDS: Uniform Hospital Discharge Data Set

ultrasound: technique using sound waves to determine the density of the outline of tissue

unbundling: assigning multiple CPT codes when one CPT code would fully describe the service or procedure

uncertain behavior: refers to the behavior of a neoplasm as being neither malignant nor benign but having characteristics of both kinds of activity

uncertain diagnosis: diagnosis documented at the time of discharge as "probable," "suspected," "likely," "questionable," "possible," or "rule out"

unilateral: occurring on one side

unlisted procedures: procedures that are considered unusual, experimental, or new and do not have a specific code number assigned; unlisted procedure codes are located at the end of the subsections or subheadings and may be used to identify any procedure that lacks a specific code

unspecified hypertension: hypertensive condition that has not been specified as either benign or malignant hypertension

unspecified nature: when the behavior or histology of a neoplasm is not known or is not specified

uptake: absorption of a radioactive substance by body tissues; recorded for diagnostic purposes in conditions such as thyroid disease

ureterectomy: surgical removal of a ureter, either totally or partially

ureterocolon: pertaining to the ureter and colon

ureterocutaneous fistula: the channel from the ureter to the exterior skin

ureteroenterostomy: creation of a connection between the intestine and the ureter

ureterolithotomy: removal of a stone from the ureter

ureterolysis: freeing of adhesions of the ureter

ureteroneocystostomy: surgical connection of the ureter to a new site on the bladder

ureteroplasty: surgical repair of the ureter

ureteropyelography: ureter and bladder radiography

ureteropyelonephrostomy: surgical connection of the ureter to a new site on the kidney

ureteropyelostomy: ureteropyelonephrostomy

ureterosigmoidostomy: surgical connection of the ureter into the sigmoid colon

ureterotomy: incision into the ureter

ureterovisceral fistula: surgical formation of a connection between the ureter and the skin

urethrocutaneous fistula: surgically created channel from the urethra to the skin surface

urethrocystography: radiography of the bladder and urethra

urethromeatoplasty: surgical repair of the urethra and meatus

urethroplasty: surgical repair of the urethra

urethrorrhaphy: suturing of the urethra

urethroscopy: use of a scope to view the urethra

urography: same as pyelography; radiographic recording of the kidneys, renal pelvis, ureters, and bladder

uveal: vascular tissue of the choroid, ciliary body, and iris

V codes: numeric designations preceded by the letter "V" used to classify persons who are not currently sick when they encounter health services

vagina: canal from the external female genitalia to the uterus

vagotomy: surgical separation of the vagus nerve

Valium: a sedative

varicocele: swelling of a scrotal vein

vas deferens: tube that carries sperm from the epididymis to the urethra

vasogram: recording of the flow in the vas deferens

vasotomy: creation of an opening in the vas deferens

vasovasorrhaphy: suturing of the vas deferens

vasovasostomy: reversal of a vasectomy

VBAC: vaginal delivery after a previous cesarean delivery

vectorcardiogram (VCG): continuous recording of electrical direction and magnitude of the heart

vein: vessel that carries unoxygenated blood to the heart from body tissues

vena caval thrombectomy: removal of a blood clot from the blood vessel (inferior vena cava, which is the vein trunk for the pelvic and abdominal area)

venography: radiographic recording of the veins and tributaries

ventricle: chamber in the lower part of the heart

version: turning of the fetus from a presentation other than cephalic (head down) to cephalic for ease of birth

vesicostomy: surgical creation of a connection of the viscera of the bladder to the skin

vesicovaginal fistula: creation of a tube between the vagina and the bladder

vesiculectomy: excision of the seminal vesicle

vesiculography: radiographic recording of the seminal vesicles

vesiculotomy: incision into the seminal vesicle

vitre/o-: prefix meaning pertaining to the vitreous body of the eye

vulva: external female genitalia including the labia majora, labia minora, clitoris, and vaginal opening

World Health Organization (WHO): group that deals with health care issues on a global basis

wound repair, complex: involves complicated wound closure, including revision, debridement, extensive undermining, and more than layered closure

wound repair, intermediate: requires closure of one or more subcutaneous tissues and superficial fascia, in addition to the skin closure

wound repair, simple: superficial wound repair, involving epidermis, dermis, and subcutaneous tissue, requiring only simple, one-layer suturing

xeroradiography: photoelectric process of radiographs

Index

Note: Page numbers followed by the letter f refer to figures and those followed by t refer to tables.

A

A codes, 181
AA modifier, for anesthesia, 98
Abbreviation(s)
  for locating CPT code, 21
  in ICD-9-CM manual, 388
Ablation
  definition of, 205
  nasal, 194
Abnormal findings, 494, 506, 587
  for outpatient, 508
Abortion
  CPT coding for, 259, 261, 262
  definition of, 263
  ICD-9-CM coding for, 483, 487, 591, 593
Abrasion
  as wound type, 148f
  for lesion removal, 156
Abscess
  definition of, 162
  in hidradenitis, 140
  nasal, incision of, 191, 192f
  of penis, 268
  of vulva, 249
  pelvic, in female, 250
  sinus tract injection for, 175
  skin, incision and drainage of, 137
  soft tissue, incision of, 173–174
Abuse
  of child or adult
    E codes for, 496, 599
    mandated tests and, 117
  of Medicare, 564–572
    definition of, 570
Accidents
  E codes for, 400, 404, 405f
    coding guidelines for, 495, 597–600
    for drugs and chemicals, 401, 402f, 503–504
  industrial, 416
Acne
  actinotherapy for, 362–363
  incision and drainage of, 137
Acquired, definition of, 637
Actinotherapy, 363, 376
Active immunization, 347
Active wound care management, 364

Acute condition
  definition of, 427
  with chronic condition, 436–437, 437f, 581–582, 584
AD modifier, for anesthesia, 98
Addiction, definition of, 637
Additional code, from ICD-9-CM, 392
Additions, to CPT manual, 7, 8f, 9
  electronic file of, 23f, 24
Add-on codes, in CPT manual, 7, 8f. *See also* Adjunct codes.
  for additional lesions, of vulva, 249
  for additional vessels, in PTCA, 230–231
  for prolonged services, 74–75
  modifier -51 and, 106
Adhesions, lysis of, 257, 258
Adjacent tissue transfers, 150–151, 150f
  for pressure ulcer, 151f, 157
Adjunct codes. *See also* Add-on codes.
  for qualifying circumstances, 95, 96f, 97
  for unusual hours or holiday, 365
Adjunctive procedures or equipment, in ICD-9-CM, 420, 421
Administration. *See also* Injection(s).
  of immune globulin, 349
  of vaccine/toxoid, 348, 349
  routes of, 369, 371, 371f, 372, 372f
Admission, 58
  definition of, 31
  from observation status, 56, 57
  to nursing facility, 71, 72
  to observation status, 57
  to partial hospital facility, 352
Adrenal glands, 288, 289f, 297
Advancement flaps, 150
Adverse effects. *See* Drug(s), adverse effects of.
AHA (American Hospital Association), 386, 417, 432, 579
AHFS (American Hospital Formulary Service), 401, 414, 416
AHIMA (American Health Information Management Association), 385f, 386, 432, 579
Alcohol
  drug interaction with, 496, 503, 599
  use of, 470–471

Alcoholism, 470
Allergen immunotherapy, 359
Allergy, 358–359
  physical examination and, 39
Allergy testing, 359
Allied health care professionals, 367
Allogenic, definition of, 162
Allogenic bone marrow, 287
Allograft, 154, 154f, 162
Alloplastic dressings, 158
Allotransplantation, 162
Alphabetic Index, in ICD-9-CM
  to diseases, 386, 388, 399–401, 400f–402f, 403, 403f, 404
    code assignment and, 432–433
    V codes in, 453–454
  to procedures, 386, 422, 422f, 424–427, 424f–426f
Alteration, as root operation, 515t, 520t
Alternative anatomic site, 13
Alternative procedure, 13
Ambulance team, physician communicating with, 67
Ambulatory Patient Classifications (APCs), 561, 562f–563f, 563–564
Ambulatory services. *See* Outpatient(s).
Ambulatory surgery
  CPT coding for, 4
  diagnosis coding for, 509, 602
  Medicare reimbursement for, 562f–563f, 563
American Health Information Management Association (AHIMA), 385f, 386, 432, 579
American Hospital Association (AHA), 386, 417, 432, 579
American Hospital Formulary Service (AHFS), 401, 414, 416
American Medical Association (AMA), 4, 6, 83, 84
American Society of Anesthesiologists (ASA), 90, 93
Amniocentesis, 260, 263
  ultrasonic guidance for, 319
A-mode ultrasound, 318, 326
Analgesia, 90